Natural Antioxidants

Chemistry, Health Effects, and Applications

Natural Antioxidants

Chemistry, Health Effects, and Applications

Editor

Fereidoon Shahidi
Department of Biochemistry
Memorial University of Newfoundland
St. John's, Newfoundland, Canada

AOCS PRESS
Champaign, Illinois

AOCS Mission Statement

To be a forum for the exchange of ideas, information, and experience among those with a professional interest in the science and technology of fats, oils, and related substances in ways that promote personal excellence and provide high standards of quality.

The paper used in this book is acid-free and falls within the guidelines established to ensure permanence and durability.

Library of Congress Cataloging-in-Publication Data

Natural antioxidants: chemistry, health effects, and applications/
editor, Fereidoon Shahidi
p. cm.
Includes bibliographical references and index.
ISBN 0-935315-77-2 (alk. paper)
1. Antioxidants. 2. Antioxidants—Health aspects. 3. Food—Vitamin content. 4. Food—Analysis. I. Shahidi, Fereidoon, 1951– .
RB170.N386 1996
616.07--dc21 96-50412
CIP

Printed in the United States of America with vegetable oil-based inks.

00 99 5 4 3 2

Preface

The food we consume contains many biomolecules that are susceptible to attack by free radicals. The free radical oxidation of food lipids by the chain reaction of lipid peroxidation is a major concern for both consumers and food manufacturers. Efforts are being made to control lipid oxidation in foods and to address the real biological significance to humans of dietary antioxidants and antioxidant supplements.

Oxidants are by-products of normal body metabolism and, if not controlled, may cause extensive damage to DNA, proteins, sugars, and lipids; they are contributors to aging and the degenerative diseases of aging such as cancer, cardiovascular diseases, cataracts, immune system decline, and brain dysfunction. Although synthetic antioxidants are generally used in foods to retain their quality, natural antioxidants such as α-tocopherol (vitamin E) and vitamin C as well as carotenoids act as antioxidant defenses in the body to combat diseases; antioxidant enzymes and selenium are also involved in this process.

Dietary antioxidants have generated particular interest as anticarcinogens and as defenses against the degenerative processes of aging. While most attention has been paid to small molecule dietary antioxidants such as tocopherol, ascorbate, and carotenoids, other food antioxidants may also augment the natural body antioxidants against oxidative damage and degenerative diseases. Thus, urate, albumin, bilirubin, carnosine, ubiquinol, flavonoids, and other phenolic compounds might play an important role as physiological and dietary antioxidants.

Antioxidants used in foods to control oxidation and prevent off-flavor development include butylated hydroxyanisole (BHA), butylated hydroxytoluene (BHT), propyl gallate (PG), and *tert*-butyl hydroquinone (TBHQ). However, concern has been expressed about their use in foods due to safety considerations. Thus, the most powerful synthetic antioxidant, namely, TBHQ is not yet allowed for food applications in Japan, Canada, and Europe, and BHA has recently been removed from the Generally Recognized As Safe (GRAS) list of compounds.

The purpose of this monograph is to provide a state-of-the-art discussion of natural antioxidants from dietary sources, their occurrence, health effects, chemistry, and methodologies. The book summarizes data on the occurrence of antioxidative compounds in cereals and legumes, oilseeds, herbs and spices, vegetables, teas, muscle foods, and other commodities. The antioxidant vitamins and enzymes are also thoroughly discussed. The potential beneficial effects of dietary antioxidants, the chemistry of food antioxidants, and methodologies to assess lipid oxidation and antioxidant activity have also been covered. The book has been organized into chapters and sections to provide a better flow of material. The monograph would be of interest to scientists, health professionals, researchers in academia, government laboratories, and industries. It may also serve as a supplementary text for senior undergraduate and graduate students in food chemistry.

Finally, I would like to express my thanks and gratitude to all of the authors for their commendable contributions which made this publication possible. Last, but not least, I thank my wife and other family members for their continued understanding of my time-consuming scientific activities, in general, and those related to the publication of this and other monographs.

F. Shahidi

Contents

	Preface	v
Chapter 1	Natural Antioxidants: An Overview *F. Shahidi*	1
Chapter 2	Natural Antioxidants—Are They a Reality? *S. Cuppett, M. Schnepf, and C. Hall III*	12
Chapter 3	Antioxidants from Cereals and Legumes *P.J. White and Y. Xing*	25
Chapter 4	Antioxidants from Spices and Herbs *N. Nakatani*	64
Chapter 5	Antioxidative Defense System in Vegetable Extracts *N. Ramarathnam, H. Ochi, and M. Takeuchi*	76
Chapter 6	Antioxidant and Biological Properties of Rosemary Components: Implications for Food and Health *E.A. Offord, F. Guillot, R. Aeschbach, J. Löliger, and A.M.A. Pfeifer*	88
Chapter 7	Natural Antioxidants from Oilseeds *V.K.S. Shukla, P.K.J.P.D. Wanasundara, and F. Shahidi*	97
Chapter 8	Carotenoids and Tocols from Palm Oil *A.S.H. Ong and Y.M. Choo*	133
Chapter 9	Antioxidants in Grapes and Wine: Chemistry and Health Effects *R.L. Williams and M.S. Elliott*	150
Chapter 10	Flavonoids as Antioxidants *C. Kandaswami and E. Middleton, Jr.*	174
Chapter 11	Antioxidative Activity of Condensed Tannins *A.D. Muir*	204
Chapter 12	Natural Antioxidants from Tea *C.-T. Ho, C.-W. Chen, U.N. Wanasundara, and F. Shahidi*	213
Chapter 13	Optimizing Lipid Stability with Natural Inhibitors *R.J. Evans*	224
Chapter 14	Vitamin Antioxidants and Disease Prevention *J.H. Weisburger*	245

Chapter 15 Endogenous Antioxidants: Role of Antioxidant Enzymes in Biological Systems 258
Y.V. Yuan and D.D. Kitts

Chapter 16 Antioxidant Activity of Carnosine, a Skeletal Muscle Dipeptide 271
E.A. Decker, W.K.M. Chan, L. Mei, G.L. McNeill-Tompkins, and S.A. Livisay

Chapter 17 Isolation of a Natural Antioxidant From Shrimp Waste 283
S.J. Li, T.A. Seymour, and M.T. Morrissey

Chapter 18 Antioxidant Properties of Maillard Reaction Products as Meat Flavor Compounds 296
M.E. Bailey, A.D. Clarke, and Y.S. Kim

Chapter 19 Controlling Oxidation and Warmed-Over Flavor in Precooked Pork Chops with Rosemary Oleoresin and Edible Film 311
D. Handley, M. Ma-Edmonds, F. Hamouz, S. Cuppett, R. Mandigo, and M. Schnepf

Chapter 20 Model Systems for Studying Pigment and Lipid Oxidation Relevant to Muscle-Based Foods 319
W.K.M. Chan, C. Faustman, and M. Renerre

Chapter 21 Prediction of Oxidative Stability of Lipids Based on the Early Stage Oxygen Consumption Rate 331
A.R. Wewala

Chapter 22 EPR Studies of Plant Polyphenols 346
W. Bors, C. Michel, K. Stettmaier, and W. Heller

Chapter 23 Application of FTIR/ATR Differential Spectroscopy for Monitoring Oil Oxidation and Antioxidant Efficacy 358
J. Sedman, A.A. Ismail, A. Nicodemo, S. Kubow, and F.R. van de Voort

Chapter 24 Measurement of Lipid Oxidation and Evaluation of Antioxidant Activity 379
F. Shahidi and U.N. Wanasundara

Chapter 25 Application of Proton Nuclear Magnetic Resonance (^{1}H NMR) Spectroscopy for Assessment of Oxidative Stability of Fats and Oils 397
F. Shahidi and U.N. Wanasundara

Index 405

Chapter 1

Natural Antioxidants: An Overview

F. Shahidi

Department of Biochemistry, Memorial University of Newfoundland, St. John's, Newfoundland, Canada.

Introduction

Antioxidants are substances that when present in foods or in the body at low concentrations compared with that of an oxidizable substrate markedly delay or prevent the oxidation of that substrate (1). Food manufacturers have used food-grade antioxidants to prevent quality deterioration of products and to maintain their nutritional value. Antioxidants have also been of interest to biochemists and health professionals because they may help the body protect itself against damage caused by reactive oxygen species and degenerative diseases.

Antioxidants are known to act at different levels in the oxidative sequence involving lipid molecules. They may act by decreasing oxygen concentration, intercepting singlet oxygen, preventing first-chain initiation by scavenging initial radicals such as hydroxyl radicals, binding metal ion catalysts, decomposing primary products to non-radical compounds, and chain-breaking to prevent continued hydrogen abstraction from substrates. The extent to which oxidation of lipids occurs also depends on the chemical structure of the fatty acids involved as well as other factors related to the storage of foods and reaction conditions.

Natural antioxidants from dietary sources include phenolic and polyphenolic compounds, chelators, antioxidant vitamins and enzymes, as well as carotenoids and carnosine. The mechanism by which these antioxidants are involved in the control of food autoxidation and rancidity prevention may be different. However, their presence in the live plants may be for the sake of protecting tissues from injurious damage. Furthermore, the beneficial effects of consuming plant foods have been ascribed, in part, to the presence of antioxidants in the plant, which is associated with counteracting risk of most cardiovascular diseases, cancer, and cataracts, among other degenerative diseases of aging.

The process of autoxidation and development of rancidity in foods involves a free radical chain mechanism proceeding via initiation, propagation, and termination steps (2). While radicals are produced in the "initiation" step, they react with unsaturated fatty acids by abstracting a hydrogen atom from their molecules in the "propagation" step. The reactions in the propagation make up a chain reaction until a "termination" reaction occurs.

Initiation: $\mathrm{LH} \xrightarrow{\text{Initiator}} \mathrm{L}^{\bullet}$

Propagation:

$$\mathrm{L}^{\bullet} + \mathrm{O_2} \rightarrow \mathrm{LOO}^{\bullet}$$

$$\mathrm{LOO}^{\bullet} + \mathrm{LH} \rightarrow \mathrm{LOOH} + \mathrm{L}^{\bullet}$$

Termination:

$$\left.\begin{array}{l} \mathrm{LOO}^{\bullet} + \mathrm{LOO}^{\bullet} \rightarrow \\ \mathrm{LOO}^{\bullet} + \mathrm{L}^{\bullet} \rightarrow \\ \mathrm{L}^{\bullet} + \mathrm{L}^{\bullet} \rightarrow \end{array}\right\} \text{non-radical products}$$

Antioxidants (AH) interfere with the above process by different mechanisms. These involve inactivation of prooxidants in the medium, such as carotenoids that scavenge singlet oxygen or chelators that inactivate metal catalysts. These reactions lead to a delay in the onset of oxidation and the extension of the induction period. Antioxidants may also donate a hydrogen atom or an electron to radicals formed from unsaturated lipids, thus imparting stability to food lipids.

$$\mathrm{LOO}^{\bullet} + \mathrm{AH} \rightarrow \mathrm{LOOH} + \mathrm{A}^{\bullet}$$

$$\left.\begin{array}{l} \mathrm{A}^{\bullet} + \mathrm{LOO}^{\bullet} \rightarrow \\ \mathrm{A}^{\bullet} + \mathrm{A}^{\bullet} \rightarrow \end{array}\right\} \text{non-radical products}$$

In the body, free radicals may be involved in a number of diseases and tissue injuries such as those of the lungs, heart and cardiovascular system, kidneys, liver, gastrointestinal tract, blood, eye, skin, muscle, brain, and the process of aging (3–5). Oxidants and radicals which mediate various disorders are mainly reactive species which are formed from triplet oxygen, water, and unsaturated lipid molecules (Fig. 1.1).

Therefore, lipid peroxidation is a problem not only in the edible oil and the food industry, but also in the human body. Excess production of oxygen radical species, particularly hydroxyl radicals, can affect lipid cell membranes to produce lipid peroxides and reactive oxygen species (ROS) which are linked to a variety of diseases as well as acceleration of the aging process (Fig. 1.2).

While hydroperoxides, referred to as primary oxidation products, are colorless and odorless when present in foods, they are labile and readily produce a number of secondary products such as alkanes, alcohols, aldehydes, and acids, some of which are highly odor-active and have low threshold values. In addition, polymers and other undesirable compounds that could affect the sensory characteristics as

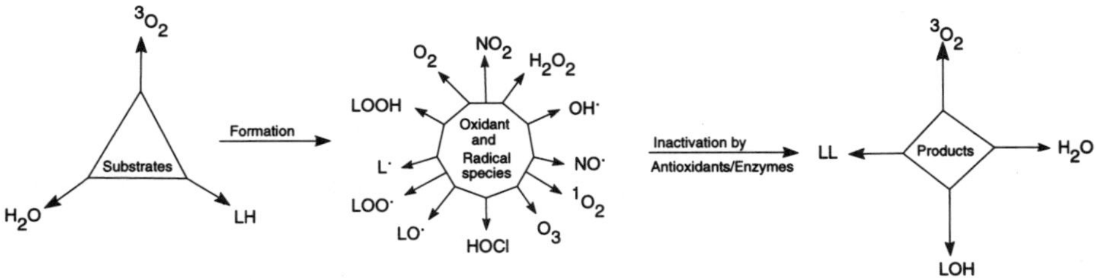

Fig. 1.1. Formation of oxidant and radical species in food and biological systems and their inactivation.

well as the safety of food products may be formed (see Fig. 1.3). Many of these secondary oxidation products are highly reactive themselves, e.g., malonaldehyde (MDA) and 4-hydroxynonenal (4-HN) (6,7). Both MDA and 4-HN are known to interact with biological and food components such as proteins, amino acids, amines, and DNA; the latter reactions are implicated in aging, mutagenesis, and carcinogenesis in the body (8–11). In foods, the above reactions are involved in changes in flavor, texture, color, and other sensory attributes as well as nutritional value of products and may lead to the destruction of essential fatty acids and lipid-soluble vitamins, in addition to being toxic by themselves. Thus, use of antioxidants in foods is recommended for controlling rancidity with its deleterious consequences. In addition, consumption of antioxidants in foods or as dietary supplements may be advised in order to influence the primary causes of atherosclerosis, cancer and degenerative diseases of the aging (12) (see Fig. 1.4).

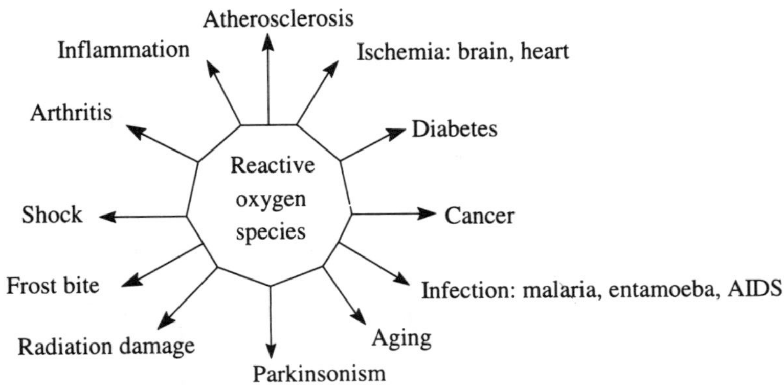

Fig. 1.2. Diseases and damages caused by reactive oxygen species; courtesy of Dr. M.-T. Huang.

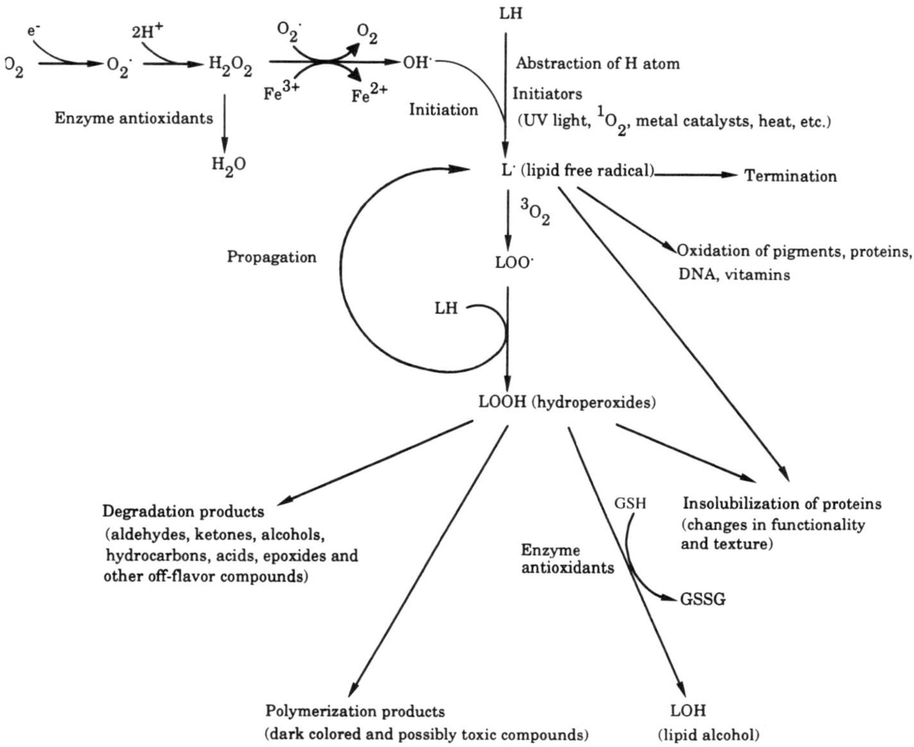

Fig. 1.3. The mechanism and consequences of lipid oxidation in food and in the body and their possible neutralization by enzyme antioxidants.

Antioxidants from Natural Sources

Plant-Based Antioxidants

Plants provide a rich source of natural antioxidants (13). These include tocopherols, vitamin C, carotenoids, and phenolic compounds. Plant phenolics are thought to protect the plants against tissue injuries as they oxidize and combine with proteins and other components. In addition, phenolic compounds in plants may serve as defense systems against herbivory (14). By-products of photosynthesis may also produce high levels of oxygen, free radicals, and reactive oxygen species (ROS) in profusion. Thus, plants use a myriad of antioxidant compounds to deal with these in order to survive. Many of these compounds have basic molecular similarities in that all have at least one aromatic ring and a hydroxyl group. These include phenolic acids, flavonoids and isoflavones, gallate esters (hydrolyzable tannins), lignans, coumarines, stilbenes, flavonones, and oligomeric proanthrocyanidins. Together, these compounds produce an array of antioxidants, which may act by different mechanisms, to confer an effec-

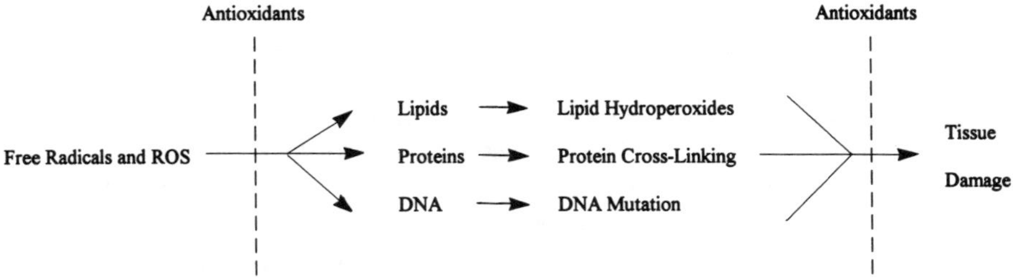

Fig. 1.4. Consequences of free radicals and reactive oxygen species (ROS) in diseases and preventive role of antioxidants.

tive defense system against free radical attack. Table 1.1 summarizes some of the natural antioxidants and their source in plant materials.

The best known natural antioxidants that have proven important in the food industry and in human health are tocopherols, vitamin C, and carotenoids (15). Herbs and spices or their extracts as well as tea extracts have also been shown to extend the shelf-life of various foods (16,17). Recent studies have led to the identification of active ingredients and antioxidant components of natural compounds, such as rosemary, rice hulls, green tea, sesame seed, canola seed, and ginger (18–24). Some of these extracts, such as those from rosemary and tea as well as mixed tocopherols and ascorbyl palmitate, have been successfully commercialized and have become popular in Japan, Europe, and recently in North America. This has happened despite higher cost of these extracts in comparison with synthetic additives. Certain vegetable oils also contain antioxidants other than tocopherols

TABLE 1.1
Natural Food Sources of Some Antioxidants

Compounds	Example of source
Vitamin E (tocopherols and tocotrienols)	Oilseeds, palm oil, nuts, eggs, dairy products, whole grains, vegetables, cereals, margarine, etc.
Vitamin C	Fruits and vegetables, berries, citrus fruits, sprouts, green peppers, potatoes, etc.
Carotenoids	Dark leafy vegetables, carrots, sweet potatoes, yams, tomatoes, cantaloupes, apricots, citrus fruits, kale, turnip greens, palm oil, etc.
Flavonoids/Isoflavones	Fruits and vegetables, oilseeds, berries, eggplants, peppers, citrus fruits, cruciferous vegetables, yams, tomatoes, onions, etc.
Phenolic acids/Derivatives	Oilseeds and certain oils, cereals, grains, etc.
Catechins	Green tea, berries, certain oilseeds, etc.
Extracts	Extracts from green tea, rosemary, sage, clove, oregano, thyme, cocoa shell, oat, rice bran, etc.

and as such might provide protection to other oils and food lipids. These include virgin olive oil, sesame oil, palm oil, cocoa lipids, rice bran oil, and oat oil. In addition, various vegetables, particularly radish, mustard, turnip, cabbage, and onions have moderate effects on stabilization of food lipids. Furthermore, a line of specialty drinks that mixes appropriate vegetable and fruit juices in desired proportions as well as those containing selected plant extracts have been introduced to the market in Japan. Although the price of these items is always higher than that of traditional drinks, consumer demand has accelerated their popularity because their potential beneficial health effects have been backed by scientific findings.

Both epidemiological and clinical studies have provided evidence that phenolic antioxidants present in cereals, fruits, and vegetables are principal contributing factors in accounting for the significantly reduced incidences of chronic and degenerative diseases encountered by populations whose diet is high in the intake of these foods (13,25). In retrospect, this is not surprising because humans have relied on plants during their evolutionary development to supplement their bodies with natural defense systems through consumption of dietary antioxidants. The authorities have now recognized these factors and in response have recommended five daily servings of fruits and vegetables and have encouraged a high intake of cereals and plant foods.

Amino Acids, Peptides and Protein Hydrolyzates as Antioxidants

Amino acids and peptides are typical metal-chelating agents frequently present in foods and found in abundance in protein hydrolyzates. In non-aqueous media, amino acids exhibit a mild antioxidant effect. Marcuse (26,27) found that 12 amino acids were present in the water phase of herring and examined their potential antioxidant effect in an emulsion of herring oil as well as in a linoleic acid model system. All amino acids, especially histidine and tryptophan, exhibit an antioxidant effect (see Table 1.2). Antioxidant activity of amino acids such as proline and lysine has also been demonstrated in bulk oils (28). However, amino acids may exert a prooxidant effect in the absence of metals or under certain other conditions such as when present in aqueous media (29,30).

Ions of copper, nickel, cobalt, and zinc readily form stable complexes with peptides by interacting with the amide nitrogens of the peptide bond (31). The stability of complexes of copper with Gly-His-Gly was extremely high and stronger than that of Gly-Gly-Gly. Meanwhile, Gly-Gly-His inhibited antioxidation of egg yolk phosphotidyl choline both in the presence of copper and in the photosensitized oxidation caused by riboflavin-5-phosphate, but the effect of β-Ala-His peptide was superior (32). A common feature appearing in most active peptides is the presence of a histidine molecule in the peptide's chemical formula. This observation gains further support from recent studies of Chen *et al.* (33) who isolated six antioxidative compounds from hydrolyzates of β-conglycinin, the 7S protein of soybean. The active peptides were composed of 5 to 16 amino acids and included

TABLE 1.2
Antioxidant Activity of Selected Amino Acids[1]

Amino acid	Concentration, M 0.001	0.01
Glutamic acid	0.92	0.74
Methionine	0.88	0.72
Alanine	0.93	0.68
Asparagine	0.88	0.66
Valine	0.87	0.57
Aspartic acid	0.86	0.56
Serine	0.81	0.47
Lysine	0.69	0.37
Tryptophan	0.45	0.31
Histidine	0.41	0.17

[1]Values represent oxygen uptake in herring oil emulsion relative to samples devoid of any amino acids. From Ref. 11.

hydrophobic amino acids, namely, valine and leucine at the *N*-terminal position and proline, histidine, or tyrosine in their sequence (see Table 1.3). These sequences were also confirmed to be present in the β-conglycinin as deduced from the nucleotide sequence. These authors did not observe any antioxidative activity when the constituent amino acids were mixed (in proportions present in the peptides) and tested in their assay media, and thus concluded that the characteristic amino acid sequences of peptides were required for them to manifest antioxidant effects. The antioxidant activity of P_3 was similar to that of BHA when tested at 10^{-6} and 10^{-4} M.

TABLE 1.3
Antioxidative Peptides of Soy 7S Protein and Egg White Albumin Hydrolyzates[1]

Peptide	Amino acid sequence
	SOY 7S PROTEIN
P_1	Val-Asn-Pro-His-Asp-His-Glu-Asn
P_2	Leu-Val-Asn-Pro-His-Asp-His-Glu-Asn
P_3	Leu-Leu-Pro-His-His
P_4	Leu-Leu-Pro-His-His-Ala-Asp-Ala-Asp-Tyr
P_5	Val-Ile-Pro-Ala-Gly-Tyr-Pro
P_6	Leu-Gln-Ser-Gly-Asp-Ala-Leu-Arg-Val-Pro-Ser-Gly-Thr-Thr-Tyr-Tyr
	EGG WHITE ALBUMIN
1	Ala-His
2	Val-His-His
3	Val-His-His-His-Ala-Asn-Glu-Asn

[1]From Refs. 32 and 33.

The antioxidant activity of histidine-containing peptides has also been reported by Uchida and Kawakishi (34) and Murase *et al.* (35). The activity of peptides examined was thought to be related to their metal-chelating ability as well as the lipid radical-trapping potential of the imidazole ring. Furthermore, the antioxidant activity of histidine-containing peptides was higher than that of histidine itself, perhaps due to the increased hydrophobicity of peptides which leads to their increased interaction with lipid fatty acids. Tyrosine moieties present in some other active peptides are thought to offer strong hydrogen donating ability.

The antioxidant peptides isolated from egg white albumin hydrolyzates were recently analyzed and confirmed the presence of histidine moieties in their structures (see Table 1.3). Recently, we have isolated a number of peptides arising from the hydrolysis of capelin, seal meat, and shrimp proteins and have found that compounds with moderate hydrophobicity were active antioxidants (e.g., 36). However, the presence of prooxidative peptides was also noted in these preparations. When added to a meat emulsion system, all hydrolyzates were effective in protecting meat against oxidation, although to different degrees.

Other effective histidine-containing antioxidative dipeptides are carnosine, homocarnosine, and anserine. Carnosine and anserine are found in relatively high amounts in muscles, and their dominance is in the white tissues where high levels of anaerobic metabolism are common (37). The antioxidant role of carnosine and anserine seems to involve singlet oxygen and free radical scavenging as well as metal chelation (38–40).

Antioxidants Activity of Phytates

Phytates are strongly negatively charged compounds found in many cereal-based foods. They are associated with proteins or metal ions and as such are capable of imparting antioxidant activity to many food systems, presumably by chelation of prooxidant metal ions. Antioxidant activity of phytic acid has been demonstrated in several model and food systems (41–43).

Phospholipids as Antioxidants

Phospholipids are obtained as by-products of oil-refining, especially from soybean. Phospholipids are known to affect lipid oxidation. Soybean lecithin and the ethanol-soluble fraction of a phospholipid are particularly effective in stabilizing lard and sunflower oil when used at a 0.1–1% level. Swift (44) found that purified phosphatidylethanolamine from cottonseed oil was a good antioxidant and increased the antioxygenic action of α-tocopherol. Later, Dalton *et al.* (45) suggested that the antioxygenic action of phospholipids was due in part to the metal-scavenging effect of the fat-soluble phosphoric acid. Therefore, use of lecithin and other phospholipids as antioxidants has been practiced (46). Löliger and Saucy (47) have patented a process in which a mixture of tocopherols, ascorbates, and lecithin was used for stabilization of bulk oils. However, use of such mixtures in emulsion-type products was ineffective (48). Many other specialized applications of phospholipids remain proprietary within the industry.

Vitamins and Enzyme Antioxidants

Vitamins may act as antioxidants in foods and in the body, both individually and in combination. Fat-soluble vitamins, such as vitamin E and vitamin A, and water-soluble vitamins such as vitamin C as well as β-carotene (vitamin A precursor) are known to exert antioxidant activity. In addition, regeneration of α-tocopherol by vitamin C is a well-known phenomenon. Due to the importance of this topic, chapter 14 has been devoted to vitamin antioxidants.

Enzyme antioxidants of interest to food and biological systems include superoxide dismutase (SOD) in different sources, catalase, glutathione and glutathione peroxidase, glutathione reductase, glutathione-5-transferase and phenol oxidase. Involvement of selenium in exerting antioxidant activity in conjunction with some enzyme antioxidants is well documented. Details of enzyme antioxidants are summarized in chapter 15.

Methodologies for Assessing Lipid Oxidation and Antioxidant Activity

Methods to assess lipid oxidation are manifold, and these may also depend on the system under investigation. Chemical, sensory, and instrumental methods are frequently employed. Therefore, monitoring of superoxide-, hydrogen peroxide-, hydroxyl radical- and peroxyl radical-scavenging effects of antioxidants is commonplace (e.g., 49–51). Assay media used may vary, depending on the type of study. In foods, both chemical and instrumental procedures are used; these include determination of peroxide value, individual peroxides, conjugated dienes, para-anisidine value, and 2-thiobarbituric acid (TBA) value (51). Sensory analysis of foods as well as analysis of total and selected volatile decomposition products of lipids may be performed (52). To monitor lipid oxidation, the loss of polyunsaturated fatty acids, especially in marine or some vegetable oils with highly unsaturated lipids, may also be followed. Meanwhile, use of novel techniques involving electron spin resonance (ESR), nuclear magnetic resonance (NMR), and infrared (IR) is of interest. In addition, employing oxygen uptake and weight gain, and use of the Rancimat, Oxidative Stability Instrument (OSI), and Oxidograph have been traditionally practiced. Several chapters in this monograph are devoted to the application of different methodologies for assessing lipid oxidation and antioxidant activity.

References

1. Halliwell, B., Aeschbach, R., Löliger, J., and Aruoma, O.I. (1995) *Food Chem. Toxicol. 33*, 601.
2. Shahidi, F., and Naczk, M. (1995) in *Food Phenolics: Sources, Chemistry, Effects and Applications*, Technomic Publ. Co., Lancaster and Basel, pp. 235–277.

3. Aruoma, O.I. (1994) *Food Chem. Toxic. 32*, 671.
4. Burr, M.L. (1994) *J. Human Nutr. Diet. 7*, 409.
5. Hennig, B., and Toborek, M. (1993) *J. Optimal Nutr. 2*, 213.
6. Benedetti, A., Comporti, M., and Estebauer, H. (1980) *Biochim. Biophys. Acta 620*, 281.
7. Benedetti, A., Ferralis, M., Casini, A.F., Pieri, S., and Comporti, M. (1980) *Biochem. Pharmacol. 29*, 121.
8. Crawford, D.L., Yu, T.C., and Sinnhuber, R.O. (1979) *J. Food Sci. 32*, 332.
9. Munkres, K.O. (1979) *Mech. Aging Dev. 10*, 249.
10. Basu, A.K., Marnett, L.J., and Romano, L.J. (1984) *Mutat Res. 129*, 39.
11. Fujimoto, K., Neff, W.E., and Frankel, E.N. (1984) *Biochim. Biophys. Acta 795*, 100.
12. Rice-Evans, C.A., and Diplock, A.T. (1993) *Free Radical Biol. and Med. 15*, 77.
13. Caragay, A.B. (1992) *Food Technol. 45*, 65.
14. Harborne, J.B. (1994) in *Polyphenols 94, Proceedings of the 17th International Conference on Polyphenols* (Brouillard, R., and Scalbert, A., eds.), pp. 19–26, INRA Editions, Paris, France.
15. Packer, L. (1996) in *Proceedings of the International Symposium on Natural Antioxidants: Molecular Mechanisms and Health Effects* (Packer, L., Traber, M.G., and Xin, W., eds.), AOCS Press, Champaign, IL, pp. 9–23.
16. Shahidi, F., Pegg, R.B., and Saleemi, Z.O. (1995) *J. Food Lipids 2*, 145.
17. Wanasundara, U.N., and Shahidi, F., *J. Am. Oil Chem. Soc.*, in press.
18. Wu, J.W., Lee, M.-T., Ho, C.-T., and Chang, S.S. (1982) *J. Am. Oil Chem. Soc. 59*, 339.
19. Ramarathnam, N., Osawa, T., Namiki, M., and Kawakishi, S. (1989) *J. Agric. Food Chem. 37*, 316.
20. Amarowicz, R., and Shahidi, F. (1996) *Food Res. Int. 29*, 71.
21. Fukuda, Y., Osawa, T., Namiki, M., and Ozaki, T. (1985) *Agric. Biol. Chem. 49*, 301.
22. Wanasundara, U., Amarowicz, R., and Shahidi, F. (1994) *J. Agric. Food Chem. 42*, 1285.
23. Jitoe, A., Masuda, T., Tengah, I.G.P., Suprapta, D.N., Gara, I.W., and Nakatani, N. (1992) *J. Agric. Food Chem. 40*, 1337.
24. Kasuga, A., Aoyagi, Y., and Sugahara, T. (1988) *Nippon Shokuhin Kogyo Gakkai-shi 35*, 828.
25. Thompson, L.U. (1994) *CRC Crit. Rev. Food Sci. Nutr. 343*, 473.
26. Marcuse, R. (1961) *Fette. Seifen Anstrichmittel. 63*, 547.
27. Marcuse, R. (1961) *Fette. Siefen. Anstrichmittel. 63*, 940.
28. Shukla, V.K.S. (1996) Presented at the 87th American Oil Chemists' Society Annual Meeting and Exposition, Indianapolis, IN, April 28–May 1.
29. Farag, R.S., Osman, S.A., Hallabo, S.A.S., and Nasr, A.A. (1978) *J. Am. Oil Chem. Soc. 55*, 703.
30. Farag, R.S., Osman, S.A., Hallabo, S.A.S., and Nasr, A.A. (1978) *Fette. Seifen. Astrichmittel 82*, 487.
31. Pokorny, J. (1987) in *Autoxidation of Unsaturated Lipids* (Chen, H.W.-S., ed.), Academic Press, London, pp. 141–206.
32. Yamashoji, S., and Kajimoto, G. (1980) *Agric. Biol. Chem. 44*, 2735.
33. Chen, H.-M., Muramoto, K., and Yamauchi, F. (1995) *J. Agric. Food Chem. 43*, 574.
34. Uchida, K., and Kawakishi, S. (1992) *J. Agric. Food Chem. 40*, 13.
35. Murase, H., Nagao, A., and Terao, J. (1993) *J. Agric. Food Chem. 58*, 300.
36. Shahidi, F. and Amarowicz, R., *J. Am. Oil Chem. Soc.*, in press.

37. Crush, K.G. (1970) *Comp. Biochem. Physiol. 34*, 3.
38. Egorov, S.Y., Kurella, E.G., Boldrynev, A.A., and Krasnovski, A.A., Jr. (1992) *Bioorg. Khin. 12*, 142.
39. Kohen, R., Yamamoto, Y., Cundy, K.C., and Ames, B. (1988) *Proc. Natl. Acad. Sci. USA 85*, 3175.
40. Brown, C.E. (1981) *J. Theor. Biol. 88*, 245.
41. Empson, K.L., Labuza, T.P., and Graf, E., *J. Food Sci. 56*, 560.
42. Graf, E., and Eaton, J.W. (1990) *Free Radical Biol. Med. 8*, 61.
43. Graf, E., Empson, K.L., and Eaton, J.W. (1987) *J. Biol. Chem. 262*, 11,647.
44. Swift, C.E., Rose, W.G., and Jamieson, G.S. (1942) *Oil and Soap 19*, 176.
45. Dalton, H.J., Schwab, A.W., Moser, H.A., and Cowan, J.C. (1948) *J. Am. Oil Chem. Soc. 25*, 385.
46. Nassner, A. (1985) *Fette. Seifen. Anstrichmittel 87*, 477.
47. Löliger, J., and Saucy, F., European Patent, EPO 326 829 B1 (1989).
48. Meyer, A.S., and Jacobsen, C. (1996) *J. Food Lipids 3*, 139.
49. Halliwell, B., and Chirico, S. (1993) *Am. J. Clin. Nutr. 57 (suppl.)*, 715S.
50. Summerfield, F.W., and Tappel, A.L. (1983) *Biochim. Biophys. Acta 740*, 185.
51. Frankel, E.N., (1993) *Trends Food Sci. Technol. 4*, 220.
52. Shahidi, F., and Pegg, R.B., *J. Food Lipids 1*, 177.

Chapter 2

Natural Antioxidants—Are They a Reality?

S. Cuppett[a], M. Schnepf[b], and C. Hall III[a]

[a]Department of Food Science and Technology; and [b]Department of Nutritional Sciences and Dietetics, University of Nebraska-Lincoln, Lincoln, Nebraska.

Introduction

The role of antioxidants in today's food system(s) is constantly expanding, given the level of processing and handling that many foods encounter on their way to the consumer. However, the consumer is becoming increasingly concerned about the use of traditional synthetic antioxidants, such as butylated hydroxyanisole (BHA) and butylated hydroxytoluene (BHT), based on concerns that these compounds may be carcinogenic (1). Therefore, research has focused on the development and utilization of antioxidants from natural sources such as plants. The purposes of this chapter are to outline the processes involved in the oxidation of foods; to discuss the mechanisms by which natural antioxidants function to inhibit lipid oxidation and extend the shelf-life of food; and to comment on the potential for using these natural antioxidants in the food system.

One of the primary reasons for consumer rejection of a food is the presence of rancidity/oxidation. Food can oxidize by two basic processes, i.e., autoxidation and photo-oxidation. To understand the mechanism which allows antioxidants to preserve foods, some time must be spent reviewing the basic mechanisms of these two forms of oxidation.

Autoxidation occurs in three steps (2); these can be summarized using the following equations:

Initiation:	$LH \longrightarrow L^\bullet$	[1]
	$L^\bullet + O_2 \longrightarrow LOO^\bullet$	[2]
Propagation:	$LOO^\bullet + L'H \longrightarrow LOOH + L'^\bullet$	[3]
Termination:	$LOO^\bullet + L'^\bullet \longrightarrow LOOL'$	[4]
	$LOO^\bullet + L'OO^\bullet \longrightarrow LOOL' + O_2$	[5]
	$L^\bullet + L'^\bullet \longrightarrow LL'$	[6]

In initiation (Equations 1 and 2) the fatty acid (LH) forms a free radical ($L^\bullet$) which then reacts with oxygen (O_2) to form the peroxy radical ($LOO^\bullet$). The oxygenation of the free radical ($L^\bullet$) to form the peroxy radical is very rapid; therefore, $LOO^\bullet$ is the primary product of autoxidation.

Propagation (Equation 3) involves the continuation and acceleration of the chain reaction begun in initiation. In this stage, the peroxy radical can abstract a hydrogen atom from an adjacent fatty acid to produce a free radical. The free radical produced ($L'^{\bullet}$) can then oxygenate, forming a peroxy radical which can accelerate the oxidation cycle.

Termination is the stage in which the free radicals (Equations 4–6) begin to react with each other and form nonradical species. Hydroperoxides (LOOH) may also decompose to produce alcohols, aldehydes, acids, ketones, and other less reactive substances. Termination completes one cycle of lipid autoxidation; however, there can be reinitiation and the cycle repeats itself. This can continue indefinitely or until oxidizable substrate is depleted.

Photo-oxidation or photosensitized oxidation occurs primarily in foods through the following mechanism (3–8):

$$^1S + h\nu \longrightarrow {}^1S^* \longrightarrow {}^3S^*$$

$$^3S^* + {}^3O_2 \longrightarrow {}^1O_2 + {}^1S \quad \text{(energy transfer)}$$

$$^1O_2 + LH \longrightarrow LOOH$$

In this mechanism, $^3S^*$, a sensitizer such as chlorophyll, absorbs ultraviolet (UV) energy ($h\nu$) and becomes excited, moving to a higher forbidden vibrational energy state ($^3S^*$). The excited sensitizer can then either (i) drop to the ground state singlet sensitizer (^1S) or, more importantly, (ii) undergo an intersystem crossing and transfer its energy to the lowest vibrational energy state of oxygen ($^3O_2$), causing the oxygen to go to a higher vibrational energy state defined as singlet oxygen ($^1O_2$) (3,7–10).

Singlet oxygen, being extremely electrophilic, can directly attack unsaturated fatty acids, due to the high electron density of the double bonds, resulting in a peroxy radical ($LOO^{\bullet}$) and, ultimately, hydroperoxides ($LOO^{\bullet}$).

$$^1O_2 + LH \longrightarrow LOO^{\bullet} \longrightarrow LOOH$$

Therefore, the rate of the photo-oxidation is a much faster reaction when compared with autoxidation. Rawls and Van Santen (5) found that singlet oxygen reacts 1000–1500 times faster than triplet oxygen.

One method for controlling the rate of lipid oxidation is by the addition of antioxidants (AO). Antioxidants have been described as "substances that, when present at low concentrations compared with those of an oxidizable substrate, significantly retards oxidation of that substrate" (11). Therefore, under this definition, metal chelating compounds can be classified as AO. The "ideal antioxidant" must meet many criteria before being used in food systems. The antioxidants must (i) be safe; (ii) not impart color, odor, or flavor; (iii) be effective at low concentrations;

(iv) survive after processing; (v) be stable in the finished product; (vi) be fat soluble; (vii) be readily available at a low cost; and, more recently, (viii) look "natural" on the label.

During the last decade, there has been heightened interest in the feasibility of utilizing natural AO in food systems; numerous reports have appeared in the literature relative to the effectiveness of AO from natural sources. A variety of plant extracts have been investigated for their antioxidant activity (AOA). Although not every system has been purified so that the active components could be identified, it has generally been shown that the AO compounds from plants are phenolic in nature and encompass such groups of compounds as tocopherols, carotenoids, phenolic acids (benzoic and cinnamic acid derivatives), flavonoids, and diterpenes.

Tocopherols

Tocopherols can be classified as either tocols or tocotrienols; within each of these two classes, there are four isomers (α,β,γ,δ), making a total of eight tocopherols. Tocopherols can act as AO by two primary mechanisms: (i) a chain-breaking electron donor (CB-D) mechanism and (ii) a chain-breaking acceptor (CB-A) mechanism (12). The second major mechanism, CB-A, includes singlet oxygen scavenging or quenching.

CB-D antioxidants compete with the unsaturated fatty acid (LH) for the lipid peroxy radical ($LOO^{\bullet}$) and, as a result, reduce the formation of the lipid radical ($L^{\bullet}$) that occurs when LH reacts with $LOO^{\bullet}$; this competition ultimately slows the propagation stage of autoxidation. Tocopherols can effectively compete with LH for the $LOO^{\bullet}$ by readily transferring a hydrogen atom to the $LOO^{\bullet}$ to produce the more stable LOOH (13). In the case of tocopherols, a hydrogen transfer occurs, resulting in a semiquinone intermediate (Fig. 2.1) which converts to tocopheryl quinone (Fig. 2.1) as the final stable end product.

The tocopheryl quinone and possibly the semiquinones can react with the $L^{\bullet}$ to produce LH, thus slowing the chain propagation stage. This type of mechanism is defined as the CB-A, and in this mechanism tocopheryl quinone competes with oxygen (triplet) for the $L^{\bullet}$ (13). Because the reactions between carbon-centered radicals ($L^{\bullet}$) and oxygen ($^3O_2$) are favored over those of the quinone oxygen and $L^{\bullet}$ reaction at normal atmospheric pressures, it is likely that this type of antioxidant activity occurs primarily in biological systems or other low oxygen pressure systems (13).

Tocopherols can also act on singlet oxygen ($^1O_2$) as a means to control oxidation processes. The oxygen-scavenging ability of tocopherols occurs through two primary methods: (i) singlet oxygen quenching and (ii) irreversible reaction with singlet oxygen to form a variety of products. The quenching mechanism is more predominant (14) and is dependent on the rate constants of the reaction between $^1O_2$ and tocopherol vs. the rate constant of $^1O_2$ being quenched to $^3O_2$ (15). Even the more acceptable mechanism explaining how tocopherols and $^1O_2$ react is not

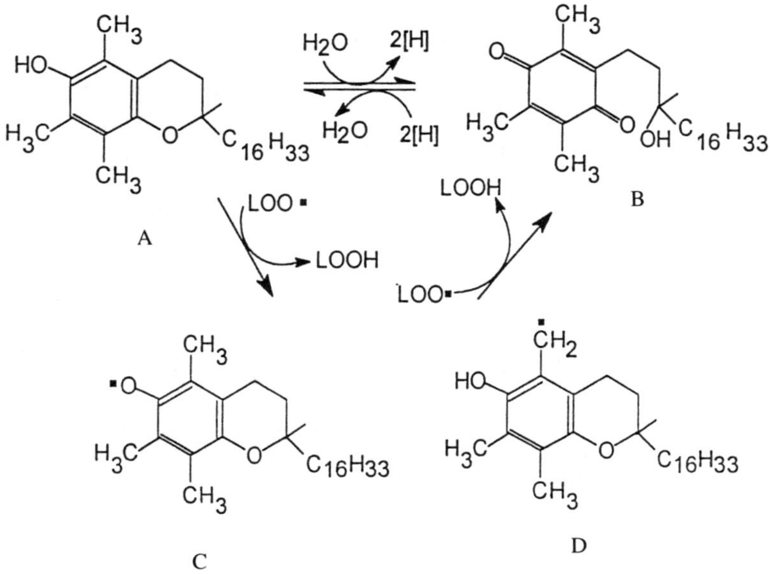

Fig. 2.1. (A) α-tocopherol oxidation to (B) α-tocopheryl quinone through semi-quinone intermediates (C,D).

clear. Clough *et al.* (14) proposed that the irreversible reaction of singlet oxygen with tocopherol results in the formation of hydroperoxydienone (Fig. 2.2) as the major end product (14). Grams *et al.* (16) found a variety of products and proposed that the 1,4-cycloaddition of oxygen to form the endoperoxides (Fig. 2.3) was the first stages of $^1O_2$ reaction with tocopherol. Clough *et al.* (14) agreed that endoperoxides could be intermediates for the hydroperoxydienone compounds found in their study.

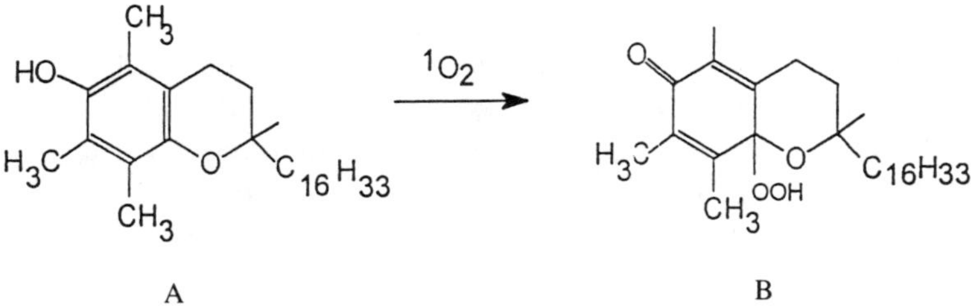

Fig. 2.2. Singlet oxidation of (A) α-tocopherol to (B) hydroperoxydienone as given by Clough *et al.* (14).

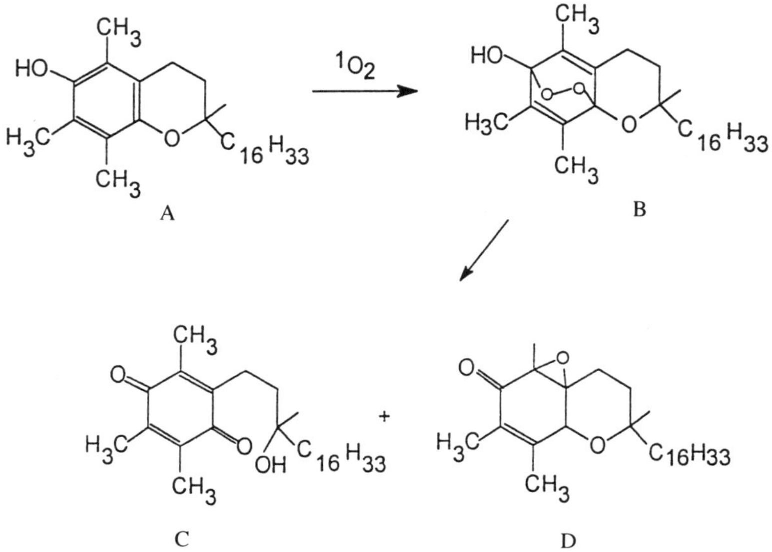

Fig. 2.3. Singlet oxidation of (A) α-tocopherol to (C) α-tocopheryl quinone and (D) quinone epoxide through (B) α-tocopherol endoperoxide as presented by Gram *et al.* (16).

Carotenes

Like tocopherols, carotenes and, in particular β-carotene are also effective $^1O_2$ quenchers. Foote and coworkers (17,18), and Farmilo and Wilkenson (19) found that the quenching of $^1O_2$ by β-carotene was due to an energy transfer from $^1O_2$ to β-carotene:

$$^1O_2 + \beta\text{-Car} \longrightarrow {}^3O_2 + 3\beta\text{-Car}$$

Foote *et al.* (20) also found that the rate of quenching was dependent on the number of conjugated double bonds. The presence of nine or more double bonds in the carotene structure greatly enhanced the quenching ability. Carotenoids with seven or fewer double bonds were not as effective, due to the inability of the conjugated chain to delocalize the unpaired electrons gained from the $^1O_2$ (20). A radical trapping mechanism has also been proposed (21,22). This mechanism relies on the delocalization of the unpaired electrons of the peroxy and free radical species over the carotenoid conjugated polyene system (21,22).

Phenolic Acids

Phenolic acids have been shown to have AO activity. The *o*-diphenols, such as caffeic, hydroxytyrosol, and oleuropein, exhibit strong AOA compared with less sterically hindered phenolic acids such as tyrosol (23). In addition, phenolic acids that are hydroxy derivatives of cinnamic acid, such as caffeic, ferulic, sinapic and *p*-coumaric acids, are more active AO than hydroxy derivatives of benzoic acid (Fig. 2.4), i.e., *p*-hydroxybenzoic, vanillic, syringic, and 3,4-dihydroxybenzoic acid (24).

Phenolic antioxidants act to inhibit lipid oxidation by trapping the peroxy radical. This can be accomplished in one of two ways:

$$LOO^{\bullet} + ArOH \longrightarrow LOOH + ArO^{\bullet} \quad [7]$$

$$LO^{\bullet} + ArO^{\bullet} \longrightarrow LOOAr \quad [8]$$

In the first mechanism (Equation 7), the peroxy radical ($LOO^{\bullet}$) abstracts a hydrogen proton from the antioxidant (ArOH) to yield an aroxyl radical ($ArO^{\bullet}$) and the

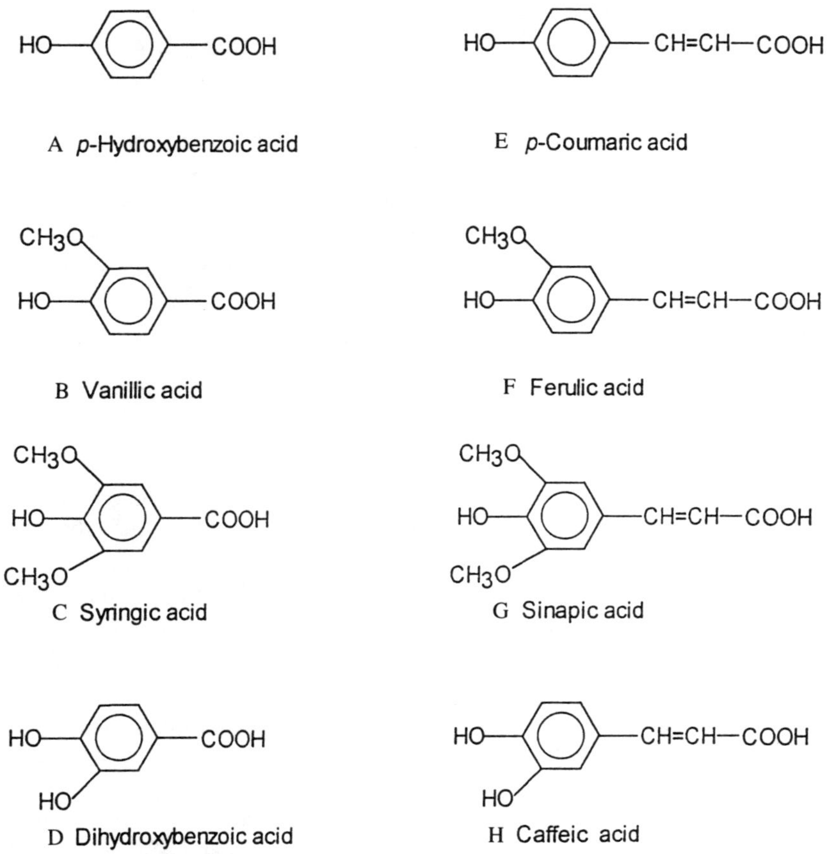

Fig. 2.4. Phenolic acids, hydroxy derivatives of benzoic acid (A–D) and of cinnamic acid (E–H).

hydroperoxide (LOOH). In the second mechanism (Equation 8), a peroxy and an aroxyl radical react by radical-radical coupling to form a nonradical product (23).

The aroxyl radical formed from the oxidation of an antioxidant can further react and can, in some instances, contribute to the production of free radicals (23).

$$ArO^{\bullet} + LOOH \longrightarrow LOO^{\bullet} + ArOH \quad [9]$$

$$2ArO^{\bullet} \longrightarrow \text{Non-radical products} \quad [10]$$

$$ArO^{\bullet} + LH \longrightarrow ArOH + L^{\bullet} \quad [11]$$

Chimi *et al* (23) reported that for sterically hindered phenols, the rates of reactions [8] and [10], which produce non-radical products, exceed the rates of reaction [9] and [11], which produce free radicals, resulting in an overall inhibition of lipid oxidation. Lack of hinderance favors reactions [9] and [11], which produce free radicals, thus decreasing the overall antioxidant activity of the phenol.

Dziedzic and Hudson (25) evaluated a series of hydroxy aromatic acids (phenolic acids) and related esters and lactones for antioxidant activity as related to structure. Based on the results of their studies, several structure-activity conclusions can be drawn. High antioxidant activity was related to the molecule containing at least two neighboring phenolic hydroxy groups; three such groups were even more desirable. In addition, a carbonyl group, such as an aromatic acid, an ester, or a lactone, enhanced activity. Activity was also increased when the carbonyl group was separated from the aromatic ring. Cinnamic acids were more effective than corresponding benzoic acids, and the most effective were the phenylacetic and phenylpropioninc acids. Steric hinderance of the phenolic hydroxyls by a neighboring inert group, such as methoxyl groups, enhanced activity.

Flavonoids

Flavonoids can act as AO by acting as hydrogen donors or by acting as chelating metals. Flavonoids can occur as glucosides (containing glucose side chains) or as aglycones (without glucose side chains).

Das and Pereira (26) studied the AOA of flavonoids and related the observed AOA to their structure(s). They found that the potency of flavonoids with polyhydroxylated substitutions was affected by the location of the hydroxyl substitution on the B ring (Fig. 2.5). Hydroxyl substitution in the *ortho* position in the B ring gave less antioxidant activity; however, hydroxyl substitution in the *ortho* position accompanied by an additional hydroxyl group in the *para* position enhanced activity. Strong antioxidant activity was found in compounds having hydroxylation in the *para* position in the B ring. In addition, it was found that a double bond between the 2 and 3 positions on the C ring contributed to antioxidant activity (Fig. 2.5). Das and Pereira (26) also found that the aglycones were stronger antioxidants than their corresponding glucosides, possibly due the lack of a free 3-hydroxy sub-

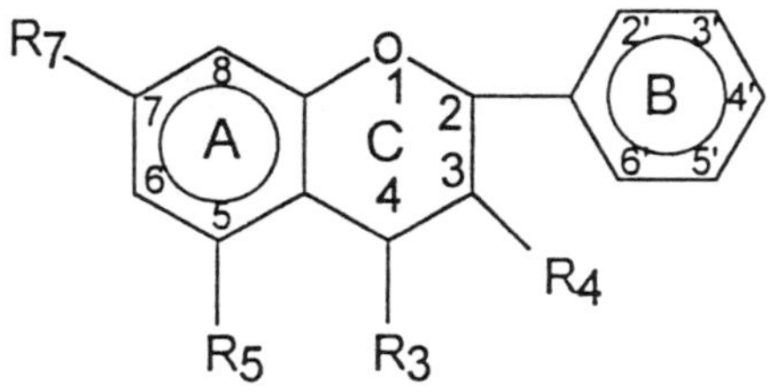

Fig. 2.5. General chemical structure of flavonoid compounds.

stitution in the C ring. This was in agreement with Hayes et al. (27) who reported that the isoflavone aglycones from soybeans exhibited greater activity than their glucoside counterparts.

Shahadi and Wanasundara (2) noted that the position and degree of hydroxylation was important in the AOA of flavonoids. They stated that an *o*-dihydroxylation of the B ring contributed to the antioxidant activity of the compound. A *p*-quinol structure on the B ring produces greater activity than the *o*-quinol; however, they also noted that *p*- and *m*-hydroxylations of the B ring do not occur in nature.

Flavonoids can also help to control the extent of lipid oxidation by chelating metal (copper) ions. Hudson and Lewis (28) studied the AOA of a series of polyhydroxy flavonoids and related their activity to their structure(s). The results of the study led to several conclusions relative to the structural features which affect the AOA of the flavonoids. First, it was noted that the molecule needed multiple hydroxy groups; a 3′, 4′-dihydroxy configuration gave strong antioxidant activity (Fig. 2.6). Second, the molecule must have a 4-carbonyl group for activity. Third, the molecule needed a free 3-hydroxy group as opposed to a 5-hydroxy group, but the presence of both 3- and 5-hydroxy groups was also effective. They projected that there was cooperation between the 4-carbonyl and the 3- or 5-hydroxy groups which acted to chelate the copper ion (Fig. 2.6).

Flavones form ligands with the cupric (Cu^{2+}) ion whereas the flavanones complex with copper ions through their enediol or enolic groups (Fig. 2.6).

Diterpenes

The AOA of phenolic diterpenes is becoming established in the literature. The most common plants being commercially exploited as sources for these natural antioxidants are rosemary and sage. Presently, there are a wide variety of rosemary extracts available for use in food systems; some carry high levels of flavor and color, while others have been bleached and/or dearomatized (29). The compounds identified as responsible for the AOA of rosemary and sage include carnosic acid, carnosol, rosmanol, epirosmanol, and isorosmanol (Fig. 2.7) (29,30).

Although carnosol and carnosic acid are reported to account for over 90% of the antioxidant activity of rosemary (11), it must be borne in mind that carnosic acid is relatively unstable. Schwarz and Ternes (29) studied the stability of carnosic acid and reported the conversion of carnosic acid to carnosol which subse-

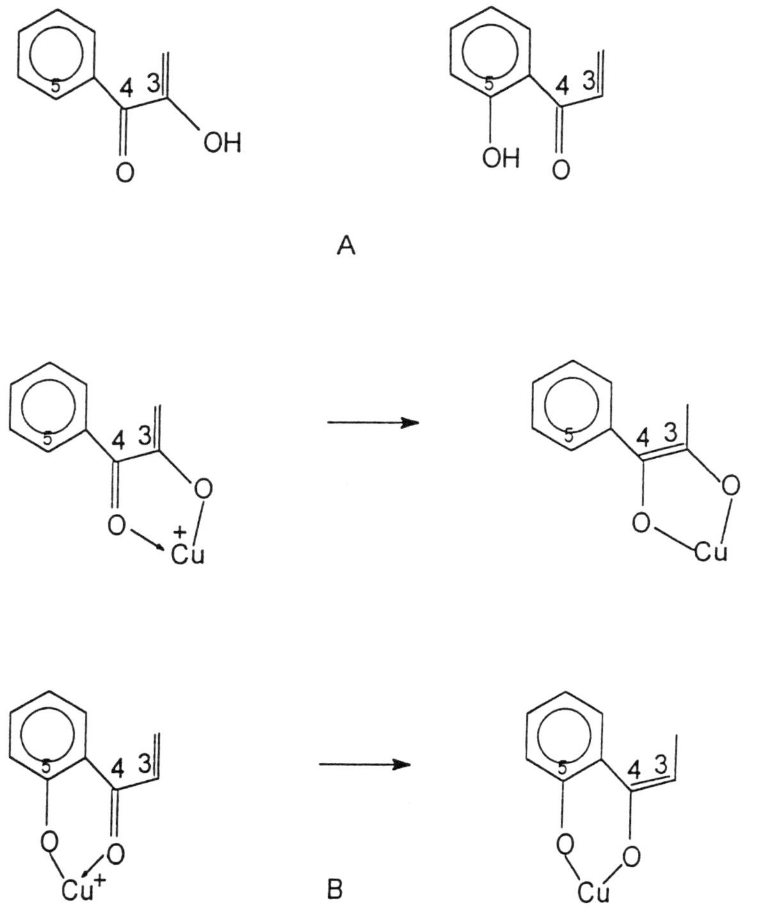

Fig. 2.6. (A) Active chelating region of flavanones and flavones and (B) the chelating mechanism for flavanones and flavones (25).

quently converted to rosmanol, 7-methylepirosmanol, and epirosmanol (Fig. 2.8). The conversion of carnosic acid to carnosol, and subsequently, rosmanol, epirosmanol and 7-methylepirosmanol, was facilitated by exposure to oxygen in the presence of light or when carnosic acid was heated in the presence of methanol. Conversion of carnosol to rosmanol was also observed in a NaOH solution containing methanol.

Because many of the commercial processes for producing rosemary extracts involve some heating in the presence of solvent, one would expect a significant conversion of carnosic acid to carnosol. The only exception may occur in extracts produced by CO_2 extraction, as in supercritical extraction. Increased levels of

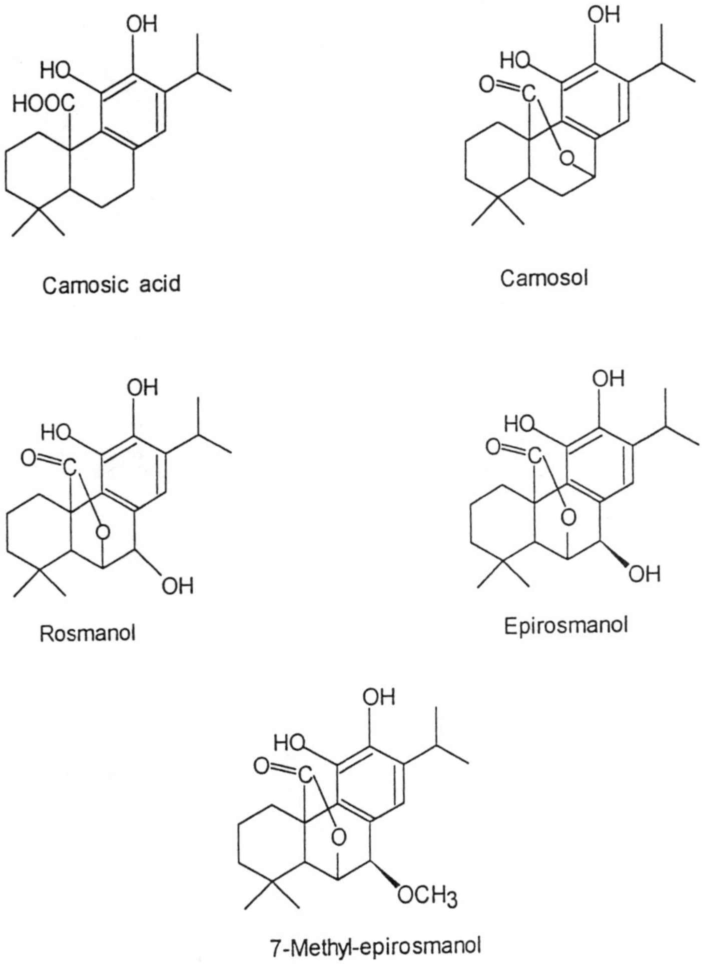

Fig. 2.7. Structure of antioxidant compounds from rosemary.

carnosol may not be undesirable because carnosol is more stable than carnosic acid; however, it does have less activity.

The interest in natural AO has led to the investigation of many plant extracts for their activity. In addition to rosemary and sage, many other spices/herbs have been studied for their antioxidant activity including thyme (32), nutmeg (33), ginger (34–36), clove (37), and oregano (38,39). Presently, intensive research is also being conducted on extracts from such plants as oats (40,41), potato peels (42–44), grapes and red wines (45), peanut hulls (46,47) and peanut kernels (48). In most of the extracts, phenolic acids and/or flavonoids have been identified as the active

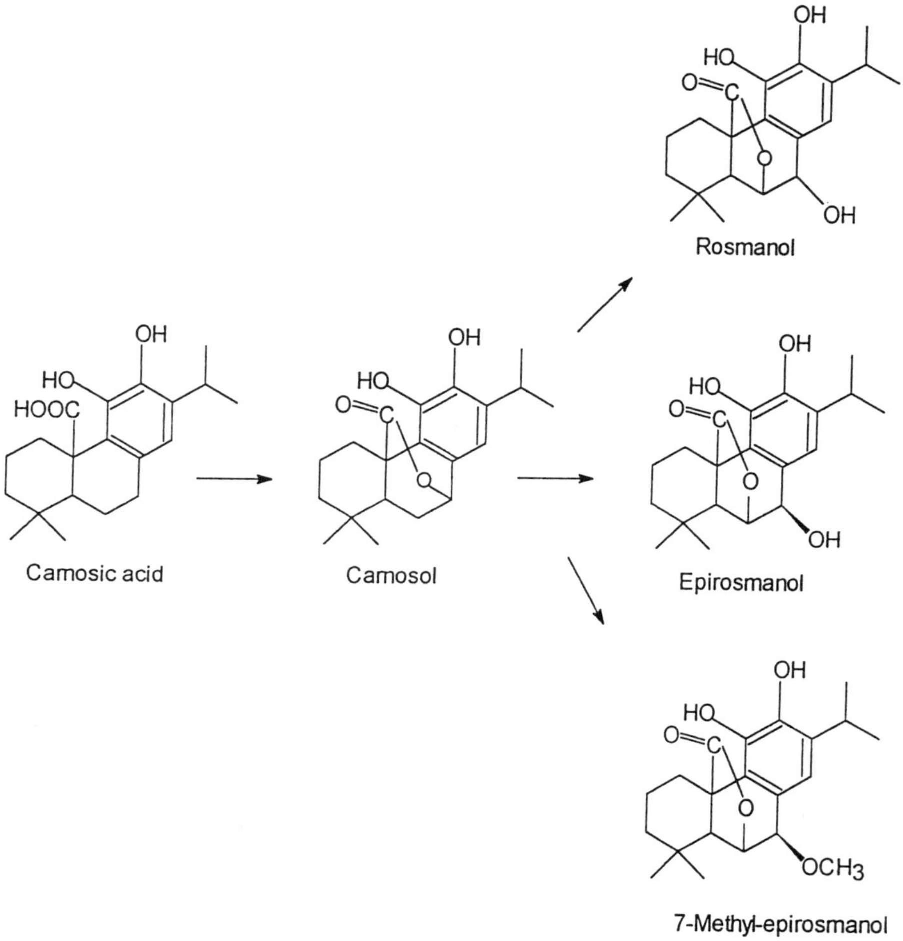

Fig. 2.8. Conversion of carnosic acid to carnosol and subsequently to rosmanol, epirosmanol, and 7-methylepirosmanol (30).

compounds. Other types of compounds have been identified in plant extracts; however, they will not be discussed here.

Conclusions

What is the future of natural antioxidants? There is no doubt that they are going to become part of the food system. One major concern that must be addressed is safety. Some data on the biological activity of some of the identified natural AO are available in the literature, but not enough is known to justify use of these compounds in foods. Because most researchers do not have the financial resources to evaluate fully the safety aspects of natural AO, then this must be done by industry and/or government. However, researchers can help narrow the list of systems/compounds to be evaluated; they can provide information on potential positive health benefits of natural compounds, including anticancer, antimutagen, and toxicological activities. Obtaining legal status for natural compounds must be a joint project between university, industry and government research.

References

1. Chen, Q., Huang, S., and Ho, C.-T. (1992) *J. Am. Oil Chem. Soc. 69*, 999.
2. Shahidi, F., and Wanasundra, P.K.J. (1992) *CRC Rev. Food Sci. and Nutr. 32*, 67.
3. Gollnick, K. (1968) in *Advances in Photochemistry* (Noyes, W.A., Hammond, G.W., and Pitts, J.N., eds.), Vol. 6, Interscience Publishers, New York, p. 1.
4. Foote, C.S. (1968) Science *162*, 963.
5. Rawls, H.R., and Van Santen, P.J. (1968) *Tetrahedron Lett. 14*, 1675.
6. Rawls, H.R., and Van Santen, P.J. (1970) *J. Am. Oil Chem. Soc. 47*, 121.
7. Chan, H.W.S. (1977) *J. Am. Oil Chem. Soc. 54*, 100.
8. Nawar, W.W. (1985) in *Food Chemistry* (Fennema, O.R., ed.), Marcel Dekker, Inc. New York, p. 139.
9. Gollnick, K., and Schenck, G.O. (1964) *Pure Applied Chem. 9*, 507.
10. Foote, C.S. (1976) in *Free Radicals in Biology* (Pryor, W., ed.), Vol. II, Academic Press, New York, pp. 85–133.
11. Aruoma, O.I., Halliwell, B., Aeschbach, R., and Loligers, J. (1992) *Xenbiotica* 2, 257.
12. Scott, G. (1985) *Chem. Br. 21*, 648.
13. Frankel, E.N. (1991) *J. Sci. Food Agric. 54*, 495.
14. Clough, R.L., Yee, B.G., and Foote, C.S. (1979) *J. Am. Oil Chem. Soc. 101*, 683.
15. Yamauchi, R., and Matsushita, S. (1977) *Agric. Biol. Chem. 41*, 1425.
16. Grams, G.W., Eskin, K., and Inglett, G.H. (1972) *J. Am. Oil Chem. Soc. 94*, 866.
17. Foote, C.S., and Denny, R.W. (1968) *J. Am. Chem. Soc. 90*, 6233.
18. Foote, C.S., Denny, R.W., Weaver, L., Chang, Y., and Peters, J. (1971) *Ann. N.Y. Acad. Sci. 171*, 139.
19. Farmilo, A., and Wilkinson, F. (1973) *Photochem. Photobiol. 18*, 447.
20. Foote, C.S., Chang, Y.C., and Denny, R.W. (1970) *J. Am. Oil Chem. Soc. 92*, 5216.
21. Burton, G.W., and Ingold, K.U. (1984) *Science 224*, 569.
22. Terao, J. (1989) *Lipids 24*, 659.
23. Chimi, H., Cillard, J., Cillard, P., and Rahmani, M. (1991) *J. Am. Oil Chem. Soc. 68*, 307.
24. Marinova, E.M., and Yanishieva, N.V. (1994) *J. Am. Oil Chem. Soc. 71*, 427.
25. Dziedzic, S.Z., and Hudson, B.J.F. (1984) *Food Chem. 14*, 45.
26. Das, N.P., and Pereira, T.A. (1990) *J. Am. Oil Chem. Soc. 67*, 255.
27. Hayes, R.E., Bookwalter, G.N., and Bagley, E.B. (1977) *J. Food Sci. 42*, 1527.
28. Hudson, B.J.F., and Lewis, J.I. (1983) *Food Chem. 10*, 47.
29. Schwarz, K., and Ternes, W. (1992) *Z. Lebensm. Unters. Forsch. 195*, 95.
30. Cuvelier, M.-E., Berset, C., and Richard, H. (1994) *J. Agric. Food Chem. 42*, 665.
31. Schwarz, K., and Ternes, W. (1992) *Z. Lebensm. Unters. Forsch. 195*, 99.
32. Miura, K., and Nakatani, N. (1989) *Agric. Biol. Chem. 53*, 3043.
33. McKee, L.H., and Harden, M.L. (1991) *Lebensm. Wiss Technol. 24*, 198.

34. Lee, Y.B., Kim, Y.S., and Ashmore, C.R. (1986) *J. Food Sci. 51*, 20.
35. Jitoe, A., Masuda, T., Tengah, I.G.P., Suptapta, D.N., Gara, I.W., and Nakatani, N. (1992) *J. Agric. Food Chem. 40*, 1337.
36. Masuda, T., and Jitoe, A. *J. Agric. Food Chem. 42*, 1850.
37. Kramer, R.E. (1985) *J. Am. Oil Chem. Soc. 62*, 111.
38. Lagouri, V., Blekas, G., Tsimidou, M., Kokkini, S., and Boskou, D. (1993) *Z. Lebensm Unters Forsch 197*, 20.
39. Vekiari, S.A., Oreopoulou, V., Tzia, C., and Thomopoulos, C.D. (1993) *J. Am. Oil Chem. Soc. 70*, 483.
40. Duve, K.J., and White, P.J. (1991) *J. Am. Oil Chem. Soc. 68*, 365.
41. Tian, L.L., and White, P.J. (1994) *J. Am. Oil Chem. Soc. 71*, 1079.
42. De Sotillo, D.R., Hadley, M., and Holm, E.T. (1994) *J. Food Sci. 59*, 649.
43. De Sotillo, D.R., Hadley, M., and Holm, E.T. (1994) *J. Food Sci. 59*, 1031.
44. Onyeneho, S.N., and Hettiarachchy, N.S. (1993) *J. Sci. Food Agric. 62*, 345.
45. Kanner, J., Frankel, E., Granit, R., German, B., and Kinsella, J.E. (1994) *J. Agric. Biol. Chem. 42*, 64.
46. Duh, P.-D., Yeh, D.-B., and Yen, G.-C. (1992) *J. Am. Oil Chem. Soc. 69*, 814.
47. Yen, G.-C., and Duh, P.-N. (1994) *J. Am. Oil Chem Soc. 42*, 629.
48. Chiou, R.Y.-Y. (1992) *J. Agric. Food Chem. 40*, 1598.

Chapter 3

Antioxidants from Cereals and Legumes

P.J. White and Y. Xing

Food Science and Human Nutrition Department, Iowa State University, Ames, Iowa.

Introduction

Autoxidation of polyunsaturated fatty acids not only lowers the nutritional value of foods (1), but is also related to membrane damage, aging, heart disease, and cancer in living organisms (2–6). Antioxidants are principal ingredients that protect food quality by retarding oxidative breakdown of lipids (7). Synthetic antioxidants, such as butylated hydroxyanisole (BHA), butylated hydroxytoluene (BHT), *tert*-butylhydroquinone (TBHQ) and propyl gallate (PG) are used widely in the food industry because of their effectiveness; generally, they are also less expensive than natural antioxidants (6–8). Concerns regarding pathological effects and carcinogenic potential of synthetic antioxidants (9) have prompted study of natural alternatives in the last few decades (7).

Natural antioxidants in foods may be from (i) endogenous compounds in one or more components of the food; (ii) substances formed from reactions during processing; or (iii) food additives isolated from natural sources (10). Most cereals and legumes contain some antioxidants, but oats and soybeans have been studied the most extensively. It has been known for most of the 20th century that certain seeds and their oils, in addition to cereals, have antioxidant properties (11). In the 1930s, Musher (12) found that rancidity in lard could be inhibited by the addition of soy flour, sesame flour, and oat flour. He obtained numerous patents on the use of oat fractions as antioxidants (13–19). Lowen *et al.* (20) demonstrated the antioxidant value of oat flour on salmon and halibut liver oils.

Types of Antioxidants Found in Cereals and Legumes

Typical compounds that possess antioxidant activity include phenols, phenolic acids and their derivatives, flavonoids, tocols, phospholipids, amino acids and peptides, phytic acid, ascorbic acid, pigments, and sterols. A general description of each of these compounds follows.

Phenols, Phenolic Acids and Their Derivatives

Phenolic compounds are widely distributed in cereals and legumes. Ferulic, caffeic, protocatechuic, *p*-hydroxybenzoic, vanillic, syringic and *p*-coumaric acids are the most common phenolic acids found in cereals. Chlorogenic, isochlorogenic, caffeic, ferulic, *p*-coumaric, syringic, vanillic and *p*-hydroxybenzoic acids commonly are present in legumes (21).

In cereals, the total free phenolic acid content rarely exceeds 0.02% of the dry weight of whole, mature, undamaged grain (22). Phenolic acids occur in the grain of cereals primarily in the bound form as conjugates with sugars, fatty acids, or proteins (23). Antioxidative activities of some ferulic acid sugar esters were found stronger than that of free ferulic acid in a microsomal lipid peroxidation system (24).

Phenolic antioxidants are primary antioxidants which act as free-radical terminators. The position and the degree of hydroxylation is of primary importance in determining antioxidant activity (10). Cuvelier *et al.* (25) tested the antioxidative efficiency of many phenolic acids and phenols and established a relationship between the structure of these molecules and their antioxidative activity. Several observations were made: (i) Apart from BHA, all of the monophenols were less efficient than the polyphenols. The introduction of a second hydroxyl group in the *ortho* or *para* position increased antioxidative activity. The antioxidative efficiency of monophenols was increased substantially by one or two methoxy substitutions at the *ortho* position relative to the hydroxyl group, but methoxy substitution was far less effective than the addition of a hydroxy group. (ii) The presence of the CH=CH-COOH group in cinnamic acids ensured greater antioxidative efficiency than the COOH group in benzoic acid. (iii) The combination of two acid phenols increased antioxidant effectiveness. Marinova and Yanishlieva (26) also compared the antioxidant properties of benzoic acid and cinnamic acid derivatives in the concentration range from 0.02 to 0.20 wt% during autoxidation at 100°C of lard and sunflower oil methyl esters. In both systems, the derivatives of benzoic acid had weaker inhibiting properties than did the corresponding analogues of cinnamic acid. Structures of some of the most common phenolic acids are shown in Fig. 3.1.

Papadopoulos and Boskou (27) tested the total polar fraction and individual phenols present in virgin olive oil for their antioxidant effect in refined olive oil. Hydroxytyrosol and caffeic acid had greater protection factors than did BHT. Protocatechuic and syringic acids also demonstrated antioxidant activity. Onyeneho and Hettiarachchy (28) noted that phenolic acids were partly responsible for the strong antioxidant activity of a freeze-dried extract of durum wheat bran.

Marinova and Yanishlieva (29) studied the antioxidant activity of 0.2–2.0 g/kg ferulic acid on purified lard triacylglycerol, at 25, 50, 75 and 100°C. The effectiveness of ferulic acid remained constant with increasing temperature. The rate of substrate oxidation decreased with increased ferulic acid concentration.

Flavonoids

Flavonoids are a group of plant phenols characterized by the carbon skeleton C_6-C_3-C_6. The basic structure of these compounds consists of two aromatic rings linked by a three-carbon aliphatic chain which normally has been condensed to form a pyran or, less commonly, a furan ring (30).

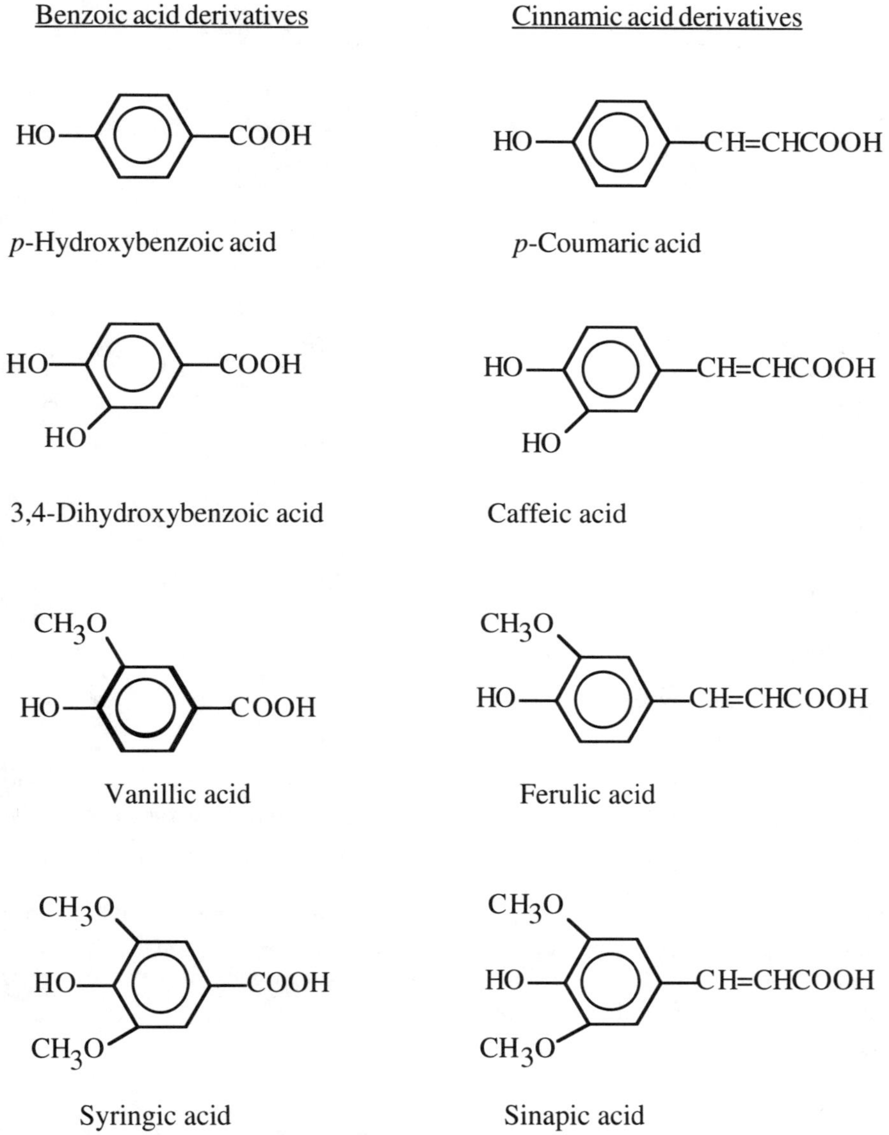

Fig. 3.1. Structures of some common phenolic acids.

Flavonoids, including flavones, flavonols, isoflavones, catechins, flavanones, and chalones, occur in all types of higher plant tissue. Flavones and flavonols are found in almost every plant, particularly in the leaves and petals, with flavonols occurring more frequently than flavones (31). The structures of some common flavonoids are shown in Fig. 3.2.

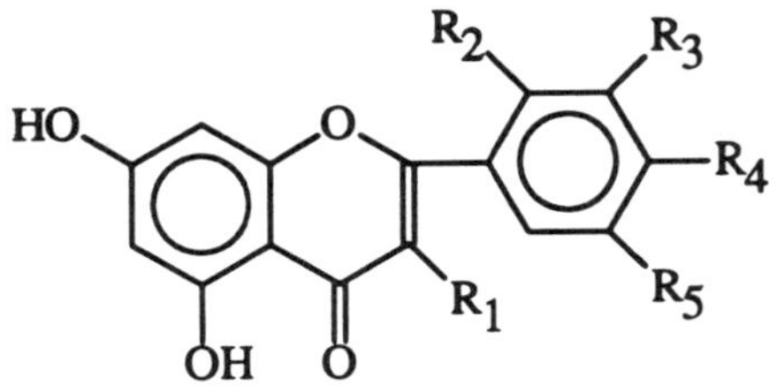

	R_1	R_2	R_3	R_4	R_5
Flavones					
Apigenin	H	H	H	OH	H
Chrysin	H	H	H	H	H
Luteolin	H	H	OH	OH	H
Flavonols					
Datiscetin	OH	OH	H	H	H
Quercetin	OH	H	OH	OH	H
Myricetin	OH	H	OH	OH	OH
Morin	OH	OH	H	OH	H
Kaempferol	OH	H	H	OH	H

Fig. 3.2. Structures of some common flavonoids.

Flavonoids occur as glycosides which, during hydrolysis with acid and heat, produce an aglycone and a sugar moiety (32). Many of the flavonoids and related compounds have strong antioxidant characteristics (30).

Heimann and co-workers (33,34) showed that quercetin, which occurs ubiquitously in natural products, is a better inhibitor of the autoxidation of ethyl linoleate than are the tocopherols or the usual antioxidants, ethyl or propyl gallate. As antioxidants, flavonoids demonstrate primary antioxidant activity (i.e., they act as free-radical acceptors and as chain-breakers) (30).

Tocols

Eight substances having vitamin E activity occur in nature (Fig. 3.3). The tocopherols have a saturated sidechain, whereas the tocotrienols have an unsaturated side chain. The various tocopherols and tocotrienols (α, β, γ and δ) differ in the methylation of the chromanol ring.

Cereals and legumes are rich sources of tocols. The contents may depend to a large extent on the variety and growing conditions of the plants and on the processing and storage of the oil (35). α-Tocopherol is the most abundant tocol in food and also the most biologically active (35,36).

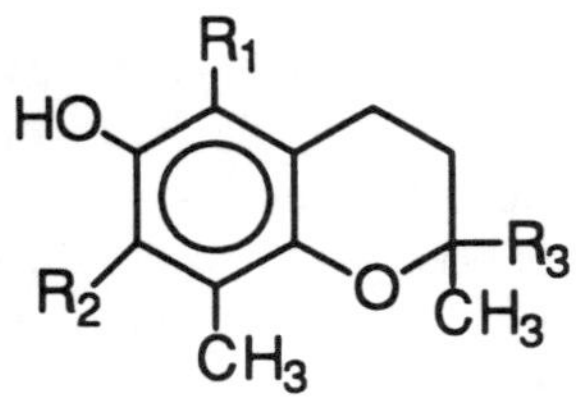

	R_1	R_2	R_3
<u>Tocopherols</u>			
α-tocopherol	CH_3	CH_3	$CH_2[CH_2CH_2CH(CH_3)CH_2]_3H$
β-tocopherol	CH_3	H	"
γ-tocopherol	H	CH_3	"
δ-tocopherol	H	H	"
<u>Tocotrienol</u>			
α-tocotrienol	CH_3	CH_3	$CH_2[CH_2CH{=}C(CH_3)CH_2]_3H$
β-tocotrienol	CH_3	H	"
γ-tocotrienol	H	CH_3	"
δ-tocotrienol	H	H	"

Fig. 3.3. Structures of tocols.

As antioxidants, tocols are important for the protection of unsaturated lipids against oxidation in biological membranes (37). The mechanism involves a reaction with chain-propagating free radicals, especially peroxyl radicals, resulting in the formation of relatively stable phenoxyl radicals (38).

The relative antioxidant activity of different tocopherols depends on temperature, lipid composition, physical state (bulk oil phase or emulsion), and tocopherol concentrations (39–44). Marinova and Yanishlieva (29) studied the antioxidant activity of 0.2–2.0 g/kg α-tocopherol on purified lard triacylglycerols at 25, 50, 75 and 100°C. α-Tocopherol was more effective in extending the induction period and reducing the rate of autoxidation as the temperature increased. The rate of substrate oxidation increased with increased α-tocopherol concentration, especially at lower temperatures. This behavior was attributed to the participation of antioxidant molecules and radicals in the autoxidation process. Antioxidant activity of the tocopherols was observed mainly in fats containing a small amount of antioxidant. The optimal effect was observed with 200 mg/kg tocopherol. The literature states that the antioxidative efficacy of tocopherols is in the following order: at 20–60°C, α > γ > β > δ; and at 80–120°C, δ > γ > α > β (43,44). For purified soybean oil, the optimum concentration of α-, γ-, and δ-tocopherols for oxidative stability was 100, 250 and 500 mg/kg, respectively, at 55°C in the dark. The tocopherols had significant prooxidant effects at higher concentrations (41).

The quantitative antioxidant effects of α-, γ- and δ-tocopherols on chlorophyll b-photosensitized oxidation of soybean oil were studied by Jung *et al.* (42). They concluded that a 1.0×10^{-3} M concentration of α-tocopherol (approximately 540 mg/kg) showed the greatest effect and that γ-tocopherol was second, followed by δ-tocopherol. α-Tocopherol and γ-tocopherol were similar in effectiveness, and δ-tocopherol had less effect at a concentration of 2.0×10^{-3} M. The three tocopherols, however, were equally effective at a concentration of 4.0×10^{-3} M. It was concluded that α-tocopherol quenched singlet oxygen to reduce the photosensitized oxidation of oil.

Huang *et al.* (40) studied the antioxidant activity of α-tocopherol and γ-tocopherol in bulk corn oil and in oil-in-water emulsions. On the basis of hydroperoxide formation, α-tocopherol showed maximum activity at 250–500 mg/kg in bulk oil, but no significant difference was observed in antioxidant activity between 250 and 1000 mg/kg in emulsions. α-Tocopherol had a slight initial prooxidant effect at 250 mg/kg or greater concentrations in bulk oil and at 500 mg/kg or greater concentrations in emulsions, whereas γ-tocopherol showed no prooxidant activity in either system. γ-Tocopherol, however, showed less antioxidant activity than α-tocopherol at 100 mg/kg, but greater antioxidant activity at higher concentrations in both systems.

The α-, γ-, and δ-tocopherols were tested with linoleic acid in an aqueous medium (45). At 0.05 mol of tocopherol/mol of linoleic acid, α-tocopherol had a prooxidant effect, whereas δ- and γ-tocopherol were antioxidants. γ-Tocopherol, however, exhibited slight antioxidant activity. When tocopherol concentration was decreased to 0.025 mol, α-tocopherol still exhibited the same prooxidant activity, and the antioxidant effects of γ- and δ-tocopherols were increased. Researchers suggested that tocopherols are oxidized in air in the order α > γ > δ and, therefore, their antioxidant activities are reversed (45).

The antioxidant effectiveness of tocopherols can be enhanced by the addition of various products usually classified as synergists. An important antioxidant activity was obtained by the association of α-tocopherol with cysteine, BHT, hydroquinone and ascorbyl palmitate (46).

Vitamin E acts as a primary antioxidant, whereas vitamin C reductively regenerates oxidized vitamin E. Finckh and Kunert (47) found that peroxidative cell damage was highly controlled by an antioxidative system of vitamins C and E. Recently, Frankel *et al.* (48) evaluated lipophilic and hydrophilic antioxidants in corn oil stripped of natural tocopherols in both bulk and emulsion systems. The lipophilic antioxidants α-tocopherol and ascorbyl palmitate were more effective in an oil-in-water emulsion system than in bulk oil, whereas the opposite was found for the hydrophilic antioxidants, Trolox C (6-hydroxy-2,5,7,8-tetramethylchroman-2-carboxylic acid, a hydrophilic carboxylic acid derivative of α-tocopherol) and ascorbic acid.

Yi *et al.* (49) studied the individual and combined effects of ascorbic acid and δ-tocopherol on the autoxidation of fish oil. The antioxidative efficiency of ascorbic acid and δ-tocopherol increased with increased concentrations, and their activities were highly synergistic. When δ-tocopherol content was varied at a fixed content of ascorbic acid, the synergistic efficiency was generally 100% or more. On the other hand, when ascorbic acid content was varied at a fixed content of δ-tocopherol, the synergistic efficiency rose sigmoidally with increasing concentration. The researchers concluded that at least 0.01–0.02% ascorbic acid was required to obtain a considerable synergistic effect with δ-tocopherol in stabilizing fish oil.

Although α-tocopherol is considered to have the greatest vitamin E activity (50), Serbinova *et al.* (51) suggested that α-tocotrienol may have 40 to 60 times greater antioxidant activity than α-tocopherol against (Fe^{2+} + ascorbate)- and (Fe^{2+} + NADPH)-induced lipid peroxidation in rat liver microsomal membranes and 6.5 times better protection of cytochrome P450 against oxidative damage. Yamaoka and co-workers (52,53) compared antioxidative activities of tocotrienol and tocopherol. They concluded that when α-tocopherol, α-tocotrienol, γ-tocopherol and γ-tocotrienol were added to a prepared dilinoleoylphosphatidylcholine (DLPC) liposome solution, the antioxidative activity of tocotrienol was greater than that of tocopherol. When incorporated into the liposomal membrane, however, the antioxidative activities of tocotrienols and tocopherol were the same and were intermediate between those of the added tocotrienols and tocopherols.

Phospholipids

Phospholipids are widely distributed in legumes and cereals. The occurrence of phospholipids in oil is important because of the detrimental effects these compounds may exert on oil stability and quality. Several studies indicated that phospholipids chelate with trace metals and carry them through the refining process. This action subsequently contributes to oil instability because of the autoxidation of unsaturated fatty acids (54–56). On the other hand, phospholipids acted as synergists with tocopherol and inhibited autoxidation of polyunsaturated fatty acids in model systems of both lard and refined soybean oil (57).

Linow and Mieth (58) found that the antioxidant activity of α-tocopherol in methyl linoleate was increased by adding 1% phosphatidylcholine (PC) or 1% phosphatidylethanolamine (PE). The addition of the phospholipids also reduced the decomposition of soybean tocopherols in linoleate oxidation. Hudson and Mahgoub (59) found that PC and PE from eggs acted as synergists with α-tocopherol and/or quercetin in the autoxidation of lard. Among PC, PE and phosphatidic acid (PA), PE was the most effective antioxidant in the autoxidation of ghee (clarified butter fat) (60).

The synergistic effects of PE in enhancing the antioxidant properties of various polyhydroxy flavones and flavanones (61), polyhydroxy isoflavones (62) and tocopherols in both lard and soybean oil (57) were demonstrated. Dipalmitoyl phosphatidylethanolamine (DPE) was a potent synergist for a wide range of primary antioxidants in edible oils at elevated temperatures, i.e., >80°C. At lower temperatures, it had very little synergistic action. At 120°C, the synergistic effect increased progressively as the concentration of the synergist increased from 0.025 to 0.25% (63). At a given level of synergist, its effect was proportionately greater at lower levels of primary antioxidant (63). In the presence of DPE, the life of PG was extended, and longer induction periods for lard were observed (64).

Hildebrand *et al.* (65) showed that the addition of tocopherols and phospholipids [PE, phosphatidylinositol (PI) and PC] increased the stability of degummed and bleached soybean oil. Phosphatidylinositol and PE were more effective than PC. The effect of the phospholipid was not simply a matter of prooxidant metal inactivation; rather, it seemed to extend the effectiveness of the tocopherol in free-radical termination.

Yuki *et al.* (66) found that PC inhibited the degradation of tocopherols and their dimers. Fujilahi and Ando (67–70) reported a similar protective activity of PC toward tocopherols in triacylglycerol oxidation. Kashima *et al.* (71) studied the antioxidant effects of phospholipids on the oxidation of refined perilla oil, tocopherol-free perilla oil (POF), and tocopherol-enriched perilla oil (POR) at 37°C. The oxidative stability of POF was markedly low, and none of the phospholipids [PC, PE or phosphatidylserine (PS)] had an antioxidant effect on POF. But the oxidation of POR was suppressed significantly by the addition of PE or PS. Phosphatidylcholine had a low antioxidant effect on POR. It seemed that the antioxidant effect of phospholipids, especially of PE and PS, was a result of the presence of tocopherols in perilla oil.

Amino Acids and Peptides

Amino acids frequently have been tested as antioxidants in oils and fats (72–78). Marcuse (72) reported that tryptophan and histidine had good antioxidant effects in methyl linoleate emulsions. Karel *et al.* (73) found that histidine, lysine, β-amino butyric acid, and cysteine had an antioxidant effect in freeze-dried model systems of methyl linoleate based on microcrystalline cellulose. Proline at 0.02% had an antioxidative effect similar to that of BHA at 0.02% in sardine oil and was five times more effective at 0.1% (74). In another study, methionine, threonine, lysine, and histidine had antioxidative effects in freeze-dried emulsions of safflower oil (75). Ahmad *et al.* (76) indicated that several amino acids, when added alone at 0.02% to crude safflower oil and to freshly prepared commercial vegetable oil composed of 50% sunflower and 50% cottonseed oil, were as effective as BHA and BHT at the same level. Seher and Löschner (77) found that a mixture of amino acids had good antioxidant activity in lard. Chen and Nawar (78) studied the positive antioxidant activity of amino acids on milk fat oxidation.

Amino acids and peptides possess both antioxidant and prooxidant activity. Marcuse (72) found that most amino acids (except cysteine) had significant antioxidative potential. In contrast, cysteine was reported to be an effective antioxidant in soybean, rice, and corn oils, lard, and tallow, and its effectiveness was ranked higher than that of methionine in olive oil (79–81). The activity of specific amino acids, whether as an antioxidant or as a prooxidant, is dependent on certain conditions such as concentration and pH. At very low concentrations, most amino acids have marked antioxidant activity, but many become prooxidative at increased concentrations. At low pH levels, most amino acids are prooxidants; higher pH levels favor antioxidant activity (72). Ahmad *et al.* (82) studied 27 amino acids and found that most had some antioxidant activity when added in aqueous solution to either safflower oil or a mixture of sunflower and cottonseed oil. But cysteine-HCl, glutamic acid (in the mixture), and glutamic acid-HCl (in safflower oil) behaved as prooxidants. Krishna and Prabhakar (83) found that the antioxidant efficacy varied with relative humidity (RH) and the individual amino acids. Arginine had a greater antioxidant efficacy at all RH values than the control. The efficacy of alanine was equal to that of arginine at RH levels of 50 and 79% but was lower at 2% RH. The presence of aliphatic, alkaline amino, hydroxyl, or thiol groups in the side chain of the amino acids increased the antioxidant efficacy at high RH levels.

Various amino acids were attached covalently to Trolox C, a lower homolog of vitamin E that has good antioxidant effectiveness. The resulting Troloxyl-amino acids had greater antioxidant effectiveness than Trolox C in a linoleate emulsion system oxidized by hemoglobin (84). Amino acids function both as primary antioxidants and as synergists with phenolic antioxidants (72). In a study of factors affecting the acceptance and stability of a soup and gravy base, Bishov *et al.* (85) observed an apparent antioxidant activity in the hydrolyzed vegetable protein (HVP) component. The sole effect of HVP and autolyzed yeast proteins (AYP) was to prolong the induction period (86). Hydrolyzed vegetable protein and AYP also can work as synergists with phenolic antioxidants (86,87). Autolyzed yeast protein (0.25%) plus 0.005% BHA (both based on oil weight in a water-corn oil emulsion) had antioxidant activity about equal to that of 0.02% BHA alone. In addition, 0.5% AYP with 0.005% BHA was more protective than was 0.02% BHA alone (87).

Phytic Acid

Phytic acid is a natural plant antioxidant constituting 1–3% by weight of many cereals and legumes (88) and typically accounting for 50–90% of the total seed phosphorus (89). The unique structure of phytic acid (Fig. 3.4) suggests tremendous chelating potential.

Many antioxidants function by reacting with activated oxygen species, thereby being consumed. Phytate, in contrast, is remarkably unreactive and extraordinarily stable. All of the antioxidant properties of phytic acid are presumably derived from its relatively high binding affinity for iron (90). This property makes phytic acid a unique and versatile food preservative. It prevents both autoxidation and hydrolysis of soybean oil (91,92) and stabilizes other lipid-containing foods against rancidity (93). Wu *et al.* (94) extracted phytic acid from wild rice and found that it had antioxidant activity in ground beef and lard.

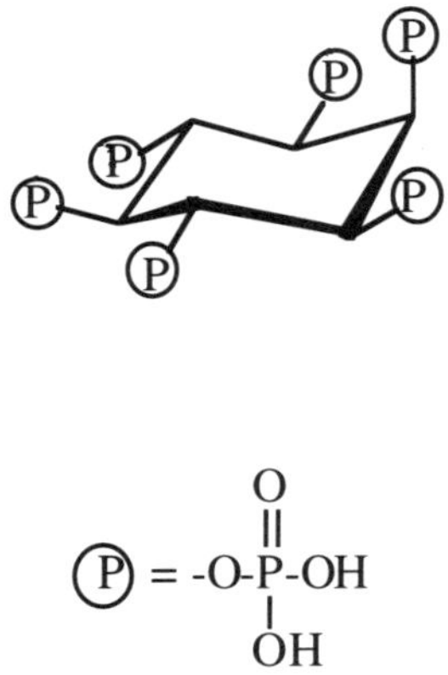

Fig. 3.4. Structure of phytic acid in dilute solution.

There is disagreement about the biological role of phytic acid. Some nutritionists consider phytic acid an antinutrient because it chelates with Ca^{2+}, Zn^{2+}, and other minerals, making them biologically unavailable. On the other hand, Graf (88) pointed out that only in rare instances has phytic acid been implicated as a direct cause of human trace-mineral deficiencies. Cationic imbalances usually occur in malnourished populations. The caloric inadequacy of their diets may have caused the phytate impairment of mineral bioavailability and its clinical symptoms. In other work, the carcinogenic effects of azoxymethane were offset significantly when experimental animals were given drinking water containing 1% sodium phytate (95). Graf and Eaton (90) concluded that dietary phytic acid may lower the incidence of colonic cancer and protect against other inflammatory bowel diseases. Its addition to foods inhibits lipid peroxidation and concomitant oxidative spoilage, such as discoloration and putrefaction.

Pigments

Carotenoids are colored pigments, a very minor constituent in cereal grains. Among the cereals, they are most abundant in corn, yellow sorghum, and millet (96). Two general classes of carotenoids, which are carotenes and xanthophylls, are primarily responsible for the yellow color of corn grain (97). Carotenoids are believed to provide antioxidant protection to lipid-rich tissues. β-Carotene and lycopene, specific carotenoids, are particularly effective at quenching singlet oxygen, which is not a free radical but is highly reactive (98). Burton and Ingold (99) found that β-carotene can behave as an antioxidant at low oxygen pressures.

In the presence of δ-tocopherol, β-carotene behaved synergistically in preventing oxidation. Apparently, tocopherols protect the β-carotene from free-radical autoxidation (100). Warner and Frankel (100) found that β-carotene at low levels (5–20 mg/kg) had a significant effect in protecting soybean oil against light deterioration, which can be attributed to the protective effect of the natural tocopherols in the soybean oil. In the dark, however, β-carotene apparently was not sufficiently protected by tocopherols, and its free-radical oxidation may account for the increased peroxide values observed under these conditions.

Many investigators consider chlorophyll a prooxidant, but a few regard chlorophyll as an antioxidant. Matsushita *et al.* (101) observed antioxidant activity in some porphyrin compounds such as pheophytin and chlorophytin. Endo *et al.* (102) investigated the effects of chlorophyll and pheophytin on the autoxidation of oils in the dark and concluded that chlorophyll existing in vegetable oils can act as an antioxidant, preventing oxidative deterioration if the vegetable oil containing chlorophyll is not exposed to light and is stored at a low temperature. Fakourelis *et al.* (103) reported that chlorophyll in the purified virgin olive oil acted as a photosensitizer for singlet oxygen formation under light.

Recently, Tsuda *et al.* (104) examined the antioxidative role of the pigments in the seed coat of pea bean. The pigment cyanidin 3-*O*-β-D-glucoside from red bean showed strong antioxidative activity in the linoleic acid system at pH 7, whereas pelargonidin 3-*O*-β-D-glucoside from red bean and delphinidin 3-*O*-β-D-glucoside from black bean exhibited no antioxidative activity at pH levels 3 and 5. These pigments are similar in structure to the flavonoids.

Sterols

Although not effective as traditional antioxidants at room temperature, sterols were reported to have antipolymerization activity in heated oils (105–110). The unsaponifiables isolated from olive, corn, wheat and *Vernonia anthelmintica* oils were effective in protecting safflower oil from oxidative polymerization during heating at frying temperature. The 4-α-methyl sterols from wheat germ oil and sterols from *Vernonia* oil were the effective agents (105). Δ^5-Avenasterol and olive oil sterol mixtures containing Δ^5-avenasterol reduced polymerization in cottonseed oil at frying temperatures (106). Δ^5-Avenasterol and fucosterol were effective at reducing polymerization at 180°C in a triacylglycerol mixture similar in composition to olive oil (107). White and Armstrong (108) studied the antipolymerization effects of Δ^5-avenasterol (separated from oat oil) in soybean oil at 180°C and found that all heated oils with added oat-sterol fractions containing Δ^5-avenasterol deteriorated more slowly than did the controls containing no sterol additions. The antipolymerization activity of the sterol at frying temperature was thought to reside in its side chain, which contains an ethylidene group (109). Yan and White (110) demonstrated that the antipolymerization activity does indeed reside in the side chain of Δ^5-avenasterol.

Vitamin C

Vitamin C (ascorbic acid), a water-soluble antioxidant, provided protection against oxidation of lipids and low-density lipoprotein (LDL) in plasma (111). It is an effective quencher of oxyradicals in the body's aqueous compartments such as blood plasma and cell cytosol (98).

Several researchers have proposed that vitamin C acts as an antioxidant-synergist with the lipid-soluble vitamin E and that both vitamins can work together as a powerful antioxidative system in cells (112). Ascorbic acid was more active in retarding rancidity than were BHA and BHT but less active than TBHQ and PG in oil systems with high tocopherol contents (113). The effects of vitamin C in combination with tocols were discussed in the section on tocols.

Antioxidants in Cereals and Legumes

The presence of all of these groups of antioxidants has been noted in many cereals and legumes. In many instances, the actual antioxidant activity was not measured. Compounds such as the phenolics were measured primarily due to the importance of their flavor, because they are quite bitter even at low levels.

Barley

Barley (*Hordeum vulgare* L.) contains a wide range of phenolic compounds in one form or another, including free and combined tyrosine, tyramine and derivatives; phenolic acids, esters and glycosides; and numerous other phenols such as lignans and substances related to lignans (114). Vanillic, ferulic, diferulic, salicylic, *p*-hydroxybenzoic, protocatechuic, *o*-, *m*- and *p*-coumaric, syringic and sinapic acids were found in barley grains (23,115,116). Ferulic and *p*-coumaric acids were quantitatively the most important phenols. The outer layers of the grain, consisting of husk, pericarp, testa and aleurone cells, contained the greatest concentrations of total phenolic acids (0.6–0.9%), whereas their concentrations were considerably lower in the endosperm layers (0.1% or less) (115). The greatest concentration of phenolic acids was observed at 19–31 d after anthesis. In the ripe seeds or seeds stored for 2–6 wk after harvesting, the concentration of free and soluble-bound phenolic acids was distinctly lower (23).

A flavonoid, 2″-*o*-glycosylisovitexin, isolated from young green barley leaves (*H. vulgare* L. var. *nudum* Hook), showed antioxidative activity almost equivalent to that of α-tocopherol in a lipid peroxidation system at a high level of 100 μg/1.5 mg of ethyl linoleate (117,118).

Barley is one of the best sources of tocols, containing all eight vitamin E isomers and having a high concentration of total tocols; however, significant genotype differences exist for most tocols in the barley species (119). Removal of the hull, aleurone, and germ by abrasion (pearling) significantly lowered the tocol concentration of the pearled barley compared with whole kernels. Barley hulls and endosperm had substantial tocol concentrations, especially tocotrienols, whereas the germ contained a large concentration of α-tocopherol (120). The pearling fraction had more total tocols than the milling fraction (121). Greater humidity during airtight storage resulted in increased oxidation of the vitamin E (122). The tocol contents of the grain and oil are shown in Table 3.1.

TABLE 3.1
Tocol Content of Barley (mg/kg)[a]

	α-T	α-T3	β-T	β-T3	γ-T	γ-T3	δ-T	δ-T3	Total	Ref
W. clean[b]	5.94	20.40	0	5.02	0.23	4.36	0.14	0.79	36.8	120
W. grain[c]	5.96	24.92	0.20	4.86	0.32	3.61	0.20	0.48	40.3	120
W. grain[d]	8.1	43.3	0.4	—	10.0	7.7	0.4	1.0	71.0	121
W. grain[e]	9.75	33.23	0.72	7.08	0.72	5.36	0.71	0.90	58.47	119
W. grain	4.6	13.0	0.2	2.7	0.7	8.4	0.2	0.7	30.5[f]	124
W. grain[g]	11.6	36.0	0.4	14.3	12.9	—	0.9	3.9	80	122
W. seed	2	11	0.4	3	0.3	2	0.1	—	18.8[f]	125
Grain	2	11	4	3	0.3	2	1	—	23.3[f]	126
Hull[c]	9.62	13.65	0.64	2.35	0.33	2.10	0.08	0.09	28.9	120
Endosperm[c]	1.05	23.40	0.06	4.49	0	3.72	0.08	0.46	33.3	120
Germ[c]	174.65	0	0	19.95	9.81	0	2.04	0	206.5	120
Flour[d]	35.4	115.8	2.0	—	21.3	28.1	0.8	2.1	205.3	121
Flour[b]	9.3	20.8	0.8	—	7.8	3.3	0.2	0.5	42.7	121
Meal	3	16	<1	6	1	6	<1	—	<34[f]	123
Oil[g]	364	1059	—	814	143	—	—	—	2380	127

[a]T = tocopherol, T3 = tocotrienol, W. = whole, Ref = reference no., — = Not detected or not reported.
[b]Milling fraction.
[c]Hand-dissected morex barley fractions.
[d]Pearling fractions.
[e]Mean of 3 locations, 12 genotypes.
[f]Total was not reported in original paper, thus calculated by author.
[g]Data recalculated by author from percentage of total content into mg/kg units.

Phospholipids accounted for 15–25% of the total lipid content in barley (128,129). Lysophosphatidylcholine (LPC), PC and PE were present in the greatest amounts. Lesser amounts of PS, PI, phosphatidyl-glycerol, diphosphatidylglycerol and a small amount of phosphatidic acid (PA) were present (130). In barley, phytic acid content was reported by different researchers to be 1% (88), 0.56% (131) and 1.15% w/w (132). In oil extracted from barley grain, β-carotene was present in concentrations ranging from 52 to 85 mg/kg, together with xanthophylls (46–65 mg/kg) and minor quantities of α-carotene and a β-carotene isomer (133).

Corn (Maize)

Many phenolics, including *p*-hydroxybenzoic, (*p*-hydroxyphenyl) acetic, vanillic, protocatechuic, syringic, *cis-p*-coumaric, *trans-p*-coumaric, *cis*-ferulic, *trans*-ferulic, caffeic and *trans*-sinapic acids, were found in corn (*Zea mays* L.) flour. *Trans*-ferulic, at 258.6 mg/kg, was the most abundant, and the two ferulic acids accounted for 85.1% of the total phenolic acids (134). These findings agreed with those of another study, which showed that *trans*-ferulic acid accounted for most of the phenolic acid content in corn (135). In corn oil, *p*-hydroxybenzoic, vanillic, caffeic, syringic, *p*-coumaric and ferulic acids were detected; ferulic acid was the most abundant at 5.79 mg/kg, followed by *p*-coumaric acid at 1.63 mg/kg (136). The alkali-labile phenolic monomer content in mature stems of corn was relatively high. Among *p*-hydroxybenzaldehyde, vanillin, *p*-hydroxybenzoic, caffeic, syringic, vanillic, *p*-coumaric and ferulic acids, *p*-coumaric acid was the most abundant (29,110 mg/kg) followed by ferulic acid (5,242 mg/kg) (137).

The concentrations of stanyl and steryl ferulates in seven hybrids were in the range of 31–70 mg/kg (138). Norton (139) isolated and identified the steryl cinnamic acid derivatives from corn bran. Ohta *et al.* (24) studied the antioxidative activity of corn bran hemicellulose fragments and found that the antioxidative activity of some ferulic-acid sugar esters was stronger than that of free ferulic acid in a microsomal lipid peroxidation system.

Much work has been done on tocols in corn. Quackenbush *et al.* (140) determined the total tocols of 125 corn inbred lines. Among these inbreds, the total tocols ranged from 0.03 to 0.33% of the oil. Karaiwanow *et al.* (141) determined the environmental influences on total tocol contents in the analyses of Russian and German lines and hybrids. No correlation appeared between α-tocopherol content and the time required to reach maturation. γ-Tocopherol, however, declined as time to reach maturity increased (142).

High-performance liquid chromatography (HPLC) is currently the preferred method for determination of the tocols. Cavins and Inglett (143) were the first to demonstrate separation of the tocols of corn oil by HPLC (144). After that, various improvements were made in the HPLC analysis of corn tocols. γ-Tocopherol was reported to be the predominant tocol in corn grain (124,142,145–147), but Weber (148) examined 15 corn inbreds and found two inbreds with α-tocopherol levels greater than levels of γ-tocopherol. The tocol contents of the corn grain and of corn oil are shown in Table 3.2.

In corn grain, the major phospholipids are PC, PI and PE; the minor phospholipids are phosphatidylglycerol, diphosphatidylglycerol, phosphatidylserine, phosphatidic acid (PA) and *N*-acylphosphatidylethanolamine (APE) (144). Phospholipids account for 6% of the total lipid content in corn grain (155). Du Plessis and Pretorius (156) studied the effects of different refining processes on the individual phospholipids. The crude corn oil of different varieties had phospholipid-phosphorus values between 145 and 361 mg/kg. For oils at further stages of refining, the values dropped to between 4.9 and 15.5 mg/kg. Degummed oils contained PC (1.1–22 mg/kg phosphorus), PE (1.5–2 mg/kg phosphorus), PI (1.6–10 mg/kg phosphorus) and PA (trace–5 mg/kg phosphorus). Further refined oils contained no phospholipids. In corn germ, phytic acid content was 6.4% (w/w); for total grain, the content dropped to 0.9% (w/w). There was no phytic acid in corn bran (88).

TABLE 3.2
Tocol Contents of Corn (mg/kg)[a]

	α-T	β-T	γ-T	δ-T	α-T3	β-T3	γ-T3	Total	Ref
Oil[b]	142.0	—	496.7	<20	—	—	—	638.7	149
Oil[c]	121	94	638	42	—	—	—	895[d]	150
Oil	223	32	790	26	0	0	0	1071[d]	151
Oil[e]	135	—	346	13.5	—	—	—	494.5[d]	152
Oil[d]	272	2.14	566	25.2	53.7	11	61.7	992[d]	153
Oil[f]	120	10	400	20	—	—	—	550[d]	154
Kernel[g]	13.5	—	46.8	—	6.4	—	16.4	83.0	148
Kernel[h,i]	17.6	—	16.1	—	6.7	—	4.4	44.8	97
Kernel[j]	14.9	—	9.1	—	7.9	—	3.3	35.3	148
Kernel[h]	23	—	22.8	—	7.4	—	5.1	58.3	148
Kernel[k]	15.5	—	16.3	—	8.8	—	2.2	42.8	148
Flakes	<1	—	1	<1	2	—	4	<9[d]	123
Seed	0.6	—	4	—	2	—	4	10.6[d]	125
Grain	13.7	—	46.1	—	—	—	—	59.8[d]	142
Grain	22.1	—	56.0	trace	6.4	—	9.9	94.4[d]	147
Grain	0.2	—	17.5	0.3	0.3	—	3.3	21.6[d]	124

[a]See Table 3.1 for abbreviations.
[b]Units, mg/L.
[c]Alkali-refined oil.
[d]Total was not reported in original paper, thus calculated by author.
[e]Mean of two replications.
[f]Refined and bleached oil.
[g]Oh43 inbred.
[h]B37 inbred.
[i]Data recalculated by author from percentage of total tocol content into mg/kg units.
[j]A632 inbred.
[k]K6 inbred.

Ten carotenoid components are present in corn grain, primarily zeaxanthin and lutein (xanthophylls) (96). Carotenoids are not evenly distributed in the corn kernel fractions but are abundant in the endosperm (96). Weber studied 15 inbreds of corn, and found a range of 16–77 mg/kg of total carotenoids on a dry weight basis. For four inbreds, total carotenoids were concentrated in the horny endosperm (83 ± 2%). After the grain was stored at room temperature for 6 mon, the mean loss of total carotenoids for the four inbreds was 42 ± 4% (97).

Usuki *et al.* (157) determined the chlorophyll and pheophytin content of three refined corn oils. The total contents varied from 95 to 162 μg/kg oil. Warner and Mounts (154) found β-sitosterol, campesterol and stigmasterol in corn oil, at levels of 269, 78 and 22 mg/100 g oil, respectively.

Millet

Phenolic acid content of teff (*Eragrostis tef*), pearl (*Pennisetum americanum*), finger (*Eleusine coracana*) and foxtail millet (*Setaria italica*) was determined by HPLC. Ferulic, coumaric, cinnamic and gentisic acids were present in greater levels than were other phenolics. Foxtail millet contained the most phenolic acids overall, but the sample was not decorticated. The decorticated grain contains fewer phenolic acids than whole kernels (158).

The major flavones in the pigments of pearl millet were identified as *C*-glycosylvitexin, vitexin and glycosylorientin (159). The *C*-glycosylflavanol content varied among millet varieties. The *C*-glycosylvitexin was 76.6 and 275.7 mg/100 g for Ghana 16152 and Ancateur samples, respectively (160).

Slover *et al.* (125) and Piironen *et al.* (123) reported γ-tocopherol to be the major tocol in millet, whereas in another study, α-tocopherol (33%), β-tocopherol (27%) and γ-tocotrienol (31%) were reported as the major tocols (161). Barnes (124) found that γ-tocopherol was the major tocol in bulrush (*P. americanum*), foxtail and finger millet, and that β-tocotrienol content was highest in common millet (*Panicum miliacium*) (Table 3.3).

The lipid content of millet (*P. americanum*) seeds was 7.2% of the seed dry weight, and phospholipids accounted for 12% of total lipid content (162). Lysophosphatidylcholine was the major phospholipid (42%) in millet seeds, with lesser amounts of PC (24%) and lysophosphatidylethanolamine (LPE, 21%) and trace amounts of phosphatidylglycerol, PA, PS and PI (162) were present. The lipid content of small millets, namely, foxtail, proso (*Panicum miliaceum*), and finger, were studied. The phospholipid content varied from 5 to 14% of the total lipids, with PC, PE and LPC the most abundant (163). In millet, phytic acid content was 0.81% w/w (131).

Oat

Oat (*Avena sativa* L.) has been identified as a source of antioxidants since the 1930s when Sidney Musher obtained numerous patents on the use of oat fractions as antioxidants. In the early 1960s, Daniels and Martin (164) isolated caffeic and

TABLE 3.3
Tocol Contents of Millet (mg/kg)[a]

	α-T	β-T	γ-T	δ-T	α-T3	β-T3	γ-T3	δ-T3	Total	Ref
Seed	0.5	trace	13	4	—	—	—	—	17.5[b]	125
W. grain	1	1	17	6	<1	—	<1	—	<27[b]	123
"Bulrush"	1.3	—	55.4	0.8	—	—	5.3	2.0	64.8[b]	124
"Foxtail"	1.9	0.4	27.8	—	0.4	—	0.6	—	31.1[b]	124
"Finger"	3.2	0.3	17.6	—	0.5	—	—	—	21.6[b]	124
"Common"	—	0.4	—	3.5	—	15.0	—	—	18.9[b]	124

[a]See Table 3.1 for abbreviations.
[b]Total was not reported in original paper, thus calculated by author.

ferulic acids from oat. They used the active oxygen method (AOM) to test the antioxidant activity of the extract. The purified oat antioxidants, which were extracted with diethyl ether, were as effective as PG and BHT. Caffeic acid, with two hydroxyl groups in the *ortho* position, was considerably more effective than ferulic acid. Daniels *et al.* (165) further fractionated the oat extract from diethyl ether. From the alkaline hydrolysis of the components in the extract, they found six esters of phenolic acid, including caffeic and ferulic acids (166,167). Later, Daniels and Martin (168) separated the oat antioxidant into 24 active fractions, with the antioxidants identified as monoesters of hexacosan-1-ol, 26-hydroxyhexacosanoic acid and 28-hydroxyoctacosanoic acid. Finally, they identified glycerol monoesters of 26-hydroxyhexacosanoic acid and 28-hydroxyoctacosanoic acid, in which the ω-hydroxy group and the two remaining hydroxyl groups of the glycerol backbone were esterified with caffeic and ferulic acids. Many possible high-molecular-weight phenolic compounds could be formed from this basic structure (169). Durkee and Thivierge (170) reported the presence of free and bound ferulic acid and other phenolics in oat seeds.

Sosulski *et al.* (134) focused on identifying the structural forms containing caffeic and ferulic acids and other phenolics in oats and other cereal grains. They categorized the major phenolics into free, soluble ester, and insoluble bound forms. The smallest number of phenolics was found in the free form, including *trans*-ferulic, syringic and caffeic acids. Of wheat, corn, rice, potato, and oats, only oats contained a measurable amount of caffeic acid. Some phenolics were found in the soluble ester form, but the greatest quantity was present in the insoluble residue, with oats containing 54.6 mg/kg *trans*-ferulic and 1.6 mg/kg caffeic acids in the insoluble bound form.

Many phenolics were found in oat groats, hulls and flour (134,170–173, and unpublished data). In hulls, ferulic, sinapic, syringic, *p*-hydroxybenzoic, *p*-coumaric, *o*-coumaric, vanillic, 3,5-dimethoxy-4-hydroxy-cinnamic acids and vanillin were identified (171,172, and unpublished data). In groats, vanillic, *p*-coumaric, *o*-coumaric, ferulic, caffeic, *p*-hydroxybenzoic acids and catechol were identified (170,173, and unpublished data). In oat flour (dehulled, debranned, and ground), *p*-

hydroxybenzoic, protocatechuic, vanillic, *trans-p*-coumaric, (*p*-hydroxyphenyl)-acetic, syringic, *trans*-sinapic, caffeic and ferulic acids were found (134).

Cherney *et al.* (137) found some alkali-labile phenolic monomers in mature stems of oats. On a dry-weight basis, *p*-coumaric was the most abundant (10,446 mg/kg) followed by ferulic acid (3,945 mg/kg). Chen *et al.* (174), using paper chromatography and thin-layer chromatography (TLC), isolated vanillin, protocatechualdehyde, and *p*-coumaric, ferulic, and caffeic acids from wild oat (*Avena fatua* L.) aqueous hull extracts.

Collins (175) examined the structures of the bound phenolic components from oat groats and hulls. Fractions of methanolic extracts of oat groats and hulls separated by anion-exchange chromatography revealed the presence of a series of anionic substituted cinnamic acid conjugates, trivially named avenanthramides. Two-dimensional TLC showed that groat extract contained more than 25 distinct avenanthramides, whereas hull extracts contained about 20. Some 15 were common to both groat and hull preparations. As derivatives of caffeic and ferulic acids, these avenanthramides are potential antioxidants. Later, Collins *et al.* (176) found a new group of phenolic acids in aqueous alcoholic extracts of both oat groats and hulls. These acids occurred as conjugates covalently linked to the amine function of several different *o*-aminobenzoic acids. Two additional derivatives of avenalumic acid also were detected: the 3′-hydroxy- and 3′-methoxy analogues. These acids are the ethylenic homologues of *p*-coumaric, ferulic, and caffeic acids.

Recently, Dimberg *et al.* (177) studied avenanthramides as a group of phenolic antioxidants in oats. They isolated two avenanthramides belonging to a group of about 40 cinnamoylanthranilic acid derivatives in oat grain: *N*-[4′-hydroxy-3′methoxy-(*E*)-cinnamoyl]-5-hydroxyantranillic acid (A1) and *N*-[4′-hydroxy-3-methoxy-(*E*)-cinnamoyl]-5-hydroxy-4-methoxyanthranilic acid (A2). The antioxidative capacities of A1 and A2 were determined by oxygen consumption in a linoleic acid system. A1 had about 20% of the activity exerted by α-tocopherol and A2 had about 60%, whereas caffeic and ferulic acids had much lower activities: 6 and 4%, respectively. A1 was preferentially located in the outer part of the grain. It seemed to be quite heat stable, at least when located within the oat tissue during steam treatment. The amount of A1 varied between 40 and 132 mg/kg grain in 10 different oat cultivars. The amount of A2 was at least 10 times lower than this.

Duve and White (6) studied the extraction of antioxidants from oats with eight solvent systems and found the greatest antioxidant activity from methanolic extracts of Noble and Ogle oats and hulls. Tian and White (173) tested the antioxidant activity of methanolic extracts of Noble groats in pure oil and in an emulsion system. The extracts had a significant antioxidant effect in most situations, with results similar to those of TBHQ.

Oat grain and oat oil contain both tocopherols and tocotrienols. Table 3.4 summarizes the compositional content. The major tocols were α-tocotrienol and α-tocopherol, but there is disagreement about the presence of δ- and γ-isomers. Several papers reported only α- and β-isomers in oat grain extracts, detected by

TABLE 3.4
Tocol Contents of Oats (mg/kg)[a]

	α-T	β-T	γ-T	δ-T	α-T3	β-T3	γ-T3	δ-T3	Total	Ref
Oil[b]	171	—	220	61	134	24	—	—	610	127
Oil[b]	33	11	0	0	89	21	12	9	175	179
Grain	5	0.9	—	—	11	2	—	—	18.9[c]	125
Grain[d]	8.13	0.90	0.91	—	14.91	0.87	—	0.21	25.94	119
Grain	4.3	0.8	—	—	11.8	1.9	—	—	18.8[c]	124
Rolled	8	1	—	—	20	3	<1	—	<33[c]	123
D groats[e]	20.0	10.9	3.4	0	55.7	5.0	0.6	4.4	40.9	182
Flour	23.0	9.7	3.9	1.1	53.8	5.3	0	3.3	27.7	182
Bran	15.1	10.0	2.3	0	63.8	5.6	0	3.1	34.8	182
Germ[f]	107.9	0	20.18	0	0	1.43	1.51	0.18	131.23	182
Endosperm[f,g]	3.48	0.08	0.65	0	34.83	2.36	0.28	0.23	41.89	182
Hulls[f,g]	0.73	0.13	0	0	1.37	0	0.32	0.14	2.68	182

[a]See Table 3.1 for abbreviations.
[b]Data recalculated by author from percentage of total content into mg/kg units.
[c]Total was not reported in original paper, thus calculated by author.
[d]Mean from 3 locations, 12 genotypes.
[e]D = dried.
[f]Hand-dissected oat (Ogle) fractions.
[g]Mean of two replications.

gas–liquid chromatography (GLC) (125), gas chromatography and mass spectroscopy (GC-MS) (178) and HPLC (124), whereas others detected the γ- and δ-isomers in addition to α- and β-isomers using TLC (179,180) or HPLC (119,181).

Peterson and Qureshi (119) studied 12 oat genotypes from three locations, and concluded that the total tocol concentrations for genotypes ranged from 19 to 30 mg/kg and for location from 21 to 32 mg/kg. Low temperatures after flowering (12°C compared with 28°C) resulted in a lower tocol content of the oat grain at maturity (182). Recently, Peterson (181) examined the effects of different storage conditions on the stability of tocols in unprocessed oat groats and several oat products. Tocols were stable for 7 mon in all products stored in airtight jars at –24°C. At room temperature, all tocols degraded in all processed products, but were stable in undried groats. Tocols degraded faster in envelopes allowing air circulation than in airtight jars at room temperature. α-Tocopherol and α-tocotrienol decreased faster than did the other homologues during room temperature storage in envelopes. Measurement of the tocol concentration of hand-dissected oat groats revealed that most of the α- and γ-tocopherols were located in the germ; tocotrienols were concentrated in the endosperm and absent from the germ.

Research into oat phospholipids can be traced back to the last century, when Stellwaag (183) estimated phospholipids by the phosphorous extractable into various solvents and reported 0.76% "lecithin" in oats. Much work has been done since that time. Aylward and Showler (184) reported the isolation of PA and PI. Tevekelev (185), Price and Parsons (155,186), Youngs *et al.* (187), Dehghan (188) and Sahasrabudhe (189) reported the composition of phospholipids and glycolipids. Among the phospholipids in oats, PC was the most abundant, accounting for 29.9% of the total (189). Phytic acid content in oats has been reported by different researchers at 0.8 (90) and 0.62% w/w (131).

In oats, the presence of two kinds of pigments, taraxanthin and xanthophyll epoxide was reported (190). Novozhilova *et al.* (190) reported 9.8–38 mg/kg, whereas Sosedov *et al.* (191) reported 104–113 mg/kg of total carotenoid content. A chlorophyll content of 77–95 mg/kg also was reported (191).

Specific sterols found in oats and other plants that have been shown to reduce polymerization of oils during frying were discussed earlier. Knight (192) reported a sterol found in oats with the trivial name of Δ^5-avenasterol (stigmasta-7,24(28)-dien-3β-ol). Idler *et al.* (193) found that β-sitosterol made up 53–56% of the total sterols in oats and that Δ^5- and Δ^7-stigmastadiene-3β-ols, the effective sterols, were present.

Rice

In the alkaline extract of rice (*Oryza sativa*) endosperm cell walls, ferulic, *p*-coumaric, and diferulic acids were detected. The amount of each compound was estimated as 9.1, 2.5 and 0.56 mg/g cell wall, respectively. Several phenolic-carbohydrate esters were isolated from the enzymatic digest of this cell wall, which included a series of ferulic acid esters of arabinoxylan fragments and also some fractions containing a high proportion of diferulic acid (194). Sosulski (134) reported the free, soluble ester, insoluble bound, and total phenolics in cereals. For rice flour, the total phenolic acid was 85.6 mg/kg, with *trans*-ferulic the most abundant at 75.1 mg/kg. Ramarathnam *et al.* (195) reported that the total phenolics from rice hull ranged from 190 to 390 mg/kg on a dry weight basis.

A family of ferulic acid esters of unsaturated triterpenoid alcohols was identified in crude rice bran oil and termed γ-oryzanols (196). The oryzanols are antioxidants and are believed to possess curative functions for various human diseases (197–199). Diack and Saska (200) separated vitamin E and γ-oryzanol components from saponified rice bran extracts by normal-phase chromatography.

A relationship between the longevity of rice seeds and the antioxidative activity of the seed coat of the husk was established (195,201). Ramarathnam *et al.* (195) found that the total phenolic level was far greater in long-life rice seed than in short-life rice seed. Methanol extracts of the rice hull from both Katakutara (long-life) and Kusabue (short-life) seeds exhibited antioxidative activity stronger than that of α-tocopherol (202). The hull extract of long-life rice seeds had a stronger antioxidant activity than that of short-life varieties (195). Isovitexin, a *C*-glycosyl flavonoid identified in long-life rice hulls, was absent in short-life rice seeds (203).

In rice grain, γ-tocopherol, γ-tocotrienol and α-tocopherol are the major tocols (Table 3.5). Refined rice oils contain fewer tocols than crude oils (204). About 7% of the tocols are in the esterified form; the rest are in the free form (205).

Miyazawa *et al.* (207) reported that the main phospholipids in rice bran were PC, PE and PI. This information agrees with the results of Hemavathy and Prabhakar (208) which showed that the major phospholipids were PC, PE, PI and PA in decreasing order of concentration. Phosphatidylglycerol, LPC, and LPE were present in small quantities. A trace of acylphosphatidylethanolamine (APE) was also detected. Hemavathy and Prabhakar (208) reported 4.5–4.9% phospholipids in the total lipid, and Choudhury and Juliano (209) reported that nonstarch lipids contained 7–10% phospholipids.

Chlorophyll and pheophytin concentrations of two refined rice bran oils were reported as 626 and 533 μg/kg oil, respectively (157).

In rice bran that contained 0.55% oil, phytic acid was 8.7% (w/w), whereas in rice bran that contained 22% oil, phytic acid was 6.55% (w/w) (131). Wild rice (*Zizania aquatica*) contained 2.2% (w/w) phytic acid (88). Wu *et al.* (94) extracted wild rice with methanol, ethanol, and ethyl acetate. The methanol and ethanol extracts showed significant activity when added to ground beef and lard. The effective isolate was identified as phytic acid.

Some researchers have reported the composition of sterols in rice bran oil and hull oil (201-215). Campesterol, stigmasterol, and β-sitosterol were the major 4-dimethyl sterols; β-sitosterol was the most abundant. Melchert (214) reported that 2% of rice bran sterols was Δ^5-avenasterol.

TABLE 3.5
Tocol Contents of Rice (mg/kg)[a]

	α-T	β-T	γ-T	δ-T	α-T3	β-T3	γ-T3	δ-T3	Total	Ref
Seed	3	—	3	0.4	tr[b]	—	5	—	11.4[c]	126
Grain	1	—	1	tr[b]	tr[b]	—	2	—	4[c]	126
Grain	0.6	—	0.8	0.2	—	—	2.6	0.2	4.4[c]	124
Polished	<1	<1	<1	<1	1	<1	3	—	<9[c]	123
Bran oil	363.9	tr[b]	P[d]	tr[b]	tr[b]	—	—	—	510	206
Germ oil	1031.2	—	348.9	184.1	—	—	—	—	1718.7	206

[a]See Table 3.1 for abbreviations.
[b]Trace.
[c]Total was not reported in original paper, thus calculated by author.
[d]Present.

Rye

The dominant form of phenolic acid in rye (*Secale cereale*) grain was ferulic acid, although isoferulic, coumaric, syringic, *p*-hydroxybenzoic and caffeic acids also were detected in minor amounts by TLC. About 80% of the *trans*-ferulic acid was found in the bran of rye (216). Stanyl and steryl ferulate also were found in rye; the total concentration was 29 mg/kg, which consisted of 15% campesteryl, 54% campestanyl and 31% sitostanyl (138). The major tocols in rye were α- and β-tocols, but γ-tocopherol also was reported (Table 3.6).

Phospholipid content was reported as 18.3% of total lipid in rye (155). The major phospholipids in rye were PI, PC and PE, which were 2.75, 0.75, and 0.12% of total lipids, respectively (217). Phytic acid in rye was 0.57% (w/w) (131).

TABLE 3.6
Tocol Contents of Rye (mg/kg)[a]

	α-T	β-T	γ-T	α-T3	β-T3	Total	Ref
Oil	714.2	(167.4)[b]		532.4	505.5	1921.1	206
Oil[e]	967	—	124	595	794	2480	127
Flour	7.9	5.6	—	8.5	9.8	31.8	206
Flour	6	3	—	4	6	19[d]	123
Seed	16	4	—	15	8	43[d]	125
Seed	8	4	6	13	9	40[d]	126
Grain	13.1	3.9	—	14.8	11.8	43.6[d]	124
Rolled	3.9	1.1	—	14.6	9.4	29.0[d]	123
Meal	10	3	—	14	11	38d	123

[a]See Table 3.1 for abbreviations.
[b]Value is the total of β-T and γ-T.
[c]Data recalculated by author from percentage of total content into mg/kg units.
[d]Total was not reported in original paper, thus calculated by author.

Sorghum

The phenolic concentrations in sorghum (*Sorghum bicolor* L. Moench) leaf blade, leaf sheath, stem, untreated stover, and residue were reported (218-221). In sorghum leaf blade and sheath, *p*-hydroxybenzoic, vanillic, *p*-coumaric, ferulic acids, *p*-hydroxybenzaldehyde, syringaldehyde and vanillin were identified, with *p*-coumaric acid the most abundant, followed by ferulic acid (218). Dimeric phenolics, such as dihydroferulic acid, also were found (218). Caffeic and syringic acids were found in stems (137), whereas some flavonoids, such as apigenin, luteolin, apigenin and luteolin 7-*O*-glucosides, butin and apigeninidin, were identified in leaf blades and sheaths. Derivatives of the following compounds also were detected: apigeninidin, luteolinidin, chalcone, flavanone and/or dihydroflavonol, cinnamic acid, apigenin and luteolin (219). One chalcone (naringinochalcone-4′-*O*-glucoside) and two flavones (naringenin and eriodictyol) were found in sorghum grain (222). Three anthocyanogen-type flavonoids (chromogens I, II, III) were found by chromatography of a methanol extract of sorghum (223).

Analysis by HPLC indicated that γ-tocopherol was the major tocol, present at a level of 11.5 mg/kg. α-Tocopherol existed in a small amount at 0.8 mg/kg on a dry weight basis (124).

Phospholipid content was reported at 10.7% of the total lipid of sorghum (155), whereas Osagie (224) reported great differences in the phospholipid content of total lipids by using different extraction solvents. Six phospholipids were separated, with lysophospholipids constituting more than 50% of the phospholipids in sorghum seed (224).

The common varieties of sorghum grain contain only a trace of carotenoids, but yellow-endosperm sorghum types have been developed which contain 5 mg/kg or more of carotenoids including lutein, zeaxanthin and β-carotene (225). Fifty percent of the carotenoid content of yellow-endosperm sorghum grain was lost when exposed to weathering after pollination (226). Phytic acid in sorghum was present at a level of 0.81% (w/w) (131).

Triticale

Little work has been done on the antioxidants of triticale (× *Triticosecale wittmack*). Maga and Lorenz (227) found *p*-hydroxybenzoic, salicylic, gentisic, protocatechuic, vanillic, syringic, *p*-coumaric, *o*-coumaric, ferulic and isoferulic acids in whole triticale and in the bran, shorts, and flour. Vanillic, ferulic and *p*-coumaric acids were the most abundant. Caffeic, sinapic, chlorogenic and isochlorogenic acids were reported only as total content; the amount present in the free form was not specified. In the case of triticale milling fractions, the highest levels were found in the bran and the lowest levels in the flour. The total concentration of stanyl and steryl ferulates in triticale was 52 μg/g, with 7% campesteryl, 54% campestanyl and 39% sitostanyl (138).

Major tocols found in triticale were α- and β-tocopherols and α- and β-tocotrienols. The contents were 9.1, 3.0, 10.3 and 15.1 mg/kg, respectively (124). The lipid content of the whole grain was about 2.4%; the phospholipid content made up 17.1% of the total lipid (155).

Wheat

Many different types of phenolic acids were found in wheat (*Triticum aestivum* L.) (134,216,221,228,229). *Para*-hydroxybenzoic, vanillic, protocatechuic, syringic, *p*-coumaric, ferulic, gentisic, caffeic, sinapic and isoferulic acids were present, with ferulic acid being the most abundant (134,216). The ferulic acid content reported by different authors varies considerably. Pussayanawin and Wetzel (229) reported 500.5 mg/kg and 41.1 mg/kg in whole wheat and flour, respectively. Sosulski *et al.* (134) reported 63.6 mg/kg ferulic acid in freshly milled flour, and 23.9 mg/kg in flour stored for 6 mon, whereas 199 ± 9 mg/kg ferulic acid was reported in wheat flour, and 1964 ± 105 mg/kg was reported in the bran (216). Approximately 80% of the *trans*-ferulic acid of the entire wheat grain was found in the bran (216). Phenolic acids in the ethanol-soluble fraction reached a maximum concentration about 9 d after germination. The amount decreased with increased age, reaching a minimum 4–5 wk later (228). In mature wheat internodes, *p*-hydroxybenzoic, vanillic, syringic, *p*-coumaric and ferulic acids, *p*-hydroxybenzaldehyde and vanillin were found in the free form (230). Stanyl and steryl ferulates were found in nine hybrids of wheat, with the total concentration varying from 62 to 123 mg/kg (138).

In durum wheat (*Triticum durum*) bran, protocatechuic, *p*-hydroxybenzoic, gentisic, caffeic, vanillic, chlorogenic, syringic, *p*-coumaric and ferulic acids were identified. Among the free phenolics, ferulic, vanillic, and *p*-coumaric acids were present in the highest amounts (28). The freeze-dried extract from durum wheat bran exhibited stronger antioxidant activity than extracts from other milling fractions. The phenolic acids seemed to be partly responsible for the antioxidant activity of the extract (28).

Two di-*C*-glycosylflavones, 6-*C*-pentosyl-8-*C*-hexosyl- and 6-*C*-hexosyl-8-*C*-pentosylapigen, were isolated from bran of hard red spring, hard red winter, durum and white wheat (231). The total flavonoid content varied from 149.1 to 289.0 mg/kg for hard red spring wheat bran, from 271.1 to 288.2 mg/kg for hard red winter wheat bran, from 291.2 to 405.7 mg/kg for durum wheat bran and 320.3 mg/kg for white wheat bran (232).

Most researchers found only the α- and β-tocols in wheat grain (124), but two reports concerned the presence of relatively large amounts of γ- and δ-tocopherols in the tocol fractions from wheat grains (233,234). In both cases, however, β-tocotrienol was not reported, even though in other studies this tocotrienol was the major tocol in the wheat grain. It may be that the tocols were misidentified in these two reports (124). A few papers reported a small portion of γ- or δ-tocopherol in germ oil or bran oil (35,50,150,179) (Table 3.7).

TABLE 3.7
Tocol Contents of Wheat (mg/kg)[a]

	α-T	β-T	γ-T	δ-T	α-T3	β-T3	Total	Ref
W. grain	10.1	6.8	—	—	3.1	25.6	45.7	206
Seed	10	7	—	—	4	28	49[b]	125
Grain	14	7	—	—	5	33	59[b]	126
Grain	9.7	3.9	—	—	2.4	19.0	35.0[b]	124
Flour[c]	16	8	—	—	3	17	44[b]	123
Bran	16	8	—	—	15	56	95[b]	123
Bran	14.9	11.1	—	—	9.1	56	91.2	206
Germ	221	86	—	<1	3	10	321[b]	123
Meal	10	5.4	—	<1	4	21	41.4[b]	123
Bran oil[d]	141	88	0	18	88	1432	1768	179
Bran rich oil[d]	899	360	—	—	225	764	2247	50
Germ oil	2153	1087	37	101	—	—	3378[b]	150
P germ oil[d,e]	2247	791	32	—	—	95	3165	50
UP germ oil[d,e]	1093	287	18	—	72	322	1791	50

[a]See Table 3.1 for abbreviations.
[b]Total was not reported in original paper, thus calculated by author.
[c]Milled fraction mainly from the aleurone tissue, 1.2–1.4% ash.
[d]Data recalculated by author from percentage of total content into mg/kg units.
[e]P = purified, UP = unpurified.

The phospholipid content of the total lipids in wheat flour was reported to be 19.5% (235). In another study, the phospholipid content of wheat grain oil was reported to be 16.5% (155), whereas the aleurone and germ lipids had phospholipid contents of 14–17%. The nonstarch endosperm lipid had a phospholipid content of 22–35%, whereas the whole kernel lipid had a phospholipid content of 30–42% (236,237). Among all of the phospholipids found, LPC was the most abundant at 60% (235). The phytic acid content was 1.1% (w/w) in wheat, and 4.8% w/w in the wheat bran (90).

Soybean

Soybeans (*Glycene max* L.) have been used as an antioxidant since the 1930s. Musher (12) reported that suspending a bag of defatted soybean flour in melted lard protected the lard from rancidity. Soybean and soy protein products (flour and grits, concentrates, and isolates) possess antioxidant activity (21). Pratt (238) found that hot water extracts of fresh and dried soybeans, soy protein concentrate and defatted soy flour possessed appreciable antioxidant activity.

Total phenolic acid content in soybean flours was reported as 73.6 mg/100 g (239) and 23.4 mg/100 g (240). Chlorogenic, isochlorogenic, caffeic, ferulic, *p*-coumaric, syringic, vanillic, *p*-hydroxybenzoic, salicylic, and sinapic acids were present in soybeans (239–241). Hydroxylated cinnamic acid derivatives (chlorogenic, isochlorogenic, and caffeic acids) possessed strong antioxidant activity in liquid-aqueous systems (30,242). Chlorogenic acid or its hydrolysis product, caffeic acid, may be the major natural antioxidant of soybeans (21).

Flavonoids of soybeans are all isoflavones (Fig. 3.5) (21). The isoflavones of soybeans occur primarily as 7-*O*-monoglucosides of three isoflavone aglycones: genistein (5,7,4′-trihydroxyisoflavone), daidzein (7,4′-hydroxyisoflavone), and glycitein (7,4′-dihydroxy-6-methoxyisoflavone) (21). These compounds have

Aglycones

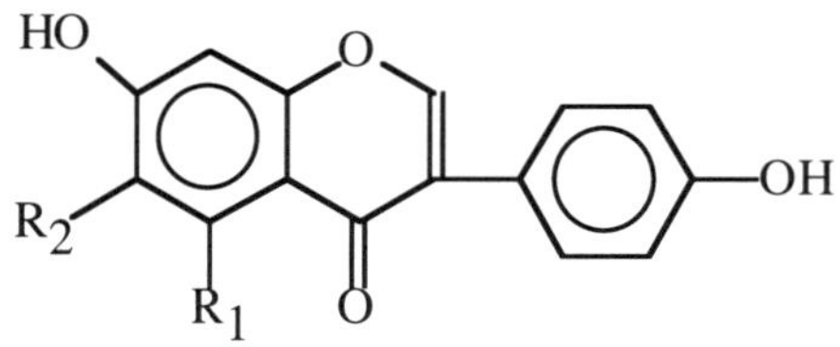

	R_1	R_2
daidzein	H	H
genistein	OH	H
glycitein	H	OCH_3

Glucosides

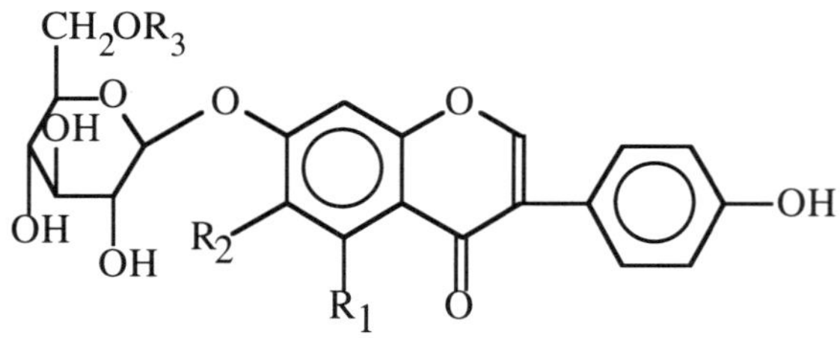

	R_1	R_2	R_3
daidzin	H	H	H
genistin	OH	H	H
glycitin	H	OCH_3	H
6″-*O*-Acetyldaidzin	H	H	$COCH_3$
6″-*O*-Acetylgenistin	OH	H	$COCH_3$
6″-*O*-Acetylglycitin	H	OCH_3	$COCH_3$

Fig. 3.5. Structures of some isoflavone isomers.

antioxidant activity and are thought to be antiestrogenic, two characteristics which may be anticarcinogenic (243). Glucosides of genistein and daidzein account for nearly 90% of the flavonoids (21).

Recently, Wang and Murphy (244) measured the amounts of 12 isoflavones in eight American and three Japanese soybean varieties using HPLC. They reported that the total isoflavone content in eight American varieties ranged from 1176 to 4216 mg/kg. The major isoflavone constituents were 6″-*O*-malonylgenistin, genistin, 6″-*O*-malonyldaidzin and daidzin. Isoflavone contents in three Japanese varieties ranged from 1,261 to 2,343 mg/kg. Compared with American varieties, Japanese varieties had greater 6″-*O*-malonylglycitin contents and greater ratios of 6″-*O*-malonyldaizin to daidzin and 6″-*O*-malonylgenistin to genistin. The same authors (245) also reported the concentration and distribution of isoflavones in 29 commercial soybean foods. Twelve isomers were quantified, three aglycones (daidzein, genistein, glycitein) and nine glucosides (daidzin, genistin, glycitin, 6″-*O*-acetyldaidzin, 6″-*O*-acetyl-genistin, 6″-*O*-acetylglycitin, 6″-*O*-malonyldaidzin, 6″-*O*-malonyl-genistin, 6″-*O*-malonylglycitin). The antioxidant activity was not lost in the preparation of soy meals, grits, concentrates, and some textured soy products (238).

The major tocols in soybean are γ- and δ-tocopherol, although α- and β-tocopherols also exist (Table 3.8). The processes of degumming, alkali refining, bleaching, and deodorization removed 31.8% of the tocopherols from crude soybean oil (246). Factors including the state of soybeans prior to extraction, high moisture content, long storage time, and bean damage all affected the tocopherol content (247).

The major phospholipids in crude soybean oils were PC, PE, PI, PA, PS and phosphatidylglycerol (250). Racicot and Handel (251) also reported the presence of LPC and LPE in crude soybean oil. The total phosphorus content ranged from 453 to 676 ppm (251). Typical phosphatide levels vary regionally and seasonally, and require monitoring by the oil processor (252).

Each step of the oil refining process reduces the phosphorus levels (252). An average of 86–98% of the phosphorus is removed during degumming (251). Damage to soybeans from pre-harvest stress, storage, and shipment has been related to an increase in nonhydratable phospholipid content of soybean oil (253). During progressive damage, the content of PC and PI decreased, whereas PA content increased (253). Mounts *et al.* (254) reported that after a 10-d storage of soy flakes, nearly 40% of their phospholipid was destroyed; PE and PC decreased, and PA increased significantly. Also, elevated temperature increased the proportion of PC and PI and decreased that of PE in soybean seeds (255).

Free amino acids and peptides are present in soybeans as a result of incomplete protein synthesis and protein degradation (256). Amino acids as nutritional supplements may contribute to antioxidant activity in products containing soybeans (21). Phytic acid content was reported at 1.4% (w/w) in whole soybeans, 1.8% (w/w) in soy flakes and 0.1% w/w in soy hulls (88), whereas other researchers reported a con-

TABLE 3.8
Tocol Concentrations of Soybean (mg/kg)[a]

	α-T	β-T	γ-T	γ-T	Total	Ref
Dry soybean	8.5	—	109.7	86.1	204.3	206
Vinton soybean	28.4	—	171	48.7	248.1[b]	248
Oil[c]	84	21	383	385	873[b]	150
Oil[d]	78	11	773	258	1120	50
Oil[e]	83	—	710	282	1075[b]	152
Oil[f]	127.6	—	728.7	221.7	1078.0	149
Oil	179	28	604	371	1182[b]	153
Oil	100	8	625	261	994[b]	151
Oil[d]	52	0	798	458	1309	179
Crude oil[d]	77	12	1062	519	1670	246
Crude oil	72.2	33.9	933	453	1490	249
Degummed oil[d]	84	11	1061	423	1579	246
Refined oil[d]	66	12	1011	456	1546	246
Bleached oil[d]	67	15	949	436	1467	246
Deodorized oil[d]	46	13	752	328	1138	246
Oil[g]	120	10	610	260	1000	154

[a]See Table 3.1 for abbreviations.
[b]Total was not reported in original paper, thus calculated by author.
[c]Alkali-refined oil.
[d]Data recalculated by author from percentage of total content into mg/kg units.
[e]Mean of two replications.
[f]Units, mg/L.
[g]Refined and bleached oil.

tent of 2.74% (w/w) phytic acid in soybean (132). Usuki *et al.* (157) reported total quantities of chlorophyll and pheophytin combined in refined soybean oil ranging from 57 to 116 μg/kg oil. Warner and Mounts (154) found β-sitosterol, campesterol and stigmasterol in soybean oil at levels of 112, 47 and 43 mg/100 g oil, respectively.

Variety Beans

The antioxidative activity of the methanolic extract of pea bean (*Phaseolus vulgaris* L.) was evaluated in a linoleic acid system; the extract exhibited strong antioxidative activity as measured by the thiocyanate method. The crude methanolic extract was partitioned between the *n*-butanol and water phases. The water phase showed strong antioxidative activity and had a synergistic effect with α-tocopherol in both food-model and liposome systems (257). A freeze-dried navy bean (*P. vulgaris* L.) hull extract was evaluated in storage studies with soy and sunflower oils and was a stronger antioxidant than a BHA-BHT mixture but was less effective than TBHQ at all levels (100, 500 and 1000 ppm) and storage conditions (26 and 37°C) (258). Drumm *et al.* (259) reported the phenolic acid contents of four market classes (navy, dark red kidney, pinto, and black turtle soup) of edible dry beans (*P. vulgaris* L.). Cinnamic, coumaric, ferulic, and sinapic acids were identified. The phenolic acids were concentrated primarily in the soluble ester fraction of plant tissues. Free phenolic acids have not been found in legume flours (260). Because the free phenolic acids are highly susceptible to oxidation, the free phenolic acids in the legume flours may have degraded before analysis (259).

Sosulski and Dabrowski (260) studied phenolic constituents in the defatted flours of 10 legume species including mung bean (*Vigna radiata*), small fababean (*Vicia faba* monor), navy bean and lima bean (*Phaseolus lunatus*). The flours contained only soluble esters, and hydrolysis revealed the presence of *trans*-ferulic, *trans*-*p*-coumaric and syringic acids in all species. Mung bean and fababean contained only 2–3 mg of phenolic acids/100 g flour; navy and lima beans contained more. Winter and Herrmann (261) found that the leaves of bush beans (variety "Fanion") had a large amount of caffeoylmalic acid as well as smaller amounts of *p*-coumaroyl-, feruloyl- and sinapoylmalic acids.

Broad bean (*Vicia faba*) leaves were reported to be rich in flavonol glycosides; they can be used as a source of such flavonoids (262). Flavonol aglycons (myricetin, quercetin, and kaempferol) were detected in the seed coat (263,264) and in the fresh broad bean (265). Five flavonoid aglycons and eight flavonol glycosides were isolated from broad bean pods. A significant increase in the concentration of both flavonoid aglycons and glycosides was observed when the pods matured and became reddish and brown (266).

In most bean varieties, only α-tocopherol and γ-tocopherol were detected, in minor amounts, in dry navy and lima beans. Total vitamin E content ranged from 0.5 to 7.7 mg/100 g in various dry beans, and was most abundant in lima beans, at 7.68 mg/100 g (206).

Phospholipid contents in four classes of dry beans ranged from 0.28 to 1.11 g/100 g lipids. The major phospholipids were PI, PA, PC and PE. Phosphatidylcholine was the most abundant, accounting for 32.48% of all phospholipids (267).

Phytate content in lima and navy beans was reported at 2.52 and 1.78% w/w, respectively, in one report (268) and at 0.84% and 1.09%, respectively, in another (131). An ethanol extract prepared from red and black bean (two varieties of pea bean) seed coats exhibited strong antioxidant activity. The pigments, cyanidin 3-*O*-β-D-glucoside (RP0) and pelargonidin 3-*O*-β-D-glucoside (RP1) from red bean and delphinidin 3-*O*-β-D-glucoside from black bean, were isolated. The RP0 exhibited strong antioxidative activity at pH 7.0, whereas the other two pigments showed strong antioxidative activity at acidic conditions (pH 3.0 and 5.0) (103). Total sterol content in four kinds of dry beans ranged from 28 to 34 mg/100 g of total lipids. Among campesterol, stigmasterol, and β-sitosterol, the last was the most abundant and ranged from 13.80 to 20.48 mg/100 g (267).

Peas

A heat-stable antioxidant component was observed to co-purify with the superoxide dismutase (SOD) activity from dried peas. The autoxidation of linoleic acid in the presence of the SOD fraction was delayed for more than 4 wk. Purified pea SOD may provide a novel, highly active, heat-stable and natural protein-bound antioxidant (269).

Peas are reported to contain a wide variety of phenolic substances. Sosulski and Dabrowski (260) found that field pea (*Pisum sativum*) and pigeon pea (*Cajanus cajan*) flours contained only 2–3 mg of phenolic acids/100 g flour, but that chickpea (*Vicer arietinum*) and cowpea (*Vigna unguiculata*) flours contained a greater amount. The flours contained only soluble esters, and hydrolysis revealed the presence of *trans*-ferulic and syringic acids in all species, whereas trans-*p*-coumaric existed only in some species and was absent in others. In another study, *p*-hydroxybenzoic, ferulic and vanillic acids were isolated from hydrolyzed and nonhydrolyzed extracts of seeds of *P. sativum* L. var. *Feltham* and var. *Lincoln*. In the Feltham variety, syringic acid was present only as the free compound, but *p*-coumaric acid occurred in both the free and bound forms (270). Elema (271) also reported the presence of caffeic, ferulic and chlorogenic acids in peas. Protocatechuic, *p*-hydroxybenzoic, vanillic, caffeic, *p*-coumaric and ferulic acids were identified and quantified in the bark, stems, and leaves of the pigeon pea. The bark and leaves contained much greater proportions of phenolic acids than the stem, and the bark contained a very high portion of free ferulic acids (272). Kaempferol and quercetin (both flavonoids) were also found in pea tissues (273).

In peas, α-, γ- and δ-tocopherols were detected, with γ-tocopherol the most abundant at 1.60 mg/100 g (274) and 2.09 mg/100 g (206). A trace of γ-tocotrienol also was reported (274).

In fresh peas, PC, PE, PI, LPC and phosphatidylglycerol were detected, with PC the most abundant followed by PE (275). The most abundant phospholipids of canned peas were PC and PI (276). In dehydrated peas, phytic acid content was reported at 0.9% (w/w) (90) and 2.2% (w/w) (132).

Peanuts

The antioxidant activity of defatted flours, protein concentrates, and protein isolates derived from peanut (*Arachis hypogaea* L.) was determined using the linoleate peroxidation model systems catalyzed by Me + Mb, Fe^{++}-EDTA (1:1), or beef homogenates (277). Dihydroquercetin (taxifolin) was identified as a flavonolic antioxidant in hot methanolic extracts of Spanish peanut (32). Strong antioxidative activity of methanolic extracts of peanut hulls also was reported (278–281). High total phenolics in peanut hulls of various maturities were associated with high antioxidant activity and with an important role in the stability of lipid oxidation (279). Total phenolic acid content was reported by different researchers as 63.6 mg/100 g (240) and 175.5 mg/100 g in peanut flour (239). Syringic, *trans-p*-coumaric, *trans*-ferulic, *trans*-caffeic and *p*-hydroxybenzoic acids were found in peanut flour, with *trans-p*-coumaric the most abundant at 146.4 mg/100 g flour (239).

The tocol content of peanuts is shown in Table 3.9. Most papers reported the presence of only α-, β-, γ- and δ-tocopherol in peanuts, but Van Niekerk *et al.* (153) also reported minor amounts of α-, β- and γ-tocotrienol.

TABLE 3.9
Tocol Contents of Peanut (mg/kg)[a]

	α-T	β-T	γ-T	δ-T	α-T3	β-T3	γ-T3	Total	Ref
Peanut	108.9	2.7	83.9	1.7	—	—	—	197.2[b]	274
Shelled	83.3	—	80.4	—	—	—	—	163.7	206
Oil[c]	170.5	—	136	6	—	—	—	312.5[b]	152
Oil	141	3.96	131	9.22	0.07[d]	3.94	0.3[d]	289.5[b]	153
Oil[e]	261.8	—	343.9	<20	—	—	—	650.7	149
Oil	139	3	189	18	0	0	0	349[b]	151
Crude oil	77.4	16.2	241	40.5	—	—	—	375	249

[a]See Table 3.1 for abbreviations.
[b]Total was not reported in original paper, thus calculated by author.
[c]Mean of two replications.
[d]Standard deviations were very high.
[e]Units, mg/L.

The major phospholipids in crude peanut oil were PC and PE, as well as PA and PI (156,282). The water-washed gums retained most of their native-state antioxidant activity. The antioxidant efficacy of water-washed gums was as good as that of synthetic antioxidants (283). The native gums, which were primarily phospholipids and glycolipids, showed increased antioxidant activity at 91% RH, whereas tocopherols did not (284). Several 4-demethylsterols were detected in peanut, including cholesterol, campesterol, stigmasterol, β-sitosterol, Δ^5-avenasterol, Δ^7-stigmasterol and Δ^7-avenasterol (285).

Conclusions

Natural antioxidants recently have gained popularity because of the belief on the part of consumers that natural food ingredients are better and safer than synthetic ones. Many natural antioxidants are found in cereals and legumes. In research studies, antioxidants often are tested alone in model systems for their antioxidative activity. In food systems, however, several kinds of antioxidants may be present, allowing complex synergistic interactions. Although some antioxidant interactions have been studied and reported here, many systems and combinations still require investigation. In addition, many of these antioxidants have not been approved as such, although they may be approved for use as flavorings. The health and safety effects of these many antioxidants demand further attention.

References

1. Farag, R.S., Badei, A.Z.M.A., and El Baroty, G.S.A. (1989) *J. Am. Oil Chem. Soc. 66*, 800.
2. Tappel, A.L. (1980) in *Free Radicals in Biology* (Pryor, W.A., ed.), Vol. IV, Academic Press, New York, pp. 1–47.

3. Pryor, W.A. (1976) in *Free Radicals in Biology* (Pryor, W.A., ed.), Vol. I, Academic Press, New York, pp. 1–49.
4. Pryor, W.A. (1984) in *Free Radicals in Molecular Biology, Aging and Disease* (Armstrong, D., Sohol, R.S., Cutler, R.G., and Slater, T.F., eds.), Raven Press, New York, pp. 13–43.
5. Cosgrove, J.P., Church, D.F., and Pryor, W.A. (1987) *Lipids 22*, 299.
6. Duve, K.J., and White, P.J. (1991) *J. Am. Oil Chem. Soc. 68*, 365.
7. Wanasundara, U.N., and Shahidi, F. (1994) *J. Am. Oil Chem. Soc. 71*, 817.
8. Sherwin, E.R., and Luckadoo, B.M. (1970) *J. Am. Oil Chem. Soc. 47*, 19.
9. Branen, A.L. (1975) *J. Am. Oil Chem. Soc. 52*, 59.
10. Pratt, D.E. (1992) in *Phenolic Compounds in Food and Their Effects on Health II, Antioxidants and Cancer Prevention* (Huang, M.-T., Ho, C.-T., and Lee, C.Y., eds.), American Chemical Society, Washington, D.C., pp. 54–71.
11. Houlihan, C.M., and Ho, C.-T. (1985) in *Flavor Chemistry of Fats and Oils* (Min, D.B., and Smouse, T.H., eds.), American Oil Chemists' Society, Champaign, pp. 117–143.
12. Musher, S. (1935) *Food Ind. 7*, 167.
13. Musher, S., U.S. Patent 2,049,017 (1936).
14. Musher, S., U.S. Patent 2,075,824 (1937).
15. Musher, S., U.S. Patent 2,176,026 (1939).
16. Musher, S., U.S. Patent 2,176,027 (1939).
17. Musher, S., U.S. Patent 2,181,765 (1939).
18. Musher, S., U.S. Patent 2,273,062 (1942).
19. Musher, S., U.S. Patent 2,355,097 (1944).
20. Lowen, L., Anderson, L., and Harrison, R.W. (1937) *Ind. Eng. Chem. 29*, 146.
21. Pratt, D.E. (1985) in *Flavor Chemistry in Fats and Oils* (Min, D.B., and Smouse, T.H., eds.), American Oil Chemists' Society, Champaign, pp. 145–153.
22. Collins, F.W. (1986) in *Oats, Chemistry and Technology* (Webster, F.H., ed.), American Association of Cereal Chemists, Inc., St. Paul, pp. 227–295.
23. Slominski, B.A. (1980) *J. Sci. Food Agric. 31*, 1007.
24. Ohta, T., Yamasaki, S., Egashira, Y., and Sanada, H. (1994) *J. Agric Food Chem. 42*, 653.
25. Cuvelier, M.-E., Richard, H., and Berset, C. (1992) *Biosci. Biotech. Biochem. 56*, 324.
26. Marinova, E.M., and Yanishlieva, N.V. (1994) *J. Am. Oil. Chem. Soc. 71*, 427.
27. Papadopoulos, G., and Boskou, D. (1991) *J. Am. Oil Chem. Soc. 68*, 669.
28. Onyeneho, S.N., and Hettiarachchy, N.S. (1992) *J. Agric. Food Chem. 40*, 1496.
29. Marinova, E.M., and Yanishlieva, N.V. (1992) *J. Sci. Food Agric. 60*, 313.
30. Pratt, D.E. (1976) in *Phenolic, Sulfur and Nitrogen Compounds in Food Flavor* (Charalambous, G., and Katz, I., eds.), ACS Symposium Series No. 26, American Chemical Society, Washington, D.C., pp. 1–13.
31. Herrmann, K. (1976) *J. Food Technol. 11*, 433.
32. Pratt, D.E., and Miller, E.E. (1984) *J. Am. Oil Chem. Soc. 61*, 1064.
33. Heimann, W., Heimann, A., Gremminger, M., and Holland, H. (1953) *Fette-Seifen-Anstrichmittel 55*, 394.
34. Heimann, W., and Reiff, F. (1953) *Fette-Seifen-Anstrichmittel 55*, 451.
35. Schuler, P. (1990) in *Food Antioxidants* (Hudson, B.J.F., ed.), Elsevier Applied Science, London and New York, pp. 99–170.

36. Wennermark, B., Ahlmén, H., and Jägerstad, M. (1994) *J. Agric. Food Chem. 42*, 1348.
37. Burton, G.W., and Traber, M.G. (1990) *Annu. Rev. Nutr. 10*, 357.
38. Goh, S.H., Hew, N.F., Ong, A.S.H., Choo, Y.M., and Brumby, S. (1990) *J. Am. Oil Chem. Soc. 67*, 250.
39. Lea, C.H., and Ward, R.J. (1959) *J. Sci. Food Agric. 10*, 537.
40. Huang, S.-W., Frankel, E.N., and German, J.B. (1994) *J. Agric. Food Chem. 42*, 2108.
41. Jung, M.Y., and Min, D.B. (1990) *J. Food Sci. 55*, 1464.
42. Jung, M.Y., Choe, E., and Min, D.B. (1991) *J. Food Sci. 56*, 807.
43. Telegdy Kováts, L., and Berndorfer-Kraszner, E. (1968) *Nahrung 12*, 407.
44. Pongracz, G. (1973) *Int. J. Vitam. Nutr. Res. 43*, 517.
45. Cillard, J., and Cillard, P. (1980) *J. Am. Oil Chem. Soc. 57*, 39.
46. Cillard, J., and Cillard, P. (1986) *J. Am. Oil Chem. Soc. 63*, 1165.
47. Finckh, B.F., and Kunert, K.J. (1985) *J. Agric. Food Chem. 33*, 574.
48. Frankel, E.N., Huang, S.-W., Kanner, J. and German, J.B. (1994) *J. Agric. Food Chem. 42*, 1054.
49. Yi, O.-S., Han, D. and Shin, H.-K. (1991) *J. Am. Oil Chem. Soc. 68*, 881.
50. Taylor, P., and Barnes, P. (1981) *Chem. Ind. 20*, 722.
51. Serbinova, E., Kagan, V., Han, D., and Packer, L. (1991) *Free Radical Biol. Med. 10*, 263.
52. Yamaoka, M., Carrillo, M.J.H., Nakahara, T., and Komiyama, K. (1991) *J. Am. Oil Chem. Soc. 68*, 114.
53. Yamaoka, M., and Komiyama, K. (1989) *J. Jpn. Oil Chem. Soc. (Yukagaku) 38*, 478.
54. Beal, R.E., Lancaster, E.B., and Brekke, O.L. (1956) *J. Am. Oil Chem. Soc. 33*, 619.
55. Lunde, G., Landmark, L.H., and Gether, J. (1976) *J. Am. Oil Chem. Soc. 53*, 207.
56. Wiedermann, L.H. (1981) *J. Am. Oil Chem. Soc. 58*, 159.
57. Hudson, B.J.F., and Ghavami, M. (1984) *Lebensm.-Wiss. u. Technol. 17*, 191.
58. Linow, F., and Mieth, G. (1976) *Nahrung 20*, 19.
59. Hudson, B.J.F., and Mahgoub, S.E.O. (1981) *J. Sci. Food Agric. 32*, 208.
60. Bhatia, I.S., Kaur, N., and Sukhija, P.S. (1978) *J. Sci. Food Agric. 29*, 747.
61. Hudson, B.J.F., and Lewis, J.I. (1983) *Food Chem. 10*, 111.
62. Dziedzic, S.Z., and Hudson, B.J.F. (1983) *Food Chem. 11*, 161.
63. Dziedzic, S.Z., and Hudson, B.J.F. (1984) *J. Am. Oil Chem. Soc. 61*, 1042.
64. Dziedzic, S.Z., Robinson, J.L., and Hudson, B.J.F. (1986) *J. Agric. Food Chem. 34*, 1027.
65. Hildebrand, D.H., Terao, J., and Kito, M. (1984) *J. Am. Oil Chem. Soc. 61*, 552.
66. Yuki, E., Morimoto, K., Ishikawa, Y., and Noguchi, H. (1978) *J. Jpn. Oil Chem. Soc. 27*, 425.
67. Fujitani, T., and Ando, H. (1981) *J. Jpn. Oil Chem. Soc. 30*, 140.
68. Fujitani, T., and Ando, H. (1982) *J. Jpn. Oil Chem. Soc. 31*, 427.
69. Fujitani, T., and Ando, H. (1984) *J. Jpn. Oil Chem. Soc. 33*, 277.
70. Fujitani, T., and Ando, H. (1985) *J. Jpn. Oil Chem. Soc. 34*, 271.
71. Kashima, M., Cha, G.-S., Isoda, Y., Hirano, J., and Miyazawa, T. (1991) *J. Am. Oil Chem. Soc. 68*, 119.
72. Marcuse, R. (1962) *J. Am. Oil Chem. Soc. 39*, 97.
73. Karel, M., Tannenbaum, S.R., Wallace, D.H., and Maloney, H. (1966) *J. Food Sci. 31*, 892.

74. Revankar, G.D. (1974) *J. Food Sci. Technol., Mysore 64*, 10.
75. Riisom, T., Sims, R.J., and Fioriti, J.A. (1980) *J. Am. Oil Chem. Soc. 57*, 354.
76. Ahmad, M.M., El-Hakim, S., and Shehata, A.A.Y. (1983) *J. Am. Oil Chem. Soc. 60*, 468.
77. Seher, A., and Löschner, D. (1986) *Fette Seifen Anstrichm. 88*, 1.
78. Chen, Z.Y., and Nawar, W.W. (1991) *J. Am. Oil Chem. Soc. 68*, 47.
79. Sliwick, J., and Siechowski, J. (1970) *Riv. Ital. Sostanze Grasse 47*, 73.
80. Enei, H., Kawaski-Shi, and Okumura, S. U.S. Patent 3,585,223 (1971).
81. Siechowaski, J. (1971) *Riv. Ital. Sostanze Grasse 48*, 365.
82. Ahmad, M.M., Al-Hakim, S., and Shehata, A.A.Y. (1983) *J. Am. Oil. Chem. Soc. 60*, 837.
83. Krishna, A.G.G., and Prabhakar, J.V. (1994) *J. Am. Oil Chem. Soc. 71*, 645.
84. Taylor, M.J., and Richardson, T. (1981) *J. Am. Oil Chem. Soc. 58*, 622.
85. Bishov, S.J., Masuoka, Y., and Henick, A.S. (1967) *Food Technol. 21*, 148A.
86. Bishov, S.J., and Henick, A.S. (1972) *J. Food Sci. 37*, 873.
87. Bishov, S.J., and Henick, A.S. (1975) *J. Food Sci. 40*, 345.
88. Graf, E. (1983) *J. Am. Oil Chem. Soc. 60*, 1861.
89. Lolas, G.M., Palamidis, N., and Markakis, P. (1976) *Cereal Chem. 53*, 867.
90. Graf, E., and Eaton, J.W. (1990) *Free Radical Biol. Med. 8*, 61.
91. Jpn. Patent 7245401; *Chem. Abstr. 80*, 2441v (1974).
92 Jpn. Patent 7245402; *Chem. Abstr. 81*, 4854b (1974).
93. Jpn. Patent 7316181; *Chem. Abstr. 79*, 145055n (1973).
94. Wu, K., Zhang, W., Addis, P.B., Epley, R.J., Salih, A.M., and Lehrfeld, J. (1994) *J. Agric. Food Chem. 42,* 34.
95. Shamsuddin, A.M., Elsayed, A.M., and Ullah, A. (1988) *Carcinogenesis 9*, 577.
96. Chung, O.K. (1991) in *Handbook of Cereal Science and Technology* (Lorenz, K.J., and Kulp, K., eds.), Marcel Deckker Inc., New York, pp. 497–553.
97. Weber, E.J. (1987) *J. Am. Oil Chem. Soc. 64*, 1129.
98. Jacob, R.A. (1994) *INFORM 5*, 1271.
99. Burton, G.W., and Ingold, K.U. (1984) *Science 224*, 569.
100. Warner, K., and Frankel, E.N. (1987) *J. Am. Oil Chem. Soc. 64*, 213.
101. Matsushita, S., and Iwami, N. (1965) *Arch. Biochem. Biophys. 112*, 467.
102. Endo, Y., Usuki, R., and Kaneda, T. (1985) *J. Am. Oil Chem. Soc. 62*, 1375.
103. Fakourelis, N., Lee, E.C., and Min, D.B. (1987) *J. Food Sci. 52*, 234.
104. Tsuda, T., Ohshima, K., Kawakishi, S., and Osawa, T. (1994) *J. Agric. Food Chem. 42*, 248.
105. Sims, R.J., Fioriti, J.A., and Kanuk, M.J. (1972) *J. Am. Oil Chem. Soc. 49*, 298.
106. Boskou, D., and Morton, I.D. (1976) *J. Sci. Food Agric. 27*, 928.
107. Gordon, M.H., and Magos, P. (1983) *Food Chem. 10*, 141.
108. White, P.J., and Armstrong, L.S. (1986) *J. Am. Oil Chem. Soc. 63*, 525.
109. Tian, L.L., and White, P.J. (1994) *J. Am. Oil Chem. Soc. 71*, 1087.
110. Yan, P.S., and White, P.J. (1990) *J. Agric. Food Chem. 38,* 1904.
111. Frei, B., England, L., and Ames, B.N. (1989) *Proc. Natl. Acad. Sci. USA 86*, 6377.
112. Tappel, A.L. (1962) *Vitam. Horm. (N.Y.) 20*, 493.
113. Dziezak, J.D. (1986) *Food Technol. 40*, 94.
114. Hockett, E.A. (1991) in *Handbook of Cereal Science and Technology* (Lorenz, K.J., and Kulp, K., eds.), Marcel Dekker Inc., New York, pp. 133–198.
115. Nordkvist, E., Salomonsson, A.-C., and Åman, P. (1984) *J. Sci. Food Agric. 35*, 657.

116. Van Sumere, C.F., Cottenie, J., De Greef, J., and Kint, J. (1972) in *Recent Advances in Phytochemistry* (Runeckles, V.C., and Watkin, J.E., eds.), Vol. 4, Appleton-Century-Crofts, Educational Division, Meredith Corporation, New York, pp. 165–221.
117. Osawa, T., Katsuzaki, H., Hagiwara, Y., Hagiwara, H., and Shibamoto, T. (1992) *J. Agric. Food Chem. 40*, 1135.
118. Kitta, K., Hagiwara, Y., and Shibamoto, T. (1992) *J. Agric. Food Chem. 40*, 1843.
119. Peterson, D., and Qureshi, A.A. (1993) *Cereal Chem. 70*, 157.
120. Peterson, D. (1994) *Cereal Chem. 71*, 42.
121. Wang, L., Xue, Q., Newman, R.K., and Newman, C.W. (1993) *Cereal Chem. 70*, 499.
122. Hakkarainen, R.V.J., Työppönen, J.T., and Bengtsson, S.G. (1983) *Acta Agric. Scand. 33*, 395.
123. Piironen, V., Syväoja, E.-L., Varo, P., Salminen, K., and Koivistoinen, P. (1986) *Cereal Chem. 63*, 78.
124. Barnes, P.J. (1983) in *Lipids in Cereal Technology* (Barnes, P.J., ed.), Academic Press, Inc., New York, pp. 33–55.
125. Slover, H.T., Lehmann, J., and Valis, R.J. (1969) *J. Am. Oil Chem. Soc. 46*, 417.
126. Slover, H.T. (1971) *Lipids 6,* 291.
127. Green, J., Marcinkiewicz, S., and Watt, P.R. (1955) *J. Sci. Food Agric. 6*, 274.
128. Parsons, J.G., and Price, P.B. (1974) *Lipids 9*, 804.
129. Price, P.B., and Parsons, J.G. (1974) *Lipids 9*, 560.
130. Parsons, J.G., and Price, P.B. (1979) *J. Agric. Food Chem. 27*, 913.
131. Lehrfeld, J. (1994) *J. Agric. Food Chem. 42*, 2726.
132. Blatny, P., Kvasnicka, F., and Kenndler, E. (1995) *J. Agric. Food Chem. 43*, 129.
133. Demchenko, A.I. (1969) *Izv. Vyssh. Ucheb. Zaved. Pishch. Tekhnol. 5*, 18.
134. Sosulski, F., Krygier, K., and Hogge, L. (1982) *J. Agric. Food Chem. 30*, 337.
135. Classen, D., Arnason, J.T., Serratos, J.A., Lambert, J.D.H., Nozzolillo, C., and Philogène, B.J.R. (1990) *J. Chem. Ecology 16*, 301.
136. Bernwieser I., and Sontag, G. (1992) *Z Lebensm Unters Forsch, 195*, 559.
137. Cherney, J.H., Anliker, K.S., Albrecht, K.A., and Wood, K.V. (1989) *J. Agric. Food Chem. 37*, 345.
138. Seitz, L.M. (1989) *J. Agric. Food Chem. 37*, 662.
139. Norton, R.A. (1994) *Cereal Chem. 71*, 111.
140. Quackenbush, F.W., Firch, J.G., Brunson, A.M., and House, L.R. (1963) *Cereal Chem. 40*, 250.
141. Karaiwanow, G., Marquard, R., and Petrovskij, E.W. (1982) *Fette Seifen Anstrichm. 84*, 251.
142. Combs, S.B., and Combs, G.F. Jr. (1985) *J. Agric. Food Chem. 33*, 815.
143. Cavins, J.F., and Inglett, G.E. (1974) *Cereal Chem. 51*, 605.
144. Weber, E.J. (1987) in *Corn, Chemistry and Technology* (Watson, S.A., and Ramstad, P.E., eds.), American Association of Cereal Chemists, Inc., St. Paul, pp. 311–349.
145. Barnes, P.J. (1983) in *Progress in Cereal Chemistry and Technology* (Holas, J., and Kratochvil, J., eds.), Vol. 1, Elsevier Scientific Publish Co., Amsterdam, pp. 195–200.
146. Cort, W.M., Vicente, T.S., Waysek, E.H., and Williams, B.D. (1983) *J. Agric. Food Chem. 31*, 1330.
147. Grams, G.W., Blessin, C.W., and Inglett, G.E. (1970) *J. Am. Oil Chem. Soc. 47*, 337.
148. Weber, E.J. (1984) *J. Am. Oil Chem. Soc. 61*, 1231.
149. Clough, A.E. (1992) *J. Am. Oil Chem. Soc. 69*, 456.

150. Boki, K., Kubo, M., Wada, T., and Tamura, T. (1992) *J. Am. Oil Chem. Soc. 69*, 232.
151. Tan, B. (1989) *J. Am. Oil Chem. Soc. 66*, 770.
152. Slover, H.T., Thompson, R.H. Jr., and Merola, G.V. (1983) *J. Am. Oil Chem. Soc. 60*, 1524.
153. Van Niekerk, P.J., and Burger, A.E.C. (1985) *J. Am. Oil Chem. Soc. 62*, 531.
154. Warner, K., and Mounts, T.L. (1990) *J. Am. Oil Chem. Soc. 67*, 827.
155. Price, P.B., and Parsons, J.G. (1975) *J. Am. Oil Chem. Soc. 52*, 490.
156. Du Plessis, L.M., and Pretorius, H.E. (1983) *J. Am. Oil Chem. Soc. 60*, 1261.
157. Usuki, R., Suzuki, T., Endo, Y., and Kaneda, T. (1984) *J. Am. Oil Chem. Soc. 61*, 785.
158. Hoseney, R.C., Varriano-Marston, E., and Dendy, D.A.V. (1981) in *Advances in Cereal Science and Technology* (Pomeranz, Y., ed.), Vol. IV, American Association of Cereal Chemists, St. Paul, pp. 71–144.
159. Reichert, R.D. (1979) *Cereal Chem. 56*, 291.
160. Akingbala, J.O. (1991) *Cereal Chem. 68,* 180.
161. Seit-Ablaeva, S.K., Nechaev, A.P., Denisenko, Y.I., and Yanotovskii, M.P. (1973) *Prikl. Biokhim. Mikrobiol 9*, 737.
162. Osagie, A.U., and Kates, M. (1984) *Lipids 19*, 958.
163. Sridhar, R., and Lakshminarayana, G. (1994) *Cereal Chem. 71*, 355.
164. Daniels, D.G.H., and Martin, H.F. (1961) *Nature 191*, 1302.
165. Daniels, D.G.H., King, H.G.C., and Martin, H.F. (1963) *J. Sci. Food Agric. 14*, 385.
166. Daniels, D.G.H., and Martin, H.F. (1964) *Chem. Ind.* (London), 2058.
167. Daniels, D.G.H., and Martin, H.F. (1965) *Chem. Ind.* (London), 1763.
168. Daniels, D.G.H., and Martin, H.F. (1967) *J. Sci. Food Agric. 18*, 589.
169. Daniels, D.G.H., and Martin, H.F. (1968) *J. Sci. Food Agric. 19*, 710.
170. Durkee, A.B., and Thivierge, P.A. (1977) *J. Food Sci. 42*, 551.
171. Taketa, F. (1957) Studies of Various Nutritional Factors in Relation to Dental Caries in the Rat, Ph.D. Thesis, University of Wisconsin, Madison.
172. Vogel, J.J. (1961) Studies on the Diet in Relation to Dental Caries in the Cotton Rat, Ph.D. Thesis, University of Wisconsin, Madison.
173. Tian, L.L., and White, P.J. (1994) *J. Am. Oil Chem. Soc. 70*, 1079.
174. Chen, F.S., Mactaggart, J.M., and Elofson, R.M. (1982) *Can. J. Plant Sci. 62*, 155.
175. Collins, F.W. (1989) *J. Agric. Food Chem. 37*, 60.
176. Collins, F.W., Mclachlan, D.C., and Blackwell, B.A. (1991) *Cereal Chem. 68*, 184.
177. Dimberg, L.H., Theander, O., and Lingnert, H. (1993) *Cereal Chem. 70,* 637.
178. Govind Rao, M.K., and Perkins, E.G. (1972) *J. Agric. Food Chem. 20*, 240.
179. Chow, C.K., Draper, H.H., and Csallany, A.S. (1969) *Anal. Biochem. 32*, 81.
180. Lásztity, R., Berndorfer-Kraszner, É., and Huszár, M. (1980) in *Cereals for Food and Beverages* (Inglett, G.E., and Munck, L., eds.), Academic Press, London, pp. 429–445.
181. Beringer, H., and Saxena, N.P. (1968) *Z. Pflanzenernaehr. Bodenkd. 120*, 71.
182. Peterson, D.M. (1995) *Cereal Chem. 72*, 21.
183. Stellwaag, A. (1890) *Landwirtsch. Ver. Stn. 37*, 135.
184. Aylward, F., and Showler, A.J. (1962) *J. Sci. Food Agric. 13*, 492.
185. Tevekelev, D. (1970) *Izv. Bulg. Akad. Nauk. Sofia Inst. Khranene 9*, 5.
186. Price, P.B., and Parsons, J. (1979) *J. Agric. Food Chem. 27*, 813.
187. Youngs, V.L., Püskülcü, H., and Smith, R.R. (1977) *Cereal Chem. 54*, 803.
188. Dehghan, M. (1979) The Relative Composition and Distribution of the Lipid in Six Common Oat Varieties and Commercial Flour, M.S. Thesis, Iowa State University, Ames.

189. Sahasrabudhe, M.R. (1979) *J. Am. Oil. Chem. Soc. 56*, 80.
190. Novozhilova, G.N., Denisenko, Y.I., Nechaev, A.P., and Shnaidman, L.O. (1968) *Prikl. Biokhim. Mikrobiol. 4*, 333.
191. Sosedov, N., Nechaev, A., Shvartsman, M., and Terent'eva, G. (1971) *Mukomol. Elevator. Prom. 11*, 39.
192. Knight, B.A. (1965) *Phytochemistry 4*, 857.
193. Idler, D.R., Nicksic, S.W., Johnson, D.R., Meloche, V.W., Schuette, H.A., and Baumann, C.A. (1953) *J. Am. Chem. Soc. 75*, 1712.
194. Shibuya, N. (1984) *Phytochemistry 23*, 2233.
195. Ramarathnam, N., Osawa, T., Namiki, M., and Tashiro, T. (1986) *J. Sci. Food Agric. 37*, 719.
196. Rogers, E.J., Rice, S.M., Nicolosi, R.J., Carpenter, D.R., McClelland, C.A., and Romanczyk, L.J. Jr. (1993) *J. Am. Oil Chem. Soc. 70*, 301.
197. Seethamaraiah, G.S., Krishnakantha, T.P., and Chandrasekhara, N. (1990) *J. Nutr. Sc. Vit. 36*, 291.
198. Yoshino, G., Kazumi, T., Amano, M., Tateiwa, M., Yamasaki, T., and Baba, S., *Curr. Ther. Res. 45*, 975 (1989).
199. Nakamur, H., *Radioisotopes 25*, 371 (1966).
200. Diack, M., and Saska, M., *J. Am. Oil Chem. Soc. 71*, 1211 (1994).
201. Osawa, T., Ramarathnam, N., Kawakishi, S., Namiki, M., and Tashiro, T., *Agric. Biol. Chem. 49*, 3085 (1985).
202. Ramarathnam, N., Osawa, T., Namiki, M., and Kawakishi, S. (1988) *J. Agric. Food Chem. 36*, 732.
203. Ramarathnam, N., Osawa, T., Namiki, M., and Kawakishi, S. (1989) *J. Agric. Food Chem. 37*, 316.
204. Tanabe, K., Yamaoka, M., Tanaka, A., Kato, A., and Amemiya, J. (1982) *Yukagaku 31*, 205.
205. Kato, A., Tanabe, K., and Yamaoka, M. (1981) *Yukagaku 30*, 515.
206. Mclaughlin, P.J., and Weihrauch, J.L. (1979) *J. Am. Diet. Assoc. 75*, 647.
207. Miyazawa, T., Yoshino, Y., and Fujino, Y. (1977) *J. Sci. Food Agric. 28*, 889.
208. Hemavathy, J., and Prabhakar, J.V. (1987) *J. Am. Oil Chem. Soc. 64*, 1016.
209. Choudhury, N.H., and Juliano, B.O. (1980) *Phytochem. 19*, 1385.
210. Itoh, T., Tamura, T., and Matsumoto, T. (1973) *J. Am. Oil Chem. Soc. 50*, 122.
211. Itoh, T., Tamura, T., and Matsumoto, T. (1973) *J. Am. Oil Chem. Soc. 50*, 300.
212. Kuroda, N., Ohnishi, M., and Fujino, Y. (1977) *Cereal Chem. 54*, 997.
213. Imai, C., Watanabe, H., Haga, N., and II, T. (1974) *J. Am. Oil Chem. Soc. 51*, 326.
214. Melchert, H.U. (1975) *Datsch. Lebensm.-Rundsch. 71*, 400.
215. Hartman, L., and Lago, R.C.A. (1976) *J. Sci. Food Agric. 27*, 939.
216. Rybka, K., Sitarski, J., and Raczynska-Bojanowska, K. (1993) *Cereal Chem. 70*, 55.
217. Zeringue Jr., H.J., and Feuge, R.O. (1980) *J. Am Oil Chem. Soc. 57*, 373.
218. Eraso, F., and Hartley, R.D. (1990) *J. Sci. Food Agric. 51*, 163.
219. Mueller-Harvey, I., and Reed, J.D. (1992) *J. Sci. Food Agric. 60*, 179.
220. Cherney, D.J.R., Patterson, J.A., Cherney, J.H., and Axtell, J.D. (1991) *J. Sci. Food Agric. 54*, 645.
221. Guenzi, W.D., and McCalla, T.M. (1966) *Agronomy J. 58*, 303.
222. Butler, L.G. (1989) in *Toxicants of Plant Origin. IV. Phenolics* (Cheeke, P.R., ed.), CRC Press, Inc., Boca Raton, pp. 95–121.

223. Yasumatsu, K., Nakayama, T.O.M., and Chichester, C.O. (1965) *J. Food Sci. 30*, 663.
224. Osagie, A.U. (1987) *J. Agric. Food Chem. 35*, 601.
225. Blessin, C.W., Vanetten, C.H., and Wiebe, R. (1958) *Cereal Chem. 35*, 359.
226. Blessin, C.W., Dimler, R.J., and Webster, O.J. (1962) *Cereal Chem. 39*, 389.
227. Maga, J.A., and Lorenz, K. (1974) *Lebensm.-Wiss. u. -Technol. 7*, 273.
228. El-Basyouni, S., and Towers, G.H.N. (1964) *Can. J. Biochem. 42*, 203.
229. Pussayanawin, V., and Wetzel, D.L. (1987) *J. Chromatography 391*, 243.
230. Lam, T.B.T., Iiyama, K., and Stone, B.A. (1990) *Phytochemistry 29*, 429.
231. Feng, Y., McDonald, C.E., and Vick, B.A. (1988) *Cereal Chem. 65*, 452.
232. Feng, Y., and McDonald, C.E. (1989) *Cereal Chem. 66*, 516.
233. Telegdy-Kovats, L., Berndorfer-Kraszner, É., and Hunyakvari, E. (1970) *Elelmezesi Ipar 24*, 302.
234. Davis, K.R., Litteneker, N., Letourneau, D., Cain, R.F., Peters, L.J., and McGinnis, J. (1980) *Cereal Chem. 57*, 178.
235. Acker, L., Schmitz, H.J., and Hamza, Y. (1967) *Ber. Getreidechemiker Tagung; Arbeitsgemein. Getreideforschung*, Granum Verlag, Detmold, pp. 30–34.
236. Hargin, K.D., Morrison, W.R., and Fulcher, R.G. (1980) *Cereal Chem. 57*, 320 (1980).
237. Hargin, K.D., and Morrison, W.R. (1980) *J. Sci. Food Agric. 31*, 877.
238. Pratt, D.E. (1972) *J. Food Sci. 37*, 322.
239. Dabrowski, K.J., and Sosulski, F.W. (1984) *J. Agric. Food Chem. 32*, 128.
240. Shahldi, F., and Naczk, M. (1992) *J. Am. Oil Chem. Soc. 69*, 917.
241. Arai, S., Suzuki, H., Fujimaki, M., and Sakurai, Y. (1966) *Agric. Biol. Chem. 30*, 364.
242. Pratt, D.E. (1965) *J. Food Sci. 30*, 737.
243. Adlercreutz, H., Fotsis, T., Bannwart, C., Wähälä, K., Mäkelä, T., Brunow, G., and Hase, T. (1986) *J. Steroid Biochem. 25*, 791.
244. Wang, H.-J., and Murphy, P.A. (1994) *J. Agric. Food Chem. 42*, 1674.
245. Wang, H.-J., and Murphy, P.A. (1994) *J. Agric. Food Chem. 42*, 1666.
246. Jung, M.Y., Yoon, S.H., and Min, D.B. (1989) *J. Am. Oil Chem. Soc. 66*, 118.
247. Chu, Y.-H., and Lin, J.-Y. (1993) *J. Am. Oil Chem. Soc. 70*, 1263.
248. Guzman, G.J., and Murphy, P.A. (1986) *J. Agric. Food Chem. 34*, 791.
249. Chase Jr., G.W., Akoh, C.C., and Eitenmiller, R.R. (1994) *J. Am. Oil Chem. Soc. 71*, 877.
250. Scholfield, C.R. (1985) in *Lecithins* (Szuhaj, B.F., and List, G.R., eds.), American Oil Chemists' Society, Champaign, IL.
251. Racicot, L.D., and Handel, A.P. (1983) *J. Am. Oil Chem. Soc. 60*, 1098.
252. Sinram, R.D. (1986) *J. Am. Oil Chem. Soc. 63*, 667.
253. Mounts, T.L., and Nash, A.M. (1990) *J. Am. Oil Chem. Soc. 67*, 757.
254. Mounts, T.L., Abidi, S.L., and Rennick, K.A. (1992) *J. Am. Oil Chem. Soc. 69*, 438.
255. Dornbos Jr., D.L., Mullen, R.E., and Hammond, E.G. (1989) *J. Am. Oil Chem. Soc. 66*, 1371.
256. Smith, A.K., and Circle, S.J. (1972) in *Soybeans, Chemistry and Technology* (Smith, A.K., and Circle, S.J., eds.), Avi Publishing Co., Westport, pp. 61,339.
257. Tsuda, T., Osawa, T., Nakayama, T., Kawakishi, S., and Ohshima, K. (1993) *J. Am. Oil Chem. Soc. 70*, 909.
258. Onyeneho, S.N., and Hettiarachchy, N.S. (1991) *J. Agric. Food Chem. 39*, 1701.
259. Drumm, T.D., Gray, J.I., and Hosfield, G.L. (1990) *J. Sci. Food Agric. 51*, 285.
260. Sosulski, F.W., and Dabrowski, K.J. (1984) *J. Agric. Food Chem. 32,* 131.

261. Winter, M., and Herrmann, K. (1986) *J. Agric. Food Chem. 34*, 616.
262. Tomás-Lorente, F., Garcia-Grau, M., Tomás-Barberán, F.A., and Nieto, J.L. (1989) *Phytochemistry 28*, 1993.
263. Herrmann, K., and Woldecke, M. (1977) *J. Sci. Food Agric. 28*, 365.
264. Nozzolillo, C., Ricciardi, L., and Lattanzio, V. (1989) *Can. J. Bot. 67*, 1600.
265. Hertog, M.G.L., Hollman, P.C.H., and Katan, M.B. (1992) *J. Agric. Food Chem. 40*, 2379.
266. Tomás-Barberán, F.A., García-Grau, M.M., and Tomás-Lorente, F. (1991) *J. Agric. Food Chem. 39*, 255.
267. Drumm, T.D., Gray, J.I., and Hosfield, G.L. (1990) *J. Sci. Food Agric. 50*, 485.
268. Harland, B.F., and Prosky, L. (1979) *Cereal Foods World 24*, 387.
269. Nice, D.J., and Robinson, D.S. (1993) *Food Chem. 48*, 353.
270. Méndez, J., and Lojo, M.I. (1971) *J. Food Sci. 36*, 871.
271. Elema, J. (1960) On the Auxin Sparing Action of Gibberellic Acid, Ph.D. Thesis, University of Utrecht, The Netherlands.
272. Nahar, N., and Mosihuzzaman, M. (1990) *J. Sci. Food Agric. 50*, 45.
273. Furuya, M., Galston, A.W., and Stowe, B.B. (1962) *Nature 193*, 456.
274. Piironen, V., Syväoja, E.-L., Varo, P., Salminen, K., and Koivistoinen, P. (1986) *J. Agric. Food Chem. 34*, 742.
275. El-Refai, A.A., Gouda, M.S., and Ammar, K.A. (1987) *Food Chem. 23*, 117.
276. Murcia, M.A., and Villalaín, J. (1993) *J. Sci. Food Agric. 61*, 345.
277. Rhee, K.S., Ziprin, Y.A., and Rhee, K.C. (1979) *J. Food Sci. 44*, 1132.
278. Duh, P.-D., Yeh, D.-B., and Yen, G.-C. (1992) *J. Am. Oil Chem. Soc. 69*, 814.
279. Yen, G.-C., Duh, P.-D., and Tsai, C.-L. (1993) *J. Agric. Food Chem. 41*, 67.
280. Yen, G.-C., and Duh, P.-D. (1993) *J. Am. Oil. Chem. Soc. 70*, 383.
281. Yen, G.-C., and Duh, P.-D. (1994) *J. Agric. Food. Chem. 42*, 629.
282. Vijayalaxmi, B., Venkob Rao, S., and Achaya, K.T. (1969) *Fette Seifen Anstrichm. 71*, 757.
283. Gopalakrishna, A.G., and Prabhakar, J.V. (1985) *J. Am. Oil Chem. Soc. 62*, 1581.
284. Gopala Krishna, A.G., and Prabhakar, J.V. (1994) *J. Am. Oil Chem. Soc. 71*, 1245.
285. Crosso, N.R., and Guzman, C.A. (1995) *J. Agric. Food Chem. 43*, 102.

Chapter 4

Antioxidants from Spices and Herbs

N. Nakatani

Department of Food and Nutrition, Osaka City University, Sumiyoshi, Osaka 558, Japan.

Introduction

One of the principal causes of food deterioration is the oxidation of fats and oils. When foods are exposed to air, oxidation reactions start to produce undesirable flavors, rancid odors, discoloration and other forms of spoilage. To prevent or retard the oxidative deterioration of foods, a variety of efforts have been undertaken. Among them, antioxidants have been used widely as additives in fats and oils, and in food processing. The most common antioxidants are tocopherols, ascorbic acid, and synthetic phenolic compounds such as butylated hydroxyanisole (BHA) and butylated hydroxytoluene (BHT) as shown in Fig. 4.1. The synthetic antioxidants are very effective and highly stable. However, their use as food additives is restricted in several countries, because of the possibility they might have undesirable effects on the enzymes of human organs. As a result, there is worldwide interest in finding new and safe antioxidants from natural sources. Our search for safe and effective naturally occurring antioxidants has been focused on edible plants, especially spices and herbs.

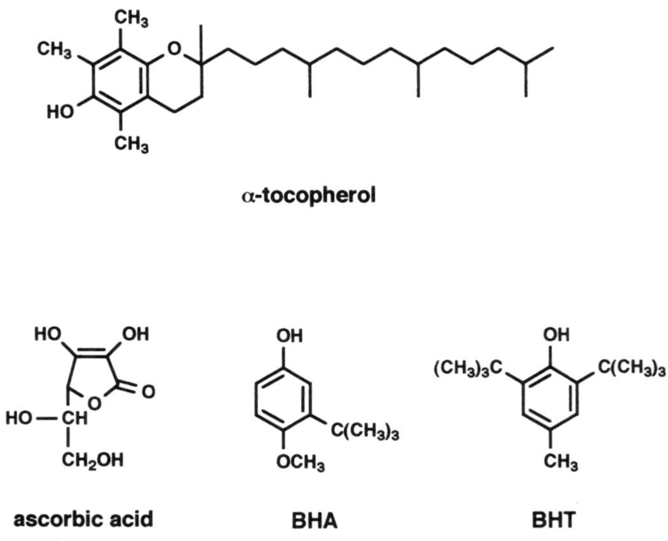

Fig. 4.1. Natural and synthetic antioxidants.

Antioxidants from Spices and Herbs

Since the prehistoric era, spices and herbs have been used not only for flavoring foods but also for their antiseptic or medicinal properties. The preservative effect of spices and herbs suggests the presence of antioxidative and antimicrobial constituents. One of the earliest reports on antioxidants from spices appeared in 1938 in a patent by Maveety (1). Some essential oils of spice such as clove oil were reported to depress rancidity of food oils. DuBois and Tressler (2) discovered antioxidant activity in pepper, sage, mace, and ginger. Chipault *et al.* (3) examined more than 70 spices and found that rosemary and sage were remarkably effective against the oxidation of lard. Oregano, thyme, nutmeg, mace, turmeric, and paprika also showed high antioxidant activity in the ground form and as extracts.

In practical use, rosemary and sage retarded oxidation in plain lard, pie crusts, mayonnaise, and French dressing, and clove showed extremely high effectiveness in oil-in-water emulsions (4). Sethi and Aggarwal (5) reported the antioxidant effects of cinnamon, turmeric, nutmeg, mace, clove, and other spices on heated peanut oil. Cort (6) compared the antioxidant activity of spice extracts with that of BHT. A number of studies on the antioxidative properties of spices and herbs followed, including those by Lewis and Watts (7) , Palitzsch *et al.* (8) and Bishov *et al.* (9). Based on these results, it may be surmised that rosemary, sage, and clove are remarkably active spices, and allspice, aniseed, basil, cardamon, cassia, cinnamon, ginger, mace, marjoram, nutmeg, oregano, pepper, savory, thyme, and turmeric are highly effective.

The next research target was to isolate the antioxidative components in spices and herbs. Herrmann (10) reported the activity of rosmarinic acid, caffeic acid, and related phenolic carboxylic acids identified in the spices belonging to the family of *Labiatae*, such as rosemary, sage, balm, majoram, and mint. Essential oils such as eugenol and isoeugenol (clove, allspice), thymol and carvacrol (thyme), and other phenolic compounds exhibited highly antioxidative activity, but these compounds are limited in practical use because of their characteristic odors. The yellow pigment of turmeric, curcumin, used as a natural food colorant in curry, possesses antioxidant ability, but its practical use is also limited as is that of capsaicin, a pungent substance in red pepper. The antioxidants obtained from spices and herbs will be described in the following sections.

Antioxidants from the Labiatae (Lamiaceae)

Rosemary (*Rosmarinus officinalis* L.). The extract of rosemary leaves exhibited the most effective activity among the herbs. Chang *et al.* (11) reported an extraction method of the active components from rosemary and sage. Thereafter, several new techniques to prepare rosemary extract or condensate followed.

These results promoted our interest in a chemical study to isolate active antioxidants in rosemary leaves. After a combination of repeated chromatographic analyses of the weakly acidic fraction of the nonvolatile part of hexane extract, four antioxidative compounds (1–4) were isolated. The chemical structures were determined by chemical and spectroscopic analyses as shown in Fig. 4.2 (12–14). The new compounds were named rosmanol (1), epirosmanol (2) and isorosmanol (3). ^1H-^1H COSY and COLOC spectra and other new techniques in nuclear magnetic resonance (NMR) spectrometry confirmed their fine structure and stereochemistry (15). Carnosol (4) had previously been isolated from sage by Brieskorn *et al.* (16). These four compounds showed remarkably high activity when evaluated in lard using the Active Oxygen Method. Among them, rosmanol (1), epirosmanol (2), and isorosmanol (3) were more than four times as effective as BHT, and carnosol (4) was twice as effective (14,17). In addition, two more active diterpenes, named rosmaridiphenol (5) and rosmariquinone (6), were isolated by Houlihan *et al.* (18,19). We found four diterpene antioxidants (1–4) including highly methylated flavonoids from sage (*Salvia officinalis* L.) (15).

Oregano (*Origanum vulgare* L.). The identification of polyhydroxybenzoic and cinnamic acids as antioxidative compounds has been reported (10,20). In our study, both the polar and nonpolar fractions of oregano leaves retarded oxidation of linoleic acid measured by the ferric thiocyanate (FTC) and thiobarbituric acid (TBA) methods. The water-soluble fraction of methanol extract of leaves was purified with column chromatography using polyamide and Sephadex LH-20 successively to give a new glycoside (7) of protocatechuic acid ester, rosmarinic acid (8) and its derivative (9), accompanied by protocatechuic and caffeic acids (21, 22). Phenolic carboxylic acids are very common in the *Labiatae* family. The antioxidant activity of compound 7 against linoleic acid oxidation in aqueous ethanolic solution, as measured by the FTC and TBA methods, was comparable to that of BHA.

Marjoram (Origanum majorana L.). Marjoram is an herb close to oregano in morphological classification but also containing phenolic compounds similar to those found in oregano. Beside simple polyphenols, 6-*O*-4-hydroxybenzoyl arbutin and 2-hydroxy-3-(3,4-dihydroxyphenyl)propionic acid showed moderate activity (15).

Thyme (Thymus vulgaris L.). Thymol and carvacrol are major aroma components of thyme leaves and both showed high antioxidant activity. Several biphenyl compounds such as compounds 10 and 11 were isolated as efficient antioxidants (23,24). These compounds are easily produced as dimerization products from thymol or carvacrol. Highly methylated flavonoids (12,13), which possessed antioxidant activity, were found in the less polar fraction (25).

Antioxidants from the Zingiberaceae

Ginger is one of the most common spices. In tropical countries, rhizomes of the family *Zingiberaceae*, such as ginger, turmeric, and other species, are cultivated and used not only for spices but also for traditional folk medicines. We examined the antioxidative activity of acetone extracts of 10 species of tropical gingers. Among them, ginger (*Zingiber officinale*) showed extremely high activity, fol-

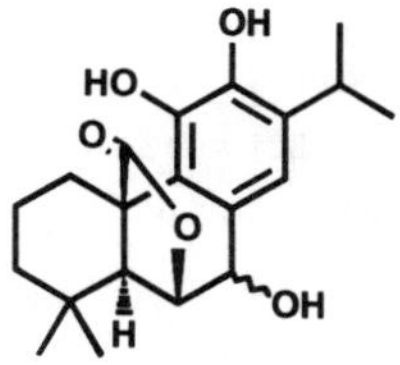

1 7α-OH
2 7β-OH

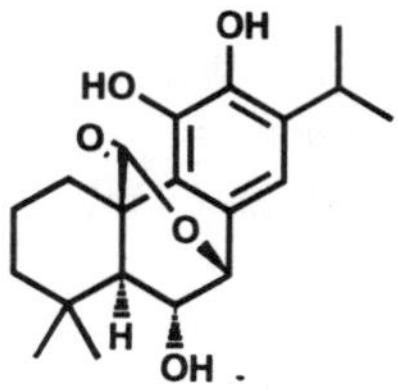

3

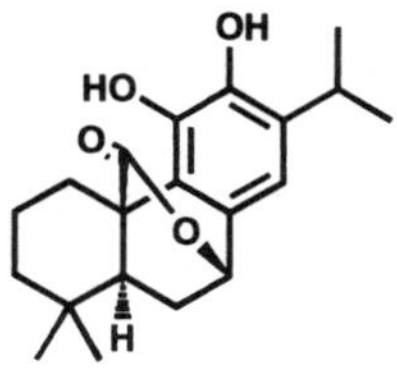

4

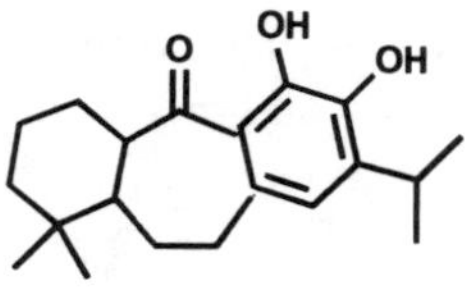

5

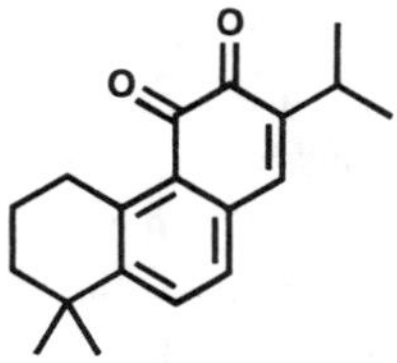

6

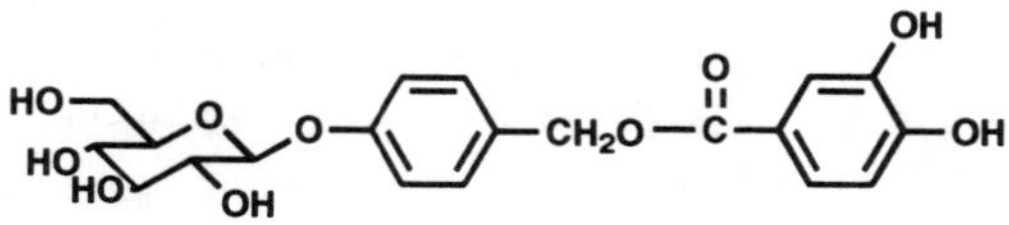

7

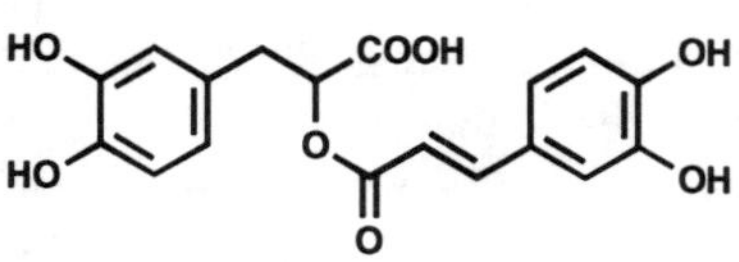

8

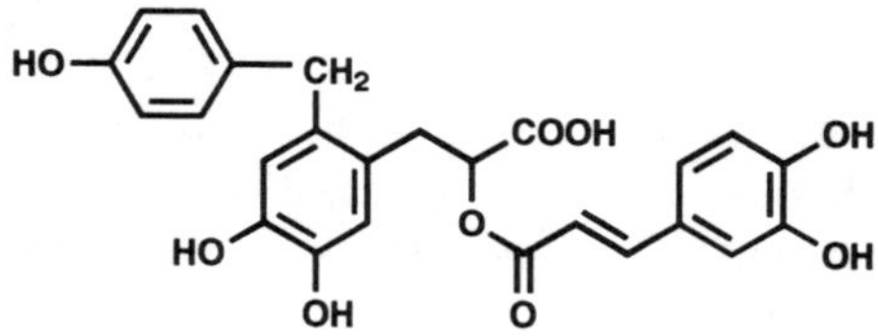

9

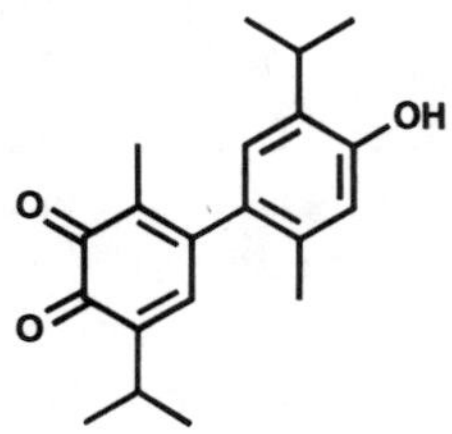

10

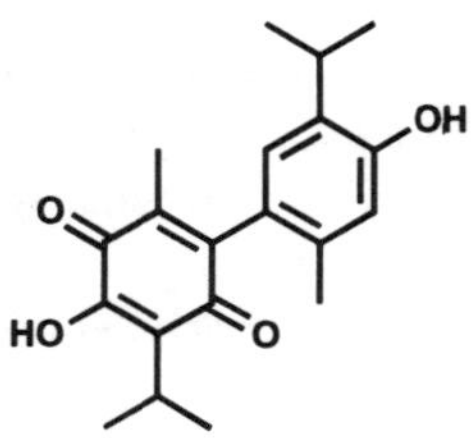

11

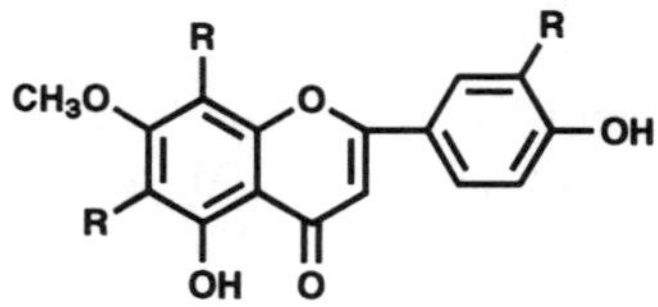

12 R=OCH_3
13 R=H

Fig. 4.2. Antioxidants from *Labiatae* family.

lowed by turmeric (*Curcuma domestica = C. longa*), *Alpinia galanga, C. xanthorrhiza, Z. cassumunar, C. mangga, and A. kepulaga*, whose activities were stronger or comparable to that of α-tocopherol (26). These results prompted us to investigate their active components.

Ginger (Zingiber officinale Roscoe). The rhizome of ginger is known to have potent antioxidant activity (27). The pungent components, gingerol, shogaol, and zingerone, were reported to show a high activity (28,29). Evaluation of the antioxidative activity indicated the presence of additional antioxidants aside from the pungent compounds. The nonvolatile fraction of dichloromethane extract of dried ginger was purified by column chromatography and high-performance liquid chromatography (HPLC) to yield more than 30 compounds, 16 which were new (30–33). These compounds can be structurally classified into two types, i.e., gingerol-related compounds and diarylheptanoids as shown in Fig. 4.3 (33). The fine structure and stereochemistry were elucidated using a new technique in NMR and mass spectrometric (MS) analyses. The antioxidant activity of the isolated compounds was measured by the FTC and TBA methods in an aqueous ethanolic solution of linoleic acid. The structure-antioxidant activity relationship of isolated compounds was examined (33,34). Figure 4.4 shows the effectiveness on the activity of gingerol-type compounds (14–17) with different side chain length at a concentration of 100 μM using the FTC method. All of these compounds showed higher activity than α-tocopherol. Higher activity is correlated with a longer side chain; that is, in the order of 14 < 15 < 16 < 17. The same tendency was observed in shogaol-type compounds (20–23). The activity of each tested compound increased as concentrations increased from 50 to 200 μM. These results suggested that side chain length is important in antioxidant activity. When compared with different substitution patterns on the benzene ring, the [6]-gingerol-type compounds bearing the same side chain, [6]-gingerol (15) with a 4-hydroxy-3-methoxyphenyl group showed remarkable activity, whereas dimethoxylated compound 18 had no activity and monohydroxy compound 19 exhibited slight effectiveness. Concerning the substitution pattern on the side chain, the activity tended to increase in the order 26 (1-ene-3,5-dione) < 15 ([6]-gingerol) < 21 ([6]-shogaol) < 24 ([6]-gingerdiol) < 25 (3R,5S-gingerdiacetate). All of these compounds displayed remarkable activity at a concentration as low as 50 μM. Among them, compound 27, bearing a furan ring on the side chain, showed the highest activity (35). Comparison of the activity among diarylheptanoids indicated similarities as the activity increased in the order of 32 (curcumin) < 28 (hexahydrocurcumin) < 29 (enone) < 30 (diol) < 31 (diacetate). These results suggested that the substitution pattern on the benzene ring and the side chain definitely played an important role in antioxidant activity.

Turmeric (Curcuma domestica L., C. longa L.). The dried rhizome of turmeric is widely used as a spice in ethnic dishes, as a coloring agent and as folk medicine. The yellow pigment, curcumin (32), and demethoxylated curcumins

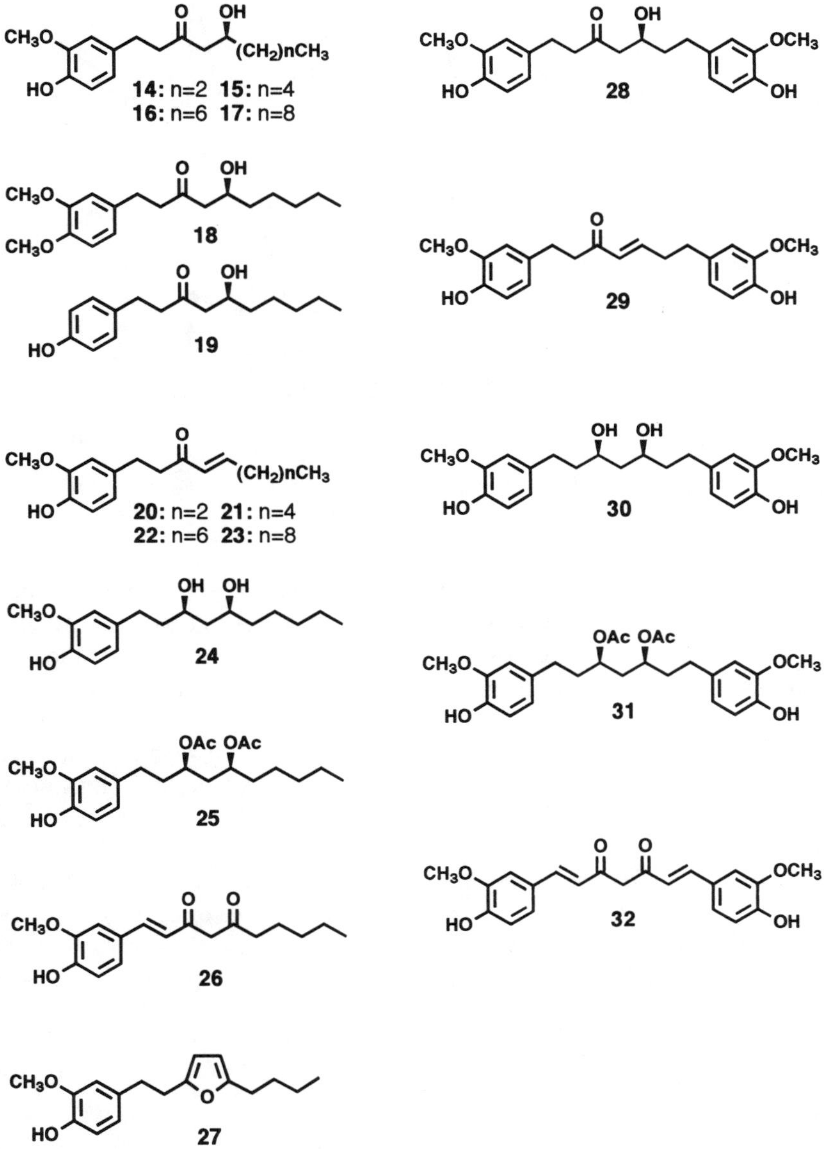

Fig. 4.3. Gingerol-related compounds and diarylheptanoids of ginger.

(33,34) shown in Fig. 4.5 are known to possess potent antioxidant activity. Each curcuminoid was 2.5 times stronger than α-tocopherol in retarding lipid oxidation (26). Quantitative analysis of curcuminoid contents and antioxidative activity for the acetone extracts of tropical gingers suggested the existence of additional antioxidants besides the known curcuminoids. The activities of the extracts of

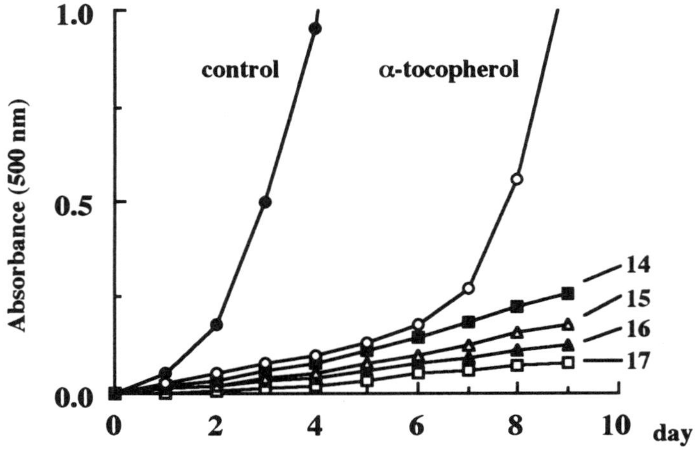

Fig. 4.4. Antioxidant activity of gingerols with different side chain lengths (ferric thiocyanate method: conc. 100 μM).

turmeric (*C. domestica*), *Alpinia galanga*, and *C. xanthorrhiza* were greater than that of α-tocopherol. The crude extracts of *Zingiber cassumuner, C. mangga, A. kepulaga, and C. aeruginosa* showed moderate activity, which was almost equal to that of α-tocopherol (26). After removal of the essential oil from moderately active extracts, the antioxidant activity of the residual parts increased. When the extract of turmeric was purified, two new and additional diarylpentanoids (35,36) were found in the rhizome (36). From the extract of *C. xanthorrhiza*, a species related to turmeric, two more antioxidative compounds were found along with three curcuminoids (37). The active fraction of another species, *Z. cassumunar*, was purified by repeated chromatography to yield six new compounds, which were determined by detailed NMR techniques (38–40). Their structures comprised a novel type of curcuminoid substituted with phenylbutenoids and were named cassumunin A-C (37–39) and cassumunarin A-C (40–42). These isolated compounds from tropical gingers exhibited not only antioxidant efficiency but also anti-inflammatory activity *in vivo* (39).

Antioxidants from Other Spices

There are several popular spices with a hot and pungent taste. Capsaicin (43) and dihydrocapsaicin, pungent principles of red pepper (*Capsicum annuum* L.), exhibit high activity against peroxidation of oils and fats. A related capsaicinoid was isolated as an additional antioxidant from chili pepper (*C. frutescence* L.) and named capsaicinol (44), as shown in Fig. 4.6. It is of interest that capsaicinol is an amide with the same skeleton as capsaicin, but without pungency (41,42).

Concerning the antioxidative activity of pepper (*Piper nigrum* L.), it had been reported that ground pepper and the extract of pepper showed low antioxidative

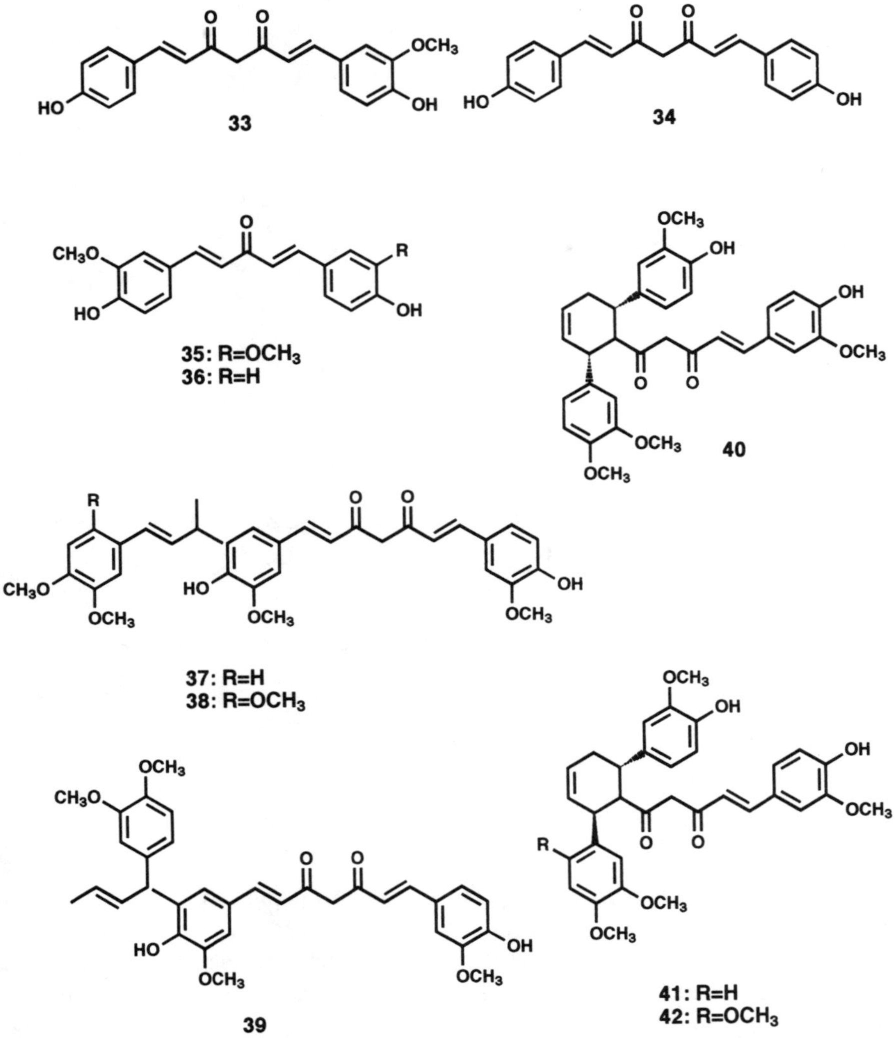

Fig. 4.5. Antioxidative and anti-inflammatory curcuminoids from tropical gingers.

activity. When the methylene chloride extract was fractionated, however, the weakly acidic fraction exhibited significant activity. Five phenolic amides such as compound 45 were isolated and their structures determined by spectroscopic method and synthesis (43,44). Their efficiency was higher than that of α-tocopherol (45). In spite of the similarity of their structures to that of piperine, a pungent principle, they showed no pungent taste and no odor. Consequently, these amides might be practically used in food systems.

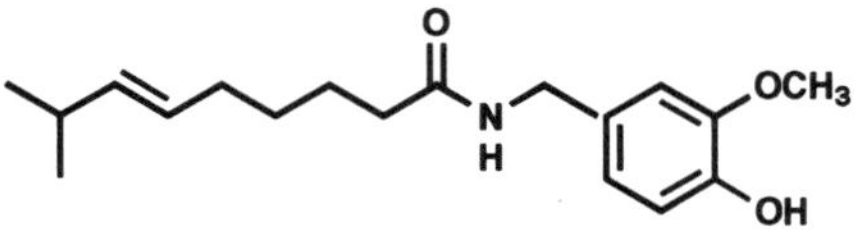

43

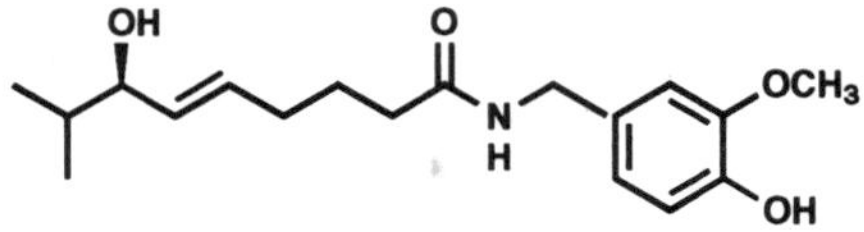

44

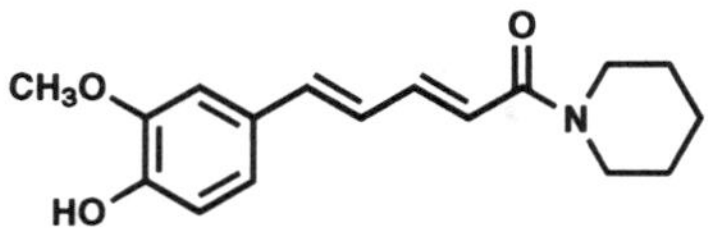

45

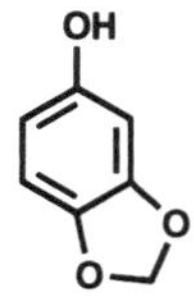

46

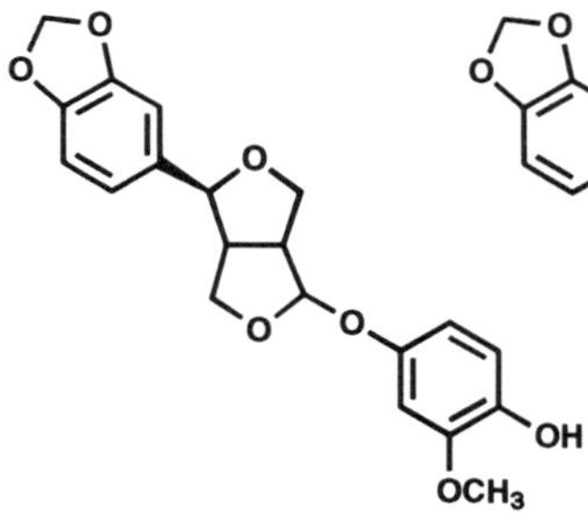

47

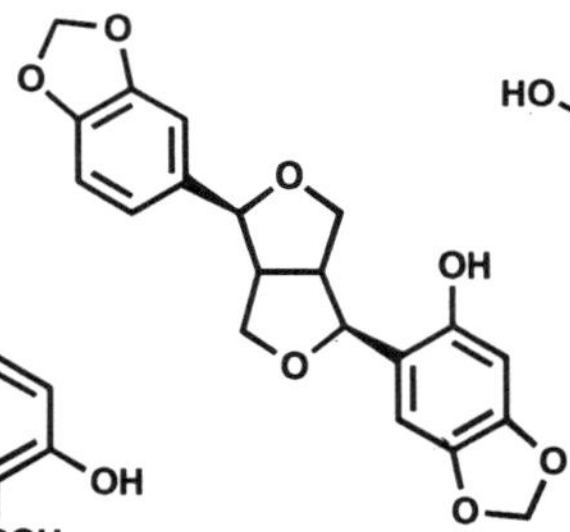

48

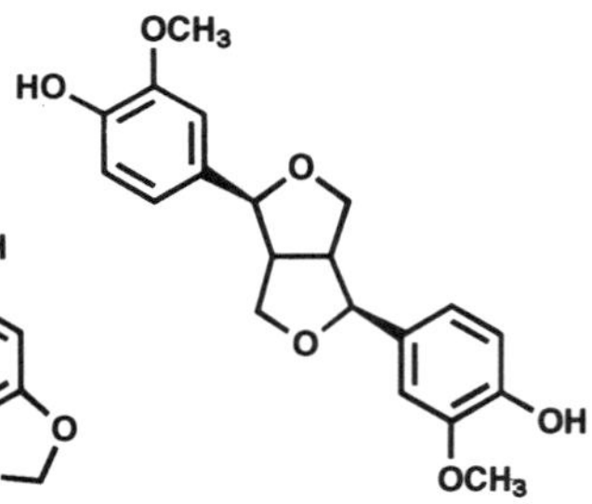

49

Fig. 4.6. Antioxidants from miscellaneous spices.

Sesame (*Sesamum indicum* L.) is one of the most popular spices and has been widely cultivated for seed oil production. Sesame seed oil has been known to exhibit higher stability to oxidative deterioration than other vegetable oils. It has been believed that sesamol (46), a phenolic compound derived from sesamolin, protects the oils from peroxidation. But only a trace amount of sesamol was found in either the seed or oil. Fukuda *et al.* (47, 48) found lignan antioxidants including sesamolinol and sesaminol in an acetone extract of sesame seed (46, 47). They also clarified the formation mechanism of a large amount of sesamolin during the refining process of oil (48). Recently, Katsuzaki *et al.* reported three novel glucosides of pinoresinol (49) from 80% ethanolic extract of defatted sesame seed meal (49).

Other Properties of Antioxidants from Spices and Herbs

Currently, natural antioxidants are receiving much attention, especially those isolated from edible plants, because they are expected to prevent not only lipid peroxidation in foods but also oxidative damage to living cells. Overproduction of active oxygen radicals in the human body causes oxygen stress in DNA and cell membranes and, consequently, induces toxic effects such as mutation, inflammation, cancer, aging, and other diseases. The self-defense system of the body against such oxidative damage may be supported by antioxidants.

It is well known that catechins from green tea leaves have a wide range of biological activities that contribute to their chemopreventive effects on tumor initiation and promotion. Ho *et al.* (50) reported that methanol extract of leaves of rosemary inhibited formation of benzo [α] pyrene (BP)-DNA adducts in mouse epidermis, skin tumor initiation by BP and 12,6-dimethylbenz[α] anthracene (DMBA), and 12-*O*-tetradecanoylphorbol-13-acetate (TPA)-induced inflammation and tumor promotion in mouse epidermis. A major constituent of rosemary antioxidants, carnosol (4), inhibited TPA-induced inflammation and tumor promotion. Huang *et al.* (32, 51) intensively studied the effect of curcumin on tumor metabolism. The anti-inflammatory activity of curcumin was evaluated by topical application on chemical-induced edema of mouse ears. Curcumin inhibited ear inflammation induced by TPA or arachidonic acid. Curcumin also was reported to inhibit both epidemal lipoxygenase and cyclooxygenase activity. Cassumunin A, B and C (37–39), new complex curcuminoids, showed stronger anti-inflammation activity toward inflammation induced by TPA on mouse ear than did curcumin (39).

Conclusions

Many new antioxidants have been isolated from natural sources and their structures determined. Spices and herbs, among foods eaten daily, are one of the most promising sources. It is expected that the results obtained from biochemical studies on antioxidants in edible plants may lead to chemoprevention of lipid peroxidation, inflammation, cancer, and aging in human organs.

References

1. Maveety, D.J., U.S. Patent 2,124,706 (1938).
2. Dubois, C.W., and Tressler, D.K. (1943) *Proc. Inst. Food Technol.*, 202.
3. Chipault, J.R., Mizuno, G.R., Hawkins, J.M., and Lundberg, W.O. (1952) *Food Res. 17*, 46.
4. Chipault, J.R., Mizuno, G.R., and Lundberg, W.O. (1956) *Food Technol. 10*, 209.
5. Sethi, S.C., and Aggarwal, J.S. (1956) *J. Sci. Ind. Res. Sect. B. 15B*, 34.
6. Cort, W.M. (1974) *Food Technol. 28*, 60.
7. Lewis, E.J., and Watts, B.M. (1959) *Food Res. 23*, 274.
8. Palitzsch, A., Schulze, H., Lotter, G., and Steichele, A. (1974) *Fleischwirtschaft 54*, 63.
9. Bishov, S.J., Masuoka, Y., and Kapsalis, J.G. (1977) *J. Food Processing and Preservation 1*, 167.
10. Herrmann, K. (1962) *Z. Lebensm. Unters. Forsch. 116*, 224.
11. Chang, S.S., Ostric-Matijasevic, B., Hsieh O.A.L., and Huang, C.L. (1977) *J. Food Sci. 42*, 1102.

12. Nakatani, N., and Inatani, R. (1981) *Agric. Biol. Chem. 45*, 2385.
13. Inatani, R., Nakatani, N., Fuwa, H., and Seto, H. (1982) *Agric. Biol. Chem. 46*, 1661.
14. Nakatani, N., and Inatani, R. (1984) *Agric, Biol. Chem. 48*, 2081.
15. Nakatani, N. (1994) in *Food Phytochemicals for Cancer Prevention II-Teas, Spices, and Herbs* (Ho, C.-T., Osawa, T., Huang, M.-T., and Rosen, R.T., eds.), ACS Symposium Series 547, Washington, DC, p. 144.
16. Brieskorn, C.H., Fuchs, A., Bredenberg, J.B., McChesney, J.D., and Wenkert, E. (1964) *J. Org. Chem. 29*, 2293.
17. Inatani, R., Nakatani, N., and Fuwa, H. (1983) *Agric. Biol. Chem. 47*, 521.
18. Houlihan, C.M., Ho, C.-T., and Chang, S.S. (1984) *J. Am. Oil Chem. Soc. 61*, 1036.
19. Houlihan, C.M., Ho, C.-T., and Chang, S.S. (1985) *J. Am. Oil Chem. Soc. 62*, 96.
20. Schulz, J.M., and Herrmann, K. (1980) *Z. Lebensm. Unters. Forsch. 171*, 193.
21. Nakatani, N., and Kikuzaki, H. (1987) *Agric. Biol. Chem. 51*, 2727.
22. Kikuzaki, H., and Nakatani, N. (1989) *Agric. Biol. Chem. 53*, 519.
23. Miura, K., and Nakatani, N. (1989) *Chemistry Express 4*, 237.
24. Miura, K., Inagaki, T., and Nakatani, N. (1989) *Chem. Pharm. Bull. 37*, 1816.
25. Miura, K., and Nakatani, N. (1989) *Agric. Biol. Chem. 53*, 3043.
26. Jitoe, A., Masuda, T., Tengah, I.G.P., Suprapta, D.N., Gara, I.W., and Nakatani, N. (1992) *J. Agric. Food Chem. 40*, 1337.
27. Hirahara, F., Takai, Y., and Iwao, H. (1974) *Eiyogakuzasshi 32*, 1.
28. Lee, I.-K., and Ahn, S.-Y. (1985) *Korean J. Food Sci. Technol. 17*, 55.
29. Fujio, H., Hiyoshi, A., Asari, T., and Suminoe, K. (1969) *Nippon Shokuhin Kogyo Gakkaishi 16*, 241.
30. Kikuzaki, H., Usuguchi, J., and Nakatani, N. (1991) *Chem. Pharm. Bull. 39*, 120.
31. Kikuzaki, H., Kobayashi, M., and Nakatani, N. (1991) *Phytochemistry 30*, 3647.
32. Kikuzaki, H., Tsai, S.-M., and Nakatani, N. (1992) *Phytochemistry 31*, 1783.
33. Kikuzaki, H., Kawasaki, Y., and Nakatani, N. (1994) in *Food Phytochemicals for Cancer Prevention II-Teas, Spices, and Herbs* (Ho, C.-T., Osawa, T., Huang, M-T., and Rosen, R-T., eds.), ACS Symposium Series 547, Washington, D.C., pp. 237–243.
34. Kikuzaki, H., and Nakatani, N. (1993) *J. Food Sci. 58*, 1407.
35. Nakatani, N., and Kikuzaki, H. (1992) *Chemistry Express 7*, 221.
36. Masuda, T., Jitoe, A., Isobe, J., Nakatani, N., and Yonemori, S. (1993) *Phytochemistry 32*, 1557.
37. Masuda, T., Isobe, J., Jitoe, A., and Nakatani, N. (1992) *Phytochemistry 32*, 3645.
38. Masuda, T., Jitoe, A., and, Nakatani, N. (1993) *Chem. Lett.*, 189.
39. Masuda, T., and Jitoe, A. (1994) *J. Agric. Food Chem. 42*, 1850.
40. Jitoe, A., Masuda, T., and Mabry, T.J. (1994) *Tetrahedron Lett. 35*, 981.
41. Nakatani, N., Tachibana, Y., and Kikuzaki, H. (1989) in *Medical Biochemical and Chemical Aspects of Free Radicals* (Hayaishi, O., Niki, E., Kondo, M., and Yoshikawa, T., eds.), Elsevier, Amsterdam, p. 453.
42. Masuda, T., and Nakatani, N. (1991) *Agric. Biol. Chem. 55*, 2337.
43. Nakatani, N., Inatani, R., and Fuwa, H. (1980) *Agric. Biol. Chem. 44*, 2831.
44. Inatani, R., Nakatani, N., and Fuwa, H. (1981) *Agric. Biol. Chem. 45*, 667.
45. Nakatani, N., Inatani, R., Ohta, H., and Nishioka, A. (1986) *Environ. Health Perspect. 67*, 135.
46. Fukuda, Y., Osawa, T., Namiki, M., and Ozaki, T. (1985) *Agric. Biol. Chem. 49*, 301.
47. Fukuda, Y., Nagata, M., Osawa, T., and Namiki, M. (1986) *J. Am. Oil Chem. Soc. 63*, 1027.

48. Fukuda, Y., Isobe, M., Nagata, M., Osawa, T., and Namiki, M. (1986) *Heterocycles 24*, 923.
49. Katsuzaki, H., Kawasumi, M., Kawakishi, S., and Osawa, T. (1992) *Biosci. Biotech. Biochem. 56*, 2087.
50. Ho, C.-T., Ferraro, T., Chen, Q., Rosen, R.T., and Huang, M.-T. (1994) in *Food Phytochemicals for Cancer Prevention II-Teas, Spices, and Herbs* (Ho, C.-T., Osawa, T., Huang, M.-T., and Rosen, R.T., eds.), ACS Symposium Series 547, Washington, D.C., pp. 2–19.
51. Huang, M.-T., Lysz, T., Ferraro, T., and Conney, A.H. (1992) in *Cancer Chemoprevention* (Wattenberg, L., Liphin, M., Boone, C.W., and Kelloff, G.J., eds.), CRC Press, Boca Raton, p. 375.

Chapter 5

Antioxidative Defense System in Vegetable Extracts

N. Ramarathnam*, H. Ochi, and M. Takeuchi

Japan Institute for the Control of Aging, Nikken Foods Co., Ltd., 723-1 Haruoka, Fukuroi-city, Shizuoka-437-01, Japan.

Introduction

Oxidative stress, induced by oxygen radicals, is believed to be a primary factor in various degenerative diseases of the central nervous system, as well as in the normal effects of aging (1,2). The reactive oxygen species formed during the normal metabolic process (Fig. 5.1) can easily initiate the peroxidation of the membrane lipids, leading to the accumulation of lipid peroxides. The peroxidation process and its secondary products, such as malondialdehyde (MDA) and 4-hydroxynonenal (4-HNE), are highly reactive. They tend to react with proteins, amines, and deoxyribonucleic acid (2). Such processes act as hosts to the degenerative diseases, and may make a significant contribution to the risks of human aging and cancer (3).

The toxic effects of normal oxygen metabolism are combated regularly by a number of endogenous antioxidant defense and protective mechanisms in the living cell. The capacity of such protective systems, however, gradually decreases with age, leading to a gradual loss of immunity to disease, malfunctioning of vital organs, and eventually resulting in death. Because such problems associated with aging and age-related diseases continue to be a burden on the health-care system in many of the developed nations, a need exists to look for new phytochemicals in conventional foods that can offer improved protection against oxygen radical-induced damages.

Animal-feeding studies in different laboratories have clearly demonstrated that cancer generally can be prevented by certain plant chemicals (4). Phytochemicals

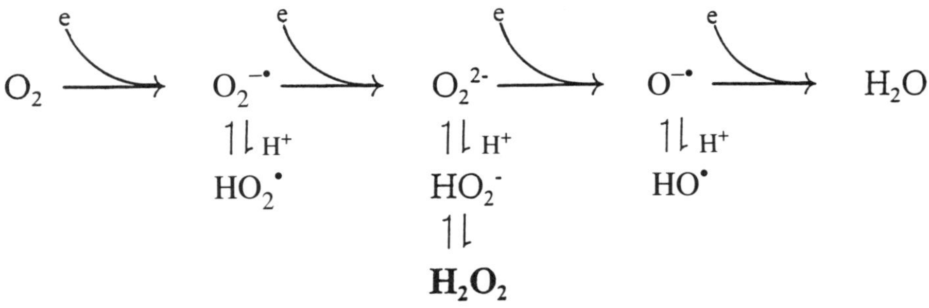

Fig. 5.1. Generation of oxidants during normal metabolic process.

*Present address: Genox Corporation, 1414 Key Highway, Baltimore, MD 21230, USA.

in fruits and vegetables that were shown to be effective in such studies have been isolated and identified (5–7). These phytochemicals are believed to function *in vivo* as complements to the endogenous antioxidants that are distributed in and around the living cells, regulating the various oxidation-reduction reactions that take place continuously inside the body.

Vegetables and fruits are abundant in vitamins, minerals, and other phytochemicals such as polyphenolic and flavonoid substances. Federal food and health agencies in many of the industrialized nations have strictly recommended a reduction in red-meat consumption, and an increase in the intake of vegetables and fruits to five or six servings a day. This is largely to increase the supplements of vitamins C and E, carotenoids, and trace minerals from natural sources such as fruits and vegetables. The recommendation to consume plant foods regularly is strongly supported by substantial epidemiologic evidence linking intake of vegetables and fruits to a decreased risk of cancer (8–10).

Vegetables such as spinach, radish, burdock, and carrot are consumed almost daily by the Japanese in their diet. In addition to providing essential nutrients, they serve as a good source for dietary fiber. Dietary fiber not only regulates the movement of the food within the intestine, but also helps in the adsorption of carcinogens, in lowering blood cholesterol levels, and in reducing risk of coronary heart disease (CHD) (11–13).

From this point of view, we believe that vegetables may play a vital role not only in lowering the incidence of cancer, but also in the control of aging and age-related diseases. It is believed that vegetables may also be enriched with novel natural defense mechanisms which are not yet known. The objective of this investigation therefore, was to prepare vegetable extracts under conventional cooking conditions and screen for the presence of antioxidant defense systems in such extracts, using *in-vitro* systems. A detailed investigation to test for the active oxygen radical scavenging potential of these extracts was also undertaken.

Vegetables Extracts

Most of the vegetables used in this study were procured from a local supermarket. A few varieties, such as purple radish, long white radish, Brussels sprout, onion, Welsh onion, and carrots, however, were grown in the experimental farm of Nikken Foods Co., Ltd. One hundred grams of each variety was chopped into small pieces and extracted for 1 h in 1 L of hot distilled water maintained at 95 ± 2°C. The contents were filtered and then concentrated under vacuum until a concentrate with a Brix value of around 30 was obtained. The concentrated samples were further freeze-dried.

Antioxidative Activities of the Vegetable Extracts

Suppression of the oxidation of 2′-deoxyribose by the vegetable extracts was investigated by the thiobarbituric acid (TBA) method of Osawa *et al.* (14). In this assay system, 2′–deoxyribose was reacted with a $HO^{\bullet}$ radical generated by ferrous sulfate chelated to ethylenediaminetetraacetic acid ($FeSO_4 \cdot 7H_2O$/EDTA) and H_2O_2, in the presence and absence of vegetable extracts. Thiobarbituric acid values of the reaction mixtures were determined at 0 time and after 4 h of reaction. α-Tocopherol and L-ascorbic acid were used as standard samples for comparison of the antioxidative activities. The assays were carried out in triplicate for each sample.

The results of the TBA analysis are summarized in Table 5.1. On the basis of the results, vegetable extracts could be categorized into three classes. Figure 5.2 illustrates the antioxidative activities of the vegetable extracts, in decreasing order, when tested at a concentration of 10 mg/mL. Vegetable extracts that retarded the oxidation of 2′-deoxyribose up to about 25% were considered to possess some degree of antioxidant properties, and hence are listed in the figure.

The first group was comprised of samples that suppressed the oxidation of 2′-deoxyribose more than 90%, these were grouped as strong antioxidants and included sweet potato extract, the Japanese mushroom (shiitake) extract, mushroom extract, and burdock extract. Sweet potato extract was effective in retarding the oxidation of 2′-deoxyribose at both tested concentrations of 10 and 1 mg/mL (5.6 and 9.4%, respectively; Table 5.1). Sweet potato is known to be a rich source of β-carotene. However, because its activity is nearly three times as strong as that of carrot extract or pumpkin extract, it is believed that the activity of sweet potato may be due to other phytochemicals such as phenolic components or anthocyanins.

While the shiitake and mushroom extracts were effective when tested at a concentration of 10 mg/mL (7.7 and 8.5% oxidation, respectively; Table 5.1), they were ineffective as antioxidants when tested at a concentration of 1 mg/mL. Extract of the traditional Japanese food article burdock restricted the oxidation of 2′-deoxyribose to 9.8% when tested at a concentration of 10 mg/mL. At a concentration of 1 mg/mL, however, burdock extract was found to be more effective than shiitake or mushroom extract. The activity of these three extracts, expressed in terms of oxidation of 2′-deoxyribose oxidation was 25.7, 27.5, and 43.5%, respectively (Table 5.1).

Weaker antioxidative activity was demonstrated by the group that allowed the oxidation of 2′-deoxyribose to occur in the range of 10–25%. This group included the extracts of potato, perilla leaf, leaves of purple radish, onion, carrot, purple radish, shallot, pumpkin, taro, cabbage, Chinese cabbage, and Welsh onion. The difference in the activities of the extract of purple radish and those of Brussels sprout, long white radish, cauliflower, and broccoli, which are also members of the same family, could be due to the presence of novel phytochemicals in the purple radish that are not yet known.

The third group included the extracts of Welsh onion, Brussels sprout, long white radish, cauliflower, broccoli, garlic, and spinach that facilitated the oxidation of 2′-deoxyribose to proceed beyond 25%. These samples have been grouped as vegetables with very weak or no antioxidant activity.

Antioxidative activities of the vegetable extracts were also determined by the high-performance thin-layer chromatography (HPTLC) method of Sano et al. (15).

TABLE 5.1
Antioxidative Activities and Active-Oxygen Radical Scavenging Potentials of Vegetable Extracts[a]

Sample	Oxidation of 2′-deoxyribose (%)		Suppression of linoleic acid ocidation	Reduction in PBN-OH signal intensity (%)		SOSA values (unit/g)
	10 mg/ML	1 mg/ML		10 mg/ML	1 mg/ML	
White radish (stem)	30.7	89.1	ND	91.6	55.7	220
White radish (leaf)	27.9	75.5	0.76	88.0	68.3	2000
Purple radish (stem)	18.6	70.3	0.49	92.4	62.4	550
Purple radish (leaf)	15.6	18.6	0.75	93.2	85.9	2860
Burdock	9.8	25.7	0.84	94.5	77.4	7500
Carrot	18.1	54.8	0.49	93.4	72.7	310
Perilla leaf	13.4	37.5	ND	94.2	82.7	43700
Sweet potato	5.6	9.4	0.77	90.5	61.8	1220
Potato	10.9	29.9	ND	92.7	89.0	880
Onion	17.5	67.4	0.71	91.9	41.5	1970
Shallot	18.9	100.0	0.58	87.7	74.1	2520
Garlic	46.6	100.0	0.68	92.0	62.9	240
Mushroom	8.5	43.5	ND	89.9	49.9	980
Cabbage	23.3	39.8	0.50	91.1	47.9	640
Broccoli	34.5	52.3	0.68	93.2	83.7	1090
Chinese cabbage	24.9	32.3	ND	92.0	69.6	430
Brussels sprout	27.7	49.0	ND	94.2	82.4	2400
Cauliflower	32.6	62.5	ND	92.7	78.7	1550
Pumpkin	18.9	49.2	0.51	94.3	74.8	320
Spinach	50.0	51.3	0.44	79.7	76.6	350
Japanese mushroom (shiitake)	7.7	27.5	0.52	94.0	70.3	690
Welsh onion	25.5	58.4	0.38	92.3	70.1	1160
Taro	19.1	29.0	0.70	92.4	88.8	900
α-Tocopherol	0	0	1.00	ND	ND	ND
L-Ascorbic acid	4.1	25.0	ND	100.0	0	170000

[a]Values are averages of three determinations.
Abbreviations: PBN, N-t-butyl-—phenylnitrone; SOSA, superoxide scavenging activity; ND, not determined.

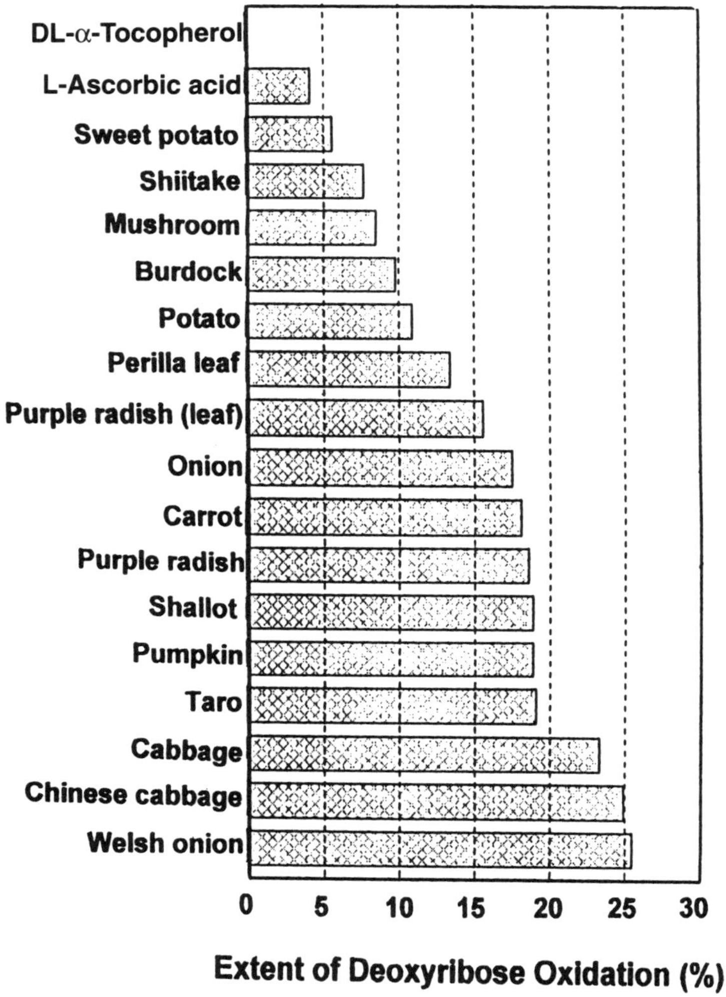

Fig. 5.2. Antioxidative activities of vegetable extracts at 10 mg/mL as determined by the thiobarbituric acid (TBA) method.

Suppression of autoxidation of linoleic acid, carried out at 80°C, in the presence and absence of vegetable extracts, was monitored on thin-layer chromatography (TLC). After spraying with 50% formic acid and 0.5% ethanolic solution of methyl indole, the plate was heated at 100°C for 1 min on a hot plate. Pink-colored spots that developed on heating were scanned with a TLC dual-wavelength flying spot scanner (model CS-9000, Shimadzu, Kyoto, Japan) at 557 nm. The percentage of inhibition of linoleic acid oxidation and the concentrations of the test samples giving 50% inhibition were determined. Samples were tested in triplicate for each assay.

The antioxidant activities of vegetable extracts determined by the HPTLC method are summarized in Table 5.1. The antioxidative activities of the vegetable concentrates, expressed in terms of α-tocopherol activity, in decreasing order, are illustrated in Fig. 5.3. It was observed that extracts of burdock, sweet potato, leaves of long white radish and purple radish, onion, and taro were nearly 70% as strong as the natural antioxidant α-tocopherol (Fig. 5.3).

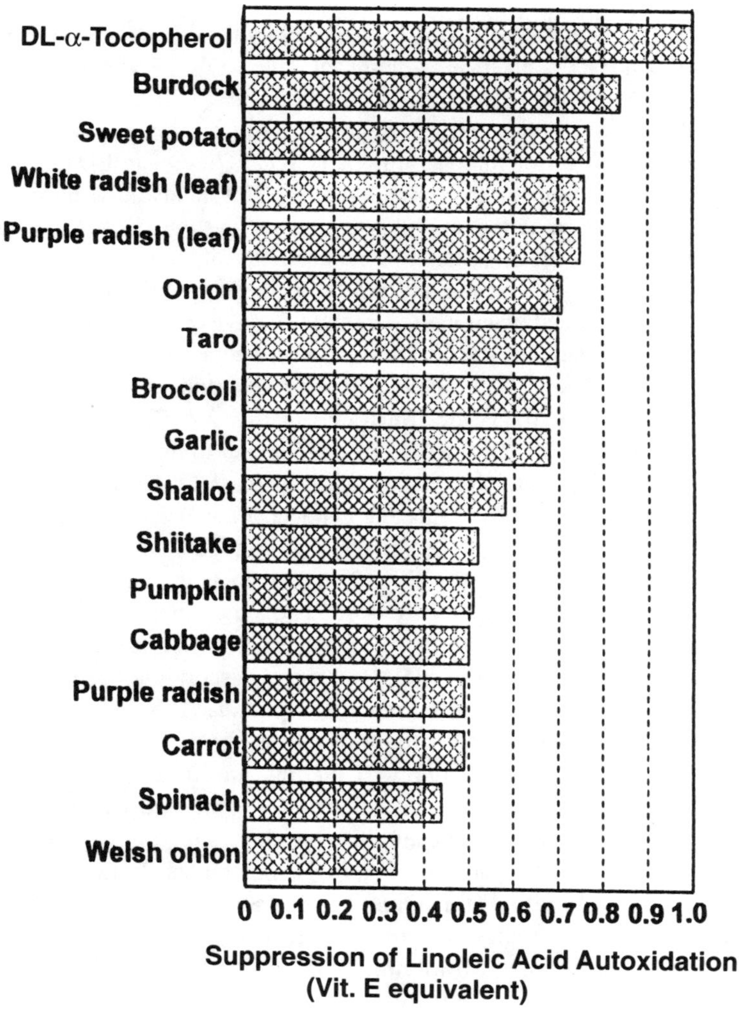

Fig. 5.3. Antioxidative activities of vegetable extracts determined by high-performance thin-layer chromatography (HPTLC).

Extracts of broccoli, garlic, shallot, shiitake (Japanese mushroom), pumpkin powder, and cabbage formed the next class of materials that exhibited a weak antioxidant activity (50–70% as strong as α-tocopherol; Fig. 5.3). Purple radish, carrot, spinach, and Welsh onion formed a third category of materials that showed very weak antioxidant activity ranging from 30–50% of that of α-tocopherol (Fig. 5.3). Extracts that showed less than 30% of the activity of α-tocopherol have been classified as substances with no antioxidant activity.

Active Oxygen Radical Scavenging Ability

Vegetable extracts were further tested for their ability to scavenge the active oxygen radicals, hydroxyl ($OH^{\bullet}$) and superoxide ($O_2^{-\bullet}$). The $HO^{\bullet}$ radical scavenging ability was determined by the use of an electron spin resonance (ESR) spectrometer (model JES-FR80, JEOL Ltd., Tokyo, Japan). Vegetable extracts were supplemented into a $HO^{\bullet}$ radical generating system consisting of FeSO4 • $7H_2O$ and EDTA. Hydrogen peroxide was added to initiate the formation of the $HO^{\bullet}$ radical. N-*t*-butyl-α-phenyl nitrone (PBN) was used as the spin-trapping agent, and the stable PBN-OH spin-adducts were then measured. Assigning the signal intensity in the case of the control (distilled water) an arbitrary value of 100, the percentage reductions in the signal intensities were calculated when the test samples were used. The values were compared with those of vitamin C used in similar concentrations as the standard.

The typical ESR signals of stable PBN-OH spin-adduct in the presence and absence of vegetable extracts are illustrated in Fig. 5.4. The ratio of the peak heights of the strongest signal of PBN-OH spin-adduct to that of the paramagnetic manganese II ion signal was first calculated in the case of the control (Fig. 5.4A; distilled water). Addition of the vegetable extracts at a concentration of 10 mg/mL reduced the signal intensity of the PBN-OH spin-adduct, lowering the relative intensity (RI) value by nearly 80% (Fig. 5.4B), whereas the addition of vegetable extracts at 1 mg/mL concentration (Fig. 5.4C) had a marginal effect in some cases. Addition of L-ascorbic acid (10 mg/mL concentration) eliminated the PBN-OH signal intensity completely (Fig. 5.4D). However, L-ascorbic acid failed to yield a similar effect when tested at a concentration of 1 mg/mL (Table 5.1).

The $HO^{\bullet}$ radical scavenging activity of the vegetable extracts, in decreasing order, when tested at a concentration of 1 mg/mL, are illustrated in Fig. 5.5, and the results, when tested at both concentrations (10 mg/mL and 1 mg/mL) are summarized in Table 5.1. It was interesting to note that all of the vegetable extracts tested in this investigation reduced the PBN-OH signal intensity far more efficiently than L-ascorbic acid tested at a similar concentration (Table 5.1; Fig. 5.5). The $HO^{\bullet}$ radical scavenging ability of burdock extract was the strongest of all, when tested at a concentration of 10 mg/mL (94.5%; Table 5.1). This extract also showed strong antioxidant activity when tested by both the TBA and HPTLC methods. Burdock extract reduced the PBN-OH signal intensity by 77.4%, when tested at a concentration of 1 mg/mL.

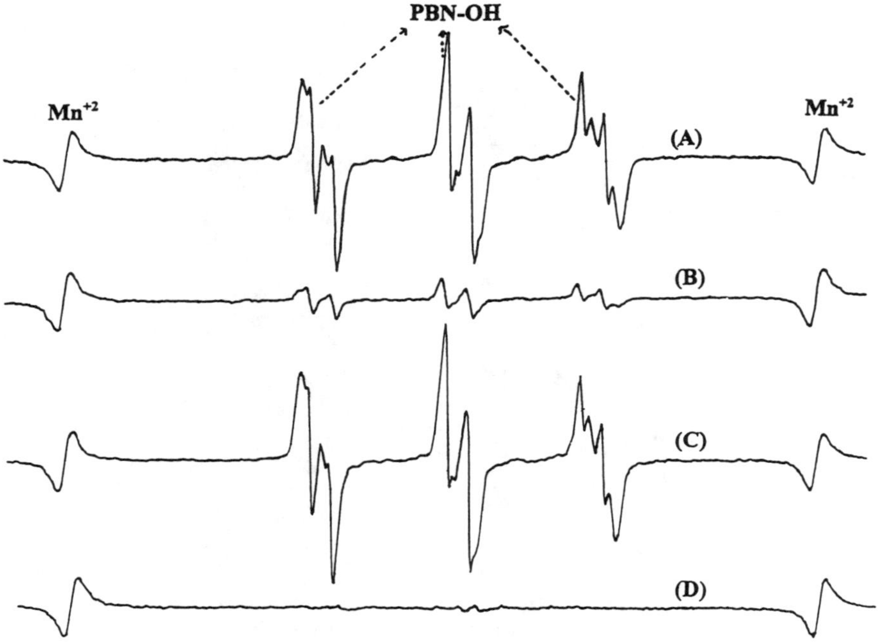

Fig. 5.4. Electron spin resonance (ESR) signals of stable N-t-butyl-α-phenylnitrone (PBN)-OH spin adducts. (A) distilled water (control); (B) after addition of vegetable extract (10 mg/mL concentration); (C) after addition of vegetable extract (1 mg/mL concentration); (D) after addition of L-ascorbic acid (10 mg/mL concentration).

Extracts of the tuber varieties potato and taro expressed the strongest $HO^{\bullet}$ radical scavenging capability when tested at a concentration of 1 mg/mL. Equally effective results were obtained in many of the tested extracts (Table 5.1). L-Ascorbic acid, when tested at this concentration, failed to demonstrate any effect. It is probable that the antimutagenic and anticarcinogenic activities of vegetable juices demonstrated by other investigators could be due to their $HO^{\bullet}$ radical scavenging potentials.

Superoxide radical scavenging activity (SOSA) values were also determined similarly using a hypoxanthine-xanthine oxidase superoxide generating system. The SOSA values of the vegetable extracts were determined by the method of Mitsuta *et al.* (16). The superoxide generated in the presence and absence of vegetable extracts was measured using 5,5-dimethyl-1-pyrroline-N-oxide (DMPO) as the spin-trapping agent. The relative intensity, the ratio of the superoxide signal intensity to that of manganese, was taken as the control value. SOSA values were determined by measuring the reduction in RI values when the samples were used at a concentration of 10 mg/mL. SOSA values were calculated by comparing the reduction of the RI values by the samples, with that of superoxide dismutase (SOD) enzyme. The $O_2^{-\bullet}$ radical scavenging activities were determined in triplicate.

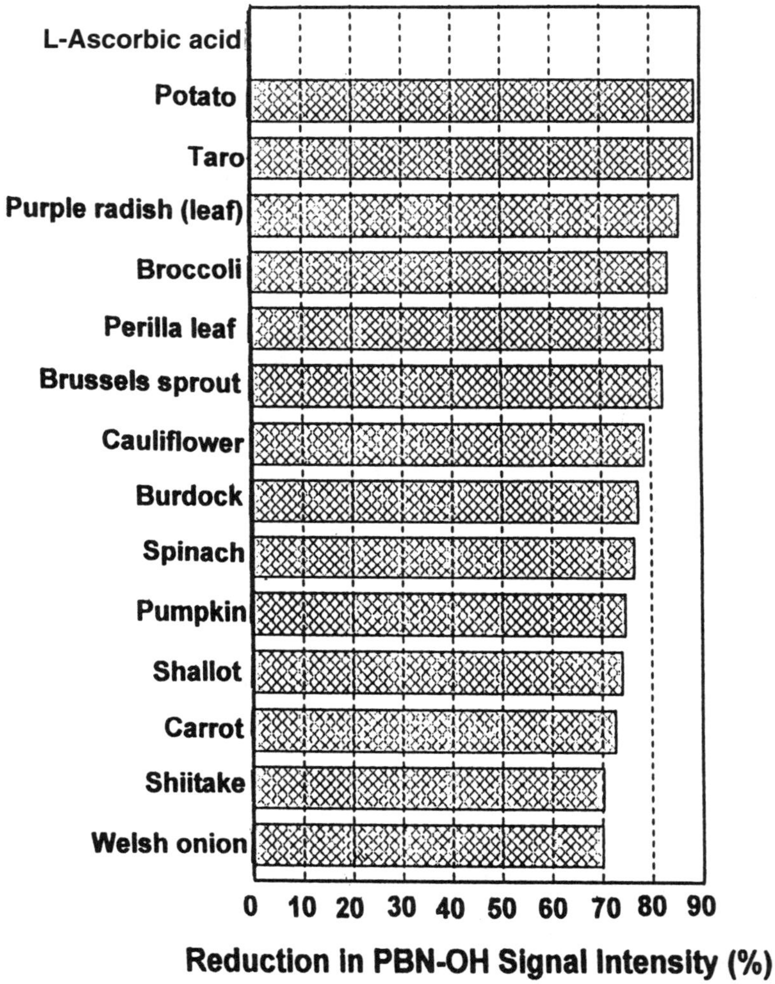

Fig. 5.5. Effect of addition of vitamin C (standard) and vegetable extracts (1 mg/mL concentration) on the N-t-butyl-α-phenylnitrone (PBN)-OH spin adduct signal intensities, determined by the electron spin resonance (ESR) method.

Superoxide scavenging activity values of the vegetable extracts are given in Table 5.1. One milligram of pure superoxide dismutase enzyme showed a SOSA value of 3500 units. L-Ascorbic acid, used as the standard, exhibited a very high value of 170,000 units/g. Of the tested concentrates, perilla leaf extract showed the highest SOSA value of 43,700 units/g (Fig. 5.6). The extract of burdock, which had demonstrated strong antioxidative activity when tested by both TBA and HPTLC methods and also had the potential to scavenge $HO^{\bullet}$ radicals quite efficiently, showed a SOSA value of 7500 units/g (Fig. 5.6; Table 5.1). Members of the *Cruciferae* species, such as Brussels sprout, cauliflower, and broccoli, had SOSA values in the range of 1000–2400 units/g (Table 5.1). However, extracts of cabbage and Chinese cabbage, which belong to the same species, had lower values of 640 and 430 units/g, respectively.

Members of the *allium* species such as shallot, onion, and Welsh onion were effective in scavenging superoxide radicals. They had SOSA values in the range of

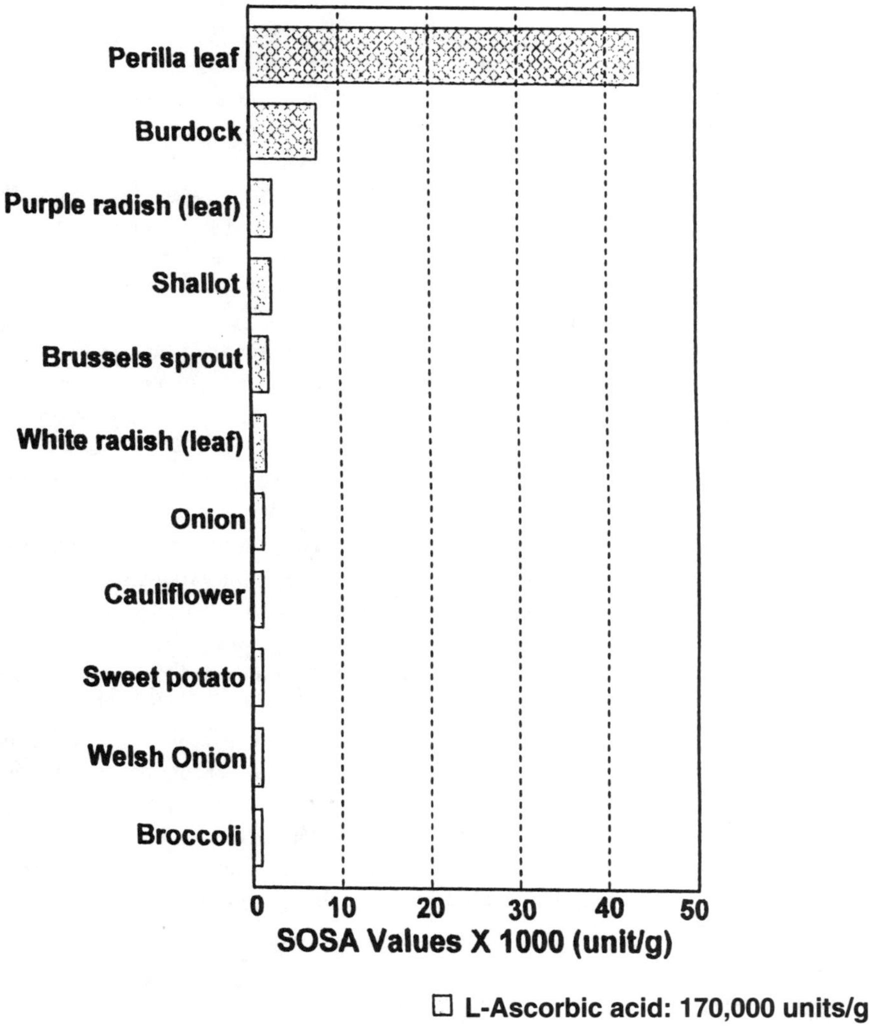

Fig. 5.6. Superoxide scavenging activity (SOSA) values (units/g) of vitamin C and vegetable extracts, determined by the electron spin resonance (ESR) method.

1100–2500 units/g (Table 5.1). However, the extract of garlic that belonged to the same family showed a very weak SOSA value of 210 units/g.

Conclusions

Free radical reactions are ubiquitous in living things. Proteins, lipids, carbohydrates, and nucleic acids are all known to be susceptible to damage by free radicals/oxides and other endogenous reactive substances. Many factors have been proposed for the aging process, such as molecular crosslinking (17), changes in immune factors (18), damage by free radicals (19), and senescence genes in the DNA (20). However, the free radical theory of aging (19) is the basis for much of the ongoing research related to molecular gerontology and aging-related diseases such as cancer, diabetes, cardiovascular diseases, and neurodegenerative diseases.

In addition, there is a concurrent increase in the search for natural antioxidants and food phytochemicals that can prevent cancer and other diseases (21). In 1945, the average life span of the Japanese was 50 for men and 53 for women. Recently published figures indicate that women in Japan can expect to live 81.4 and men 75.6 years (22). Many factors such as improvement in public sanitation, introduction of antibiotics, and improvement in the awareness of health and eating habits through proper education have been implicated as being responsible for these improvements in life span. The current focus of attention, which is to improve the health aspect of old age in Japan, however, combines the best of western food and traditional Japanese food (22).

In view of this, the present investigation, as the first of a series of planned studies, was conducted to screen traditional Japanese food for its antioxidant and oxygen radical scavenging effects. Vegetables have always occupied a special place in the Japanese diet, and the consumption of processed vegetable products has continued to increase in recent years. The present investigation has revealed for the first time the importance of the biofactors of vegetables as potential free radical scavengers, and as a useful source for the formulation of an antioxidant-supplemented diet. In assessing the antioxidant potential of natural food factors, it is essential to take into consideration, as demonstrated in this study, the overall contribution of such components in the prevention of oxidation of the lipids, proteins, sugars, and as scavengers of active oxygen radicals. Attempts are being made to reveal the chemical nature of the antioxidant defense system and free radical scavenging mechanism of the vegetable extracts. In addition, *in vivo* studies are being planned to tap the potential applications of vegetables in the design of novel health foods.

References

1. Harman, D. (1992) *Mutat. Res. 275*, 257–266.
2. Kehrer, J.P. (1993) *Crit. Rev. Toxicol. 23*, 21–48.
3. Marnett, L.J., Hurd, H.K., Hollstein, M.C., Levin, D.E., Esterbauer, H. and Ames, B.N. (1985) *Mutat. Res. 148*, 25–34.

4. Huang, M.-T., Ferraro, T., and Ho, C.-T. (1994) in *Food Phytochemicals for Cancer Prevention. I. Fruits and Vegetables* (Huang, M.-T., Osawa, T., Ho, C.-T., Rosen, R.T., eds.), American Chemical Society, Washington, DC, pp. 2–16.
5. Boone. C.W., Kelloff, G.J., and Malone, W.E. (1990) *Cancer Res. 50*, 2–9.
6. Wattenberg, L.W. (1983) *Cancer Res. 43*, 2448–2453s.
7. Wattenberg, L.W. (1992) *Cancer Res. 52*, 2085–2091s.
8. Block, G., Patterson, B., and Subar, A. (1992) *Nutr. Cancer 18*, 1–29.
9. Steinmetz, K.A., and Potter J.D. (1991) *Cancer Causes Control* 2, 325–357.
10. Steinmetz, K.A., and Potter J.D. (1991) *Cancer Causes Control* 2, 425–442.
11. Ripsin, C.M., Keenan, J.M., and Jacobs, D.R. Jr. (1992) *JAMA 267*, 3317–3325.
12. Kushi, L.H., Lew, R.A., and Stare, F.J. (1985) *N. Engl. J. Med. 312*, 811–818.
13. Morris, J.N., Marr, J.W., and Clayton, D.G. (1977) *Br. Med. J. 2*, 1307–1314.
14. Osawa, T., Katsuzaki, H., Hagiwara, Y., Hagiwara, H., and Shibamoto, T. (1992) *J. Agric. Food Chem. 40*, 1135–1138.
15. Sano, M., Abe, M., Yoshino, K., Matsuura, T., Sekino, T., Saito, S.-I., and Tomita, I. (1986) *Chem. Pharm. Bull. 34*, 174–178.
16. Mitsuta, K., Mizuta, Y., Kohno, M., Hiramatsu, M., and Mori, A. (1990) *Bull. Chem. Soc. Jpn. 63*, 187–191.
17. Bjorksten, J. (1968) *J. Am. Geriat. Soc. 16*, 408–427.
18. Walford, R.L. (1969) *The Immunological Theory of Aging*, Munksgaard, Copenhagen.
19. Harman, D. (1956) *J. Gerontol. 11*, 298–300.
20. Hayflick, L. (1987) in *Modern Biological Theories of Aging* (Warner, M.R., Butler, R.N., Sprott, R.L., Schneider, E.L., eds.), Raven Press, New York, pp. 21–34.
21. Ho, C.-T,; Osawa, T., Huang, M.-T., and Rosen, R.T., eds. (1994) *Food Phytochemicals for Cancer Prevention,* Vols. I and II, American Chemical Society, Washington, DC.
22. Ochi, H. (1983) in *East Meets West: Super Nutrition from Japan* (Castillo, E., ed.), Ishi Press International, Mountain View, p. 3.

Chapter 6

Antioxidant and Biological Properties of Rosemary Components: Implications for Food and Health

E.A. Offord, F. Guillot, R. Aeschbach, J. Löliger, and A.M.A. Pfeifer

Nestlé Research Centre, CH-1000 Lausanne 26, Switzerland.

Introduction

Plant phenols and polyphenolic compounds are widespread components of the human diet found in vegetables, fruits, soybeans, cereals, tea, coffee, and natural herb and spice extracts (1,2). Some examples include vitamins C and E, flavonoids (quercetin, rutin), hydroxycinnamic acids (chlorogenic, caffeic and ferulic acids), phenols in green tea (catechins) and black tea (thearubigin, theaflavin), and antioxidants from spices such as rosemary (carnosol, carnosic acid), thyme (thymol, carvacrol), and ginger (6-gingerol, zingerone). The interest of the food industry in phenolic antioxidants is related primarily to their antioxidant activity resulting in increased shelf-life of food products. However, these compounds also show important biological activity *in vivo* and may be beneficial in combating diseases related to excessive oxygen radical formation exceeding the antioxidant defense capacity of the human body. Certain pathological processes are a consequence of the action of reactive oxygen species; for example, atherosclerosis is linked to lipid peroxidation, aging and cataract formation to protein oxidation, and some cancers result from DNA modifications following damage induced by radicals. Antioxidant polyphenols have broad, mainly positive effects that may counteract many of these adverse reactions because of their ability to terminate radical reaction chains, scavenge active oxygen species, and trap elecrophiles. The health aspect of natural dietary antioxidants is therefore an important issue in nutrition and is of interest not only to the food industry but also to the consumer, particularly due to the safety concern (real or imagined) with regard to synthetic compounds. Caution is nevertheless required because natural does not always equal beneficial. The use of polyphenolic antioxidants by the food industry with the aim of producing optimal food for better health requires extensive research to optimize the composition and concentration of natural polyphenols in food. This will require proof of their antioxidant effect *in vivo*, their bioavailability and toxicological properties, and the molecular and cellular mechanisms contributing to their biological activities.

In this chapter, we focus our attention on natural polyphenolic compounds extracted from the leaves of the plant *Rosmarinus officinalis* L. We first describe the antioxidant properties of rosemary and its application to food stabilization and then go on to show its biological effects in cell model systems, with some interesting implications for human health.

Purification and Characterization of Rosemary Antioxidants

The leaves of the plant *Rosmarinus officinalis* L. are best known as a spice and flavoring agent. However, antioxidants have been extracted from this plant in significant quantities (3–5). The interest in exploiting these antioxidant properties for the stabilization of food is relatively recent and is linked to the increasing trend to favor natural rather than synthetic antioxidants. The advantage of rosemary as a natural source of antioxidants is the ready availability of the raw material and its high antioxidant potential. Crude and refined extracts of *Rosmarinus officinalis* L. are now commercially available in powder and liquid form at different concentrations of the active components (FIS S.A., Châtel-St.-Denis, Switzerland). To overcome the problems of odor, color and taste associated with rosemary components, a more refined rosemary extract (RE-S) has been developed and used in chemical and biological studies (6). In the first step, the essential oils of rosemary are removed by steam distillation or selective solvent extraction. The residue containing the active antioxidant components is further treated with hexane to remove the wax and with ethanol to extract the antioxidants. The final preparation is almost without odor and color. Protocols have been further developed to isolate pure molecules associated with the antioxidant activity of rosemary. The structures of these compounds are shown in Fig. 6.1.

The phenolic diterpenes, carnosol and carnosic acid, make up about 15% of RE-S and account for over 90% of its antioxidant activity (7). Rosmarinic acid has antioxidant activity and is found at a concentration of 1 or 2% in the fresh extract. The triterpenic acids ursolic acid (25%), oleanolic acid (10%), and betulinic acid (15%) are major components of RE-S but are not strong antioxidants. However, they may contribute to the anticarcinogenic properties of rosemary as described below (8–10). Other constituents of rosemary include the triterpines, betulin and amyrin (8–10%), sugars (8%), flavonoids, and other phenolics (2–4%). Minor constituents such as rosmanol, isorosmanol, rosmaridiphenol, and rosmariquinone also have antioxidant activity (11–13).

Antioxidant Activity of Rosemary Components in Food

During storage of prepared or dehydrated food, lipid autoxidative degradation products, e.g., hydroperoxides, malondialdehydes, aldehydes, ketones, and hydroxy fatty acids may occur if the food is not properly protected by antioxidants. These products not only result in unpleasant flavors but may also pose a health risk (14). Lipid oxidation is an autocatalyzed radical chain reaction induced by free radicals (15). The function of antioxidants, synthetic or natural, in food matrices is to act as radical scavengers. Polyphenolic antioxidants possess a relatively reactive

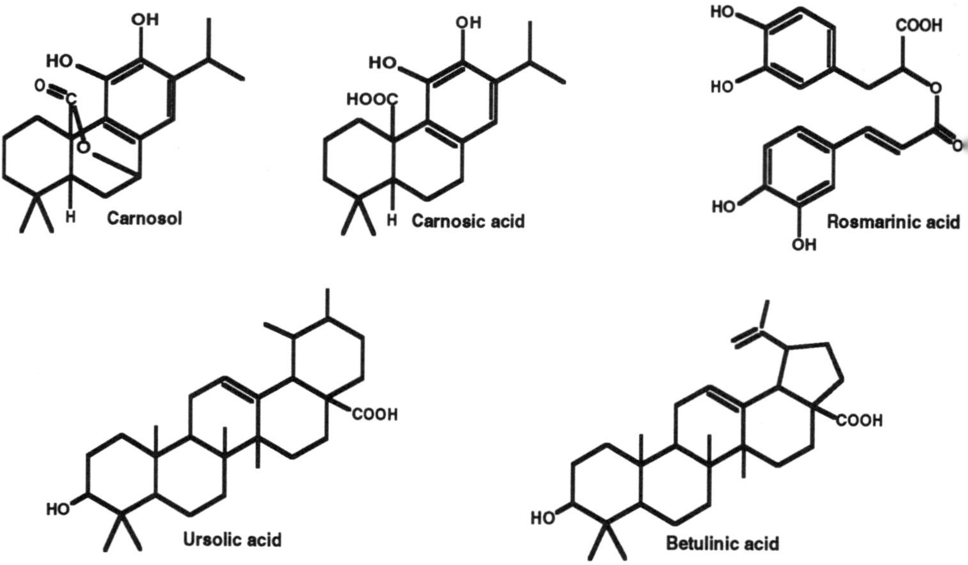

Fig. 6.1. Structures of polyphenolic compounds isolated from *Rosmarinus officinalis* L.

phenolic hydrogen atom which functions as a donor, allowing the formation of the antioxidant phenoxy radical.

Rosemary extract has been shown to act as an effective antioxidant in several food systems, especially in animal fats and vegetable oils (3–5). With the Rancimat test, in which fats and oils are oxidized under elevated temperatures and accelerated aeration, the induction time of lard was longer in the presence of rosemary extract or its most active antioxidant components, carnosol and carnosic acid, and had stronger antioxidant activities than BHT and BHA (16). Another way to assess lipid peroxidation in foods is by headspace gas chromatographic analysis of volatile hydrocarbons, such as pentane, which are released after thermal decomposition of lipid peroxides. Pentane is a secondary degradation product of linoleic acid oxidation. RE-S was shown to effectively stabilize wheat, rice, oat, or potato flakes stored at 20°C and frozen ground pork patties stored at –20°C (2,17). RE-S activity was compared with green tea and the synthetic antioxidants BHT/BHA. At a concentration of 500 or 1000 ppm in the pork preparation, RE-S showed an antioxidant activity similar to BHT/BHA.

Antioxidant Activity of Rosemary Components in Lipid and Nonlipid Systems

The antioxidant properties of carnosol and carnosic acid were studied in lipid and non-lipid systems in collaboration with Aruoma *et al.* (7). The results may be summarized as follows: both carnosic acid and carnosol were shown to be effective scavengers of peroxyl ($CCl_3O_2^{\bullet}$) radicals generated by radiolysis of a mixture of propan-2-ol and CCl_4, with carnosic acid 10 times more effective than carnosol. Both carnosol and carnosic acid effectively scavenged $HO^{\bullet}$ radicals as shown by their ability to inhibit degradation of the sugar deoxyribose in an aqueous mixture of ferric ion/EDTA and ascorbic acid. Carnosic acid also appeared to scavenge H_2O_2, whereas carnosol was inactive. Carnosic acid was able to scavenge hypochlorous acid (HOCl), a compound produced in the body at sites of inflammation and which can attack biological membranes. Carnosol and carnosic acid were powerful inhibitors of non-enzymatic peroxidation of rat liver microsomes and ox brain phospholipid liposomes in the presence of $FeCl_3$ and ascorbic acid. These results together demonstrate the high antioxidant capacity of carnosol and carnosic acid which may be beneficial not only in combating degeneration of foods through oxidation but also to health in scavenging free radicals that are implicated in human disease.

Antimutagenicity in Bacteria

The possible antimutagenic property of antioxidants used in food products was examined because oxygen species are known to be involved in cancer development (18). The antimutagenic activity of rosemary components was investigated in the standard *in vitro* Ames test with the bacterial tester strain *Salmonella typhimurium* TA102 which is known to be highly sensitive to reactive oxygen species (19). Mutagenicity was induced by the generation of oxygen radicals by *tert*-butylhydroperoxide (*t*-BuOOH). Therefore, any antimutagenic property must be attributed to the antioxidant activity of the tested compounds. The antioxidant fraction of RE-S consisted of carnosic acid (88%) and carnosol (12%) and made up 10–15% of the whole extract. RE-S and carnosic acid significantly and in a dose-dependent manner reduced the *t*-BuOOH-induced mutagenicity. This antimutagenic effect was obtained with a concentration of ~10 times lower than that necessary for ascorbic acid. Carnosol had only a weak inhibitory effect in this system. The stronger antimutagenic property of carnosic acid compared with carnosol and ascorbic acid was attributed to its more efficient radical-scavenging property. As mentioned above, carnosic acid was also found to be 10 times more efficient than carnosol as a scavenger of tricholoromethyl radicals (7). RE-S, carnosic acid, or carnosol had no prooxidant effects. Mutagenicity experiments *in vitro* allow only limited extrapolations to the biological activity of polyphenolic antioxidants due to the low defense system and the differences in metabolism in prokaryotes; thus, we developed some mammalian *in vitro* systems for more predictive screening of anticarcinogenic compounds.

Antigenotoxicity in Human Bronchial Cells

Carcinogenesis is a multistage process consisting of initiation, promotion, and progression. Protection against the various stages of carcinogenesis is one of the important findings obtained with phenolic antioxidants such as teas and rosemary (20). In animal models, examples of intervention of rosemary at the tumor initiation stage include the inhibition of binding of benzo(a)pyrene [B(a)P] or 7,12-dimethylbenz (a)anthracene (DMBA) metabolites to mouse epidermal DNA or to rat mammary epithelial DNA (10,21). We have developed a model in the human bronchial epithelial cell line, BEAS-2B (22), to study the mechanisms by which rosemary components inhibit B(a)P-DNA adduct formation. Inhibition of the initiation stage of carcinogenesis may occur by reducing phase I metabolism or increasing detoxification by phase II enzymes (23). RE-S, carnosol, or carnosic acid inhibited the genotoxicity of B(a)P by employing both of these mechanisms (24). Cells were exposed to RE-S (6 μg/mL) or an equivalent concentration of carnosol or carnosic acid for 1 h before coincubation with 1.5 μM B(a)P for 6 h. DNA adduct formation, measured by the incorporation of tritiated B(a)P metabolites into DNA, was inhibited in a dose-dependent manner by these treatments (Fig. 6.2). In parallel, cytochrome P450 1A1 (CYP1A1) activity, measured with the substrate 7-ethoxyresorufin, was also inhibited in a dose-dependent manner (Fig. 6.2). The inhibition of CYP1A1 activity was explained, at least in part, by inhibition of CYP 1A1 mRNA expression (24). Rosemary components therefore block the metabolic activation of B(a)P to its DNA-binding metabolite by inhibiting the expression and activity of the principal enzyme involved in the activation process. Furthermore, carnosol (1 μg/mL) induced the

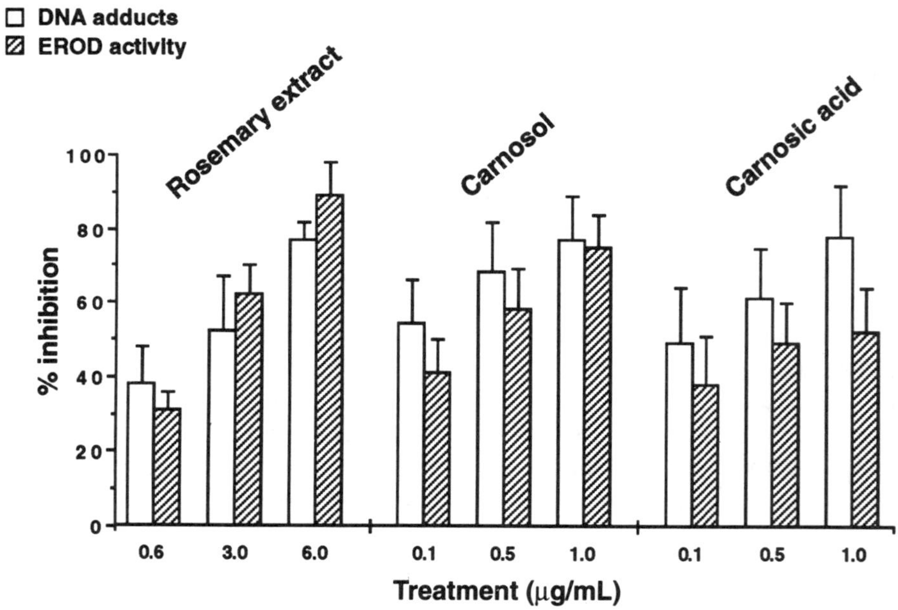

Fig. 6.2. Antigenotoxicity effect of rosemary and its constituents in BEAS-2B cells: parallel inhibition of B(a)P-DNA adduct formation and CYP1A1 (7-ethoxyresorufin) activity. At least four independent experiments were performed for each test condition. The details are described in the text.

expression of the phase II enzyme glutathione *S*-transferase (GST) involved in the detoxification of the proximate carcinogenic metabolite of B(a)P (25,26). A second phase II enzyme, NAD(P)H:quinone reductase (QR) was also induced by carnosol. This enzyme catalyzes the detoxification of reactive quinone intermediates. In rats fed rosemary at 0.25–1.0% of their diet, DMBA-DNA adduct formation was inhibited and the activities of liver GST and QR enzymes were induced three- to four-fold (27). Our results in BEAS-2B cells therefore correlate well with *in vivo* data. The induction of phase II detoxifying enzymes is a mechanism whereby many chemopreventive agents exert their beneficial effects (28). Therefore, rosemary components may be effective protectors against a wide range of carcinogens, making them promising candidates for chemopreventive programs.

Antitumor-Promoting Activity in Murine JB6 Cells

The selective clonal expansion of initiated cells by increased resistance to the cytotoxic effects of phorbol esters and reactive oxygen species appears to be one of the mechanisms involved in tumor promotion. The protective effect of phenolic antioxidants against tumor promotion may be due to the removal of oxygen radicals and/or the modulation of gene expression during tumor promotion, e.g., inhibition of ornithine decarboxylase activity (ODC) or protein kinase C (PKC). Indeed, Huang *et al.* (10) reported that application of rosemary extract to mouse skin had strong inhibitory effects on 12-*O*-tetradecanoylphorbol-13-acetate (TPA)-induced inflammation, ODC activity, and tumor promotion, as well as on arachidonic acid-induced inflammation. Carnosol and ursolic acid were the active components of this extract. The lipoxygenase pathways of arachidonic acid metabolism produce reactive oxygen species which may play a role in inflammation and tumor promotion. Chen *et al.* (16) showed that rosemary extracts inhibited soybean 15-lipoxygenase activity with IC_{50} values ranging from 1.3 to 2.6 µg. Carnosol was a more effective lipoxygenase inhibitor than was carnosic acid, and ursolic acid showed a significant inhibitory effect. Because soybean lipoxygenase bears many similarities to the mammalian lipoxygenase enzyme (29), these results further suggest that rosemary components have the potential to act as antitumor promoting agents. Antitumor-promoting activity in mouse skin has also been demonstrated for betulinic acid and oleanolic acid (8,9).

The JB6 epidermal cell model is analogous to late stage promotion in mouse skin (30). JB6 cells, established from mouse epidermis, retain differentiation markers and respond to tumor promoters by an increase in ODC, PKC, fos and myc, and growth in soft agar (31). We chose the inhibition of growth in soft agar as a screening system for the antipromoting activity of rosemary components in the JB6 promotable clone 41 (31). JB6 cells (10,000 cells/6-cm petri dish) were suspended in growth medium (Eagle's minimum essential medium without phenol red, 5% fetal calf serum), containing 0.33% agar with or without the phorbol ester TPA (12-*O*-tetradecanoylphorbol-13-acetate; 10 ng/mL) and in the presence or absence of rosemary components. The cells were layered onto a preestablished semisolid medium (0.33% agar containing TPA and/or antioxidants as above). Fourteen days after seeding, the colonies were stained with a 1 mg/mL solution of MTT [3-(4,5-dimethylthiazol-2yl)-2,5-diphenyltetrazoliumbromide] diluted in culture medium. The semisolid medium was then rinsed with a protamine sulfate buffer. The colonies were later counted using an image counter/analyzer.

Carnosic acid and carnosol inhibited promotion induced by TPA in a dose-dependent manner (Fig. 6.3). One hundred nanograms carnosic acid or carnosol resulted in 30 and 50% inhibition, respectively, 500 ng caused a reduction of 60%,

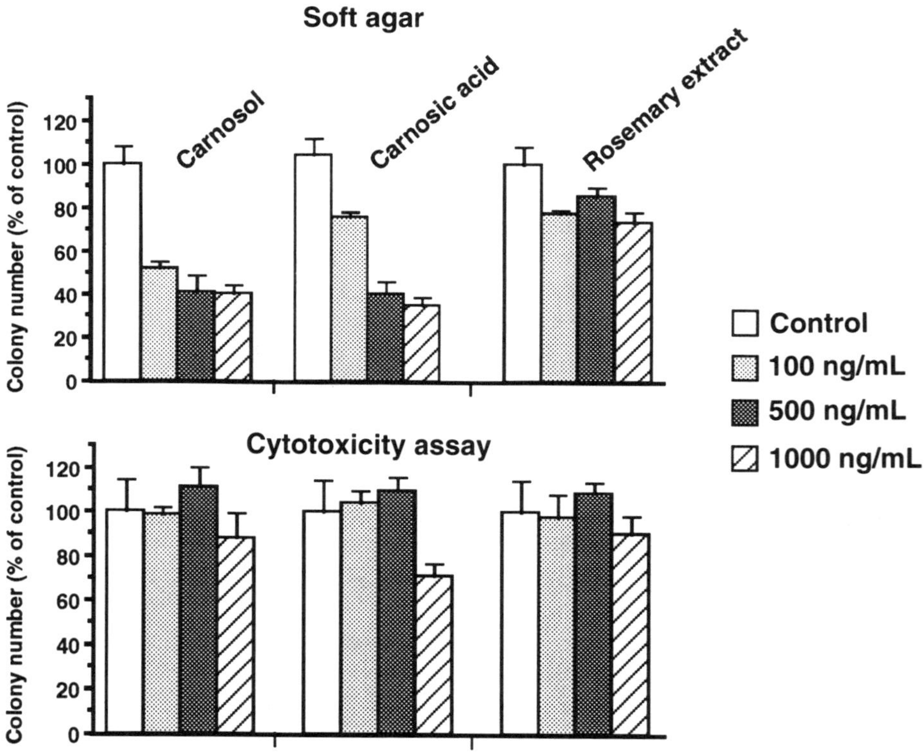

Fig. 6.3. Antipromoting effect of rosemary and its constituents in the JB6 (cl41) cell model. The upper graph shows the inhibition of TPA-induced growth in soft agar by carnosol, carnosic acid, and whole rosemary extract, as described in the text. Inhibition of anchorage-independent growth was calculated as follows:

$$\%\ \text{inhibition} = 100 - \left[\frac{\text{number of colonies in test plate (TPA + RE-S)} \times 100}{\text{number of colonies with TPA alone}}\right]$$

The lower graph shows the results of a colony-forming efficiency assay in which JB6 cells (500 cells/6-cm petri dish) were incubated for 14 d in the presence or absence of rosemary antioxidants. Colonies were then stained with a crystal violet/formaldehyde solution and counted. No cytotoxicity was observed with the rosemary antioxidants in the dose range used for the soft-agar studies.

and with 1000 ng there was only a small further reduction. The whole RE-S demonstrated biological activity corresponding to the concentration of carnosic acid and carnosol in the extract. This suggests that these components are predominantly responsible for the antipromoting effect. Ursolic acid (100–1000 ng) had no effect on TPA-induced colony formation, whereas 1000 ng of betulinic acid or rosmarinic acid led to 30% inhibition. No prooxidant, promoting, or cytotoxic effects were observed with the rosemary components within the dose range used (Fig. 6.3). These *in vitro* results correlate well with those found *in vivo* for the inhibition of TPA-induced tumor promotion by RE-S, carnosol, and carnosic acid. Some differences were seen for the other constituents of rosemary such as ursolic acid which was inhibitory *in vivo* but not *in vitro*.

In conclusion, our results and those of others suggest that phenolic antioxidants, such as those found in rosemary, may have a further application in the food industry besides those of traditional flavoring and stabilizing agents because their chemopreventive properties may lead to beneficial effects on human health.

Acknowledgments

We would like to thank P. Cerutti and P. Amstad for their encouragement and helpful advice throughout the anticarcinogenic studies and for supplying us with the JB6 cells.

References

1. Pratt, D.E. (1992) in *Phenolic Compounds in Food and Their Effects on Health II: Antioxidants & Cancer Prevention* (Huang, M.-T., Ho, C.-T., and Lee, C.Y., eds.), ACS Symposium Series 507, Washington, DC, pp. 54–71.
2. Löliger, J., and Wille, H.J. (1993) *Oils & Fats International 9*, 18–22.
3. Chang, S.S., Biserka, O.-M., Hsieh, O.A.L., and Huang, C.-L. (1977) *J. Food Sci. 42*, 1102.
4. Bracco, U., Löliger, J., and Viret, J.-L. (1981) *J. Am. Oil Chem. Soc. 58*, 686.
5. Wu, J.W., Lee, M.H., Ho, C.T., and Chang, S.S. (1982) *J. Am. Oil Chem. Soc. 59*, 339.
6. Aeschbach, R., and Philippossian, G., European Patent 88113185.8 (1988).
7. Aruoma, O.I., Halliwell, B., Aeschbach, R., and Löliger, J. (1992) *Xenobiotica 22*, 257.
8. Tokuda, H., Ohigashi, H., Koshimizu, K., and Ito, Y. (1986) *Cancer Lett. 33*, 279–285.
9. Yasukawa, K., Takido, M., Matsumoto, T., Takeuchi, M., and Nakagawa, S. (1991) *Oncology 48*, 72.
10. Huang, M.-T., Ho, C.-T., Wang, Z.Y., Ferraro, T., Lou, Y.-R., Stauber, K., Ma, W., Gerogiadis, C., Laskin, J.D., and Conney, A.H. (1994) *Cancer Res. 54*, 701.
11. Inatani, R., Nakatani, N., and Fuwa, H. (1983) *Agric. Biol. Chem. 47*, 521.
12. Houlihan, C.M., Ho, C.-T., and Chang, S.S. (1984) *J. Am. Oil Chem. Soc. 61*, 1036.
13. Houlihan, C.M., Ho, C.-T., and Chang, S.S. (1985) *J. Am. Oil Chem. Soc. 62*, 96.
14. Addis, P.B., and Warner, G.J. (1991) in *Free Radicals and Food Additives* (Aruoma, O.I., Halliwell, B., eds.), Taylor & Francis Ltd., London, pp. 77–119.
15. Kappus, H. (1991) in *Free Radicals and Food Additives* (Aruoma, O.I., Halliwell, B., eds.), Taylor & Francis: London, pp. 59–75.

16. Chen, Q., Huang, S., and Ho, C.-T. (1992) *J. Am. Oil Chem. Soc. 69*, 999.
17. Löliger, J. (1991) in *Free Radicals and Food Additives* (Aruoma, O.I., Halliwell, B., eds.), Taylor & Francis: London, pp. 121–150.
18. Cerutti, P. (1985) *Science 227*, 375.
19. Minnuni, M., Wolleb, U., Mueller, O., Pfeifer, A., and Aeschbacher, H.U. (1992) *Mut. Res. 269*, 193.
20. Ho, C.-T., Ferraro, T., Chen, Q., Rosen, R.T., Huang, M.-T. (1994) in *Food Phytochemicals for Cancer Prevention II* (Ho, C.-T., Toshihiko, O., Huang, M.-T., and Rosen, R.T., eds.), ACS Symposium Series 547, Washington, D.C., pp. 2–19.
21. Singletary, K.W., and Nelshoppen, J.M. (1991) *Cancer Lett. 60*, 169.
22. Reddel, R.R., Ke, Y., Gerwin, B.I., McMenamin, M.G., Lechner, J.F., Su, R.T., Brash, D.E., Park, J.B., Rhim, J.S., and Harris, C.C. (1988) *Cancer Res. 48*, 1904.
23. Morse, M.A., and Stoner, G.D. (1993) *Carcinogenesis 14*, 1737.
24. Offord, E.A., Macé, K., Ruffieux, C., Malhoë, A., and Pfeifer, A.M.A. (1995) *Carcinogenesis 16*, 2057–2062.
25. Robertson, I.G.C., Guthenberg, C., Mannervik, B., and Jernström, B. (1986) *Cancer Res. 46*, 2220.
26. Swedmark, S., Romert, L., Morgenstern, R., Jenssen, D. (1992) *Carcinogenesis 13*, 1719.
27. Singletary, K.W., and Gutierrez, E. (1993) *FASEB J. 7*, A866 (abstract).
28. Kensler, T.W., Davidson, N.E., Groopman, J.D., Roebuck, B.D., Prochaska, H.J., and Talalay, P.T. (1993) in *Antimutagenesis and Anticarcinogenesis Mechanisms III* (Bronzetti, G., ed.), Plenum Press, New York, pp. 127–136.
29. Percival, M.D. (1991) *J. Biol. Chem. 266*, 10058.
30. Colburn, N.H., Former, B.F., Nelson, K.A., and Yuspa, S.H. (1979) *Nature 281*, 589.
31. Gindhart, T.D., Nakamura, Y., Stevens, L.A., Hegameyer, G.A., West, M.W., Smith, B.M., and Colburn, N.H. (1985) in *Carcinogenesis* (Mass, M.J.E., ed.), Raven Press, New York, pp. 341–366.

Chapter 7

Natural Antioxidants from Oilseeds

V.K.S. Shukla[a], P.K.J.P.D. Wanasundara[b], and F. Shahidi[a,b]

[a]International Food Science Centre A/S, Sønderskovvej 7, 8520 Lystrup, Denmark; and [b]Department of Biochemistry, Memorial University of Newfoundland, St. John's, Newfoundland, Canada

Introduction

Atmospheric oxygen is an essential requirement for most living organisms including higher plants. Oxygen in the atmosphere is present in the stable triplet biradical ($^3O_2$), in the ground state. Once inside the living cell it can be transformed by a four-electron reduction process to water, thus producing the superoxide radical (O_2^-), hydroxyl radical (HO•) and hydrogen peroxide (H_2O_2) as reactive intermediates. Singlet oxygen is formed from ground state triplet oxygen by the action of various sensitizers such as plant pigments. The major inter- and extracellular components such as proteins, unsaturated lipids, deoxyribonucleo acid (DNA), and ribonucleic acid (RNA) are the main target molecules for active oxygen species.

Participation of active oxygen species and free radicals in a variety of diseases such as tumor formation, cancer, and the aging process in the human body has been of great concern. The oxidative damage caused by the active oxygen species and free radicals on membrane lipids of cells leads to cancer and also aging. The formation of oxidized DNA bases by active oxygen species can act as both a cancer initiator and a promoter. The formation of oxidized DNA bases may lead to mutagens, a characteristic of initiation of cancer by oxidants and other carcinogens.

Oxidation of unsaturated lipids initiated by free radicals is a major cause of food quality deterioration and leads to several other chemical reactions that negatively affect food quality. The products of lipid oxidation are known to be important health risk factors. The efficient antioxidative defense mechanism of living cells protects healthy cell membranes from active oxygen species and free radicals. Self-defense systems against the toxic effects of oxygen free radicals may be supported by antioxidative compounds taken as foods, cosmetics, and medicine. Therefore, the antioxidative compounds provided by the diet may enrich the antioxidative status of living cells and thus reduce the damage, particularly in the elderly. Several types of antioxidants are added to foods to prevent lipid oxidation-mediated quality deterioration. However, a recent concern in the food industry is the use of natural antioxidants in foods.

There are several plant constituents that may act as antioxidants to counteract the action of oxygen-containing free radicals and other excited molecules mediated by active oxygen. This antioxidative defense mechanism of plants is due to enzymes (catalase, peroxidase, glutathione, and superoxide dismutase), carotenoids, peptides, and other nitrogen-containing compounds (alkaloids, chlorophyll derivatives) and phenolic compounds (such as flavonoids, phenolic acids, lignans, and tocopherols). Plant seeds must be adequately protected against active oxygen and probably contain very effective antioxidative compounds to maintain viability (1).

Different types of oil-bearing seeds have been used since antiquity for human consumption and other essential needs. Within the last two decades, both traditional and nontraditional oilseeds have been scrutinized carefully for their antioxidative compounds, especially for use in foods and as a source of natural antioxidants.

Phenolic Compounds

Phenolic compounds constitute one of the most widespread and diverse groups of secondary plant metabolites. Oilseeds generally contain phenolic compounds of various chemical nature, including flavonoids, lignans, lignins, phenolic acids, and tannins. Phenolic-type compounds are the most widely reported antioxidative compounds in oilseeds and are present in considerable amounts in mature seeds.

Flavonoids. Flavonoids occur widely in the plant kingdom and are present in almost all parts of the plant. The basic structure of a flavonoid molecule consists of two aromatic rings linked by a three-carbon aliphatic chain (C_6-C_3-C_6) which is condensed to form a pyran or, less commonly, a furan ring (2) (Fig. 7.1). Different oxidation levels of the central pyran ring differentiate chemical activity of flavonoids. In the case of chalcones, the central pyran ring is open. The flavones (Fig. 7.1A), flavonols (Fig. 7.1B), monomeric flavanols (Fig. 7.1F), and chalcones (Fig. 7.1E) are commonly found in plants and may possess antioxidative activity. Flavonoids are usually present as glycosides, with a sugar moiety linked to hydroxyl groups (referred to as *O*-glycosyl flavonoids) or through carbon-carbon bonds (referred to as *C*-glycosyl flavonoids).

Pratt and Watts (3) and Pratt (2,4) have considered flavonoids as primary antioxidants that act as free radical acceptors and chain breakers. Besides those activities, flavonols are known to chelate metal ions, at the 3-hydroxy-4-keto group and/or 5-hydroxy-4-keto group (when the A-ring is hydroxylated at the 5th position; Fig. 7.1B). An *o*-quinol group at the B-ring can also demonstrate metal chelating activity (5). The ability of flavonoids to form complexes with cupric ion (Fig. 7.2) has also been demonstrated by ultraviolet (UV) spectral studies. Such complexations may contribute to the antioxidative action of flavonoids (6). Chelation of metal ions renders them catalytically inactive and prevents initiation of autoxidation of unsaturated lipids.

It has been well established that the position and degree of hydroxylation are of primary importance in determining antioxidant activity of flavonoids. The *o*-dihydroxylation of the B-ring contributes to the antioxidant activity. The *p*-quinol

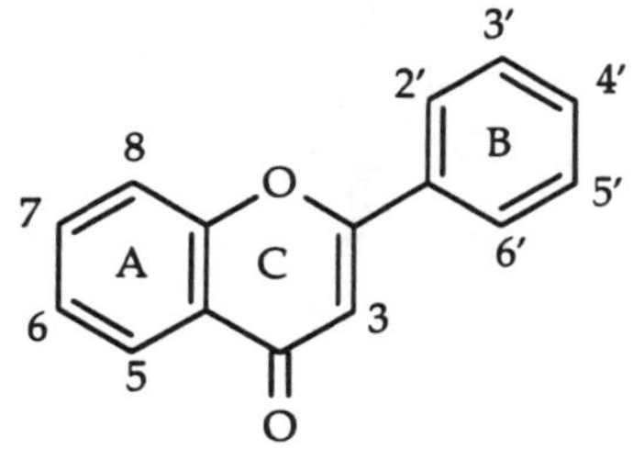

(a) Flavones

Apigenin - 5,7,4′-tri-OH
Fisetin - 3,7,3′,4′-tetra-OH
Luteolin - 5,7,3′,4′-tetra-OH
Robinetin - 3,7,3′,4′,5′-penta-OH

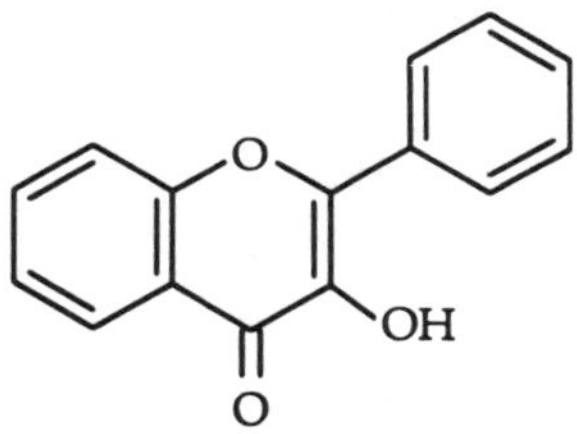

(b) Flavonols

Kaempferol - 3,5,7,4′-tetra-OH
Myricetin - 3,5,7,3′,4′,5′-hexa-OH
Morin - 3,5,7,2′,4′-penta-OH
Quercetin - 3,5,7,3′,4′-penta-OH
Rutin - 3-O-rutinose, 5,7,3′,4′-tetra-OH

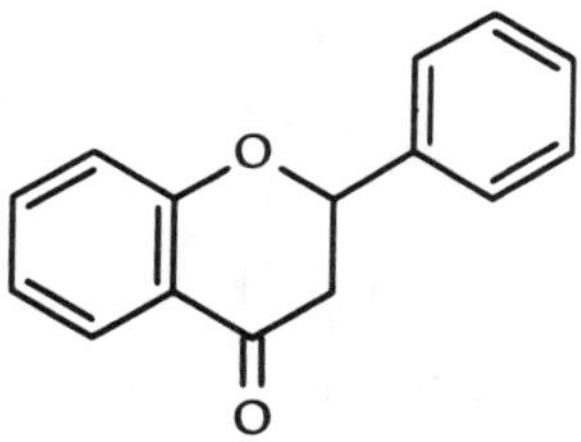

(c) Flavanones

Hespiritin - 5,7,3′-tri-OH
Eriodictyol - 5,7,3′,4′-tetra-OH
Naringenin - 5,7,4′-tri-OH
Naringin - 7-rhamnoglucose, 5,4′-di-OH

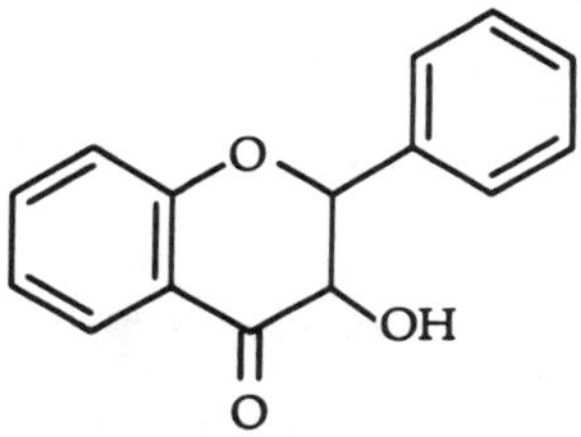

(d) Flavononols

Taxifolin - 3,5,7,3′,4′-penta-OH

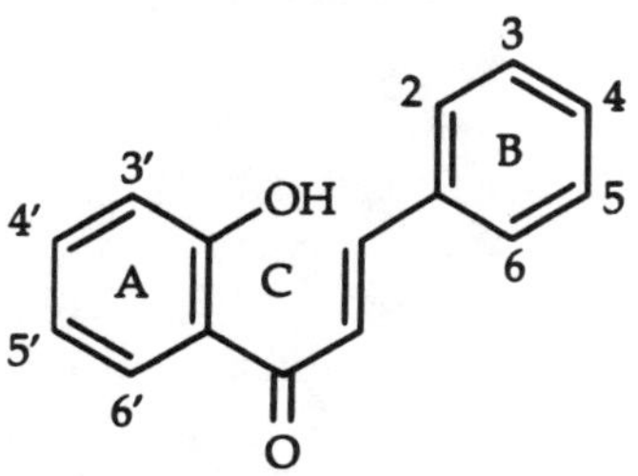

(e) Chalcones

Butein - 2,4,3′,4′-tetra-OH
Okanin - 2,3,4,3′,4′-penta-OH

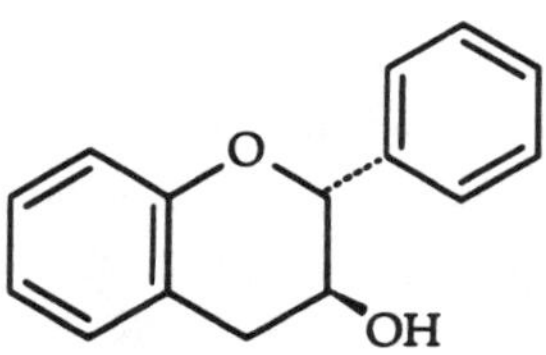

(f) Flavan-3-ol

(-)Epicatechin - 3,5,7,3′,4′-penta-OH

Fig. 7.1. Chemical structures of flavonoids.

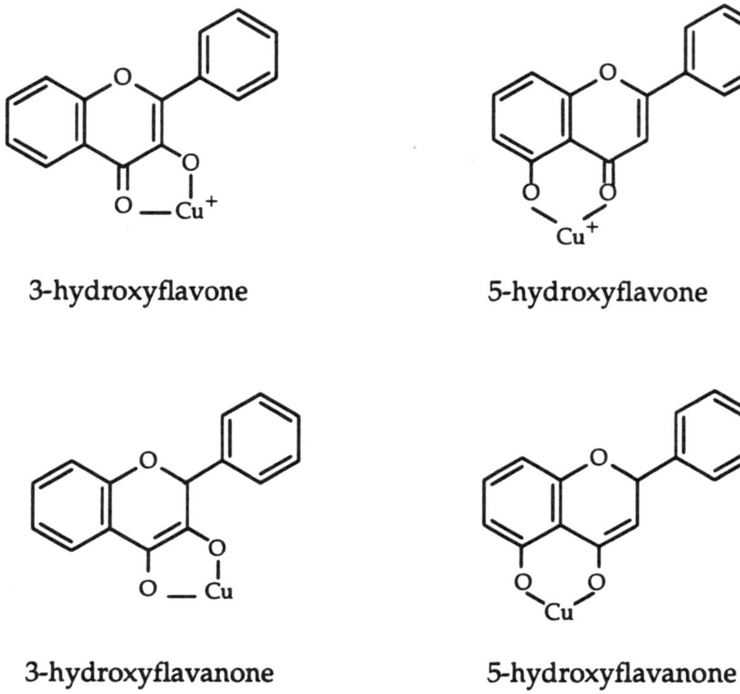

Fig. 7.2. Formation of metal chelates with flavones and flavonones.

structure of the B-ring has been shown to impart even greater activity than *o*-quinol; however, *p*- and *m*-hydroxylations of the B-ring do not occur naturally (5). All flavonoids with 3′, 4′-dihydroxy configuration possess antioxidant activity. It has also been documented that at least two, and even better, three neighboring phenolic hydroxy groups (catechol or pyrogallol structure) and a carbonyl group in the form of an aromatic ester or lactone or a chalcone, flavanone, or flavone are the essential molecular features required to achieve a high level of antioxidant activity (7).

Hydroxylation of the B-ring is the major consideration for antioxidant activity. The additional hydroxy group at the 5′ position of the robinetin (Fig. 7.1A) and myricetin (Fig. 7.1B) molecules has been shown to enhance their antioxidative activity in comparison with the corresponding flavones which do not possess the 5′ hydroxy group, such as fisetin (Fig. 7.1A) and quercetin (Fig. 7.1B). Both naringenin and hesperitin (Fig. 7.1C), have only one hydroxy group in the B-ring and possess little antioxidant activity (5). Other important features include the presence of a carbonyl group at position 4 and a free hydroxy group at position 3 and/or 5 (7).

Uri (8) has reported the importance of hydroxylation of other sites for antioxidative potential of flavonoids. It has been shown that the *o*-dihydroxy grouping on one ring and *p*-dihyroxy grouping on the other (e.g., 3,5,8,3′,4′- and 3,7,8,2′,5′-pentahydroxy flavones) produce very potent antioxidants, whereas 5,7-dihydroxylation of the A ring apparently has little influence on the antioxidant activity of the compound. Therefore, quercetin (Fig. 7.1B) and fisetin (Fig. 7.1A) have almost the same activity, whereas myricetin possesses an activity similar to that of robinetin (5).

Chalcones are natural precursors of flavones and flavanones and are readily cyclized under acidic conditions. The 3,4-dihydroxychalcones are particularly effective, and chalcones are more effective antioxidants than their corresponding flavanones. The effectiveness of 3,4-dihydroxychalcones (butein and okanin, Fig. 7.1E) depends on the formation of resonance-stabilized free radicals (7) (Fig. 7.3A).

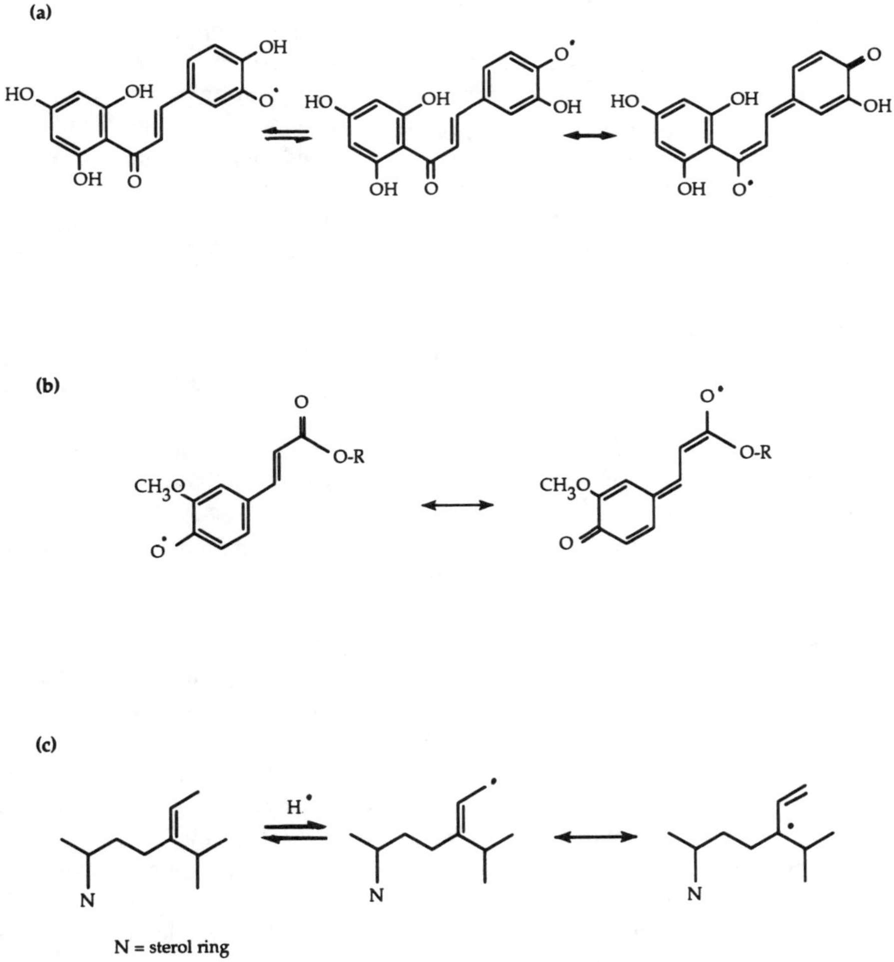

Fig. 7.3. Resonance stabilized structures formed by (A) chalcones, (B) cinnamic acid, and (C) sterols.

In the isoflavones, it is clear that both hydroxy groups in the 4′ and 5 positions are needed for antioxidant activity of the molecule as in genistein. Even 6,7,4′-trihydroxyisoflavone is marginally active in comparison with apigenin (Fig. 7.1A) which is quite active as an antioxidant. The resonance-stabilized quinoid structures of isoflavones show that the carbonyl group at position 4 loses its functionality, thus explaining the superior antioxidant activity of genistein compared with apigenin. Naturally occurring isoflavones, which are mainly found in plants of *Leguminoseae* family, have shown synergistic activity with phospholipids such as phosphotidyl ethanolamine (9).

Lignans. Lignans are widely found in all parts of plants and include compounds with great chemical diversity. By definition, lignans are dimers of phenylpropanoid (C_6-C_3) units linked by the central carbons of their side chains (10). According to their oxygenation, four major groups of linear lignans are found, namely, lignan or butane derivatives, lignanolides or butanolide derivatives, monoepoxylignans or tetrahydrofuran derivatives, and biepoxylignans or derivatives of 3,7-dioxabicyclo-(3,3,0)-octane (Fig. 7.4). Cyclized lignans or cyclolignans occur as tetrahydronapthalene or naphthalene derivatives (11) (Fig. 7.4). Lignan-type compounds isolated from plants and oilseeds have shown good antioxidant properties.

Phenolic acids. Phenolic acids are formed *via* the shikimic acid pathway during disposal of aromatic amino acids, namely, phenylalanine and tyrosine. Phenolic acids found in plants have the basic chemical structure of C_6-C_1 (benzoic acids) and C_6-C_3 (cinnamic acids) (Fig. 7.5). Both types of phenolic acids usually occur in conjugated or esterified form, sometimes as depsides such as chlorogenic acid (3-caffeoyl-quinic acid) (Fig. 7.5).

Phenolic acids can act as free radical acceptors and chain breakers, thus providing very efficient antioxidant activities in biological systems. According to Chimi *et al.* (12) and Pokorny (13), monophenols are less efficient antioxidants than polyphenols, the introduction of a secondary hydroxyl group in the *ortho* or *para* position increases the antioxidant activity of hydroxylated phenolic acids. Therefore, protocatechuic and caffeic acids, which are *o*-diphenols, are more efficient antioxidants than their respective monophenols, *p*-hydroxybenzoic and *p*-coumaric acid. Gallic acid with three hydroxyl groups is more active than protocatechuic acid; however, the presence of more than three hydroxyl groups on a given aromatic nucleus does not improve the antioxidative efficacy (13).

Substitution of one or two methoxy groups at the *ortho* position relative to the hydroxyl group markedly increases the antioxidant activity of phenolic acids. Therefore, sinapic acid is a more efficient antioxidant than ferulic acid, which is more efficient than *p*-coumaric acid. For the same reason, syringic acid is more active than vanillic and *p*-hydroxy benzoic acids (14). It is well established that *ortho* substitution with electron donor alkyl or methoxy groups increases the stabil-

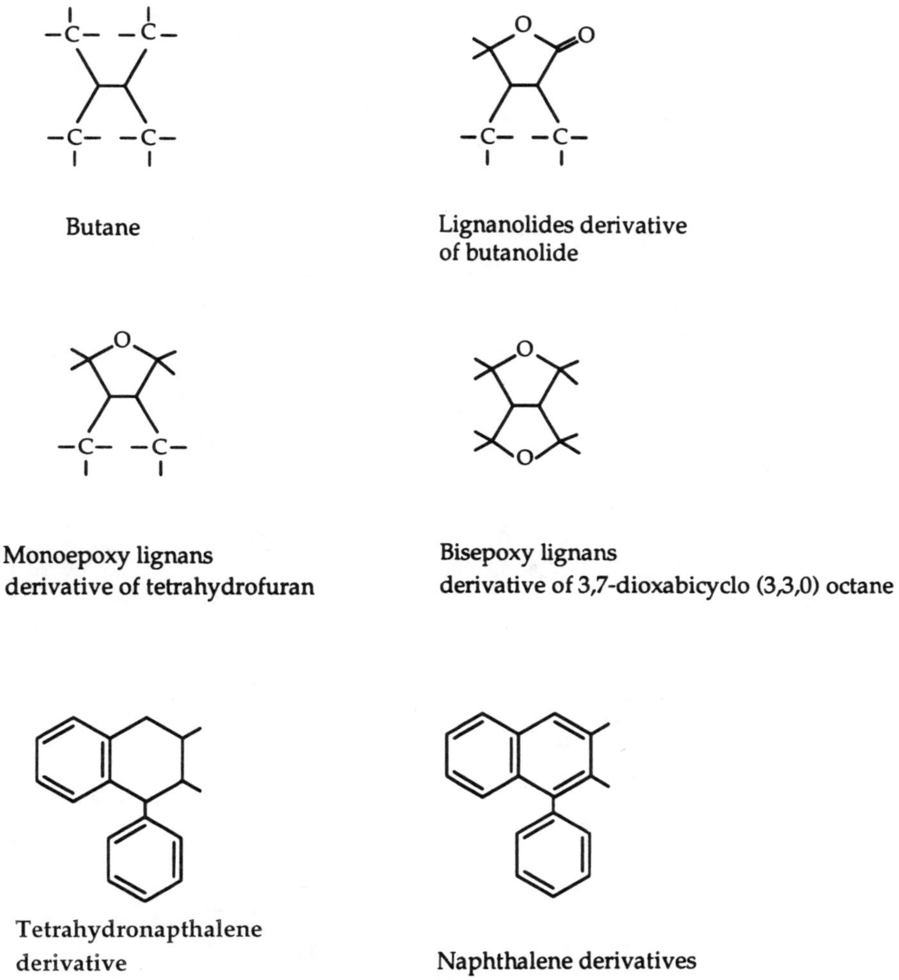

Fig. 7.4. Basic chemical structures of lignans.

ity of the aryloxy radical and thus the antioxidant activity. However, methoxy substitution is far from being equivalent to the addition of a hydroxyl group; for example, ferulic and vanillic acids remain substantially more active than caffeic and protocatechuic acids, respectively (12,13,15).

The presence of the CH=CH-COOH group in cinnamic acids ensures greater efficiency of antioxidative ability than the COOH group in benzoic acids. In fact, caffeic, *p*-coumaric, ferulic and sinapic acids are more active than protocatechuic, *p*-hydroxybenzoic, vanillic, and syringic acids, respectively. It may be the participation of the C=C bond which helps in stabilizing the radical by resonance (Fig. 7.3B). On

(a)

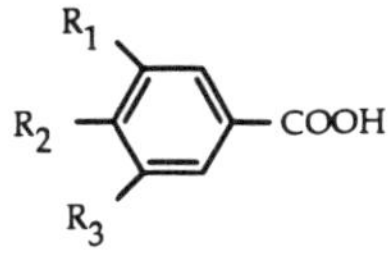

Acid	R_1	R_2	R_3
p-Hydroxybenzoic	H	OH	H
Protocatechuic	H	OH	OH
Vanillic	CH_3O	OH	H
Syringic	CH_3O	OH	CH_3O
Gallic	OH	OH	OH

(b)

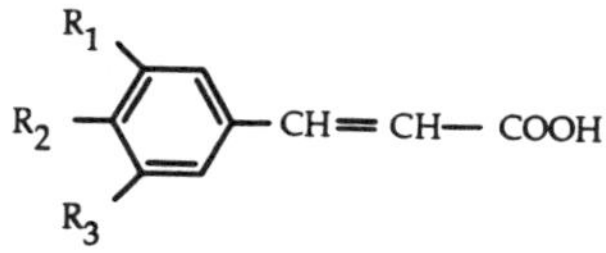

Acid	R_1	R_2	R_3
p-Coumaric	H	OH	H
Caffeic	H	OH	OH
Ferulic	CH_3O	OH	H
Sinapic	CH_3O	OH	CH_3O

(c)

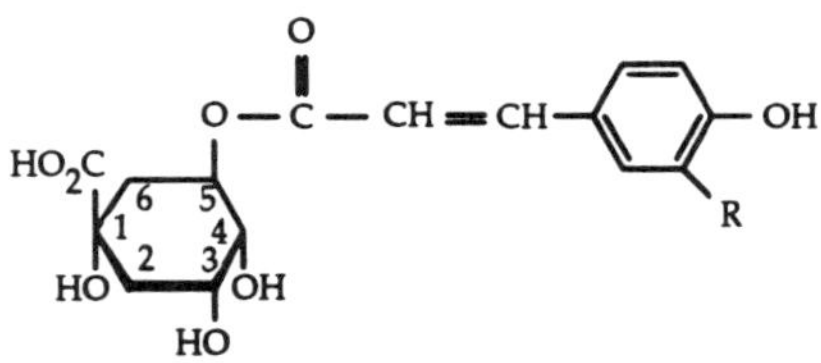

Acid	R
5-*p*-Coumaroylquinic	H
5-*p*-Caffeoylquinic	OH
5-*p*-Feruloylquinic	CH_3O

Fig. 7.5. Chemical structures of phenolic acids: (A) benzoic acids (B) cinnamic acids, and (C) chlorogenic acids.

the other hand, the presence of a single COOH group exhibits a negative role on antioxidative activity (14).

Alkyl esterification does not modify antioxidative activity because gallic acid and its propyl ester show similar potencies. The antioxidant activity of phenolic acids and their esters depends on the number of hydroxyl groups in the molecule, and this would be strengthened by steric hindrance. Hydroxylated cinnamic acids were found to be more effective than their benzoic acid counterparts. Generally, phenolic acids exist in plants as glycosides by esterification of the acid group with a sugar, and such a bulky group may further enhance the antioxidative potency of the molecule (14).

Tannins. Tannins are complex phenolic compounds having molecular weights in the range of 500–6000 Da (16,17). Tannins comprise a considerable amount of the hulls and seed coats of oligenous seeds. They can be classified as condensed or hydrolyzable, based on their structural type and reactivity towards hydrolytic agents/acids (18,19). Hydrolyzable tannins produce gallic acid (gallotannins) and/or a hexahydroxydiphenic acid that spontaneously converts to ellagic acid (ellgitannins) upon acid hydrolysis. However, condensed tannins are formed by polymerization of flavan-3-ols or flavan-3,4-diols (20).

Tocopherols. Tocopherols occur widely in plant tissues and are monophenolic as well as lipophilic compounds. Tocopherols and tocotrienols, collectively referred to as tocols, are classified into α, β, γ, or δ, depending on the number and position of the methyl groups attached to the chromane rings (Fig. 7.6). In tocopherols, the side chain is saturated whereas in tocotrienols it is unsaturated. Tocopherols are important biological antioxidants with vitamin E activity. α-Tocopherol, which exhibits maximum vitamin E activity, prevents oxidation of lipids *in vivo* including polyunsaturated fatty acids and lipid components of cells and organelle membranes. The antioxidative activity is reported to decrease from δ to α (21).

The antioxidant activity of tocopherol is based mainly on the tocopherol-tocopheryl quinone redox system (Fig. 7.7A). Tocopherols are free radical scavengers and quench lipid free radicals, thus generating a neutral lipid molecule and a tocopheryl semiquinone radical. Two tocopheryl semiquinone radicals may form a methyl tocopheryl quinone and α-tocopherol molecule which also exhibits antioxidant activity (Fig. 7.7B). Ishikawa and Yuki (22) and Schuler (23) have reviewed the antioxidant activities of oxidized tocopherols.

Enzymes, Amino Acids, Peptides and Other Nitrogen-Containing Compounds

Amino acids, enzymes, peptides amines, alkaloids, and chlorophyll derivatives perform significant defense activity in living cells. Although enzymes, discussed below, efficiently counteract active oxygen species, their activity as natural antioxidants in mature oilseeds has not been reported.

Tocopherol

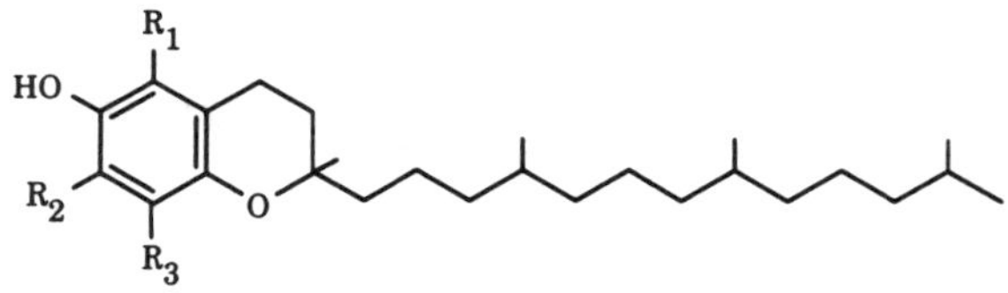

Tocotrienol

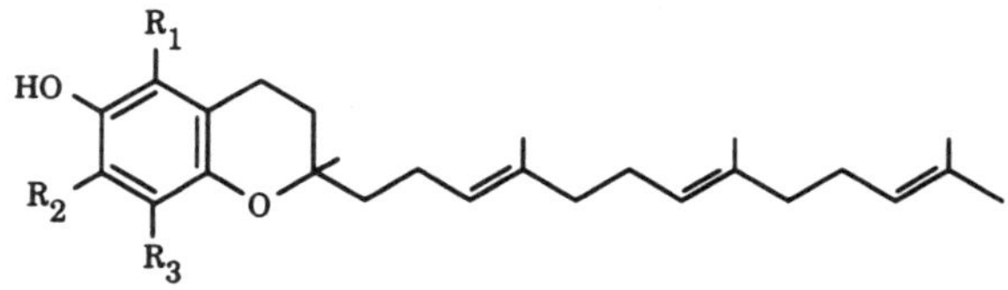

Tocol		R_1	R_2	R_3
Tocopherol	α	CH_3	CH_3	CH_3
	β	CH_3	H	CH_3
	γ	CH_3	CH_3	CH_3
	δ	CH_3	H	CH_3
Tocotrienol	α	CH_3	CH_3	CH_3
	β	CH_3	H	CH_3
	γ	CH_3	CH_3	CH_3
	δ	CH_3	H	CH_3

Fig. 7.6. Chemical structures of tocopherols and tocotrienols.

Catalase and Peroxidases. Catalase, which is a metalloenzyme, is the most efficient enzyme which promotes redox reaction leading to the formation of water and oxygen from hydrogen peroxide. Hydrogen peroxide itself is not particularly reactive towards most biologically important molecules; however, it may serve as an intracellular precursor for more reactive oxidants such as HO• (1). Although catalase is rather specific for H_2O_2, it also reacts with a limited number of organic hydroperoxides, such as CH_3OOH, and uses them to carry out oxidative reactions on acceptor molecules while simultaneously reducing the peroxidic substrates (24). Peroxidases which are also present in plants function in a similar manner (1).

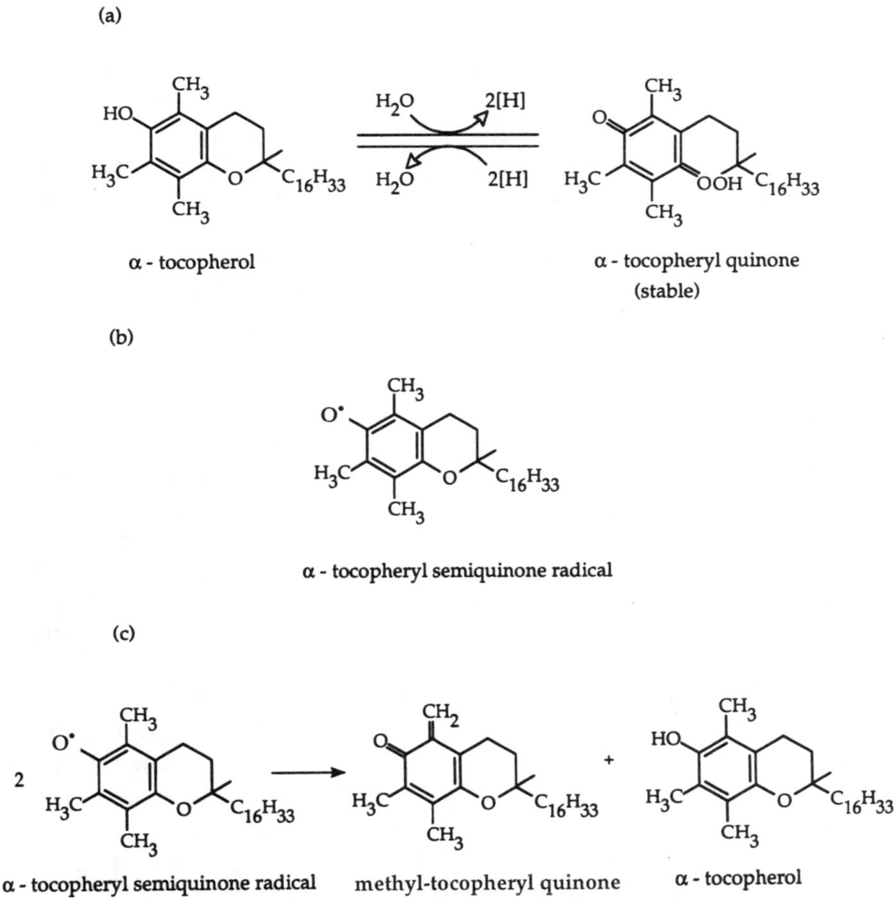

Fig. 7.7. Formation of tocopherol–tocopheryl quinone redox system.

Superoxide Dismutase (SOD). There are many processes that occur in plant cells for converting O_2 to its radical anion reduction product, $O_2^{\bullet -}$ (superoxide anion). Superoxide, similar to H_2O_2, is not directly reactive towards most organic compounds but may give rise to more reactive oxygen species with potentially higher toxicities. Superoxide dismutase (SOD) catalyzes the conversion of $O_2^{\bullet -}$ to H_2O_2 and O_2. It has been suggested that both SOD and catalase provide important functions in protecting plant leaves from deleterious effects of membrane lipid destruction (25).

Glutathione. Glutathione (GSH) is a tripeptide with a thiol group and is found in very high concentrations in many cells. It reacts with oxidants such as H_2O_2 to form a disulphide (GSSG) and other intracellular oxidants such as $^1O_2$, $O_2^{\bullet -}$ and $HO^{\bullet}$ (1).

Amino Acids. Amino acids in the free form and peptides are present in seeds as a result of incomplete protein synthesis or possibly due to partial protein degradation (26). Marcuse (27,28) has reported that a number of amino acids, with the exception of cysteine, had antioxidative effects which were dependent on the experimental conditions. In a suitable environment, extremely low amino acid concentrations may exhibit strong antioxidative effects but at high concentrations may become prooxidative. The antioxidative property of methionine was also concentration dependent (29). Peptides and amino acid mixtures also show antioxidant activity synergistic with α-tocopherol. Marcuse (27) hypothesized that amino acids are good metal chelators; however, Bishov and Henick (30) reported that other mechanisms might also be involved.

Alkaloids and Amines. Basic nitrogen compounds of plants are potent inhibitors of various oxidative processes. Indole alkaloids such as strychnine and brucine can inhibit $^1O_2$ by physical quenching due to their rigid structures (1). Lipid peroxidation induced by radioactive cobalt irradiation or ferrous ion was inhibited by the bis-benzyl isoquinoline alkaloid, cepharanthine (31). Caffeine also shows antioxidative activity against oxidation of linoleic acid, comparable to that of butylated hydroxyanisole (BHA) and butylated hydroxytoluene (BHT) (32). It has been established that caffeine can act as a hydroxy radical scavenger (33). The hydrophobic cationic alkaloids are more likely to interact with phospholipids and other anionic components of cell membranes and therefore, can be potent antioxidants (34,35).

Tertiary amines, such as trimethylamine, are very effective quenchers of peroxy radicals. The radicals derived from amines have very large termination rate constants, thus contributing to the efficient cessation of radical chain reactions (36). Polyamines, such as spermine, are related to simple acyclic alkaloids found in legumes, and show scavenging activity towards superoxide radicals at concentrations of 0.01–0.03 M. This ability of spermine has been suggested to be related to its well-known membrane stabilizing activity (1).

Chlorophyll Derivatives. Although both chlorophyll and pheophytin promote oxidation of lipids in the light, they are inhibitors of autoxidation under dark conditions. Chlorophyll *a* and pheophytin *a* appear to react with peroxy radicals but are unreactive towards lipid hydroperoxides (37). Furthermore, the pheophorbide derivatives, chlorophyllone *a* (38), pheophytin *a* (39), and pyropheophytin *a* (40), have been isolated as antioxidative compounds of marine plants. These pigments are derived from chlorophyll metabolism and are present in various plants or may originate during processing (degradations products during cooking, canning). The porphyrin ring of these pigments has been suggested as being important in structure-activity relationship studies (40).

Other Compounds

Ascorbic Acid. Ascorbic acid (vitamin C) is a well-known biological antioxidant and exists in rather high concentrations in plants, especially chloroplasts.

Ascorbate can reduce $O_2^{\bullet -}$ (41) and may react with $^1O_2$ (42). Vitamin C inhibits the peroxy radical-initiated oxidation of methyl linoleate in methanol/*t*-butanol at 37°C. Vitamin C also acts as a chain-breaking scavenger for peroxy radicals and acts synergistically with vitamin E (43). However, ascorbic acid has not been reported as an ingredient in most of the mature and dry oilseeds discussed here.

β-Carotene and Other Carotenoids. β-Carotene may act as an antioxidant by quenching singlet oxygen and converting it to triplet oxygen. Kellogg and Fridovich (44) showed that β-carotene inhibits lipid oxidation that was initiated by xanthine oxidase; this inhibition might be due to its effect on singlet oxygen. It has also been observed that β-carotene can inhibit lipid oxidation initiated under photooxidizing conditions (45). The presence of carotenoids in oilseeds and their oils may help to protect them against formation of singlet oxygen by blocking light transmission through oil which has been obtained from such oilseeds. Due to their multiple conjugated double bond system, carotenoids, particularly the 4-oxo derivatives such as astaxanthin and canthaxanthin, are also able to scavenge free radicals (46).

Phytic Acid. Phytic acid (*myo*-inositol-1,2,3,4,5,6-hexakis-dihydrogen phosphate) (Fig. 7.8) is an abundant plant constituent which could comprise up to 5% by weight of dried legumes, cereals, oilseeds, pollens, and nuts (47). The phytic acid molecule contains 12 replaceable protons, of which six can be strongly dissociated (48); therefore, it is very reactive towards positively charged groups such as metal cations. Phytic acid is usually found as salts of calcium or magnesium in

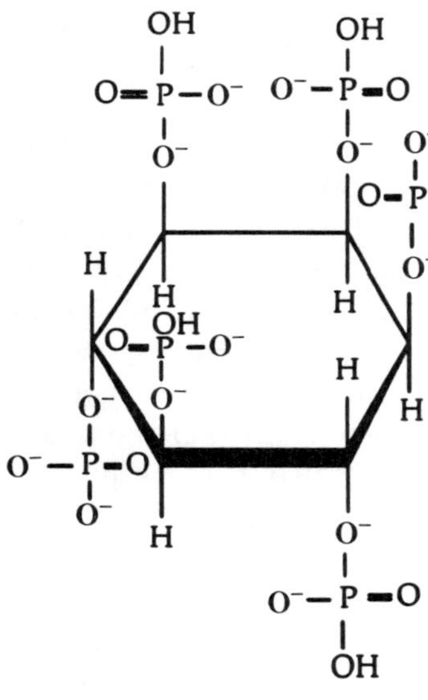

Fig. 7.8. Chemical structure of phytic acid.

plants. In this regard, phytic acid, by virtue of chelating free iron, is a potent inhibitor of iron-driven hydroxyl radical ($HO^{\bullet}$) formation (49). Hydroxyl radical generation mediated by iron requires the availability of at least one coordination site that is open or occupied by a readily dissociable ligand such as water. Although most iron chelates retain a reactive coordination site, Fe^{3+}-phytate is unique in not retaining a reactive coordination site and consequently it fails to support $HO^{\bullet}$ generation (49,50). Furthermore, phytic acid provides an exclusive trivalent oxidation state that blocks the necessary redox cycling of iron required in many oxidation reactions. Therefore, phytic acid may serve as an antioxidant in the plant cell environment besides its function as a storage of phosphorus, cations, glucouronates (cell wall precursor), or high energy phosphoryl groups (51). Empson *et al.* (52) have reported possible antioxidative activity of pure phytic acid in retarding warmed-over flavor development that could be useful in food systems.

Phospholipids. Phospholipids compose the structural lipids of the plant cell membrane. Phospholipid content of seed oil can be up to 10% of total lipids depending on the type of seed (53). Several studies have indicated that phospholipids chelate trace metals, thus acting as a secondary antioxidant, and subsequently increase oxidative stability of the oil (54,55). Acidic phospholipids such as phosphotidylinositol can form inactive complexes with metals but not with phosphotidylcholine or phosphatidylethanolamine (13). However, it has been well established that phospholipids can act as synergists with tocopherol (56) and flavonoids (7). Therefore, it has been suggested that phospholipids may act as antioxidants by releasing protons and bringing about rapid decomposition of hydroperoxides without the formation of free radicals (57,58). It should also be noted that surface activity of phospholipids at the air-oil interface or water-oil interface might also be involved in antioxidative activity of phospholipids in bulk oils and emulsion systems.

Sterols. Sterols are components of the unsaponifiable fraction of plant lipids. Sterols (Δ^5-avenasterol, fucosterol, citrostadienol) are reported to have antipolymerization activity in heated oils (59,60,61), but some are ineffective as antioxidants. It has been suggested that donation of a hydrogen atom from the allylic methyl group in the side chain of sterols (Fig. 7.3C), followed by isomerization in a relatively stable tertiary allylic free radical represents the mode of activity of sterols as antioxidants (60). Sterols obtained from wheat germ (4-α-methyl sterol), Vernonia oil, and oat germ (Δ^5-avenasterol) have been shown to have antipolymerizing effects in heated vegetable oils (59,60,62). This activity of sterols at frying temperatures is suggested to reside in the side chain of the sterol molecule which contains an ethylidine group (60,62).

Compounds Derived During Processing. Some oilseeds are subjected to roasting for use as snacks (e.g., sesame, peanut) as snacks or before oil extraction (e.g., sesame). Heating of oilseeds prior to oil extraction may also be carried out to inactivate enzymes in the seeds such as myrosinase in rapeseed. Oilseeds may also be used for production of protein hydrolysates for incorporation into different food formulations. Some oilseeds are also incorporated directly into foods such as bakery products (e.g., flax, sesame).

The high temperatures reached during roasting and baking result in the formation of Maillard reaction products. Melanoidins and compounds with reductone structures are reported to possess antioxidative activity (64–66). Maillard reaction products have been found to possess metal chelating properties (67,68) and to effectively convert hydroperoxides to non-radical products (69). The antioxidative effect of reductones has been attributed to a radical chain breaking mechanism due to the donation of a hydrogen atom (70). Strong antioxidative activities were also found in the systems containing low-molecular weight sugars and dicarbonyl compounds such as methylglyoxal, glyceraldehyde, dihydroxyacetone (71), and dehydroxyascorbic acid (72).

Small molecular weight peptides of soybean protein hydrolysates prepared by enzymic hydrolysis also exhibit antioxidative activity (30). Antioxidative activity of chlorophyll degradation products that are usually generated during thermal processing of green plant tissues has been discussed under chlorophyll derivatives. Some other compounds in oilseeds may also undergo chemical transformation during thermal processing or fermentation and produce substances with potent antioxidant activity (e.g., sesame, soybean).

Methods of Screening Antioxidative Compounds of Oilseeds

The general hypothesis for screening oilseeds for antioxidative compounds is that such seeds must protect their oil against oxidation by possessing effective antioxidants. Therefore, it might be realistic to assume that more unsaturated seed oils contain strong antioxidative components. There is no single solvent system that is suitable for the extraction and isolation of all antioxidative compounds due to their diverse chemical nature. Solubility of these chemical compounds in aqueous solvents is expected, because it is a required factor for their antioxidant activity in the cell as well as lipid-containing foods. Therefore, use of polar solvents such as aqueous ethanol or methanol for extraction of oilseed antioxidants is commonly practiced. Repeated extraction for a longer time (12–18 h) is recommended, sometimes at an elevated temperature (45–65°C), which may also inactivate any enzymes that may degrade antioxidative compounds (e.g., polyphenol oxidase). It is necessary to remove any lipids present in the plant tissues for effective extraction of these compounds. However, there is an exception for tocopherols, phospholipids, and other lipophilic compounds that are usually extracted into nonpolar solvents due to their non-polar nature. The extracts always contain a mixture of compounds of different chemical classes and, therefore, purification steps are necessary to remove unwanted substances.

The antioxidant activity of the oilseed extracts or isolated compounds can be estimated quantitatively by determining primary or secondary products of lipid oxidation. Generally, the delay in hydroperoxide formation or production of secondary autoxidation products by chemical or (rarely) sensory methods can be used. These procedures can be applied to intact foods, their extracts, or model systems.

Studies on foods can be performed under normal storage conditions or under accelerated oxidation such as the active oxygen method (AOM), Schaal oven test, oxygen uptake/absorption, oxygen bomb calorimetry, or by using the fully automated Rancimat or Oxidative Stability Instrument (OSI) (73,74). The extension of the induction period by addition of an antioxidant has been related to antioxidant efficacy which is sometimes expressed as antioxidant index or protection factor (74).

Formation of hydroperoxides is measured by an iodometric titration of released iodine by hydroperoxides and is generally expressed as peroxide value. Colorimetric determination of hydroperoxides with Fe-thiocyanate is also widely used to determine the extent of hydroperoxide formation (76). Of the available methods for measuring hydroperoxide decomposition products, determination of aldehydic compounds [e.g., 2-thiobarbituric acid (TBA), or 2-thiobarbituric acid reactive substances (TBARS) test, or *p*-anisidine test), measurement of total carbonyls, or a related carbonyl compound and assessment of off flavors and off odors due to the formation of volatile decomposition products of hydroperoxides in foods by objective and subjective means are extensively used. Schiff bases produced by carbonyl compounds of lipid oxidation and amino compounds added to the system give luminescence that can be used to measure the extent of formation of secondary oxidation products (77). Gas chromatography–mass spectrometry (GC–MS) with fast atom bombardment (FAB) to determine lipid oxidation products is very sensitive (66). Electron spin resonance (ESR) spectroscopy lends itself especially to detection of free radicals; however, this would be less practical for lipid oxidation measurement due to the short life of free radicals. Chemical methods of determining lipid oxidation products and antioxidative activity have been reviewed elsewhere in this book.

Model systems for testing the antioxidant activity of oilseed meals and extracts have been used extensively. Peroxidation catalyzed by metmyoglobin, Fe^{2+}-EDTA, or fresh beef homogenate has been used for screening antioxidative activity of methanolic extracts of various oilseeds by Rhee and coworkers (78,79). Based on the carotene discoloration method developed by Marco (80) and Miller (81), Taga and coworkers (82) have described a relatively easy procedure for determining antioxidant activity. This procedure involves colorimetric measurement of β-carotene bleaching at 470 nm in an aqueous emulsion of linoleic acid containing an antioxidative compound. Castro-Martinez *et al.* (83) have used the same principle of β-carotene bleaching activity but evaluated it on agar plates containing antioxidant and related the antioxidative activity to intensity and persistence of the β-carotene color. Osawa and Namiki (84, 85) have reported a method based on colorimetric determination of hydroperoxides formed in an ethanolic linoleic acid system containing antioxidants using the color reaction of $FeCl_2$ and thiocyanate. A method involving separation of individual components on a fluorescent thin-layer chromatography (TLC) plate and visualizing them by spraying with tocopherol-free soybean oil solution under UV light at 254 nm was described by Chang and co-workers (86). However, it is important to note that the relative activity of antioxidants varies with the substrate and conditions used for evaluation (74).

The activity of the antioxidant tested by chemical methods offers no information on its behavior in biological systems. Therefore, *in-vitro* methods that link chemical and biological methods have been developed to replace animal models in assessing antioxidative activity of plant extracts and their isolated compounds. Namiki and Osawa (87) have described two of these model systems to evaluate the antioxidant efficacy against induced peroxidation, using biological membranes with a high content of phospholipids composed of highly unsaturated fatty acids. In one system, the suppressive effect of antioxidants on peroxidation induced by *tert*-butyl peroxide on ghost membranes of rat erythrocyte is measured as a 2-thiobarbituric acid (TBA) value. Kato *et al.* (88) have used high doses of UV B light to induce lipid oxidation in a similar system containing rabbit erythrocyte membrane. The other system contains highly unsaturated fatty acids and is known to be oxidized in biological systems in the presence of reduced nicotinamide adenine dinucleotide phosphate (NADPH) and cytochrome P-450 reductase. Oxidation of unsaturated fatty acids could occur by initiation with perferryl ion formed by direct reduction of adenine diphosphate (ADP)-chelated iron with NADPH-cytochrome P-450 reductase and molecular oxygen (ADP-Fe^{2+}/NADPH system) or by the reduction of oxygen to superoxide. Alternatively, initiation of hydroperoxide formation may be promoted by EDTA-chelated Fe^{2+} ion, which can directly form EDTA-Fe^{3+} by NADPH-cytochrome P-450 reductase or indirectly by superoxide (ADP-Fe^{3+}/EDTA-Fe^{3+}/NADPH system). The extent of oxidation is measured as a TBA value (66). Adrimyacin-induced lipid oxidation in the same rat liver microsome model can also be used (89,90).

Antioxidative Compounds Identified from Specific Oilseeds

Canola/Rapeseed (Brassica napus, B. campestris)

Canola or low erucic acid rapeseed is widely grown around the world for its oil. The oil is used primarily for edible purposes, and the seed meal is an inexpensive protein supplement and a replacement for soybean meal in animal feeds.

Canola seeds contain considerable amounts of phenolic compounds compared with other oilseeds. The total content of phenolic acids of defatted rapeseed flour is about 623–1281 mg/100 g (91–93). Sinapic acid is the predominant phenolic acid found in canola and occurs in the free, esterified, and glycosidic as well as insoluble-bound forms. Minor phenolic acids are *p*-hydroxybenzoic, vanillic, gensitic, protocatechuic, syringic, *p*-coumaric ferulic and caffeic acids (91,94). Canola hulls contain a considerable amount of condensed tannins whereas cotyledons possess few tannins (95,96). The acetone extractable condensed tannins of rapeseed hulls were composed of leucocyanidin units (97).

Antioxidant activity of free phenolic acids, sinapic acid, and sinapine obtained from ethanolic extract of rapeseed (variety, Jantar) has been observed by Nowak *et al.* (98) in a β-carotene-linoleate model system. The free phenolic acid fraction showed the highest antioxidant activity with sinapic acid and sinapine having the least activity.

Ethanolic extract of canola seeds exhibited antioxidant activity in a meat model system (99) and canola oil (100,101); the effect in canola oil was stronger than that of BHA and BHT (100). Fractionation of the dried crude canola extract by Sephadex LH-20 column chromatography according to phenolic and sugar contents and UV absorbance gave seven fractions. Fraction IV, which showed the highest antioxidative potency in a β-carotene-linoleate model system, contained moderate amounts of phenolics (101). Further screening of antioxidative activity in this fraction and identification revealed that the compound with the strongest antioxidant activity was 1-*O*-β-D-glucopyranosyl sinapate (102) (Fig. 7.9).

The tocopherol content of canola oil is appreciably less than that of soybean oil, but its α-tocopherol content exceeds that of corn and sunflower oils (103). Yuki and Ishikawa (104) reported that 64% of total tocopherols were retained after heating of the oil at temperatures simulating deep fat frying. Canola oil is also rich in chlorophyll and pheophytin (5–25 ppm); however, these compounds are removed during the bleaching process (105).

The phytic acid content of canola/rapeseed is higher than most other oilseeds. The whole seed is reported to contain 2–4% phytic acid, 2–5% in defatted meal, 5–7% in protein concentrates, and <1–9.8 in protein isolates, depending on the method of protein isolation (106).

Mustard (Brassica juncea)

Mustard seed is used as a condiment and also for edible oil extraction. Low-pungency mustard flour, obtained by inactivating the enzyme myrosinase, is used as a filler ingredient in some processed meat products (107).

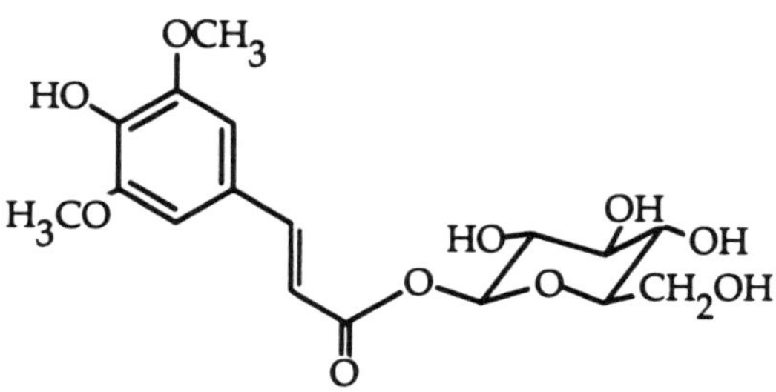

Fig. 7.9. Chemical structure of antioxidative flavonoid glycoside identified in canola seeds.

Yamaguchi *et al.* (108) reported that mustard powder (whole seed) has strong antioxidant activity and shows synergism with seed tocopherols. Inactivation of myrosinase by heat treatment or defatting improved the antioxidative activity of mustard flour. Oil and protein isolated from mustard seeds possessed weaker antioxidant activity than whole-eed flours.

The low-pungency mustard flour (107) and its aqueous methanolic extracts exhibited good antioxidant properties in a meat model system (109,110). Ethanolic extracts of low-pungency mustard flour were separated by Sephadex LH-20 column chromatography and their antioxidant activity was determined using a β-carotene-linoleate model system. Three different fractions were separated based on the UV absorbance and contents of sugars and total phenolics. The highest antioxidant activity was observed for fraction I which also contained the highest amount of phenolic compounds. Further studies on fraction I revealed that the strongest antioxidative component was a trihydroxy phenolic compound whose detailed structure has not yet been elucidated (111).

Mustard seeds contain considerable amounts of phenolic acids similar to levels in rapeseed and canola. The most abundant phenolic acids in mustard were trans-sinapic and *p*-hydroxybenzoic; *cis*-sinapic and *trans*-ferulic acids were also present in considerable quantities (94). Mustard seed also contained α-, γ-, and δ-tocopherols (112).

Flaxseed (Linum usitatissimum L.)

Flaxseed oil has been used mainly for industrial purposes. However, it has also been used for edible and medicinal purposes in certain cultures around the world. Traditional flaxseed oil contains 55–70% α-linolenic and 12–18% linoleic acids and is highly prone to oxidation (113).

Aqueous ethanolic (95%) extracts of flaxseed meal exhibited moderate antioxidant properties as evaluated in a β-carotene-linoleate model system. Chromatographic separation of ethanolic extract of flaxseed gave four fractions in which the highest antioxidant activity was observed in fraction I which contained moderate amounts of phenolic compounds. Fractions I, II, and III had a maximum UV absorbance at 290 nm, and fraction IV exhibited a band at 284 nm. All of these fractions gave a shoulder absorbance at 302–308 nm, which may indicate that they are not phenolic acids alone. Further separation of fraction I on TLC plates indicated that flaxseed lignans might be involved (101,114,115). Flaxseed lignan has been identified as seicoisolariciresinol diglucoside (116) (Fig. 7.10), which can generate the mammalian lignans enterodiol and enterolactone once hydrolyzed by intestinal microfloral enzymes (117). Various biological activities including the anticarcinogenic ability of flaxseed lignans have been reported (118). Antioxidative activity of secoisolariciresinol is expected to be strong because its chemical structure is very similar to nordihydroguaiaretic acid (NDGA) (Fig. 7.10) which is known to be a strong antioxidant.

The phenolic acid content of flaxseed was considerably lower than that of other oilseeds (92, 94, 119). *Trans*-ferulic was the predominant phenolic acid in

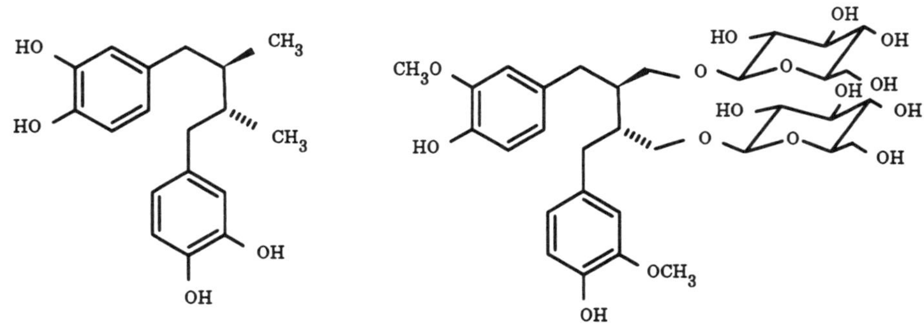

Nordihydroguaiaretic acid (NDGA) **Secoisolariciresinol diglucoside**

Fig. 7.10. Lignans of flaxseed.

flaxseed and *trans*-sinapic, *trans*-*p*-coumaric, *trans*-caffeic, and *p*-hydroxybenzoic acid were found in smaller amounts (93). The content of condensed tannins in flaxseed was comparatively low compared with that of canola seeds (119). Major sterols of flaxseed oil have been identified as β-sitosterol, campesterol and Δ^5-avenasterol. Stigmasterol, Δ^7-stigmasterol, and brassicasterol were present in minor quantities (120). Major tocopherols of flaxseed were β- and γ-tocopherols, whereas δ-tocopherol was present in minute amounts and α-tocopherol was not detected (120). The phytic acid content of defatted flaxseed meal was 2.4–2.7% (119,121).

Chia (Salvia hispanica L.)

Seeds of the chia plant have long been used as a food component by American Indians and Mexicans. The seed contains 25–35% extractable oil which is rich in polyunsaturated fatty acids. Methanolic and aqueous extracts of chia seeds possessed antioxidant activities as determined against β-carotene bleaching. The major antioxidant activity in the nonhydrolyzed extract was due to flavonol glycosides, chlorogenic, and caffeic acids. The hydrolyzed extracts contained caffeic acid and flavonol aglycones, namely, kempferol, quercetin, and myricetin (82).

Cottonseed (Gossipium hirsutum L.)

Cottonseed is a co-product of the cotton fiber industry and is a good source of oil. Virtually the entire production of cottonseed oil is used for the manufacture of salad/cooking oil, shortening or margarine. Gossypol-free cottonseed flour is used to prepare protein ingredients for human consumption (103).

Methanolic extracts of glandless cottonseed meal and protein isolates have shown antioxidative activity against autoxidation of metmyoglobin, Fe^{2+}-EDTA model system, and beef homogenate (79). Methanolic extracts of cottonseed were found to possess antioxidant activity in a β-carotene-linoleate model system (122).

Separation of antioxidative compounds was accomplished by thin-layer, paper and gas–liquid chromatography, and spectral analyses revealed that quercetin (Fig. 7.1B) was the major flavonoid present. The glycosyl substitution of the flavonoids is found as glucose and rhamnose; therefore, rutin is the major quercetin glycoside present in cottonseed.

Gossypol, a major phenolic compound present in cottonseed meal, has been known to possess male antifertility activity when administered orally; however, no studies have been reported about its antioxidative ability. Cottonseed does not contain high amounts of phenolic acids compared with other oilseeds. Predominant phenolic acids of cottonseed (glanded and glandless) include *trans*-ferulic, trans-*p*-coumaric, *p*-hydroxybenzoic, and *trans*-caffeic acids in decreasing order of abundance (94).

Olive (Olea europaea L.)

Olive oil is very popular among inhabitants of Mediterranean countries and is obtained by mechanical pressing of the mesocarps of the olive fruit. Olive oil is used mainly as a salad oil. Unrefined oil (acidity 1–3%) is referred to as virgin olive oil and contains a considerable amount of phenolic compounds expressed from the fruit. Because of its high oleic acid (53–86%) content and antioxidative compounds, olive oil has exceptional stability even during deep frying (103,123).

According to Nergiz and Unal (124), phenolic compounds which are present in virgin olive oil are almost completely destroyed during the refining process. These phenolic compounds could be extracted from the oil into aqueous methanol, but their chemical structure has not yet been completely identified. However, several phenolic acids, namely, *p*-coumaric, syringic, vanillic, ferulic, caffeic, *p*-hydroxybenzoic, and protocatechuic acids have been identified in virgin olive oil according to their abundance (124). Among the phenolic compounds present, other than phenolic acids, are 4-hydroxyphenylethanol (tyrosol), 3,4-dihydroxyphenylethanol (hydroxytyrosol), and a number of unidentified esters and glycosides (12,125,126). Using these individual *o*-diphenol compounds (e.g., hydroxytyrosol and caffeic acid) at various levels (15–200 ppm), pronounced stabilizing effects were demonstrated when refined olive oil as used (127–129). Another study has shown that the antioxidant activity of these *o*-diphenolic compounds in olive oil is much greater than that of α-tocopherol (130).

Peanut (Arachis hypogaea)

The kernel of the peanut is used for oil extraction and as an ingredient in different food products such as peanut butter, salted peanut, candies, and desserts. Peanut oil is used extensively as a salad oil.

Methanolic extracts of peanut protein isolate and concentrate have shown antioxidative activity in a metmyoglobin-Fe^{++}-EDTA model system (79). The work by Pratt and Miller (131) reported that hot methanolic extracts of peanut kernels (Spanish variety) contained antioxidative activity as determined by their resistance to β-carotene bleaching. The active component was identified as dihydroquercetin (taxifolin) (Fig. 7.1D). Peanut flour also contained about 175 mg/100 g of total phenolic acids which consisted of *trans-p*-coumaric, syringic, *trans*-ferulic, *trans*-caffeic, and *p*-hydroxybenzoic acid in decreasing order of abundance (94). Recently, hulls of peanuts were investigated for their antioxidative compounds (132–135).

Methanolic extracts of peanut hulls (Spanish variety, cultivar Tainan) exhibited very strong antioxidative activity, equal to that of BHA as determined by peroxide value and inhibition of β-carotene bleaching. Further separation and structural determination revealed that luteolin (Fig. 7.1A) was the active antioxidative flavonoid present in peanut hulls (129). The methanolic extract of peanut hulls demonstrated very good thermal stability by maintaining 85% of its antioxidant activity when heated to 185°C for 2 h (134) and acted as a free radical and active-oxygen radical scavenger (135). The content of luteolin and total phenols in peanut hulls increased with the maturity of the seeds and hulls (133). According to Daigle *et al.* (136), immature peanut hulls/shells contained predominantly eriodictyol (Fig. 7.1C), whereas mature hulls/shells were rich in luteolin. Tannins of peanut were concentrated in the skin and hulls (137) and were composed of 17% procyanidin by weight, of which 50% were low molecular weight, ethyl acetate-soluble oligomers of catechin and epicatechin (138).

Peanut oil contains α-, β-, γ-, and α-tocopherol (139–142) and minute quantities of α-, β-, and γ-tocotrienols (139). Antioxidant activity of native gums (phospho- and glycolipids) has been identified, and gums are considered as being responsible for the good oxidative stability of raw peanut oil even at a relative humidity of 91% (143). Defatted peanut meal contained 1.5–1.7% phytic acid whereas peanut protein isolates contained about 1% phytic acid (144).

Sesame (*Sesamum indicum*)

Sesame seed and oil are traditional food and medicinal ingredients in several cultures around the world, especially in the Orient. The high resistance of sesame oil to oxidation has long been known. Sesame seed is a popular snack and confectionery ingredient, probably due to its sweet taste.

Antioxidative compounds of sesame seeds have been identified as lignophenols and carboxyphenols (66,145–150) (Fig. 7.11). Sesame seed contains bis-epoxylignans sesamin (0.2–0.5%) and sesamolin (0.2–0.3%). Acetone extract of sesame seed contained sesamolinol and sesaminol (151,152). After treating defatted sesame seed flour with β-glucosidase, it was revealed that the ligno- and carboxyphenols exist as their glucosides which release their aglycones (147). Recently, two new pinoresinol diglucosides (KP1 and KP2) (Fig. 7.12) (153) and a triglucoside (KP3) (Fig. 7.12) (149) that exhibited strong antioxidant activity in a rabbit erythrocyte membrane ghost system have been isolated from sesame seed and identified (154). The acetone extract of ground sesame seed which possessed strong antioxidant activity, as determined by the thiocyanate method, contained

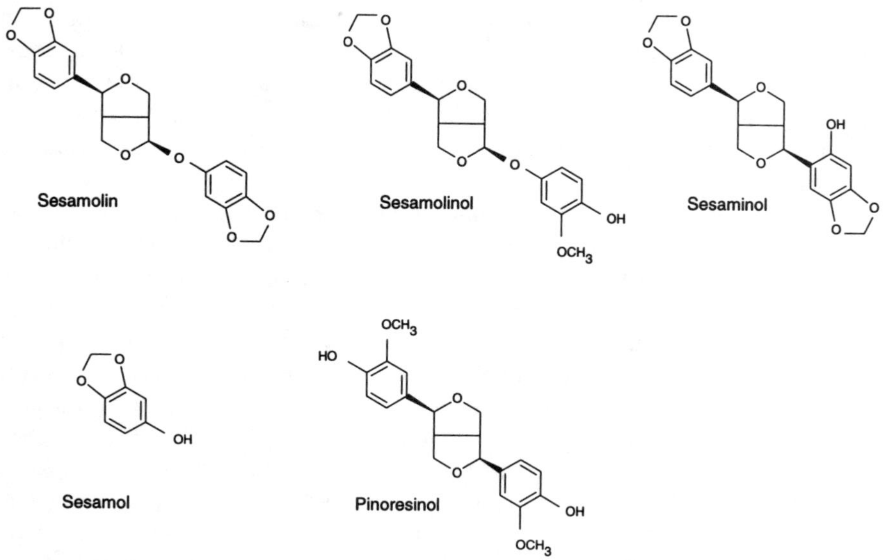

Fig. 7.11. Antioxidative lignans found in sesame seed and oil.

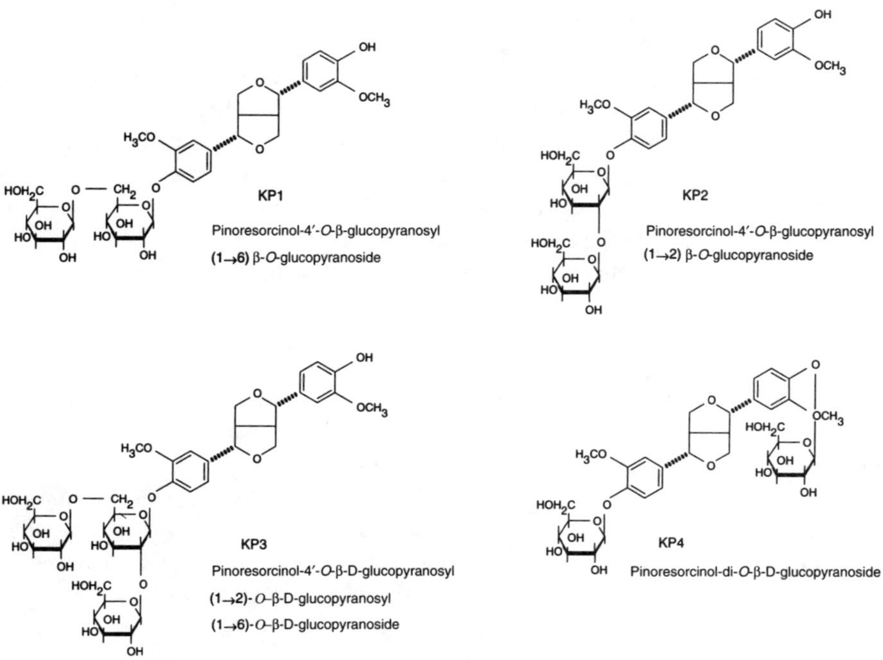

Fig. 7.12. Pinoresinol glucosides of sesame seed.

sesaminol, sesamolinol, sesaminol, and *trans*-ferulic acid (147,149). According to Dabrowski and Sosulski (94), 80% ethanolic extract of sesame seed yielded trans-caffeic, *trans-p*-coumaric, and *trans*-ferulic acids in decreasing order of abundance. However, according to Kozlowska *et al.* (92), vanillic, syringic, sinapic, and *o*-coumaric acids were also present in sesame seed and could be extracted into 80% methanol.

Antioxidants of sesame seed oil have been investigated separately due the high oxidative stability of the oil and foods fried in it. Sesame oil is obtained from both roasted and unroasted seeds. Oil from unroasted sesame seed is obtained by expeller pressing and refined by alkaline treatment, bleaching with acid clay, and deodorizing. However, oil from roasted seed is only filtered only to remove contaminants (66). Sesamolinol (151) and sesaminol (155) were found in sesame seed and oil (Fig. 7.11). Sesaminol is found in high quantities (0.5–1.0 mg/g) in purified unroasted oil but is present in sesame seed only in minor quantities (156). This difference was proved to be due to a chemical change occurring during the refining process. At the bleaching step, a drastic change in the amounts of sesamin, episesamin, sesamolin, sesamol, and sesaminol occurs (155). Fukuda *et al.* (154–156) have suggested that sesaminol was formed from sesamolin under anhydrous conditions in the presence of an acid (acid clay used for bleaching) catalyst at high temperatures. Sesamolin is first decomposed to sesamol to form an oxonium ion, and then the carbon-carbon bond is formed; thus the hypothesis is that sesaminol is formed from sesamolin by intermolecular group transformation (157). Figure 7.13 provides suggested changes that occur in sesamolin during the refining of sesame oil.

Sesamol was completely destroyed when heated at 180°C for 4 h, but sesamol remained partially (40.5%) intact after heating for 6 h at the same temperature (158). The degree of browning and oxidative stability of roasted seed oil was increased at higher roasting temperatures. However, the amount of sesamol which was produced upon degradation of sesamolin during roasting of seed did not increase considerably with roasting temperature (159).

Fresh oils obtained from coated and dehulled sesame seeds of Egyptian (Giza 24) and Sudanese (Gabaly Abiad) varieties contained sesamin, 649.1, 610.0 and 579.7 mg/100 g oil and sesamolin 183.3, 168.1, and 349.2 mg/100 g oil, respectively. γ-Tocopherol was the only tocopherol detected in the oils. Roasting, (200°C, 20 min), steaming (100°C, 20 min), roasting (200°C, 15 min) combined with steaming (7 min), and microwaving (2450 MHz, 15 min) of seeds reduced the sesamin content drastically, especially in the oil from dehulled seeds. Storage of these oils under Schall oven test conditions (65°C, 35 d) showed a decrease in both sesamin and sesamolin contents. The decrease in sesamolin content was greater during the storage period for all oils probably due to the degradation of sesamolin to sesamol during the thermal treatment. Roasting combined with steaming treatment gave a lesser reduction in sesamin, sesamolin, and γ-tocopherol contents (160).

Sesamolin is the characteristic lignan of sesame seed and serves as the precursor to strong antioxidants. Screening of sesame seed varieties for their content of

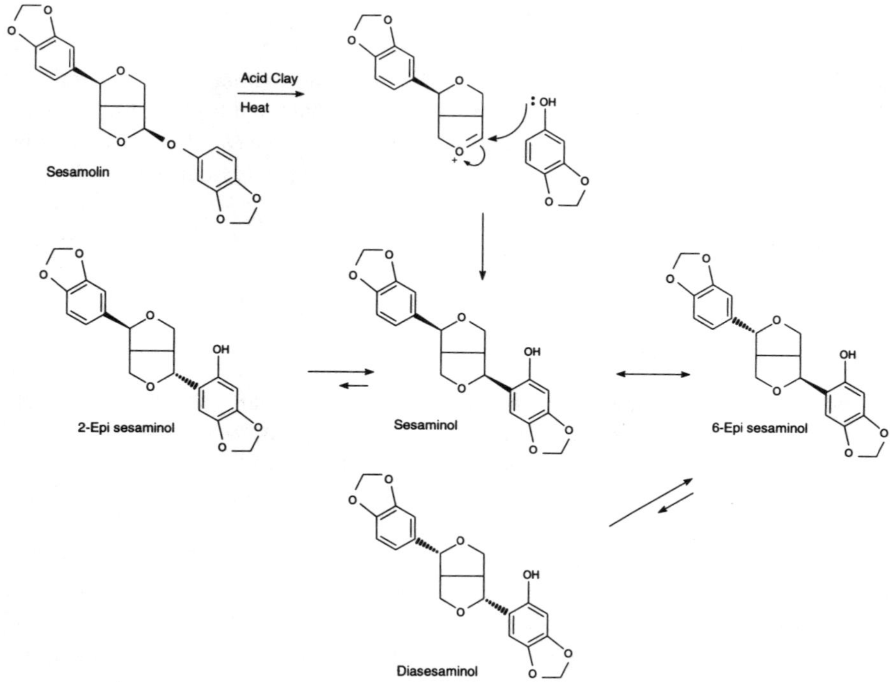

Fig. 7.13. Formation of sesaminol from sesamolin during oil refining process.

sesamolin revealed, however, that while sesame seeds contained more sesamolin than black seed varieties, the ratio of sesamolin to sesamin was higher in black seeds than in white seeds (159).

The high stability of oil from roasted sesame seeds has not been attributed to any one compound. γ-Tocopherol, minor amounts of sesamol, and Maillard reaction products generated during roasting, may be responsible for the excellent oxidative stability of this oil (161). It has also been found that decomposition of tocopherol at 185°C for 6 h is less when sesaminol is present, thus suggesting a synergism of sesaminol with γ-tocopherol. It has been suggested that sesaminol and sesamol are free radical scavengers (158). Pinoresinol glucosides (KP1, KP2 and KP3) (Fig. 7.12) are very strong antioxidants in the ethanol-soluble (80%, vol/vol) components of sesame seed. All three of these glucosides are considered as antioxidant precursors because they can be hydrolyzed by the β-glucosidases of intestinal bacteria and release pinoresinol, which is lipid-soluble and acts as a potent antioxidant for the protection of membrane lipids (150).

The callus cells of sesame obtained by tissue culture produced a large biomass of cells in a short time and also exhibited potent antioxidant activity as assessed by rabbit erythrocyte ghost membrane (152). The aqueous methanolic (80%) extracts of the suspension cell cultures were used to isolate the strongest antioxidative compounds. The antioxidative compound in the 40% methanol-eluted fraction was identified as acteoside (3,4-dihydroxy-β-phenethyl-*O*-α-rhamnopyranosyl (1-3)-4-*O*-caffeoyl-β-glucopyranoside) (Fig. 7.14A) and had antioxidant activity similar to that of BHA. The fraction eluted by 60% methanol contained SI-1 (3,4-dihydroxy-β-phenyl-*O*-ethylcarboxyl-*O*-α-L-rhamnopyranosyl (1-3)-4-*O*-caffeoyl-β-glucopyranoside) (Fig. 7.14B) which was a stronger antioxidant than acteoside. The antioxidative activity of these polyphenol glycosides is suggested to be due to the presence of two caffeoyl moieties combined with glucoside (162). Sesame seed is also reported to contain a high level of phytic acid (163).

Soybean (Glycene max L.)

Soybean is cultivated mainly for its seeds, used commercially as human food and livestock feed and for the extraction of oil. The highest domestic consumption of soybean is in Asia where it has been a basic food item for centuries. Soybean is used for production of a variety of protein food products which are used for different nutritional and functional purposes.

The ability of full-fat soybean flour to extend the storage life of lard (164), ghee (165), frozen pastry (166), dehydrated pork-corn scrapple (167), frozen raw or precooked ground pork (168), and corn-soy extruded blends (169) has been reported. Aqueous extracts of fresh and dried soybeans, soy protein concentrates and defatted soy flour had appreciable antioxidant activity (78).

Total phenolic acid content of soy flour varied from 23.4 to 73.6 mg/100 g and included chlorogenic, isochlorogenic, caffeic, ferulic, *p*-coumaric, syringic, vanillic, *p*-hydroxybenzoic, salicylic, and sinapic acids (94,170). Chlorogenic and isochlorogenic acids were present in the ratio of 1:10, and such hydroxycinnamic acid derivatives have been shown to be partly responsible for the antioxidant activity of lipid-aqueous systems (4).

Contrary to most other oilseeds, soybean contains isoflavones (Fig. 7.15). Isoflavones occur as glucosides of daidzein (7,4′-dihydroxyisoflavone), genistein (5,7,4′-trihydroxyisoflavone), and glycitein (7,4′-dihydroxy, 6-methylisoflavone) (171–173). The respective glucosides are identified as daidzin, genistin, and glycitin. According to Naim *et al.* (174), 99% of the isoflavones of soybean seeds and defatted flours are present as 7-*O*-glycosides, 64% genistein, 23% daidzein, and 13% glycitein 7-*O*-monoglucosides. Because sugars confer water solubility to the molecule, these glycosidic forms of isoflavones may be the major antioxidative compounds of water extracts of soybean seed and flour (2).

In fermented soybean, tempeh (175), and soy protein hydrolysates (176), these three isoflavones occur as their aglycones. The comparatively high oxidative stability of tempeh compared with unfermented soybean and the stability of oil-containing foods that include soy protein hydrolysates are attributed mainly to the activity of aglycone isoflavones. The glucosides are split into aglycones and sugars *via* the action of β-glucosidase of *Rhizopus oligosphorus* during fermentation or

(a)

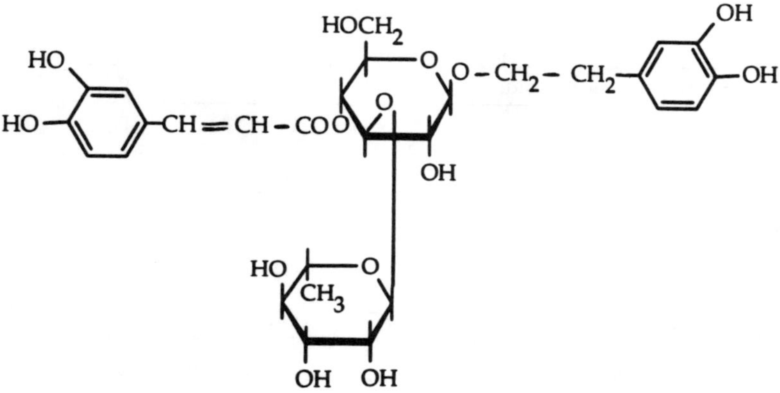

3,4-dihydroxy-β-phenethyl-*O*-α-L-rhamnopyronosyl-(1-3)-4-*O*-caffeoyl-β-glucopyranoside

(b)

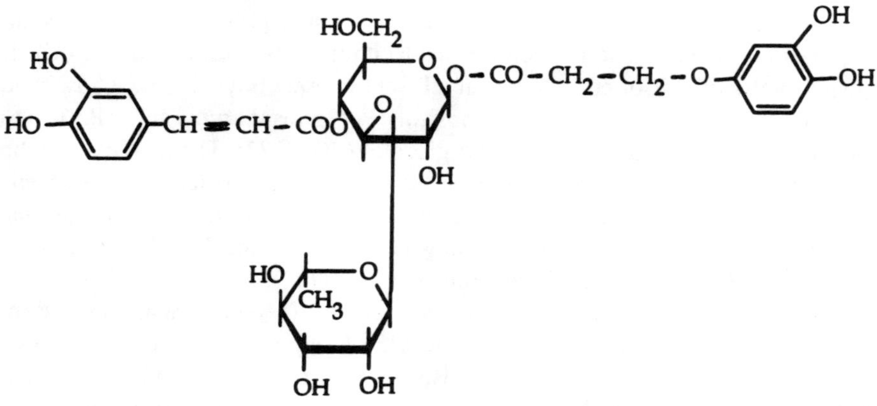

3,4-dihydroxy-β-phenyl-*O*-ethylcarboxyl-*O*-α-L-rhamnopyronosyl-(1-3)-4-*O*-caffeoyl-β-glucopyranoside

Fig. 7.14. Chemical structures of antioxidative phenol glycosides isolated from callus cultures of sesame.

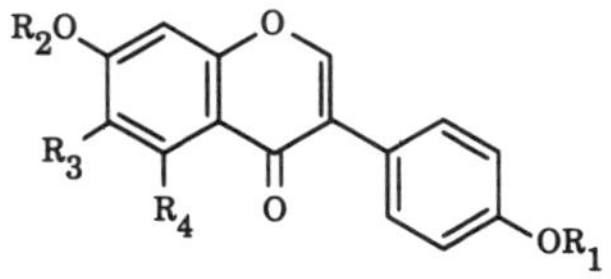

Isoflavone/isoflavone glycoside	R_1	R_2	R_3	R_4
Daidzin	H	Glu	H	H
Daidzein	H	H	H	H
Genistin	H	Glu	H	OH
Genistein	H	H	H	OH
Glycitin-7-*O*-glucoside	H	Glu	OCH_3	H

Fig. 7.15. Chemical structures of soybean isoflavones and their glucosides.

acid-heat treatments occurring in the preparation of protein hydrolysates (177). This may be the reason for the increased content of the lipophilic aglycones, daidzein and genistein, which are the main antioxidative components of tempeh and miso (178) (Fig. 7.15). In addition, melanoidins (179) and peptides (180) are also presumed to exhibit antioxidant activity in miso. However, the content of free isoflavones of natto (fermented steamed soybean with *Bacillus natto*) is slightly increased due to fermentation, but the activity of the antioxidants of the water-soluble fraction was increased significantly (181).

Soybean contains considerable amounts of phospholipids and is a source material for the production of commercial lecithin (phosphotidyl choline; PC). The major phospholipids of crude soybean oil were phosphotidyl choline, phosphatidyl ethanolamine (PE), phosphatidyl inositol (PI), phosphatidic acid (PA), phosphatidyl serine (PS), and phosphatidyl glycerol (PG) (182). The total phospholipid content of soybean was reported to be 30 ppm (183). Purified lecithin obtained from soybean was ineffective as an antioxidant and may in fact be prooxygenic (184). Major tocopherols of soybean oil were α, δ, and γ-tocol; however, during oil processing, 32% of the total tocopherols were lost (183).

It has been shown that hydrolyzed soy proteins (peptide and amino acid mixtures) can act as primary antioxidants (30,185). Using a freeze-dried model system with tocopherol-free corn oil, it was shown that the fraction with a molecular weight of 700–1500 and >1500 Da of hydrolyzed soy protein had inferior antioxidant activity compared with the fraction with a molecular weight <700 Da (185). It is possible that isoflavones and other compounds with antioxidant activity may also contribute to the antioxidant activity of soy protein hydrolysates in the fraction with a molecular weight of <700 Da. It was also shown that peptide-amino acid mixtures and amino acids, *per se*, act synergistically with α-tocopherol (29).

Warner and Mounts (186) have reported the presence of β-sitosterol, campesterol, and stigmasterol in soybean oil. Phytic acid content of raw soybean seed was 1.4%, whereas fermented product tempeh contained 0.95% phytic acid (187).

Oil Palm (Elaeis guineensis Jacq.)

Oil palm is one of the important sources of edible oils in tropical countries and is the second most widely consumed edible oil in the world after soybean (103). Palm oil contains equal proportions of saturated and unsaturated fatty acids, whereas palmitic and oleic acids comprise 75–95% of total fatty acids.

Palm oil contains large amounts of tocopherols and tocotrienols, up to 800 ppm in total (188). The tocotrienol-rich fraction obtained from palm oil was shown to reduce lipid oxidation activities in liver tissues of palm oil-supplemented rats (189). The α- and γ-tocopherols predominate in palm oil and are present at 300 and 500 ppm, respectively (190), but their content may be reduced during processing (191).

The deep red color of palm oil is due to the presence of carotenoids, and their content may reach up to 2000 ppm (192). The carotenoids of palm oil include mainly α- and β-carotenes with lesser amounts of γ-carotene, lycopene, and xanthophylls (193,194). β-Carotene obtained from palm oil was able to prevent accumulation of lipid peroxidation products in induced oxidation of liver homogenates (195).

The sterol content of palm oil is relatively low; the predominant sterols are β-sitosterol (74%), stigmasterol (8%), and campesterol (14%), whereas cholesterol comprises about 1% of total sterols (196). The total sterol content of palm oil is reduced during refining (193).

Corn (Zea mays L.)

Corn is cultivated for both food and feed purposes. Corn oil is produced as a by-product of commercial corn processing. The germ, which can be separated and used for extraction, contains up to 37% oil, by weight (103).

Ohata *et al.* (197) reported the antioxidative activity of corn bran hemicellulose and found that sugar esters of ferulic acid were the strongest antioxidative compound present. Among the phenolic acids found in corn flour and oil, ferulic acid was most abundant (198,199).

Total tocol content of corn oil ranged from 0.03 to 0.33%, with γ-tocopherol predominating (200,201). Phospholipids accounted for up to 6% of total lipids of corn oil and were composed of PC, PI and PE (202,203). Carotenoids of corn were primarily zeaxanthin and lutein, which are found abundantly in the endosperm (204). Among the sterols found in corn oil, β-sitosterol, campesterol, and stigmasterol predominated (186).

Rice (Oryza sativa L.)

Rice is the second largest cereal grain produced in the world. Rice bran, which is a co-product in the rice milling process, contains 17–23% oil which can be extracted and used for edible purposes (103).

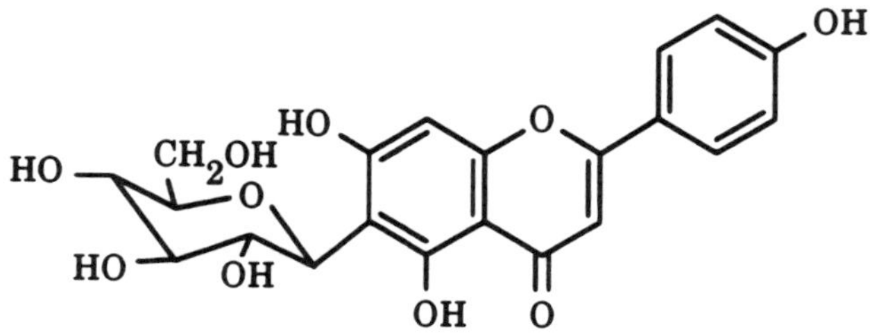

Fig. 7.16. Major antioxidative compound isolated from rice hulls.

The methanolic extracts of rice hulls of long-life (Katakutara) and short-life (Kusabue) varieties exhibited superior antioxidant activities compared with α-tocopherol. The strong antioxidative compound found in the long-life varieties has been characterized as isovitexin (Fig. 7.16), a C-glycosyl flavonoid (205).

Crude rice bran oil contains a mixture of ferulic acid esters of triterpenoid alcohol which are referred to as γ-oryzanols and exhibit antioxidant activity (206). Rice flour contains phenolic acids in which trans-ferulic acid was predominant (198). γ-Tocopherol, γ-tocotrienol, and α-tocopherol are major tocols of rice grain; however, their contents were reduced during the refining process (207). The major phospholipids of rice bran oil are phosphatidyl choline, phosphotidyl ethanolamine, phosphatidyl inositol, and phosphatidic acid. Among the sterols of rice bran oil, β-sitosterol, campesterol, and stigmasterol were the major components (208).

Conclusions

Antioxidative compounds of oilseeds can be of great value as natural antioxidants. The safety of these compounds has been proven by prolonged and continuous use. Antioxidants of oilseeds can be considered in two ways. They can be used to prevent oxidation of foods containing unsaturated lipids, thus replacing synthetic antioxidants. Similarly, these compounds, once incorporated into living cells, enhance the antioxidative status of the body, thus improving its defense capability against oxidative damage.

References

1. Larson, R.A. (1988) *Phytochem. 27*, 969.
2. Pratt, D.E. (1972) *J. Food Sci. 37*, 322.
3. Pratt, D.E., and Watts, B.M. (1964) *J. Food Sci. 29*, 27.
4. Pratt, D.E. (1965) *J. Food Sci. 30*, 737.
5. Pratt, D.E., and Hudson, B.J.F. (1990) in *Food Antioxidants* (Hudson, B.J.F., ed.), Elsevier Applied Science, London, pp. 171–192.
6. Hudson, B.J.F., and Lewis, J.I. (1983) *Food Chem. 10*, 47.
7. Dziedzic, S.Z., and Hudson, B.J.F. (1983) *Food Chem. 11*, 161.

8. Uri, N. (1961) in *Autoxidation and Antioxidants* (Lundbert, W.O.), Interscience Publishers, New York.
9. Dziedzic, S.Z., and Hudson, B.J.F. (1983) *Food Chem. 12*, 205.
10. Haworth, R.D. (1936) *Ann. Rep. Prog. Chem. 33*, 266.
11. McRae, W.D., and Towers, G.H.N. (1984) *Phytochem. 23*, 1207.
12. Chimi, H., Sadik, A., Le Tutor, B., and Rahmani, M. (1988) *R. Fr. Des Crops. Gras. 35*, 339.
13. Pokorny, J. (1988) in *Autoxidation of Unsaturated Lipids* (Chan, H., ed.), Academic Press, London, pp. 141–206.
14. Cuvelier, M.-E, Richard, H., and Berset, C, (1992) *Biosci. Biotech. Biochem. 56*, 324.
15. Cort, W. (1974) *Food Technol. 10*, 60.
16. Gustavson, K.H. (1956) *The Chemistry of Tanning Process*, Academic Press, New York.
17. Foo, L.Y., and Porter, L.J. (1980) *Phytochem. 19*, 1747.
18. Haslam, E. (1966) *Chemistry of Vegetable Tannins*, Academic Press, New York.
19. Roux, D.G., Ferreira, D., and Botha, J.J. (1980) *J. Agric. Food Chem. 28*, 216.
20. Haslam, E. (1979) *Phytochem. 16*, 1625.
21. Dziezak, J.D. (1986) *Food Technol. 9*, 94.
22. Ishikawa, Y., and Yuki, E. (1975) *Agric. Biol. Chem. 39*, 851.
23. Schuler, P. (1990) in *Food Antioxidants* (Hudson, B.J.F., ed.), Elsevier Applied Science, London, pp. 99–170.
24. Stern, K.A. (1936) *J. Biol. Chem. 114*, 473.
25. Dhindsa, R.S., Plumb-Dhindsa, P., and Thorpe, T.E. (1981) *J. Expt. Bot. 126*, 93.
26. Smith, A.K., and Circle, S.J. (1972) in *Soybean, Chemistry and Technology* (Smith, A.K., and Circle, S.J., eds.), AVI Pub. Co., West Port, pp. 339.
27. Marcuse, R. (1960) *Nature, 186*, 866.
28. Marcuse, R. (1962) *J. Am. Oil Chem. Soc. 39*, 97.
29. Siechowski, J. (1971) *Rev. Ital. Sost. Grasse 48*, 502.
30. Bishov, S.J., and Henick, A.S. (1975) *Food Technol. 40*, 345.
31. Tajima, K., Sakamoto, M., Okada, K., Mukai, K., Ishizu, K., Sakurai, H., and Mori, H. (1983) *Biochem. Biophys. Res. Commun. 115*, 1002.
32. Tanizawa, H., Toda, S., Sasuka, Y., Taniyama, T., Hayashi, T., and Takino, Y. (1984) *Chem. Pharm. Bull. 32*, 2011.
33. Shi, X., Dalal, N.S., and Jain, A.C. (1991) *Food Chem. Toxicol. 29*, 1.
34. Nagai, J., Tanaka, M., Hibasami, H., and Ikeda, T. (1981) *J. Biochem. (Tokyo) 89*, 1143.
35. Terce, F., Tocanne, J.F., and Laneele, G. (1982) *Eur. J. Biochem. 125*, 203.
36. Howard, J.A., and Yamada, T. (1981) *J. Am. Oil Chem. Soc. 103*, 7102.
37. Endo, Y., Usuki, R., and Kaneda, T. (1985) *J. Am. Oil Chem. Soc. 62*, 1375.
38. Sakata, K., Yamamoto, K., and Ishikawa, H. (1990) *Tetrahedron Lett. 31*, 1165.
39. Nishibori, S., and Namika, K. (1988) *Nippon Kaseigaku Kaishi, 39*, 1174.
40. Cahyana, A.H., Shuto, Y., and Kinoshita, Y. (1992) *Biosci. Biotech. Biochem. 56*, 1533.
41. Nishikimi, M. (1975) *Biosci. Biophys. Res. Commun. 63*, 463.
42. Koch, E. (1968) *Tetrahedron, 24*, 6295.
43. Niki, E., Saito, T., and Kamiya, Y. (1983) *Chem. Lett.*, 631.
44. Kellogg, E.W. III, and Fridovich, I. (1975) *J. Biol. Chem. 250*, 8812.
45. Clements, A.H., Van den Engh, R.H., Frost, D.T., and Hoogenhout, K. (1973) *J. Am. Oil Chem. Soc. 50*, 325.

46. Pokorny, Y. (1991) *Trends Food Sci. Technol. 3*, 223.
47. Cheryan, M. (1980) *CRC Crit. Rev. Food Sci. Nutr. 13*, 296.
48. Barre, R., Courtois, J.E., and Wormser, G. (1954) *Bull. Soc. Chim. Biol. 36*, 455.
49. Graf, E., Mahony, J.R., Bryant, R.G., and Eaton, J.W. (1984) *J. Biol. Chem. 259*, 3620.
50. Graf, E., Empson, K.L., and Eaton, J.W. (1987) *J. Biol. Chem. 262*, 11647.
51. Scott, J.J., and Loewus, F.A. (1986) in *Phytic Acid, Chemistry and Applications* (Graf, E., ed.), Pilatus Press, Minneapolis, pp. 23–42.
52. Empson, K.L., Labuza, T.P., and Graf, E. (1991) *J. Food Sci. 56*, 560.
53. Belitz, H.D., and Grosch, W. (1987) *Food Chemistry*, Springer Verlag, Berlin, p. 144.
54. Brandt, P., Hollstein, E., and Franzke, C. (1973) *Lebensmittel Ind. 20*, 31.
55. Gordon, M.H. (1990) in *Food Antioxidants* (Hudson, B.J.F., ed.), Elsevier Applied Science, London, pp. 1–18.
56. Hudson, B.J.F., and Ghavami, M. (1984) *Lebensmi.-Wiss. u. Technol. 17*, 191.
57. Tai, P.T., Pokorny, J., and Janicek, G. (1974) *Z. Lebensm. Unters. Forsch. 156*, 257.
58. Pokorny, J., Poskocilova, H., and Davidek, J. (1981) *Nahrung 25*, K29.
59. Sims, R.J., Fioriti, J.A., and Kanuk, M.J. (1972) *J. Am. Oil Chem. Soc. 49*, 298.
60. Gordon, M.H., and Magos, P. (1983) *Food Chem. 10*, 141.
61. Yan, P.S., and White, P.J. (1990) *J. Agric. Food Chem. 38*, 1904.
62. Boskou, D., and Morton, I.D. (1976) *J. Sci. Food Agric. 27*, 928.
63. Tian, L.L., and White, P.J. (1994) *J. Am. Oil Chem. Soc. 71*, 1084.
64. Kirigaya, N., Kato, M., and Fujimaki, M. (1968) *Agric. Biol. Chem. 32*, 287.
65. Yamaguchi, N., Koyama, Y., and Fujimaki, M. (1981) *Prog. Food Nutr. Sci. 5*, 429.
66. Namiki, M. (1990) *CRC Crit. Rev. Food Sci. Nutr. 29*, 273.
67. Gomyo, T., and Horikosshi, M. (1976) *Agric. Biol. Chem. 40*, 33.
68. Kajimoto, G., and Yoshida, H. (1975) *Yukagaku 24*, 297.
69. Eichner, K. (1981) *Prog. Food Nutr. Sci. 5*, 441.
70. Lundberg, W.O. (1961) *Autoxidation and Antioxidants*, Vol. 1, Interscience Publishing Co., New York.
71. Kawashima, K., Itoh, H., and Chibata, I. (1977) *J. Agric. Food Chem. 25*, 202.
72. Namiki, M., Shigeta, A., and Hayashi, T. (1982) *Agric. Biol. Chem. 46*, 1199.
73. Kahl, R., and Hidelberg, A.G. (1986) *Food Chem. Toxicol. 24*, 1007.
74. Kochhar, S.P., and Rossell, J.D. (1990) in *Food Antioxidants* (Hudson, B.J.F., ed.), Elsevier Applied Science, London, pp. 19–64.
75. Shahidi, F., and Wanasundara, P.K.J.P.D. (1992) *CRC Crit. Rev. Food Sci. Nutr. 32*, 67.
76. Mitsuda, H., Yasumoto, K., and Iwami, K. (1966) *Eiyo to Shokuryo 19*, 210.
77. Tappel, A.L. (1980) in *Free Radicals in Biology* (Pryor, W.A., ed.), Vol. 4, Academic Press, Orlando, p. 1.
78. Rhee, K.S., Ziprin, Y.A., and Rhee, K.C. (1979) *J. Food Sci. 44*, 1132.
79. Rhee, K.S., Ziprin, Y.A., and Rhee, K.C. (1981) *J. Food Sci. 46*, 75.
80. Marco, G.J. (1968) *J. Am. Oil Chem. Soc. 45*, 594.
81. Miller, E.E. (1971) *J. Am. Oil Chem. Soc. 48*, 91.
82. Taga, M.S., Miller, E.E., and Pratt, D.E. (1984) *J. Am. Oil. Chem. Soc. 61*, 928.
83. Castro-Martinez, R., Pratt, D.E., and Miller, E.E. (1986) in *Proceedings of World Conference on Emerging Technologies in Fats and Oil Industry* (Baldwin, A.R., ed.), American Oil Chemists' Society, Champaign, pp. 392–400.

84. Osawa, T., and Namiki, M. (1981) *Agric. Biol. Chem. 45*, 735.
85. Osawa, T., and Namiki, M. (1981) *J. Agric. Food Chem. 33*, 775.
86. Chang, N.H., Liu, H.X., and Cheng, A.C. (1983) *J. Food Sci. 48*, 658.
87. Namiki, M., and Osawa, T. (1986) in *Antimutagenesis and Anticarcinogenesis Mechanism* (Shankel, D.M., Hartman, P.E., Kada, T., and Hollaender, A., eds.), Plenum Press, pp. 131–155.
88. Kato, T., Murakami, M., Tanimura, H., Mimura, A., and Takahara, Y. (1992) *Proc. Ann. Mtg. Soc. Fermentat. Technol.* (Japan), p. 213.
89. Sugioko, K., and Nakano, M. (1982) *Biochem. Biophys. Acta 713*, 333.
90. Land, E.J., Mukherjee, T., Swallow, A.J., and Bruce, J.M. (1983) *Arch. Biochem. Biophys. 225*, 116.
91. Krygier, K., Sosulski, F.W., and Hogge, L. (1982) *J. Agric. Food Chem. 30*, 334.
92. Kozlowzka, H., Rotkiewicz, D.A., Zadernowski, R.L., and Sosulski, F.W. (1983) *J. Am. Oil Chem. Soc. 60*, 1119.
93. Naczk, M., and Shahidi, F. (1989) *Food Chem. 31*, 159.
94. Dabrowski, K.J., and Sosulski, F.W. (1984) *J. Agric. Food Chem. 32*, 128.
95. Blair, R., and Reichard, R.D. (1984) *J. Sci. Food Agric. 35*, 29.
96. Naczk, M., Nichols, T., Pink, D., and Sosulski, F.W. (1994) *J. Agric. Food Chem. 42*, 2196.
97. Leung, J., Fenton, T.W., Meuller, M.M., and Clandinin, D.R. (1979) *J. Food Sci. 44*, 1313.
98. Nowak, H., Kujawa, K., Zadernowski, R., Roczniak, B., and Kozlowska, H. (1992) *Fat Sci. Technol. 94*, 149.
99. Shahidi, F., and Saleemi, Z. (1993) in *Proceedings of Thirty-Eighth International Congress of Meat Science and Technology*, Calgary, Alberta, Canada.
100. Wanasundara, U.N., and Shahidi, F. (1995) *J. Am. Oil Chem. Soc. 71*, 817.
101. Shahidi, F., Wanasundara, U.N., and Amarowicz, R. (1995) in *Food Flavors, Generation, Analysis and Process Influence* (Charalambous, G., ed.), Elsevier Applied Science, London, pp. 1087–1099.
102. Wanasundara, U.N., Amarowicz, R., and Shahidi, F. (1994) *J. Agric. Food Chem. 42*, 1285.
103. Salunkhe, D.K., Chavan, J.K., Adsule, R.N., and Kadam, S.S. (1992) *World Oilseeds, Chemistry, Technology and Utilization*, Van Nostrand Reinhold, AVI, NY, pp. 249–279.
104. Yuki, E., and Ishikawa, Y. (1976) *J. Am. Oil Chem. Soc. 53*, 673.
105. Koseoglu, S.S., and Lusas, E.W. (1990) in *Canola and Rapeseed* (Shahidi, F., ed.), Van Nostrand Reinhold, AVI, NY, pp. 123–148.
106. Thompson, L.U. (1990) in *Canola and Rapeseed* (Shahidi, F., ed.), Van Nostrand Reinhold, AVI, NY, pp. 173–192.
107. Shahidi, F., Wanasundara, P.K.J.P.D., and Hong, C. (1992) in *Phenolic Compounds in Food and Their Effects on Health, I* (Ho, C.-T., Leu, C.Y., and Huang, M.-T., eds.), American Chemical Society, Series 506, Washington, D.C., pp. 214–222.
108. Yamaguchi, N., Kandoo, M., Ikeda, K., and Kijima, I. (1984) *Nippon Shokuhin Kogyo Gakkaishi 31*, 114.
109. Saleemi, Z.O., Wanasundara, P.K.J.P.D., and Shahidi, F. (1993) *J. Agric. Food Chem. 41*, 641.
110. Shahidi, F., Yang, Z., Saleemi, Z.O., and Omar, S. (1993) *J. Food Lipids 1*, 89.

111. Shahidi, F., Wanasundara, U.N., and Amarowicz, R. (1994) *Food Res. Int. 27*, 489.
112. Slover, H.T. (1970) Lipids, 6, 291.
113. Dybing, C.D., and Lay, C. (1981) in *Hand Book of Biosolar Resources, Vol. II* (Zaborsky, O.R., ed.), CRC Press, Boca Raton, pp. 71–85.
114. Amarowicz, R., Wanasundara, U., Wanasundara, J., and Shahidi, F. (1993) *J. Food Lipids 1*, 111.
115. Amarowicz, R., Wanasundara, P.K.J.P.D., and Shahidi, F. (1994) *Nahrung 38*, 520.
116. Brekke, J.E., and Klosterman, H.J. (1956) *Proc. North Dakota Agric. Sci. 10*, 18.
117. Borreillo, S.P., Setchell, K.D., Axelson, M., and Lawson, A.M. (1985) *J. Appl. Bacteriol. 58*, 37.
118. Harris, R.K., and Haggerty, W.J. (1993) *Cereal Foods World 38*, 147.
119. Wanasundara, P.K.J.P.D., and Shahidi, F. (1994) *Food Chem. 49*, 39.
120. Conte, L.S., Lercker, G., Capella, P., and Catena, M. (1979) *Riv. Ital. Sost. Grasse. 56*, 339.
121. Bhatty, R.S., and Cherdkiatgumchai, P. (1990) *J. Am. Oil. Chem. Soc. 67*, 79.
122. Whittern, C.C., Miller, E.E., and Pratt, D.E. (1984) *J. Am. Oil. Chem. Soc. 61*, 1075.
123. Satue, M.T., Huang, S.W., and Frankel, E.N. (1995) *J. Am. Oil Chem. Soc. 72*, 1131.
124. Nergiz, C., and Unal, K. (1991) *Food Chem. 39*, 237.
125. Montedoro, G., Servili, M., Baldioli, M., and Miniati, E. (1992) *J. Agric. Food Chem. 40*, 1571.
126. Tsimidou, M., Papadopoulos, G., and Boskou, D. (1992) *Food Chem. 45*, 141.
127. Chimi, H., Cillard, J., Cillard, P., and Rahmani, M. (1991) *J. Am. Oil Chem. Soc. 68*, 307.
128. Nergiz, C. (1991) *Riv. H. Sost. Grasse. 68*, 553.
129. Papadopoulos, G., and Boskou, D. (1991) *J. Am. Oil. Chem. Soc. 68*, 669.
130. Blekas, G., Tsimidou, M., and Boskou, D. (1995) *Food Chem. 52*, 289.
131. Pratt, D.E., and Miller, E.E. (1984) *J. Am. Oil Chem. Soc. 61*, 1064.
132. Duh, P.-D., Yeh, D.-B., and Yen, G.-C. (1992) *J. Am. Oil Chem. Soc. 69*, 814.
133. Yen, G.-C., Duh, P.-D., and Tsai, C.-L. (1993) *J. Agric. Food Chem. 41*, 67.
134. Yen, G.-C., and Duh, P.-D. (1993) *J. Am. Oil Chem Soc. 70*, 383.
135. Yen, G.-C., and Duh, P.-D. (1994) *J. Agric. Food Chem. 42*, 629.
136. Daigle, D.J., Conkerton, E.J., Sanders, T.H., and Mixon, A.C. (1988) *J. Agric. Food Chem. 36*, 1179.
137. Sanders, T.H. (1977) *Peanut Sci. 4*, 51.
138. Karchesy, J., and Hemingway, R.W. (1986) *J. Agric. Food Chem. 34*, 966.
139. Van Niekerk, P.J., and Burger, A.E.C. (1985) *J. Am. Oil Chem. 62*, 531.
140. Tan, B. (1988) *J. Am. Oil Chem. Soc. 66*, 770.
141. Pirronen, V., Syväoja, E.L., Varo, P., Salminen, K., Koivistooinen, P. (1986) *J. Agric. Food Chem. 34*, 742.
142. Chase, Jr., E.R., Akoh, C.C., Eitenmiler, R.R. (1994) *J. Am. Oil Chem. Soc. 71*, 877.
143. Gopalakrishna, A.G., and Probhakar, J.V. (1994) *J. Am. Oil Chem. Soc. 71*, 1245.
144. Seo, A., and Morr, C.V. (1985) *J. Food Sci. 50*, 262.
145. Budowski, P., Menezenes, F.G.T., and Doller, F.G. (1950) *J. Am. Oil Chem. Soc. 27*, 377.
146. Budowski, P. (1964) *J. Am. Oil Chem. Soc. 41*, 260.
147. Fukuda, Y., Osawa, T., Namiki, M., and Ozaki, T. (1985) *Agric. Biol. Chem. 49*, 301.
148. Katsuzaki, H., Kawasumi, M., Kawakishi, S., and Osawa, T. (1992) *Biosci. Biotech. Biochem. 56*, 2087.

149. Katsuzaki, H., Kawakishi, S., and Osawa, T. (1993) *Heterocycles. 36*, 933.
150. Katsuzaki, H., Kawakishi, S., and Osawa, T. (1994) *Phytochemistry 35*, 773.
151. Osawa, T., Nagata, M., Namiki, M., and Fukuda, Y. (1985) *Agric. Biol. Chem. 49*, 3351.
152. Nagata, M., Osawa, T., Namiki, M., and Fukuda, Y. (1987) *Agric. Biol. Chem. 51*, 1285.
153. Osawa, T., Ide, A., Su, J.-De, and Namiki, M. (1987) *J. Agric. Food Chem. 35*, 802.
154. Fukuda, Y., Nagata, M., Osawa, T., and Namiki, M. (1986) *J. Am. Oil Chem. Soc. 63*, 1027.
155. Fukuda, Y., Osawa, T., and Namiki, M. (1981) *Nippon Shokuhí Kogyo Gakkaishi 28*, 461.
156. Fukuda, Y., Isobe, M., Nagata, M., Osawa, T., and Namiki, M. (1986) *Heterocycles 24*, 923.
157. Osawa, T., Kumon, H., Namiki, M., Kawakishi, S., and Fukuda, Y. (1990) in *Mutagens and Carcinogens in the Diet* (Pariza, M.W., Aeschbacher, H.U., Felton, J.S., and Sato, S., eds.), Wiley-Liss. Inc., pp. 223–238.
158. Fukuda, Y., Osawa, T., Kawakishi, S., and Namiki, M. (1994) in *Food Phytochemicals in Cancer Prevention, II* (Ho, C.-T., Osawa, T., Huang, M.-T., and Rosen, R.T., eds.), American Chemical Society, Series 547, pp. 264–274.
159. Fukuda, Y., Osawa, T., Kawakishi, S., and Namiki, M. (1988) *Nippon Shokuhin Kogyo Gakkashí 35*, 483.
160. Shahidi, F., Amarowicz, R., Abu Gharbia, H.-A., and Shehata, A.A.Y. (1996) *J. Am. Oil Chem. Soc.*, in press.
161. Fukuda, Y., Nagata, M., Osawa, T., and Namiki, M. (1986) *Agric. Biol. Chem. 50*, 857.
162. Mimura, A., Takebayashi, K., Niwano, M., Takahara, Y., Osawa, T., and Tokuda, H. (1994) in *Food Phytochemicals in Cancer Prevention, II* (Ho, C.-T., Osawa, T., Huang, M.-T., and Rosen, R.-T., eds.), American Chemical Society, Series 547, Washington, D.C., pp. 281–294.
163. De Boland, A.R., Garner, G.B., and O'Dell, B.L. (1975) *J. Agric. Food Chem. 23*, 1186.
164. Musher, S. (1935) *Food Ind. 7*, 167.
165. El-Sokkary, A.M., and Ghoneim, M.A. (1951) *Ind. J. Dairy Sci. 4*, 123.
166. Overman, A. (1947) *Food Res. 12*, 365.
167. Morgan, A.F., and Watts, B.M. (1948) U.S. Patent, 2,457,063.
168. Neil, J.E., and Page, L. (1956) *Food Technol. 10*, 315.
169. Bookwalter, G.M., Knolek, W.F., Black, L.T., and Griffin, E.L. (1971) *J. Food Sci. 36*, 1026.
170. Arai, S., Suzuki, H., Fujimaki, M., and Sakurai, Y. (1966) *Agric. Biol. Chem. 30*, 364.
171. Walz, E. (1931) *Chem. Abs. 25*, 5675.
172. Walter, E.D. (1941) *J. Am. Chem. Soc. 63*, 3273.
173. Naim, M., Gestetner, B., Kirson, I., Birk, Y., and Bondi, A. (1973) *Phytochem. 12*, 169.
174. Naim, M., Gestetner, B., Zilkah, S., Birk, Y., and Bondi, A. (1974) *J. Agric. Food Chem. 22*, 806.
175. Murakimí, H., Asakawa, T., Terao, J., and Matsushita, S. (1984) *Agric. Biol. Chem. 48*, 2971.

176. Pratt, D.E., Pietor, C.D., Porter, W.L., and Giffee, J.W. (1981) *J. Food Sci. 47*, 24.
177. Hayes, R.E., Bookwalter, G.N., and Bagley, E.B. (1977) *J. Food Sci. 42*, 1527.
178. Esaki, H., Onozaki, H., and Osawa, T. (1994) in *Food Phytochemicals for Cancer Prevention I,* edited by Huang, M.-T., Osawa, T., Ho, C.-T., and Rosen, R.T., eds.), American Chemical Society, Washington, D.C., pp. 353–360.
179. Yamaguchi, N., and Fujimaki, M. (1973) *Nippon Shokuhin Kogyo Gakkaishi 20*, 507.
180. Okamoto, M., Homma, S., and Fujimakí, M. (1982) *Kaseigaku Zashi 33*, 585.
181. Esaki, H., Nohara, Y., Onozaki, H., and Osawa, T. (1990) *Nippon Shokuhin Kogyo Gakkashi 37*, 474.
182. Scholfield, C.R. (1985) in *Lecithins* (Szuhaj, B.F., and List, G.R., eds.), American Oil Chemists' Society, Champaign, pp. 2–10.
183. Jung, M.Y., Yoon, S.H., and Min, D.B. (1989) *J. Am. Oil Chem. Soc. 66*, 118.
184. Olcott, H.S., and Matill, H.A. (1936) *Oil Soap. Chicago 13*, 98.
185. Bishov, S.J., and Henick, A.S. (1972) *Food Technol. 37*, 873.
186. Warner, K., and Mounts, T.L. (1990) *J. Am. Oil Chem. Soc. 67*, 827.
187. Harland, B.F., and Oberlears, D. (1977) *Cereal Chem. 54*, 827.
188. Jacobsberg, B., Deldime, P., and Gapor, A.B. (1978) *Oleagineux 28*, 25.
189. Nesaratnam, K., Devasaugayam, T.P.A., Singh, B.B., and Basiron, Y. (1993) *Biochem. Mol. Biol. Int. 30*, 159.
190. Bernidini, E. (1984) *Oils and Fats Refining, Vol. II*, B.E. Publishing House, Rome.
191. Wong, M.L., Timms, R.E., and Goh, E.M. (1988) *J. Am. Oil Chem. Soc. 65*, 258.
192. Patterson, H.B.W. (19XX) *Handling and Storage of Oilseeds, Oils, Fats and Meals*, Elsevier Applied Science, London.
193. Goh, E.M., and Gee, P.T. (1986) *J. Am. Oil Chem. Soc. 63*, 226.
194. Ng, J.H., and Jan, B. (1988) *J. Chromatogr. Sci. 26*, 463.
195. Serbinova, E., Choo, M., and Packer, L. (1992) *Biochem. Int. 28*, 881.
196. Itoh, T., Tamura, T., and Matsumodo, T. (1973) *J. Am. Oil Chem. Soc. 50*, 122.
197. Ohata, T., Yamasaki, S., Egashing, Y., and Sanada, Y. (1994) *J. Agric Food Chem. 42*, 653.
198. Sosulski, F., Krygier, K., and Hogge, L. (1982) *J. Agric. Food Chem. 30*, 337.
199. Classen, D., Arnason, J.T., Serratos, J.A., Lambert, J.D.H., Nozzolilla, C., and Philogéne, B.J.R. (1990) *J. Chem. Ecol. 16*, 301.
200. Grams, G.W., Blessin, C.W., and Inglett, G.E. (1970) *J. Am. Oil Chem. Soc. 47*, 337.
201. Combs, S.B., and Combs, G.F. Jr. (1985) *J. Agric. Food Chem. 33*, 815.
202. Price, P.B., and Parsons, J.G. (1975) *J. Am. Oil Chem. Soc. 52*, 490.
203. Weber, E.J. (1987) in *Corn, Chemistry and Technology* (Wadson, S.A., and Ramstod, P.E., eds.), Am. Assoc. Cereal Chem. Inc., St. Paul, pp. 311–349.
204. Chung, O.K. (1991) in *Handbook of Cereal Science and Technology* (Lorenz, K.J., and Kulp, K., eds.), Marcel Dekker Inc., NY, pp. 497–553.
205. Ramarathnam, N., Osawa, T., Namiki, M., and Kawakishi, S. (1989) *J. Agric. Food Chem. 37*, 316.
206. Rogers, E.J., Rice, S.M., Nicolosi, R.J., Darpenter, D.R., McClelland, C.A., and Romanczy, C.J. Jr. (1993) *J. Am. Oil Chem. Soc. 70*, 301.
207. Tanabe, K., Yamaoka, M., Tanaka, A., Kato, A., and Amemiya, J. (1982) *Yukaguku 31*, 205.
208. Gaydou, E.M., and Raonizafinimanana, R. (1980) *J. Am. Oil Chem. Soc. 57*, 141.

Chapter 8

Carotenoids and Tocols from Palm Oil

A.S.H. Ong[a] and Y.M. Choo[b]

[a]Malaysian Palm Oil Promotion Council; and [b]Palm Oil Research Institute of Malaysia, Kuala Lumpur, Malaysia.

Introduction

The palm oil industry has grown to become a very important agricultural-based industry in Malaysia. The total quantity of oils and fats produced in the world in 1993 was about 85 million metric tons of which palm oil is the second largest, accounting for about 16%. In terms of exports, palm oil is the market leader, constituting about 36% of world trade in oils and fats. Malaysia produces about 53% of the global palm oil output and accounts for 66% of the net world export trade of palm oil. It is projected that in the year 2000, palm oil production will reach 17.5 million metric tons with exports reaching 14.4 million metric tons. Malaysia is expected to produce over 8 million metric tons, an increase of 31% within the decade.

Composition

Palm oil is obtained from the flesh surrounding the seed, simply by cooking, meshing, and pressing (1). In this process, the seeds are separated, and, after cracking and removing the shell, the kernel can be processed to yield palm kernel oil. Palm kernel oil comprises about 10% of the total oil yield and has different composition and uses from palm oil. In fatty acid composition, palm oil occupies an intermediate position among natural fats. Its saturated fatty acid content is 50%; the rest is made up of monounsaturated and polyunsaturated fatty acids. By virtue of its fatty acid composition, palm oil is semisolid, containing mainly palmitic, oleic, and linoleic acids which are the most common components of all food fats. Palm kernel oil, on the other hand, is rich in lauric acid and is interchangeable with coconut oil in most of its applications; it is more flexible, however, because it is more unsaturated than coconut oil. Crude palm oil, besides its fatty acid composition, also contains 1% minor components (2). A diagrammatic presentation of crude palm oil minor components is given in Fig. 8.1.

Carotenoids and Tocols

Carotenoids form a class of C_{40} polyunsaturated hydrocarbons (carotenes) and their oxygenated derivatives (xanthophylls). These compounds impart a rich

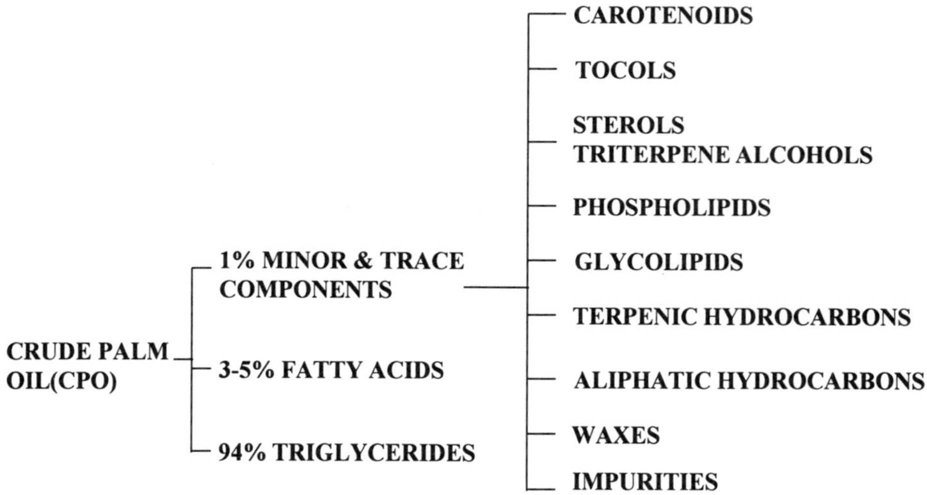

Fig. 8.1. Constituents of crude palm oil.

orange-red color to the oil (3). Crude palm oil is one of the richest natural plant sources of carotenes with a concentration of 500–700 ppm. It has 15 times more retinol equivalents than carrots and 300 times more than tomatoes. Analysis shows that α- and β-carotenes constitute ~90% of the total carotenoid content; the rest are δ-carotenes, γ-carotene, phytofluene, phytoene, zeacarotene, lycopene, neurosporene, and α- and β-zeacarotenes (4,5). Because the production of palm oil from Malaysia is projected to reach over 8 million metric tons by the year 2000, the potential availability of carotenes in the year 2000 is about 4800 metric tons.

The tocopherols and tocotrienols are found in crude palm oil at concentrations of 600–1000 ppm. The main constituents are γ-tocotrienol (44%), α-tocopherol (22%), δ-tocotrienol (12%), the remainder is made up of α- and β-tocotrienols, γ- and δ-tocopherols (6).

Nutritional Benefits of Carotenoids and Tocols in Palm Oil

In human nutrition, carotenoids play an important role as a source of provitamin A. β-Carotene, especially, is the most nutritionally active carotene as provitamin A. It is converted in the gastrointestinal tract into vitamin A. Vitamin A, of course, plays an important role in regulating vision, growth, and reproduction. It is essential for the normal cellular differentiation of most epithelia, including those of the skin, bronchi and trachea, stomach, intestine, uterus, kidney, and other organs.

The FAO/WHO recommendations on fats and oils in human nutrition stated that "in countries where vitamin A deficiency is a health problem, the use of red palm oil, wherever readily available should be encouraged" (7). Study has shown that red palm oil, besides providing caloric density to the oil, is also the richest natural source of β-carotene and is able to combat vitamin A deficiency in the developing countries (8–10). Human studies have also indicated strongly that carotenoids possess antioxidant properties and may protect against certain types of cancer. It has been postulated that β-carotene offers significant protection against cancer (11). This has sparked much interest, and numerous reports have now appeared to shed new light on this question. An inverse association between serum β-carotene and the risk of squamous cell carcinoma of the lung has been found (12). It was also reported that β-carotene inhibited oral tumors when applied topically or given as a dietary supplement (13).

The antitumor effects of palm carotenes (PC) were studied by examining the development of chemically induced skin cancer and viral-induced lymph cancer in HRS/J female hairless mice. Palm carotene was found to possess antitumorigenic effects, and the inhibition of subcutaneous lymphoma was concentration dependent, i.e., 0.3% PC > 0.1% PC > 0.05% PC. All of the palm carotenes inhibited epithelial papilloma formation as well (14). In another study, it was also reported that a natural carotene sample obtained from palm oil suppressed the promoting stage of two-stage carcinogenesis of mouse skin, and also inhibited the proliferation of human malignant tumor cells such as neuroblastoma GOTO cells, stomach cancer HGC-27 cells, and pancreatic cancer PANC-I cells (15). Among the major constituents of palm carotene, α-carotene demonstrated a stronger antiproliferative effect than β-carotene.

A study by Murakoshi *et al.* (16) on experimental mice also demonstrated that α-carotene had a higher potency than β-carotene in suppressing liver carcinogenesis, and that a mixture of natural carotenes extracted from palm oil had stronger activity than that of α- or β-carotene. In addition, palm oil carotene showed a stronger activity than that of α- and β-carotene in inhibiting skin carcinogenesis in DMBA-initiated mice.

Recently, it has been shown that carotenoids can act as biological antioxidants (17,18). Antioxidant protection activities of carotenoids in biological systems include quenching of singlet oxygen and reaction with peroxy- or alkoxy-radicals (19–21). A study on antioxidant activity of a palm oil carotene fraction in rats has shown an inverse correlation between tissue carotenoid level and accumulation of lipid peroxidation products and that α-carotene > lycopene > β-carotene (22).

Vitamin E functions primarily as an antioxidant, especially to prevent oxidation and peroxidation of polyunsaturated fatty acid units of membrane phospholipid (within and on the plasma membrane of cells) (23). This works against injury to cell membranes, as in red blood cell fragility in humans. It is also implicated in preventing photooxidative damage to the lens and thus in preventing cataract formation. It has been suggested that the antioxidant properties of vitamin E prevent/delay the onset of various degenerative diseases such as aging, cancer, arthritis, damage to cells caused by air pollution, and also in preventing coronary heart diseases (24).

The nutritional benefits of palm vitamin E (palm vitee) have been studied in human as well as animal models. The hypocholesterolemic effect of palm vitee has been studied by various researchers. It was found in one study that the concentrations of serum total cholesterol (–15%), LDL cholesterol (–8%), apoprotein B (–10%) and thromboxane (–25%) decreased significantly in 15 hypercholesterolemic subjects fed 200 mg palm vitee capsules/d (25). Another study on nine healthy volunteers taking one capsule of palm vitee per day also showed a reduction of serum cholesterol (reduction range –5–35.9%) and LDL cholesterol (reduction range 0.9–37%) (26). The effect of palm oil vitamin E on isolated Langendorff perfused rat hearts has also been studied, and results indicated that palm vitee containing a mixture of tocotrienols and tocopherols may be more efficient than α-tocopherol alone in protecting the heart against oxidative stress induced by ischemia-reperfusion (27).

Large population studies have analyzed the relationship between antioxidant nutrients such as carotenoids and vitamin E and degenerative diseases. A continuing study among 22,000 male physicians in the U.S. yielded an interim finding that those taking a supplement of β-carotene reduced the occurrence of major cardiovascular events by almost 50% (28). An inverse correlation between plasma vitamin E levels and mortality from ischemic heart disease was reported in a cross-cultural epidemiology study (29).

Carotenoids

Sources of Carotenoids

Various analytical methods have been used for the determination of the carotenoid profile of crude palm oil. Column chromatography was used in earlier studies using different adsorbents, and reverse-phase high-performance liquid chromatography (HPLC) has been shown to have several advantages for the separation of carotenoids in the oil.

Table 8.1 shows the carotenoid contents of various palm oil extracts (4). A carotenoid-rich oil can be obtained from palm pressed fiber, a palm oil by-product which is presently burned as a fuel in palm oil mills. The pressed fiber was found to contain about 5–6% of residual oil with a carotenoid concentration of 4000–6000 ppm, and the carotenoid content of the residual oil in the pressed fiber of the hybrid oil palm fruit is even higher (6000–7000 ppm).

Carotenoids from commercial crude palm oil are concentrated during the extraction and fractionation processes. A system of palm oil extraction based on a double-pressing technique has been implemented by several mills in Malaysia. The expected advantages of double pressing over the conventional single-stage pressing include lower oil loss in fiber, higher kernel extraction rate, less wear on the screw worm and cages, and reduction of contamination of the kernel oil with crude palm oil. More interestingly, the oil produced from the second pressing has a high-

TABLE 8.1
Carotenoid Contents of Palm Oil Extracts[a]

Palm oil extract	Carotenoid content (ppm)
Crude palm oil	630–700
Crude palm olein	680–760
Crude palm stearin	380–540
Second pressed oil	1800–2400
Residual oil from fiber	4000–6000

[a]Total carotenoids estimated at 446 nm.
Source: Ref. 4.

er concentration of carotenoids. This could be due to the fact that the first pressing in a double-pressing process is carried out at a lower pressure (to avoid cracking of the nut), and oil relatively higher in carotenoids than that from the second pressing is extracted. After removal of the nuts, the fiber is then subjected to a higher pressure and more carotenoids are extracted out of the mesocarp, together with the residual oil from the first pressing.

Carotenoids are also being concentrated in the industrial process called fractionation. Palm oil is a semisolid fat at ordinary room temperature. Fractionation is carried out to extend the uses of palm oil; the products obtained are the liquid oil (olein, 70–80%) and the solid fat (stearin, 20–30%). The carotenoid content in the palm olein (lower melting) fraction is enriched by 10–20%, as shown in Table 8.1.

Recovery and Extraction of Carotenoids

The carotenes on the market at present are chemically synthetic β-carotene, carotene extracted from carrots, and carotene extracted from algae Dunaliella. The carotenoid composition of the various carotenes is shown in Table 8.2. The demand for natural carotenes is such that customers are willing to pay a premium for them because they are valued for their perceived safety. Figure 8.2 shows the major commercial uses of β-carotene in the global market in which they are widely used as a food colorant.

Because carotenoids are likely to grow in importance and value, the recovery of carotenoids from palm oil and its by-products is important. In addition, some studies are also being carried out to recover and concentrate palm-based carotenoids for

TABLE 8.2
Carotenoid Compositions of Various Carotenes

	α-C	β-C	Others
Carrot carotene	30–50%	40–60%	10–15%
Synthetic β-carotene		100%	
Dunaliella carotene	6–10%	84–90%	
Palm oil carotene	30–35%	60–65%	5–10%

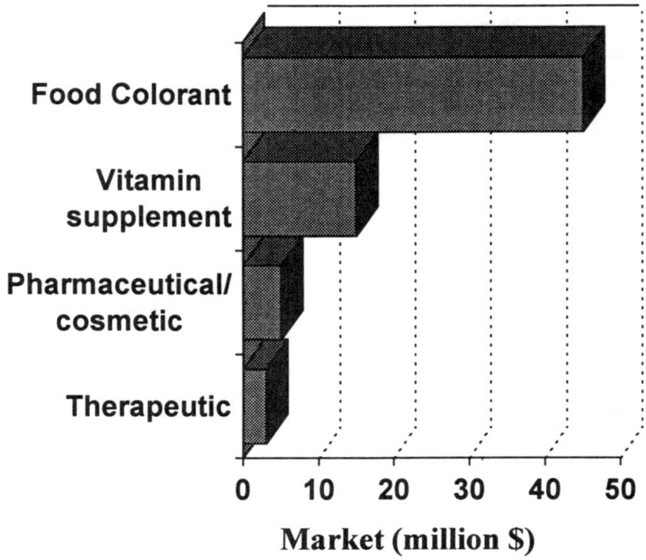

Fig. 8.2. Major commercial uses of β-carotene (1989 global market). *Source:* Ref. (36).

pharmaceutical purposes. Numerous extraction methods have been developed to recover the carotenoids from crude palm oil (Table 8.3). Most of the reported methods are difficult, costly, or inefficient.

Concentration of Carotenoids Via Alkyl Esters Route. However, a process for the concentration and recovery of carotenoids *via* the alkyl esters of palm oil route has been successfully developed by PORIM (30–34). Volatile palm oil methyl

TABLE 8.3
Carotenoid Concentrates from Various Methods[a]

Method	Carotenoid content (ppm)	Recovery (%)
Vacuum distillation[b]	>20,784	<46
Molecular distillation[b]	>80,000	>80
Adsorption[b]		
C_{18}	8000–9000	>90
Carbon	5000–7000	<50
Molecular distillation of crude palm oil	1290–1990	
Adsorption from crude palm oil (activated carbon)	3700–5600	<80

[a]Total carotenoids estimated at 440 nm. *Source*: Ref (4).
[b]Through methyl ester route.

esters have been prepared on a large scale as an oleochemical or diesel substitute. This process of conversion of crude palm oil into methyl esters involves mild reaction conditions; the valuable minor components such as carotenoids and vitamin E would remain intact in the alkyl esters, thus providing a unique opportunity for the recovery of these minor components.

The first stage of the process involves distillation steps including molecular distillation of alkyl esters. This has been proven successful in producing a carotenoid concentrate of >80,000 ppm on both the laboratory and pilot plant scale (34). The major carotenes in the concentrate are α- and β-carotenes. The second stage involves column chromatography with an adsorbent to give a carotene fraction (35). The concentration of this carotene fraction ranged from 90–100% (Tables 8.4, 8.5). The carotene fraction can then be diluted to produce the desired commercial carotene concentrate in various concentrations (1–30%) for various applications.

Lion Corporation of Japan has made efforts to recover carotenes from palm oil since the 1970s. They have developed a process which is also via the methyl ester route (36) (Fig. 8.3). Crude palm oil is converted into methyl esters by transesterification with methanol at low temperature which results in little, if any, loss of carotenes. In the second step, methyl esters are mixed in an organic solvent, and then the mixture is separated into a carotene-rich layer and a decolorized methyl esters layer. The methyl esters are used for oleochemical purposes while the carotenes may be further concentrated from the carotene-rich layer by ordinary means. Finally, the carotenes are purified by liquid chromatography with hexane. The palm oil carotenes contain more than 95% of carotenoids (60–70% of β-carotenes, 30–35% α-carotenes and small amounts of γ- and δ-carotenes).

Carotech has also developed an integrated process for recovery of carotenoids and tocotrienols from crude palm oil, again *via* the alkyl esters route (37). Fatty acids in a vegetable oil are subjected to alcoholic esterification to form an ester-rich layer including fatty acid alkyl esters, carotenoids, and tocotrienols. The ester-rich layer is exposed to solvolytic micellization to form a carotenoid-rich layer. The ester-rich layer is separated from the carotenoid-rich layer. The carotenoids in the carotenoid-rich layer are concentrated and can be adsorptively separated from the carotenoid-rich layer. Fatty acid alkyl esters are separated from the ester-rich layer to form a tocotrienol-rich layer.

TABLE 8.4
Carotene Content of Various Palm Products

	Content
Palm oil	600 ppm
Alkyl esters	600 ppm
Carotene concentrate	10,000–80,000 ppm
Carotenes	>90%

TABLE 8.5
Carotene Composition (%) of Palm Oil and Carotene Concentrates

Carotene	Concentrate	Crude Palm Oil
Phytoene	1.5	1.3
Phytofluene	0.3	0.1
cis-β-Carotene	0.9	0.7
β-Carotene	49.9	56.0
α-Carotene	33.3	35.1
cis-α-Carotene	5.5	2.5
γ-Carotene	1.7	0.7
ζ-Carotene	1.3	0.3
δ-Carotene	0.6	0.8
Neurosporene	0.1	0.3
β-Zeacarotene	1.3	0.7
α-Zeacarotene	0.4	0.2
Lycopene	3.4	1.3
Total (ppm)	80,560	673

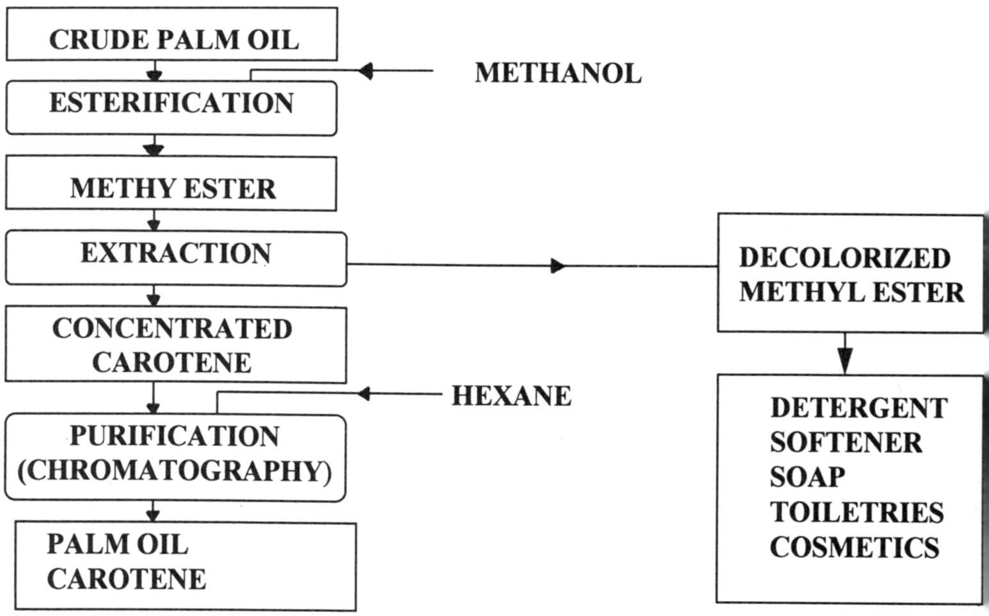

Fig. 8.3. Lion Corporation procedure for producing palm oil carotene.

TABLE 8.6
Carotene Composition (%) of Deacidified and Deodorized Red Palm Oil and Crude Palm Oil

Carotene	Red Palm Oil	Crude Palm Oil
Phytoene	2.0	1.3
Phytofluene	1.2	0.1
cis-β-Carotene	0.8	0.7
β-Carotene	47.4	56.0
α-Carotene	37.0	35.1
cis-α-Carotene	6.9	2.5
γ-Carotene	1.3	0.7
ζ-Carotene	0.5	0.3
δ-Carotene	0.6	0.8
Neurosporene	trace	0.3
β-Zeacarotene	0.5	0.7
α-Zeacarotene	0.3	0.2
Lycopene	1.5	1.3
Total (ppm)	545	673

Red Palm Oil. A process has also been developed by PORIM (38,39) to produce deacidified and deodorized red palm oil from the degummed palm oil with more than 80% of the original carotenes as well as the vitamin E still intact. This red palm oil is of similar excellent quality to the refined, bleached and deodorized (RBD) palm oil that is normally traded but contains no carotenes. The process involves two stages, i.e., pretreatment of the crude palm oil followed by deodorization and deacidification by molecular distillation. The pretreatment is carried out in a conventional manner using phosphoric acid followed by bleaching earth. This allows impurities and oxidative products in the crude oil to be removed. The deodorization and deacidification are carried out using a molecular distillation unit at temperatures <165°C and a pressure of 20–35 × 10^{-3} torr. Analysis by HPLC shows that the profile of carotenes is not destroyed during the process (Table 8.6), and the quality of red palm oil has also been found to be good (Table 8.7). Sensory evaluation carried out on red palm oil also showed it to be of very good quality and comparable to RBD palm oil.

The commercial production of red palm oil involves the capital investment in a molecular distillation unit which includes a vacuum system. The other costs involved are the power supply, water supply for cooling, and storage tanks. The cost of production, based on a 5-year investment plan is given in Table 8.8.

Unitata has also developed a process to produce carotene-enriched red palm oil. This is a chemical process which involves chemical neutralization of the free fatty acids, followed by pretreatment, then deodorization using conventional methods to remove the odor. The quality of the product obtained from this process is

TABLE 8.7
Quality Parameters of Red Palm Oil

	Level
Carotenes	>80% intact
Tocopherols and tocotrienols	>80% intact
Free fatty acids	<0.1%
Peroxide value	<0.2 meq/kg
Phosphorus content	<2 ppm
Moisture and impurities	<0.1%

Source: Ref. (39).

similar to the RBD palm oil, containing not less than 250 ppm of carotenes and 800 ppm of vitamin E. The oil produced has been marketed bearing the tradename NUTROLEIN (Nair, P., private communication).

Tocols

Source of Tocols

Tocols refer to tocopherols and tocotrienols; the tocotrienols, which are similar to tocopherols in molecular structure except that there are three double bonds in the isoprenoid side chain, are widely distributed in the plant kingdom. In general, they are found in such cereals as wheat, barley, rye, and rice, and in some oils, such as palm oil and rice bran oil as well as in rubber (*Hevea brasiliensis*) latex (6). The vitamin E content of palm oil and other edible oils is shown in Table 8.9. Palm oil has an abundance of tocotrienols compared with other oils.

Table 8.10 shows the various sources of tocopherols from palm oil and its products. Tocopherols accumulated in the palm fatty acid distillate (PFAD) after physical refining can be as high as 0.8% or greater so that the PFAD is viewed as a good source of natural tocopherols and tocotrienols. In fractionation or fractional crystallizations, tocopherols tend to remain in the liquid or olein fractions, thus rendering the solid fractions deficient in antioxidants.

Palm Vitamin E Isolation. The palm fatty acid distillate (PFAD) contains 0.4–0.8% tocopherols and tocotrienols, with the tocotrienols present as a major

TABLE 8.8
Cost of Producing Red Palm Oil

Plant capacity (T/y)	10,000	30,000
Pretreatment (RM/t)	17.00	17.00
Molecular distillation (RM/t)	99.00	96.30
Total cost of red palm oil (RM/kg) (includes cost of crude palm olein)	1.259	1.2374

Abbreviation: RM, Malyasian Ringet.

TABLE 8.9
Total Tocopherols and Tocotrienols of Oils and Fats[a]

Oils and fats	α-T (ppm)	β-T (ppm)	γ-T (ppm)	δ-T (ppm)	% T	α-T3 (ppm)	β-T3 (ppm)	γ-T3 (ppm)	δ-T3 (ppm)	% T3	Total T + T3 (ppm)
	Tocopherols								Tocotrienols		
Palm oil	256	—	316	70	55	143	32	286	69	45	1172
Palm oil	279	—	61	—	31	274	—	38	69	69	1081
Palm oil	152	—	—	—	17	205	—	439	94	83	890
Soybean oil	101	—	593	264	100	—	—	—	—	0	958
Safflower oil	387	—	174	240	100	—	—	—	—	0	801
Corn oil	112	50	602	18	100	—	—	—	—	0	782
Cottonseed oil	389	—	387	—	100	—	—	—	—	0	776
Sunflower oil	487	—	51	8	100	—	—	—	—	0	546
Peanut oil	130	—	216	21	100	—	—	—	—	0	367
Cocoa butter	11	—	170	17	99	2	—	—	—	1	200
Olive oil	51	—	—	—	100	—	—	—	—	0	51
Coconut oil	5	—	—	6	31	5	1	19	—	69	36
Palm kernel oil	13	—	—	—	38	21	—	—	—	62	34
Lard	12	—	7	—	73	7	—	—	—	27	26

[a]*Source:* Ref. 41–44.

TABLE 8.10
Tocols in Palm Oil[a]

	Content (ppm)
Crude palm oil	600–1000
Crude palm olein	800–1000
Crude palm stearin	250–350
Palm fatty acid distillate	150–8500
RBD palm oil	356–630
RBD palm olein	468–673
Palm kernel oil	80–100[b]
Palm leaflet	1400–2800[c]
Fiber oil	1200–3000[d]
Second pressed oil	1600–1800[d]

[a]*Source*: Ref. (45–46).
[b]*Source:* Ref. (47).
[c]*Source*: Ref. (48).
[d]*Source:* unpublished data.

component. The bulk of the PFAD is free fatty acids. A complete composition of PFAD is given in Table 8.11. The concept of isolating the tocopherols and tocotrienols (palm vitamin E) is based on the conversion of free fatty acids, partial glycerides, and triacylglycerols into methyl esters; distillation yields a concentrate of palm vitee (40). Purification of the concentrate yields tocopherols and tocotrienols.

The purification of the crude mixture is effected by crystallization during which sterols are separated, followed by ion exchange chromatography, in which

TABLE 8.11
Composition of Palm Fatty Acid Distillate (PFAD)

Free Fatty Acids	81.7%
Acylglycerols	14.4%
Triacylglycerols	4.1%
Diacylglycerols	7.6%
Monoacylglycerols	2.7%
Sterols	0.34%
Cholesterol	0.004%
Campesterol	0.092%
Stigmasterol	0.032%
β-Sitosterol	0.212%
Hydrocarbons	1.47%
Squalene	0.76%
Others	0.71%
Tocopherols +	
Tocotrienols	0.48%
Others	1.6%

RAW MATERIAL
PALM ACID DISTILLATE
(0.5%)
↓
ESTERIFICATION PROCESS
(0.5%)
↓
DISTILLATION PROCESS
(10%)
↓
CONCENTRATION AND PURIFICATION PROCESS
(70% - 80%)
↓
VITAMIN E
(100%)

Fig. 8.4. Concentration of palm vitamin E at different production stages.

the tocopherols and tocotrienols are separated from squalene. Palm vitee is then washed, dried, and purified by molecular distillation. Finally, it is deodorized before being dissolved in super olein prior to encapsulation. The process flow of isolation of palm vitee is shown in Fig. 8.4. The concentration of vitamin E at different stages of the process is given in Fig. 8.5. The pilot plant is capable of producing vitamin E with the following results: purity, 95–99%; overall yield, 65%; and production, 5–6 kg/batch.

Economic Viability Evaluation. It has been shown that it is technically feasible to produce tocopherols and tocotrienols from PFAD, and preliminary economic assessment of the process has been attempted. Vitamin E extraction is a concentration process from the 0.5% vitamin E content of the feed material, PFAD, to 99% purity. There are eight processing steps, and based on the two capacities of 25,000 and 50,000 metric tons PFAD per year, the plant investment amounts to RM49.86 and RM75.50 million, respectively (1989 estimates). The material, utility and labor costs are estimated based on the pilot plant experience. The effect of variation of selling prices on project feasibility is shown in Table 8.12.

The economic analysis indicated that for 50,000 metric tons of plant capacity for PFAD or 162,500 kg of vitamin E, the project is feasible when the selling price is maintained at about RM200/kg for an investment of 75.5 million ringgit. For 25,000 metric tons of plant capacity for PFAD or 81,250 kg of vitamin E, the pro-

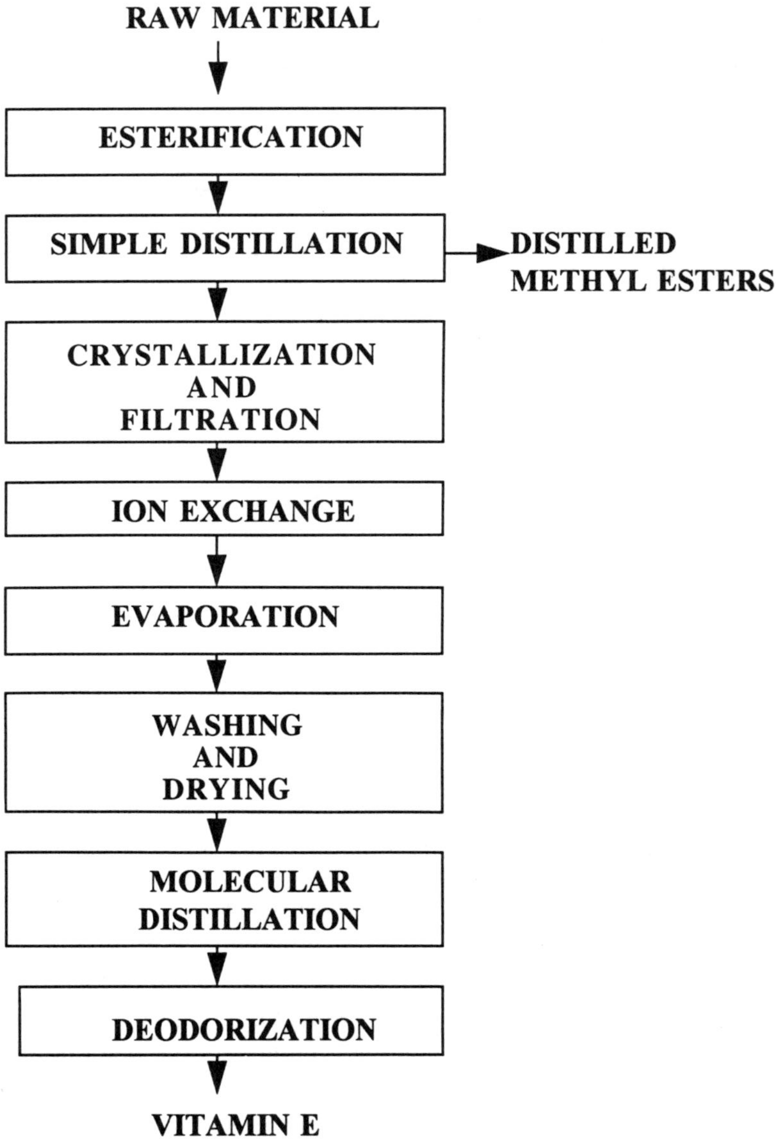

Fig. 8.5. Vitamin E pilot plant production process.

ject is marginally feasible if the selling price of vitamin E can be maintained at RM200 or more; some of the costs may be further reduced such as depreciation of the plant and material (PFAD). Nevertheless, a detailed analysis, including a market study, is required before these processes could be fully commercialized.

TABLE 8.12
Viability of Vitamin E Production from Palm Oil

Vitamin E price (RM/kg)	Investment (RM million)	Production capacity[a] (metric tons PFAD)	Payback period (y)
125.00	75.00	50,000	over 20
150.00	75.00	50,000	11.5
200.00	75.00	50,000	1.5
250.00	75.00	50,000	<1
Capacity sensitivity			
150.00	49.80	25,000	not viable
150.00	114.5	100.00	3
Capacity sensitivity at high vitamin E price			
200.00	49.80	25,000	5
200.00	114.5	100,000	<1
Investment sensitivity			
150.00	62.2	50,000	5.5
150.00	52.2	50,000	3

[a]PFAD, Palm fatty acid distillate.

Conclusions

Natural palm oil provides the richest plant source of carotenoids and tocotrienols. The nutritional benefits of carotenoids and palm vitamin E have been supported by research findings. Currently, three commercial processes for the extraction of carotenoids are available, that is, the processes developed by PORIM, Carotech and Lion Corporation. Two methods for production of carotene-enriched palm oil are available, one by PORIM and the other by Unitata. The technology for the isolation of palm vitee (the tocopherols and tocotrienols) from PFAD, developed jointly by PORIM and MITI, Japan, is ready for commercialization.

Acknowledgments

The authors would like to thank the Chief Executive Officer of Malaysian Palm Oil Production Council and the Director-General of Palm Oil Research Institute of Malaysia for support and encouragement.

References

1. Ong, S.H., Choo, Y.M., and Ooi, C.K. (1995) in *Developments in Oils and Fats* (Hamilton, R.J., ed.) Blackie Academic and Professional, London, pp. 153–189.
2. Goh, S.H., Choo, Y.M., and Ong, A.S.H. (1985) *J. Am. Oil. Chem. Soc. 62*, 237.
3. Ong, A.S.H., and Tee, E.S. (1992) in *Methods in Enzymology* (Packer, L., ed.), Vol. 13, Academic Press, New York, pp. 142–167.
4. Choo, Y.M. (1994) *Food Nutr. Bull.*, 15.
5. Yap, S.C., Choo, Y.M., Ooi, C.K., Ong, A.S.H., and Goh, S.H. (1991) *Elaeis 3*, 369.

6. Ong, A.S.H. (1993) in *Vitamin E in Health and Diseases* (Packer, L., and Fuchs, J., eds.), Marcel Deckker, Inc., New York, pp. 1–8.
7. FAO/WHO (1993) in *Recommendation on Fats and Oils in Human Nutrition*, press release, December.
8. Rukmini, C. (1994) *Food Nutr. Bull. 15*, 126.
9. Roels, O.A., Djaeni, S., Trout, M.E., Lauw, T.G., Heath, A., Poey, S.H., Tarwotjo, M.S., and Suhadi, B. (1963) *Am. J. Clin. Nutr. 12*, 380.
10. Lian, O.K., Tie, L.T., Rose, C.S., Prawiranegara, D.D., and Gyorgy, P. (1976) *Am. J. Clin. Nutr. 20*, 1267.
11. Peto, R., Doll, R., Buckley, J.D., and Sporn, M.B. (1981) *Nature 290*, 201.
12. Menkes, M.S., Comstock, G.W., Vuilleumer, J.P., Helsing, K.J., Rider, A.A., and Brookmeyer, R. (1986) *New. Engl. J. Med. 5*, 305.
13. Suda, D., Schwartz, J., and Shklar, G. (1986) *Carcinogenesis 7*, 711.
14. Tan, B. (1992) *Nutr. Res. 12, Suppl. 1*, S163.
15. Nishino, P.H., Takayasu, J., Iwashima, A., Murakoshi, J., and Imanishi, E.J. (1989) *C.R. Soc. Biol. 183*, 85.
16. Murakoshi, M., Nishino, H., Satomi, Y., Takayasu, J., Hasegawa, T., Tokuda, H., Iwashima, A., Okuzumi, J., Iwasaki, R., Kitano, H., Tanaka, Y., and Inagaki, T. (1993) paper presented at the 10th International Symposium on Carotenoids, Norway.
17. Burton, G., and Ingold, K. (1984) *Science 224*, 569.
18. Palozza, P., and Krinsky, N. (1992) in *Methods in Enzymology* (Packer, L., ed.), Vol. 213, Academic Press, New York, pp. 403–420.
19. Di Mascio, P., Kaiser, S., and Sies, H. (1989) *Arch. Biochem. Biophys. 274*, 532.
20. Weitberg, A., Weitzman, S., Clark, E., and Stossel, T. (1985) *J. Clin. Invest. 75*, 1835.
21. Tsuchiya, M., Scita. G., Freisleben, H.J., Kagan, V., and Packer, L. (1992) in *Methods in Enzymology* (Packer, L., ed.), Vol. 213, p. 460.
22. Serbinova, E.A., and Packer, L. (1994) *Food Nutr. Bull. 15*, 138.
23. Serbinova, E.A., and Packer, L.C. (1994) *Food Nutr. Bull. 15*, 138.
24. Packer, L. (1993) *Vitamin E in Health and Disease* (Packer, L., and Fuchs, J., eds), Marcel Dekker, Inc., New York, pp. 977–983.
25. Qureshi, A.A., Qureshi, N., Wright, J.J.K., Shen, Z., Kramer, G., Gapor, A., Chong, Y.H., De Witt, G., Ong, A.S.H., Peterson, D.M., and Bradlow, B.A. (1991) *Am. J. Clin. Nutr. (Suppl.) 53*, 1021S.
26. Tan, D.T.S., Khor, H.T., Low, H.S., Ahmad, A., and Gapor, A. (1991) *Am. J. Clin. Nutr. 53*, 1027S.
27. Serbinova, E., Khwaja, S., Cotudoic, J., Ericson, J., Tomes, Z., Gapor, A., Kagan, V., and Packer, L. (1992) *Nutr. Res. 12*, S203.
28. Hennekens, C.H., and Eberlein, K.A. (1985) *Prev. Med. 14*, 165.
29. Gey, K.F., Purka, P., Jordan, P., and Moser, H.K. (1991) *Am. J. Clin. Nutr. 53*, 326S.
30. Choo, Y.M., and Goh, S.H., U.K. Patent No. 2148897 (1987); Malaysian Patent No. PI8702770 (1989).
31. Choo, Y.M., and Ong, A.S.H. (1989) U.K. Patent No. 2161809.
32. Ong, A.S.H., Choo, Y.M., Cheah, K.Y., and Bakar, A., Australian Patent No. 42519/89 (1992); Malaysian Patent No. PI8801234 (1992).
33. Choo, Y.M., Goh, S.H., and Khor, H.T., U.K. Patent No. 2188057 (1990).
34. Ong, A.S.H., Choo, Y.M., and Ooi, C.K., U.S. Patent No. 5019668 (1991); Malaysian

Patent No. PI8900779 (1989); European Patent No. 89305826-3 (1992); Australian Patent No. 36320/89 (1992); Japanese Patent No. 1-153561 (1989).

35. Ooi, C.K., Choo, Y.M., Ma, A.N., and Yap, S.C., Patent pending (1994).
36. Anon. (1992) *INFORM 3*, 210.
37. Barrie, T., and Saleh, M.H. (1992) U.S. Patent No. US005157132A.
38. Ooi, C.K., Choo, Y.M., and Ong, A.S.H., Australian Patent No. 31084/89 (1992); Malaysian Patent No. PI8800447 (1988); Indonesia Patent No. 13413 (1992).
39. Choo, Y.M., Ma, A.N., Yap, S.C., Ooi, C.K., and Yusof, B. (1993) *Palm Oil Dev. 19*, 30.
40. Gapor, A., Leong, W.L., Ong, A.S.H., Kawada, T., Watanabe, H., and Tsuchiya, N. (1988) Australian Patent No. 8260.
41. Slover (1971) *Lipids 6*, 291.
42. Whittle, and Pennock, J.F. (1976) *Analyst 92*, 423.
43. Gunstone, F.D., Harwood, J.L., and Padley, F.B. (1986) in *The Lipid Handbook*, Chapman and Hall, London, p. 108.
44. Glover, H.T., Lehman, J., and Vallis, R. (1969) *J. Am. Oil. Chem. Soc. 46*, 417.
45. Tan, B.K., and Oh, C.H. (1981) *PORIM Techn. 3*.
46. Gapor, A., Berger, K.G., Hashimoto, T., Kato, A., Tanabe, K., Mamuro, H., and Yamaoka, M. (1983) in *Proceedings of The Palm Oil Product Technology in the Eighties* (Pushparajah, E., and Rajadurai, M., eds.), The Corporation Society of Planters, Kuala Lumpur, pp. 145–156.
47. Jabobsberg, B. (1974) in *Proceedings of First MARDI Workshop on Oil Palm Technology*, Kuala Lumpur, Malaysia.
48. Gapor, A., Kato, A., and Ong, A.S.H. (1986) *J. Am. Oil Chem. Soc. 63*, 330.

Chapter 9

Antioxidants in Grapes and Wine: Chemistry and Health Effects

R.L. Williams and M.S. Elliott

Old Dominion University Enological Research Facility, Department of Chemistry/Biochemistry, Old Dominion University, Norfolk, Virginia 23529.

Introduction

Natural proanthocyanidins can be found in a great many plants and plant products. These polyphenolic substances have been well characterized with regard to their origin, diversity of structure, and potential health effects. This chapter will attempt to bring together certain aspects of this fascinating class of natural organic materials in an effort to demonstrate the versatility and breadth of reactivity that have been noted in the literature.

Structure and Occurrence

Natural proanthocyanidins have been studied for the past century as components of leaves, fruits, and flowers (1,2). These polyphenolic compounds are characterized by a C_{30} flavonoid system with three distinct ring components. The biosynthesis of the parent precursor flavan-3-ols , (+)-catechin and (-)-epicatechin, arises from the Shikimate-Chorismate pathway (3,4) by a sequence of unique reductions and condensation steps in the plant involving the *trans* and *cis* flavan-3,4-diols. These transient diols subsequently condense *via* enzyme-catalyzed reactions to give a series of dimeric, trimeric and oligomeric proanthocyanidins or procyanidins in which ring C is joined to ring A with another monomer unit in either a 4,8 or 4,6 linkage. Perhaps the most widely studied sequence of proanthocyanidins or procyanidins, with regard to grapes and wine, is the condensed proanthocyanidin B series which includes the dimers B_1 through B_4 (Fig. 9.1). The biogenesis of these condensed proanthocyanidins has been reviewed by Herget (5).

These proanthocyanidins have long been associated with nonspecific protein interaction and the classical tanning process; however, in the context of this chapter, these compounds can be considered as essential components of a wine's flavor and aging potential. These compounds are known to interact with the protein components of saliva and produce the characteristic astringency associated with young red wines. Their inherent antioxidant capacity is also responsible for their contribution to the aging potential of fine red wines.

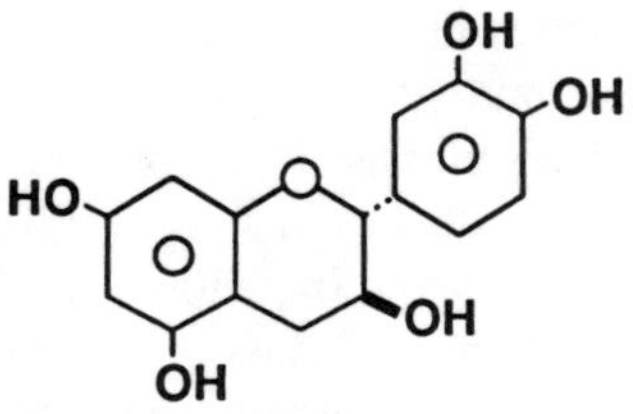

(1)

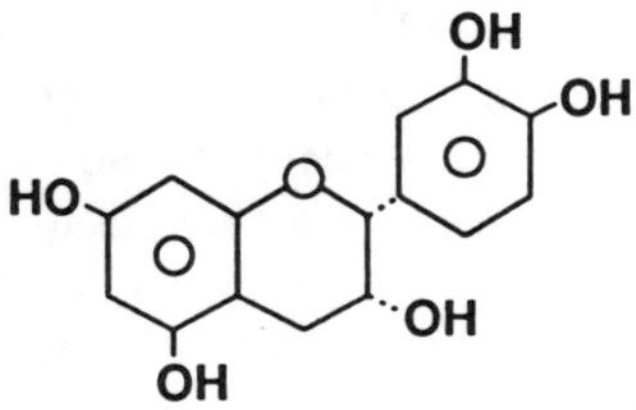

(2)

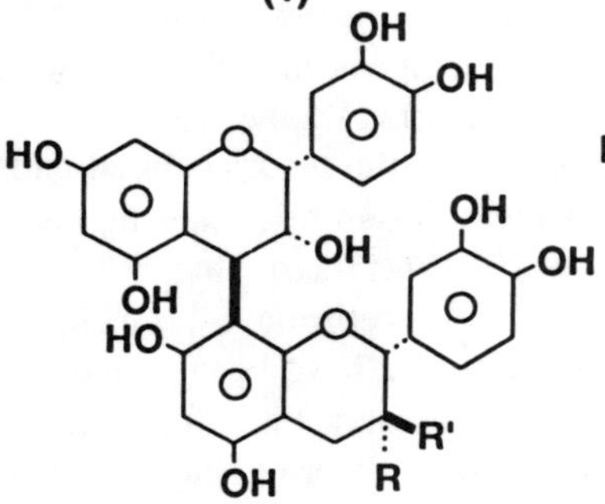

(3) = B_1; R' = OH, R = H
(4) = B_2; R' = H, R = OH

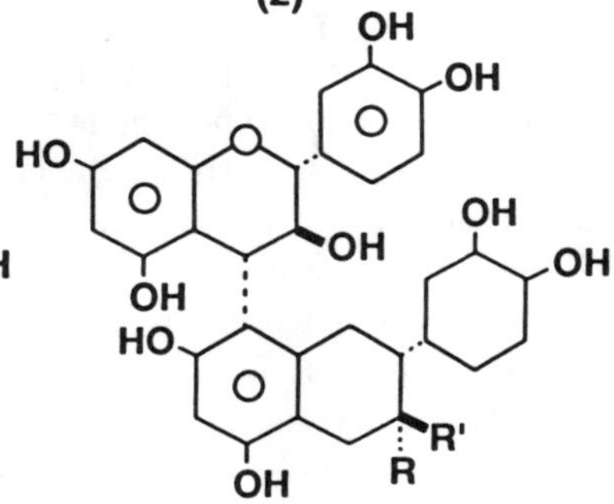

(5) = B_3; R' = OH, R = H
(6) = B_4; R' = H, R = OH

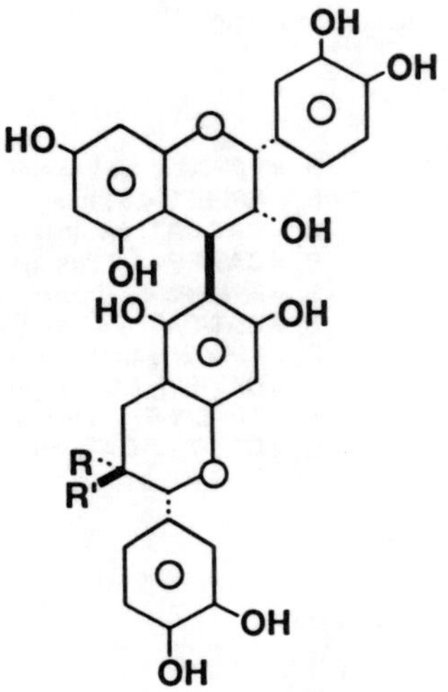

(7) = B_7; R' = OH, R = H
(8) = B_5; R' = H, R = OH

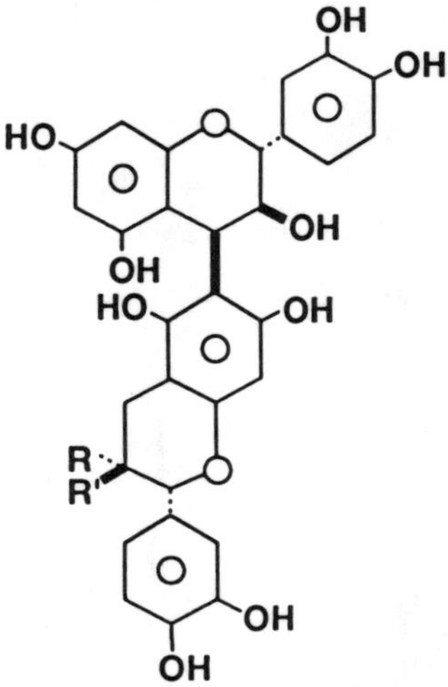

(9) = B_6; R' = OH, R = H
(10) = B_8; R' = H, R = OH

Fig. 9.1. Grape seed and wine proanthocyanidins.

Red wines have been shown to contain much higher levels of these proanthocyanidins (6–9) than white wines, due to the classic method of fermentation and maceration of red wines (Fig. 9.2). The highest level of these oligomeric proanthocyanidins can be found in the seeds of most grape varieties. Smaller quantities of these materials can be isolated from grape skins and stems (6,10); however, the pulp of the grape is essentially devoid of proanthocyanidins. The proanthocyandin content of various wines and grape seeds has been studied extensively by Bourzeix (6,11), Da Silva (12,13), Oszmianski and Lee (14,15), and Singleton (16). Among the red grape varietals, the Pinot Noir has been shown to possess the highest content of proanthocyanidins (6) whereas the Pinot Blanc apparently exhibits one of the highest levels of proanthocyandins in the white grape varietals (7). More recently, this laboratory has produced a new, seed-enhanced white wine which has been shown to contain polyphenolic levels comparable to some red wines (17).

The transfer of these polyphenolic compounds from the grape seed into wines and the interaction of anthocyanins and these proanthocyanidins have been described by Singleton and coworkers (18,19). The flavor thresholds of these polyphenolics and related compounds such as quercetin have been reported by Delcour *et al.* (20). Certain of the proanthocyanidins have been actively synthesized in the laboratory *via* the reduction of dihydroquercetin and subsequent acid catalyzed condensation of the transient 3,4-diol with either (+)-catechin or (-)-epicatechin (21–23). This synthetic approach leads to the formation of the dimeric 4,8 proanthocyanidins B_3 and B_4 together with the 4,6 dimers B_6 and B_8. Subsequent condensation of the B_3 dimer with (+)-catechin gives the 4,8,4,8 trimer known as C_2 while condensation of B_4 with (-)-epicatechin gave the trimer C_1.

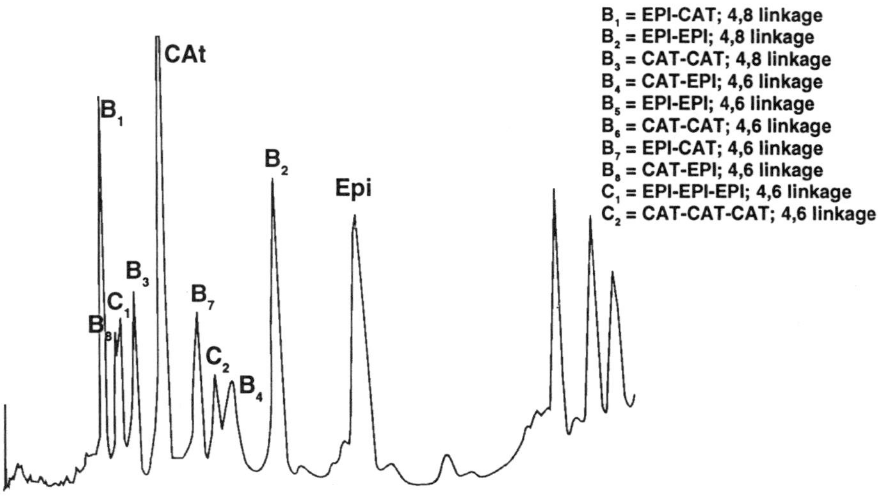

Fig. 9.2. Red wine and white wine proanthocyanidin levels.

Chromatographic Methods for Analysis of Proanthocyanidins

Thin-Layer Chromatography (TLC). A wide variety of plant materials containing these proanthocyanidins have been examined by TLC methods. Two-dimensional paper chromatographic methods have been used for some time to identify the B series of dimeric proanthocyanindins together with the trimers C_1 and C_2 (24). The various compounds are generally visualized with an acidic vanillin spray or with ultraviolet light. The chromatographic methods for the analysis of proanthocyanidins have been reviewed by Karchesy *et al.* (25).

High-pressure liquid chromatography (HPLC) has become quite popular for the analysis of the proanthocyanidins in wine and grape seed components. The most common chromatographic conditions include the use of a C_{18} or C_8 reverse-phase chromatographic column with an acetonitrile/water or acetic acid/water elution gradient which is monitored at 280 nm (26,27). Prepurification of wine samples was accomplished using C_{18} Sep-Paks to remove the acidic phenolic components (28); however, there is evidence that this method leads to considerable loss of proanthocyanidins bound to the Sep-Pak. For the analysis of wine samples, we found it unnecessary to use the Sep-Paks and prefer to do direct sample analysis without purification of the sample except for filtration through a 4-μm filter. We have developed a very satisfactory analytical procedure for the analysis of wine with a C_{18}AQ HPLC column. This column allows for a more efficient separation of the oligomeric proanthocyanidins using an acetonitrile/water gradient monitored at 280 nm (29) (Fig. 9.3).

The analysis of grape seeds for proanthocyanidin content requires an initial isolation procedure which allows for the removal of the higher molecular weight components. Our laboratory had used a modified extraction procedure based on the earlier work of Michaud *et al.* (30). Fresh grape seeds are ground in a blender and then extracted with a 3:1 mixture of acetone/water. The slurry is filtered to remove the solid material and the acetone is removed *in vacuo*. The resulting aqueous layer is then salted out with sodium chloride to precipitate the high molecular weight fractions which are removed by filtration. The resulting aqueous layer is extracted several times with ethyl acetate, and the combined organic layers are then dried with magnesium sulfate. Removal of the ethyl acetate *in vacuo*, and subsequent trituration with chloroform, produces the solid oligomeric fraction of proanthocyanidin dimers and trimers (31). To extract certain of the more interesting flavonoids, such as the less soluble quercetin molecule, one has to consider using a more polar extraction solvent or a more lipophilic solvent to replace the ethyl acetate in the second extraction step.

The HPLC analysis of most red wines and red grape varietals shows that there are over twenty individual proanthocyanidin components present in these natural mixtures. Ten to twelve of these components have now been identified (13,29) and many have been isolated for biological studies. Grape seed extract is similarly comprised of over twenty compounds, and the HPLC profile of the wine and grape seed extract is basically identical in most respects. An analysis of several over-the-

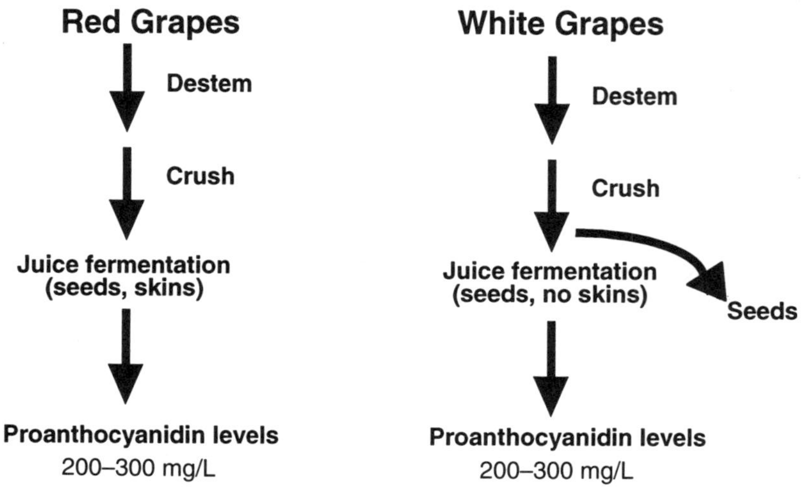

Fig. 9.3. Semi-Prep C_{18} AQ high-performance liquid chromatography (HPLC) of seed extract. Abbreviations: epi, epicatechin; cat, catechin.

counter drugs described as natural antioxidants from grape seeds also shows the same proanthocyanidin profile by HPLC analysis (Fig. 9.3).

Proanthocyanidins and Their Potential Health Effects

Overview. It should not be surprising to find that the proanthocyanidins have become of interest to medicinal chemistry, considering the wealth of natural products that have found their way into the recent literature. In view of the potential of the proanthocyanidins to complex with both proteins and carbohydrates (32,33), it would seem very likely that these condensed tannins might exhibit some intriguing biological activity. A variety of potentially important enzymes and glycoproteins, which might act as drug receptors, could be likely targets for interaction with these polyphenolic species.

Masquelier (34,35) was perhaps one of the first to recognize the potential of this class of compounds, referring to them as pycnogenols, or proanthocyanidols. In one of his early papers (36), the basic therapeutic potential of the pycnogenols was described. Among the many different types of biological activity ascribed to these grape seed components were vascular protecting activity, anti-cancer activity, anti-histaminic activity, anti-viral activity, anti-caries activity, free radical scavenging antioxidant activity, and anti-inflammatory activity.

Although there have been many other scientific papers describing the potential health effects of these proanthocyanidins, no one event has had more of an impact on the possible role of proanthocyanidins or procyanidins and health than the now famous "French Paradox" disclosure. The first suggestion that there might be some components in red wine that have some beneficial health effects can be traced to the work of St. Leger (37). In 1972, St. Leger made reference to the unusually low level of ischemic heart disease found in the French population that consumed moderate levels of red wine. St. Leger suggested at that time that there must be active ingredients in red wine that provide some degree of protective influence on the cardiovascular system. We now associate this protective influence with the proanthocyanidins present in red wine.

This anomaly was confirmed by Renaud (38) in 1992 using data from the World Health Organization's (WHO) study of ischemic heart disease as it relates to a wide variety of physical and dietary factors within the world's population (Fig. 9.4). The French Paradox was thus disclosed, and the world immediately became aware of the potential health effects of moderate wine consumption. Subsequently, however, the importance of the proanthocyanidins has been superseded by the role of alcohol as a possible protective agent against cardiovascular disease. This protective influence may be attributed to a hemostatic effect which may lead to a decrease in platelet reactivity and a lowering in the occurrence of atherosclerotic lesions (38).

Proanthocyanidins and Cardiovascular Disease

Although there appear to be some positive health benefits associated with moderate alcohol intake, the functional versatility and complexity of the proanthocyanidins and their interaction with proteins and carbohydrates suggest a greater scope of possible biological activity than of alcohol alone. Undoubtedly, some of the beneficial effects associated with moderate red wine consumption, and the corresponding intake of high levels of proanthocyanidins, can be attributed to the potential antioxidant activity of these compounds.

Chronic heart disease is often associated with problems of fatty acid metabolism as well as excessive lipid peroxidation of low density lipoprotein (LDL) both of which result in considerable damage to the vasculature (Fig. 9.5). The production of high levels of lipid hydroperoxides (LOOH) can perhaps be attributed to relatively low levels of endogenous antioxidants such as vitamin E. Lipid hydroperoxides have also been implicated in the eventual generation of thromboxane from arachidonic acid *via* cyclooxygenase. Thromboxane is known to lead to enhanced platelet aggregation which in turn leads to arterial blockage and thrombosis. Radical scavengers such as vitamin E and vitamin C are quite effective in reducing the levels of LOOH and thus protecting the cardiovascular system. This protective mechanism could be enhanced by the cellular uptake of natural, exogenous antioxidants such as the proanthocyanidins.

Proanthocyanidins as Natural Antioxidants: Biological Implications

Reactive oxygen species are oxygen free radicals that can be produced by a variety of enzymatic reactions *in vitro* and *in vivo*. The production of the reactive oxygen

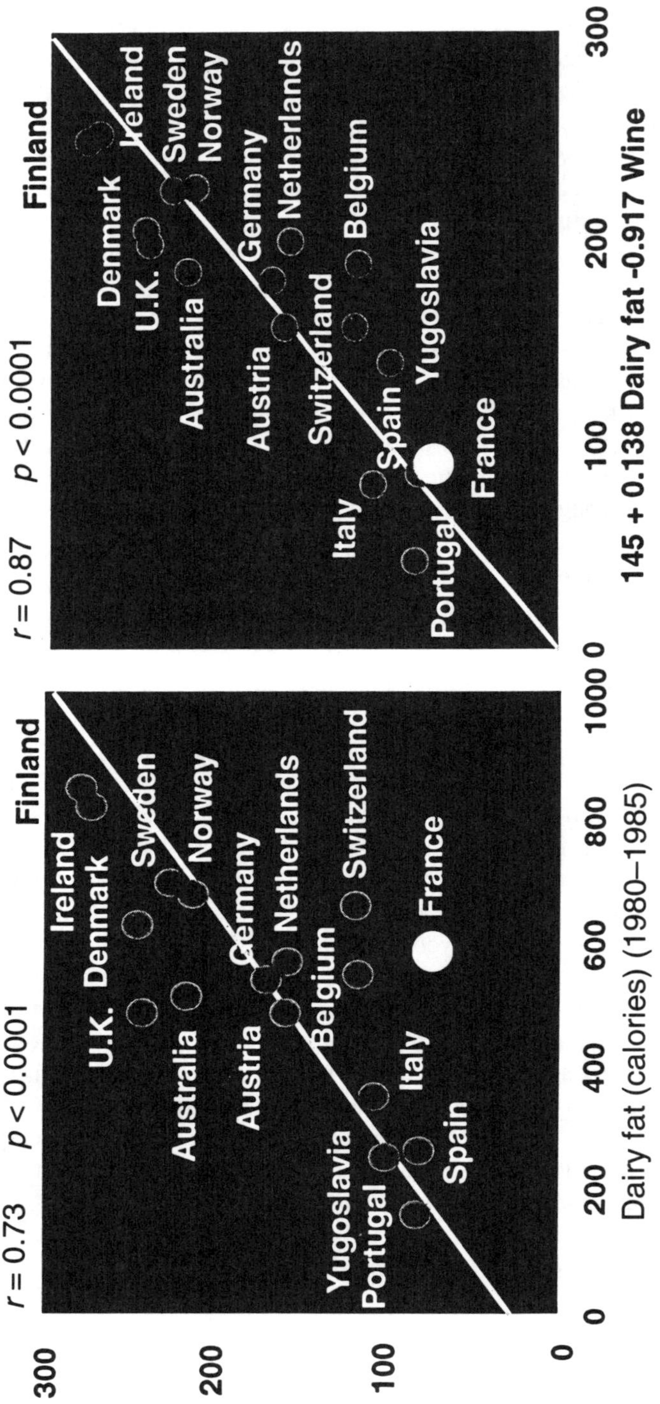

Fig. 9.4. French Paradox.

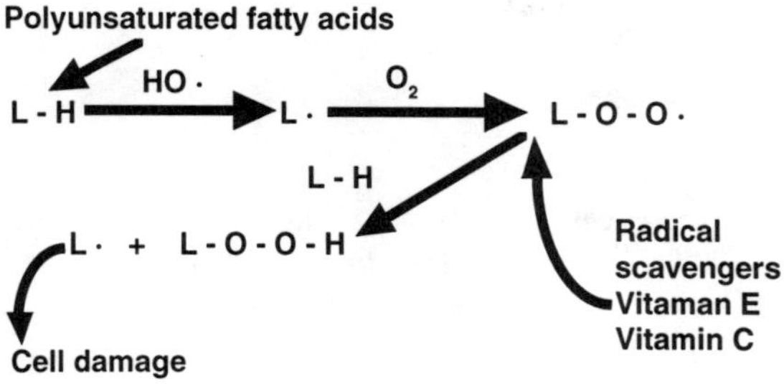

Fig. 9.5. Lipid peroxidation of LDL.

species (ROS) is best described as a chain reaction in which highly reactive oxygen free radical anions and hydroxyl free radicals are produced in several very discrete steps. Figure 9.6 describes the production of the ROS using a xanthine/xanthine oxidase (X/XO) system.

The formation and subsequent reactivity of the ROS induce what has been called oxidative stress. This process results from the interaction of the ROS with proteins which may lead to changes in transport phenomena, or the interaction with nucleic acids and subsequent cellular mutations. Reactions of the ROS with glutathione may lead to changes in cell viability, and interaction with LDL leads to changes in the membrane integrity of the vasculature and possible heart disease (Fig. 9.7). Natural antioxidants that can interact with or scavenge these ROS are found throughout nature and a review of natural antioxidants from plant materials was published in 1992 (39). Natural antioxidants have been found in soy products, certain types of algae, various seed oils including grape seed oil, a whole variety of vegetables as well as fruits, and in certain spices and herbs. We can now include grape seeds and wine as a source of natural antioxidant agents. The structural components responsible for this antioxidant activity are varied and include certain amino acids, carotenoids and the flavonoids (Fig. 9.8). These antioxidants can be further organized as preventative (intracellular enzymes such as catalase or superoxide dismutase, SOD), chain breaking, or complementary in nature (40) (Fig. 9.9). The proanthocyanidins belong to the complementary category in that they are

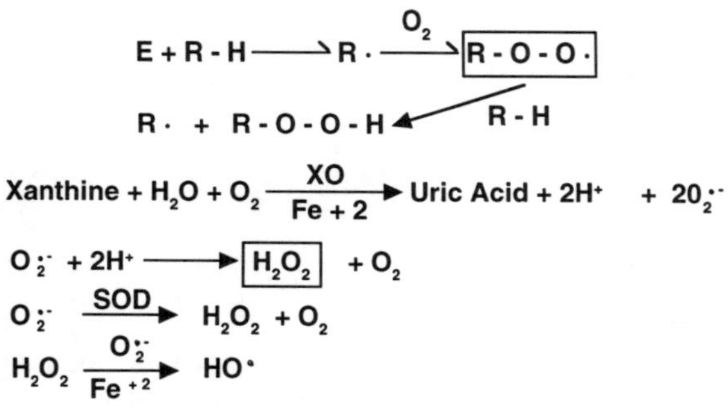

Fig. 9.6. Production of reactive oxygen species (ROS).

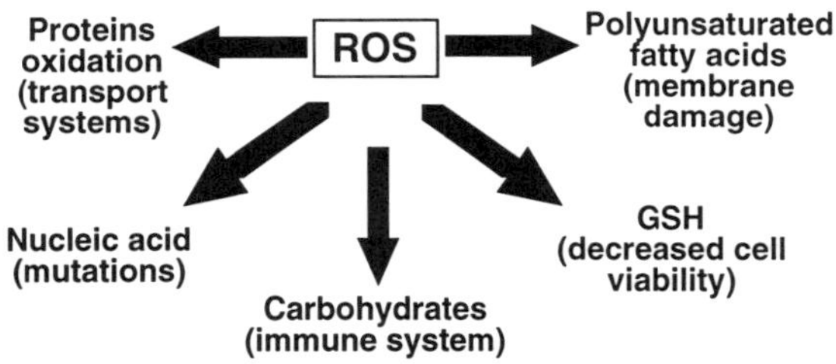

Fig. 9.7. Results of oxidative stress from reactive oxygen species (ROS).

believed to function extracellularly. The antioxidant mechanism associated with vitamin E and other phenolic antioxidants involves the abstraction of the phenolic hydrogen from ring A and the subsequent stabilization of the phenoxide free radical by resonance contributions from the tetrahydropyran oxygen (41) (Fig. 9.10).

Da Silva *et al.* (42) demonstrated the free radical scavenging ability of various grape seed components against superoxide and hydroxyl radicals. Using a polarographic measurement of total oxygen consumption in a xanthine/xanthine oxidase system, these researchers showed that several of the proanthocyanidin B dimers were very effective free radical scavengers. Dimers B_1, B_2 and B_3 were all found to be more effective free radical scavengers than the monomeric (+)-catechin and (-)-epicatechin. They also concluded that the degree of polymerization of the proanthocyanidin was not important with regard to superoxide radical scavenging ability. The presence of a gallate ester a the 3′ position greatly enhances the antioxidant capacity of these substituted species. B_2-3′-*O*-Gallate was found to be the most potent free radical scavenger in this study (Fig. 9.11).

In an earlier study, Ariga *et al.* (43,44) described the antioxidative scavenging properties of B_1 and B_3 against peroxyl free radicals. These studies showed that the dimeric proanthocyanidins were much more effective as antioxidants than other commercially available antioxidants such as ascorbic acid, gallic acid, and vitamin E. The concurrent electron spin resonance (ESR) studies of the oxidative scavenging capacity of these dimers suggests that B_3 is capable of trapping a maximum of eight radicals per molecule. This would suggest that the proanthocyanidins are

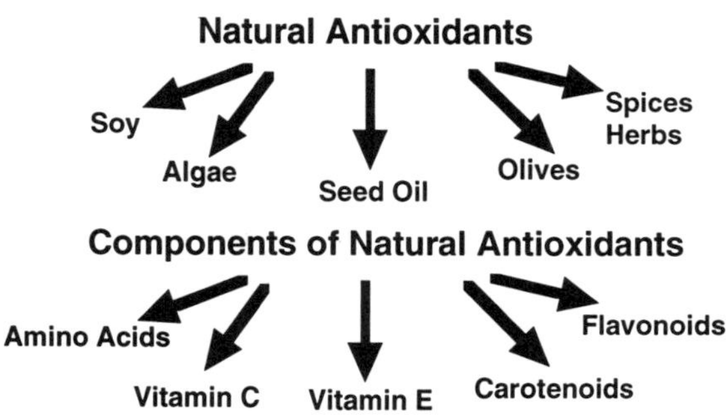

Fig. 9.8. Natural antioxidant sources and components.

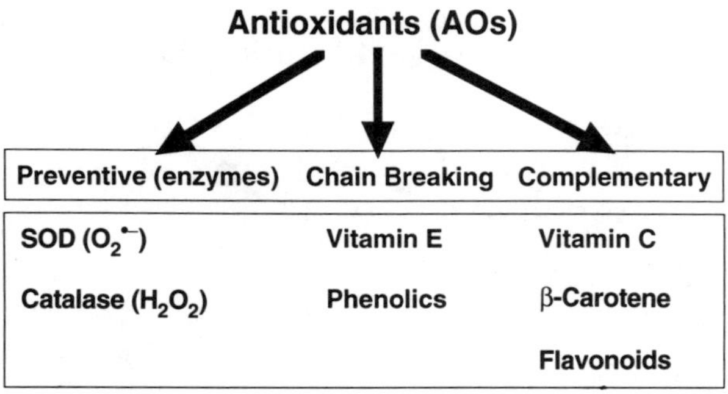

Fig. 9.9. Classification of antioxidants. Abbreviations: SOD, superoxide dismutase. *Source:* Ref. (40).

indeed very effective scavengers for the peroxyl radicals which are closely associated with lipid peroxidation. This research has led to a recent patent for a natural antioxidant based on the proanthocyanidin structure (45).

Recently, V. Hu *et al.* (46) have described the development of a structure-activity-relationship (SAR) within the proanthocyanidin family. Using a hypoxanthine/xanthine oxidase free radical generating system, these authors measured the IC_{50} values for free radical scavenging of twelve flavonoids (Fig. 9.12). The results of this study suggest that the scavenging ability of the agents increased with the number of hydroxy groups on ring B of the proanthocyanidin structures. It was also demonstrated that alkylation or glycosolation of the C_3 hydroxyl position led to lower radical scavenging capacity which is in agreement with the earlier work of Sichel *et al.* (47). It was also shown that the free radical scavenging activity was highest when the C_2–C_3 bond of the flavonoid was saturated and when the C_4 position was not a carbonyl function. Not surprisingly, epigallocatechine showed the highest free radical scavenging capacity with superoxide radicals.

Recent Studies on the Antioxidant Capacity of Wine

If one examines the relative composition of red wine and white wine, we find that the major difference is associated with the levels of phenolics present in each wine. Red wines contain over 20 times the levels of the proanthocyanidins and certain

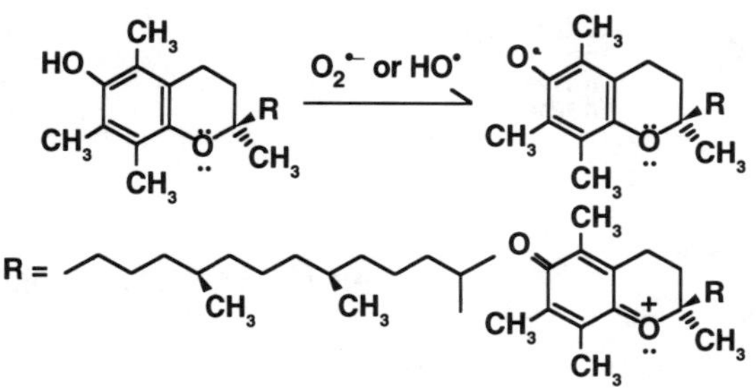

Fig. 9.10. Vitamin E antioxidant mechanism. *Source*: Ref. (41).

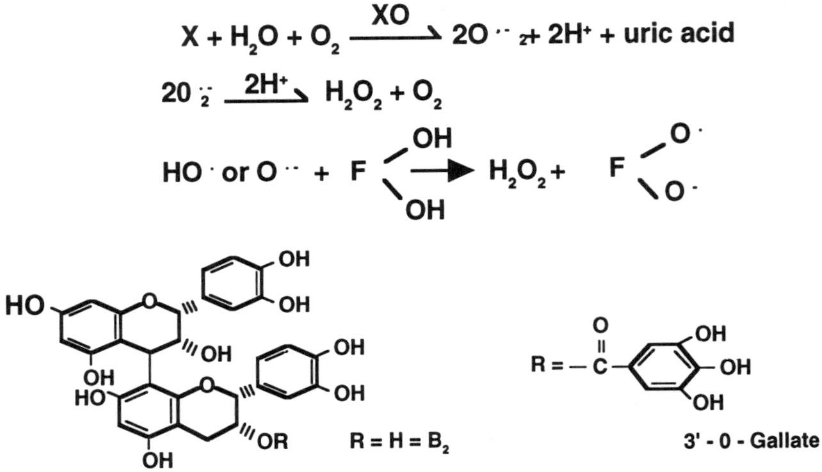

Fig. 9.11. Free radical scavenging action of proanthocyanidins from grape seed. *Source*: Ref. (42).

flavanones compared with white wines due to the effects of the method of fermentation of red wines on the seeds and skins. Some of the more common wine and grape seed components of interest as natural antioxidants are shown in Fig 9.13 together with the proanthocyanidins in Fig. 9.1. Cheynier *et al.* (48) have recently described the isolation and identification of twenty different oligomeric proanthocyanidins from grape seeds using a thiolytic microdegradation method and subsequent HPLC analysis of the degradation products. Twelve of these proanthocyanidins have never been identified from grape seed extracts and include three 4,6 dimers, B_5, B_6, and B_8. Four new trimeric proanthocyanidins were identified by HPLC, together with five new proanthocyanidins which were esterified with gallic acid at the 3 or 3′ position.

In 1993, Frankel *et al.* (49) demonstrated that red wine concentrate was able to effectively inhibit the copper-catalyzed oxidation of LDL *in vitro*. At 10 µmol/L, the red wine concentrate was shown to be more effective (86% inhibition) than an

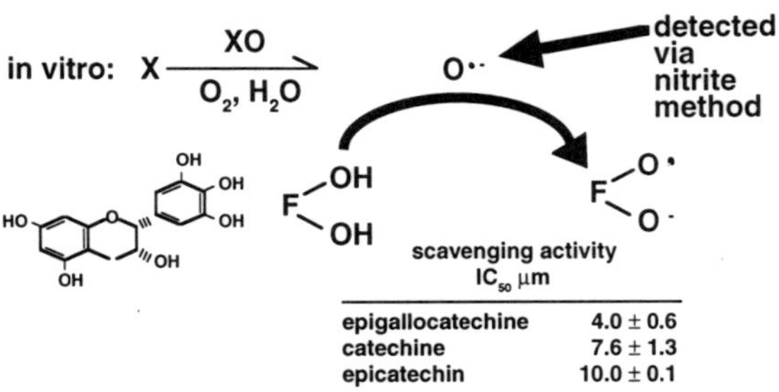

Fig. 9.12. SAR relationship of flavonoids and superoxide. *Source:* Ref. (46).

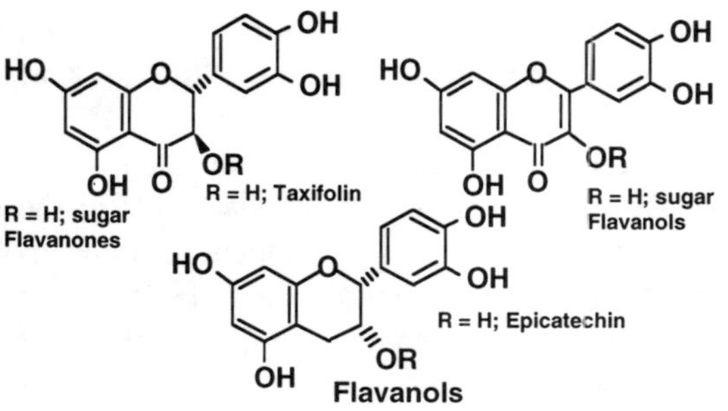

Fig. 9.13. Wine and grape seed proanthocyanidins.

equal concentration of vitamin E (59% inhibition). No HPLC analysis of the wine was given, but it must be assumed that the antioxidant effectiveness of the red wine concentrate was due to the combined capacity of the many proanthocyanidins present in this wine.

In a 1995 study, Whitehead *et al.* (50) described their research in the development of an assay to examine the effects of various natural antioxidants on serum antioxidant capacity (SAOC). Using a chemiluminescent technique, they were able to monitor the effectiveness of the natural antioxidants in red wine and white wine compared with high doses of vitamin C. Human subjects were given equivalent volumes of red and white wines (300 mL), and their SAOC was monitored over a period of 1–2 h. Other volunteers were given high doses of vitamin C (1000 mg). The results of this study showed that ingestion of red wine caused an increase in the SAOC of 18% within the first hour, whereas white wine caused only a 4% increase in SAOC. As expected, vitamin C was more effective than either wine, and the researchers observed a 22% increase in SAOC with vitamin C within the first hour.

This study and all studies related to the effects of the proanthocyanidins on such factors as SAOC or free radical scavenging capacity or cell growth invariably will be dependent on the accessibility or lipophilicity of the specific proanthocyanidins. Recently, Waterhouse (51) has shown, using HPLC techniques, that only about 20% of ingested (+)-catechin is capable of reaching the plasma after the consumption of 300 mL of red wine. Furthermore, the maximum levels of catechin found in the plasma were reached after 3 h postingestion and declined thereafter. The effective dose of proanthocyanidins necessary to bring about the desired positive health effects is still a very elusive question.

Perhaps one of the most striking experiments to date, one that attempts to relate the effectiveness of the proanthocyanidins in wine to potential health benefits, has been described by Demrow *et al.* (52). In this study, anesthetized dogs were subjected to a mechanically induced thrombus-forming paradigm in which the platelet-mediated thrombus led to a cyclic flow reduction in coronary blood flow (CFR). The CFR were apparently eliminated or reduced in relatively short periods of time by the intravenous and intragastric administration of diluted red wine and diluted grape juice. Although white wine was used in this study, it did not have any significant effects on the CFR, presumably due to the low levels of proanthocyanidins and other flavonoids.

The HPLC analysis of the red wine used in this experiment showed unusually high levels of quercetin (76 mg/L). No mention was made of the levels of the proanthocyanidins except that the red wine had 2.7 times the amount of unidentified compounds, presumed to be flavonoids, than the commercial grape juice. An HPLC analysis of the grape juice showed it to contain 86 mg/L of quercetin and 82 mg/L of rutin, the glycoside of quercetin; however, most commercial grape juices are in fact enriched with high levels of vitamin C. The surprising reduction in CFR resulting from the infusion of diluted grape juice may therefore reflect the antioxidant action of enhanced vitamin C levels in the plasma.

Since the disclosure of the French Paradox and the implications that have been presented with regard to the positive health benefits of moderate wine consumption, red wines have received a great deal of attention in comparison with white wines. The higher levels of proanthocyanidins and other flavonoids found in red wines suggest that they have a greater antioxidant potential than white wines. This laboratory has now produced a white wine which is exceptionally high in proanthocyanidins. Although white wines are not traditionally fermented on the skins or seeds like red wines, such an exposure to the proanthocyanidin-rich seeds would provide a way of increasing or enhancing the proanthocyanidin levels.

In 1992, this laboratory began a study whose goal was the development of a seed-enhanced white wine with greater positive health potential. The first experimental seed-enhanced chardonnay was produced by fermenting 18 L of fresh chardonnay juice on 800 g of fresh chardonnay seeds (53). After 17 d of fermentation and maceration on the seeds, the resulting wine exhibited over 280 mg/L of proanthocyanidins including (+)-catechin, (–)-epicatechin and the dimers B_1 through B_4. This level of proanthocyanidins is exceptionally high for any white wine and is well within the range of most red wines. On bottle aging, however, this new seed-enhanced wine showed signs of haze formation and developed a deep yellow color and an off taste. These negative attributes may well reflect the saturation point of such proanthocyanidins in a white wine and the subsequent production of a protein/proanthocyanidin haze.

In 1993, a second seed-enhanced chardonnay wine was produced by seven Virginia wineries. These wineries were given different levels of chardonnay seeds (150–500 g) in an effort to determine the optimum level of seeds to achieve an acceptable product. Eighteen liters of these experimental wines were fermented for different periods of time ranging from 10–40 d. The levels of developing proanthocyandins were monitored by HPLC, and the resulting wines exhibited proanthocyanidin levels ranging from 50–98 mg/L. Although the levels of proanthocyanidins in these wines were considerably lower than those observed in the 1992 seed-enhanced wine, none of the 1993 wines experienced any problems with haze production or color. The levels of proanthocyanidins achieved by this seed-enhancement procedure were considerably higher than those found in any commercial chardonnay (typically 10–35 mg/L) that we have been able to analyze to date. These seed-enhanced wines were evaluated by the winemakers and were found to be quite acceptable as experimental, unfinished wines.

In 1994, four Virginia wineries produced 224 L of seed-enhanced chardonnay wine which had been fermented in French oak on 6 kg of chardonnay seeds. These wines exhibited proanthocyanidins levels ranging from 122–139 mg/L and were judged to be of higher quality and character than any of the previous seed-enhanced wines (17). Figure 9.14 depicts the gradual rise in proanthocyanidins levels in one of the seed-enhanced wines over the period of analysis. Figure 9.15 describes a typical proanthocyanidin profile in the final seed-enhanced wine produced from 6 kg of seeds in 224 L of juice. This profile is rather characteristic of the levels of proanthocyanidins in all of the wines in which B_2 levels exceed (+)-catechin which was higher than B_1 and (–)-epicatechin; B_3 levels were usually higher than B_4. It was generally agreed by the winemakers that these wines benefited from their exposure to French Oak which tended to offset the sensory impression of these relatively high levels of proanthocyanidins in a white wine. This new, seed-enhanced white wine is currently being evaluated in human subjects with regard to its potential effects on the cardiovascular system and inhibition of platelet aggregation.

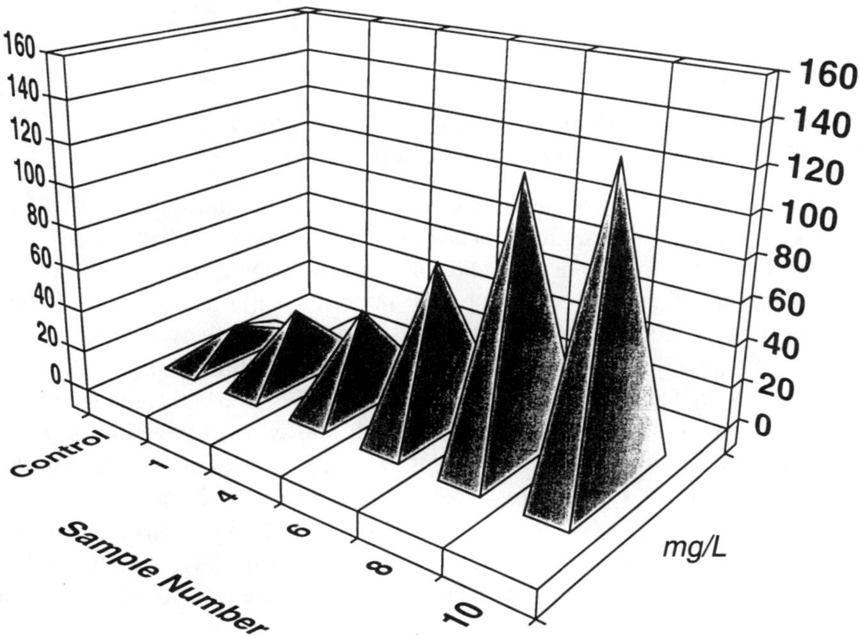

Fig. 9.14. Development of proanthocyanidins in 1994 seed-enhanced chardonnay wine.

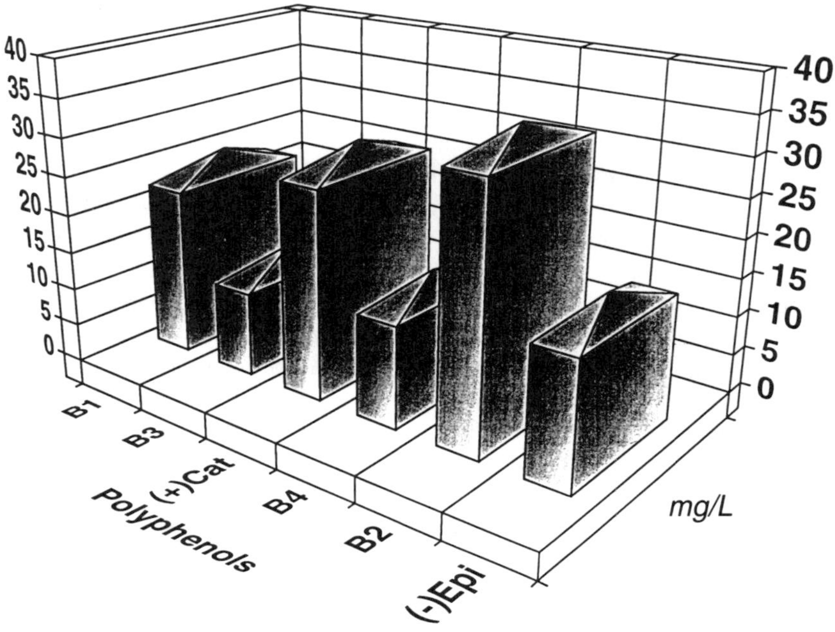

Fig. 9.15. Profile of proanthocyanidins in seed-enhanced chardonnay. Abbreviation: epi, epicatechin.

Biological Activity of Proanthocyanidins in Cell Culture: Human Fibroblast Cell Culture Studies: Cell Growth

The interaction of various organic compounds with human fibroblast cells in culture has been used for years as a means of determining the effects of different agents on cell viability and as an indicator of possible cytotoxicity. Cell growth studies using these cells in culture provide important information regarding the impact of organic agents on cellular metabolism and the growth cycle. This laboratory initiated studies on the effects of the proanthocyanidins in wine and grape seed extract on human fibroblast cells in culture in 1993. The cells are maintained in minimum essential media supplemented with 500 units of penicillin-streptomycin and 10% neonatal calf serum. Confluent cell cultures are subcultured by trypsinization, diluted 1:4 into fresh media and seeded into 25-cm^2 polystyrene flasks. Each passage is the equivalent of two population doublings, and this method is used to approximate the age of the culture. Typically, these fibroblast cultures will survive 20–25 subculturings, which is equivalent to 40–50 population doublings prior to senescence.

When human fibroblast cells were exposed to the proanthocyanidins isolated from grape seeds, including (+)-catechin, (–)-epicatechin, dimers B_1 through B_4, taxifolin, quercetin, and crude seed extract, we observed a 10–15% increase in cell growth in the 1–10 ng/mL level for the B dimers and the crude seed extract. However, at higher doses, these same compounds produced a gradual decline in cell growth. Quercetin was most striking in that it was apparently quite cytotoxic even at rather low dose levels (0.1 ng/mL) (Fig. 9.16). At the higher doses of all of the proanthocyanidins, there were very definite morphological or phenotypic changes in the fibroblast cell structure (54). There was a loss of the well-defined spindle-like morphology in the treated cells compared with the controls, as well as an apparent increase in the cytosolic volume. At the much higher dose levels, there appears to be evidence of significant cellular/nuclear damage and that the nucleus was actively degrading (apoptosis).

When the human fibroblast cells were treated with a single dose of 50 μg/mL over a period of 7 d, the cells responded with a general decrease in cell growth compared with the controls. Quercetin at this concentration was shown to be cytotoxic after the first day of treatment (Fig. 9.17).

Free Radical Scavenging Activity in Cell Culture: Antioxidant Activity

Cultured human fibroblasts are routinely used in free radical scavenging studies associated with aging and various dysfunctions that arise from free radical damage to cellular components (55). Generally, a correlation can be made between the longevity of human fibroblast cells in culture under oxidative stress and the age of

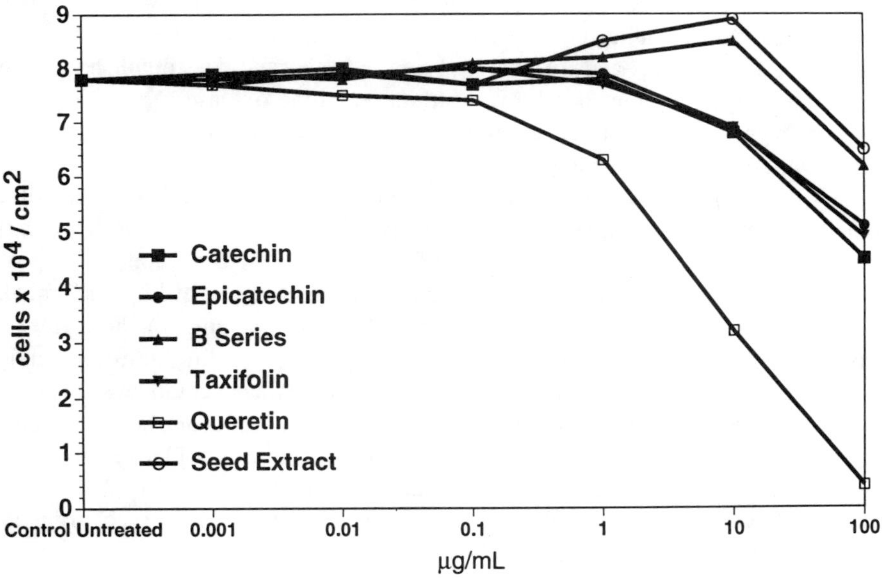

Fig. 9.16. Human fibroblast cell exposure to proanthocyanidins (1 ng/mL–100 μg/mL).

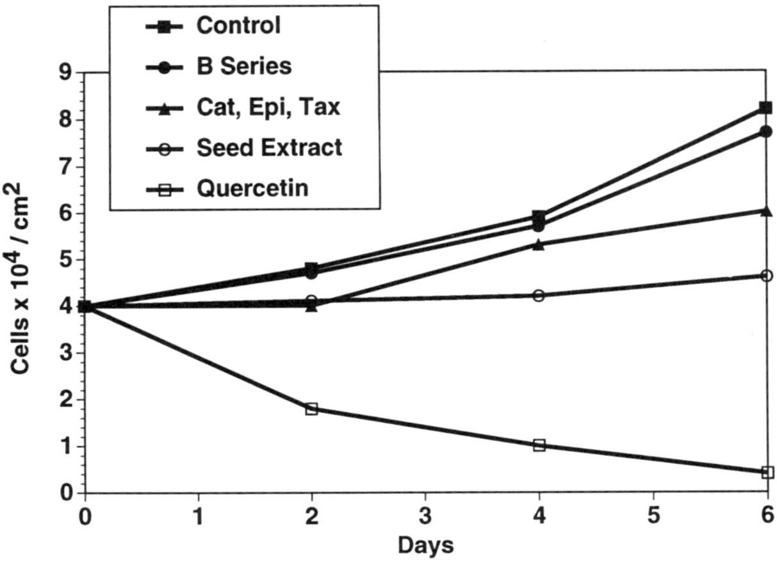

Fig. 9.17. Human fibroblast study at 50 µg/mL proanthocyanidins. Abbreviations: cat, catechin; epi, epicatechin; tax, taxifolin.

the tissue from which the cell culture was established. A human skin fibroblast model has been developed to screen potential antioxidants and free radical scavengers (56). This assay relates prospective antioxidant's protective capabilities against free radical-induced cell death and growth inhibition. The generation of superoxide free radicals and the hydroxyl free radicals can be accomplished using a cellular enzyme system involving xanthine-xanthine oxidase (X/XO) (57). A similar enzymatic system has been used to study the free radical scavenging activity of a variety of proanthocyanidins *in vitro* (42).

Using this particular paradigm, we have begun a series of antioxidant studies in cell culture with human fibroblasts to determine the effectiveness of the proanthocyanidins in oxidative stress (58). The oxidative stress conditions were produced with 10^{-3} and 10^{-2} units/mL of xanthine oxidase and 500 µM hypoxanthine. Human fibroblast cells were pretreated for 1 h with 50 µg/mL of the different proanthocyandins, (+)-catechin, (–)-epicatechin, B_1, quercetin, taxifolin, crude seed extract, and vitamin C (Fig. 9.18). Oxidative cell damage could be seen at the higher levels of xanthine oxidase treatment compared with controls; however, none of the proanthocyandins appeared to protect the cells from this oxidative damage at 50 µg/mL. In fact, there appears to be enhanced cellular damage in all cases in which cells were treated with the proanthocyanidins. Quercetin is especially ineffective and profoundly cytotoxic at this dose level.

Using a single level of xanthine oxidase (10^{-3} units/mL XO), the fibroblast cells were pretreated with a range of concentrations of the vitamin C and the vari-

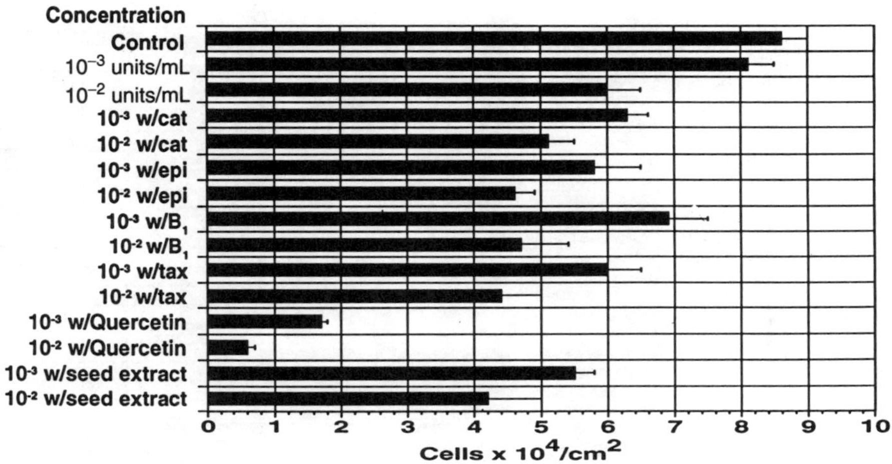

Fig. 9.18. Hypoxanthine-xanthine oxidase, oxidative stress study with human fibroblast cells in culture. Abbreviations: cat, catechin; epi, epicatechin; tax, taxifolin.

ous proanthocyanidins from 0.01–100 μg/mL of each agent (Fig. 9.19). Although vitamin C effectively protects the cells against this oxidative stress, the only proanthocyanidins which exhibited any relevant protective influence were (+)-catechin and (–)-epicatechin. This protective influence was seen only at a very high concentration for these two agents (100 μg/mL) (Figs. 9.19 and 9.20). Taxifolin was the

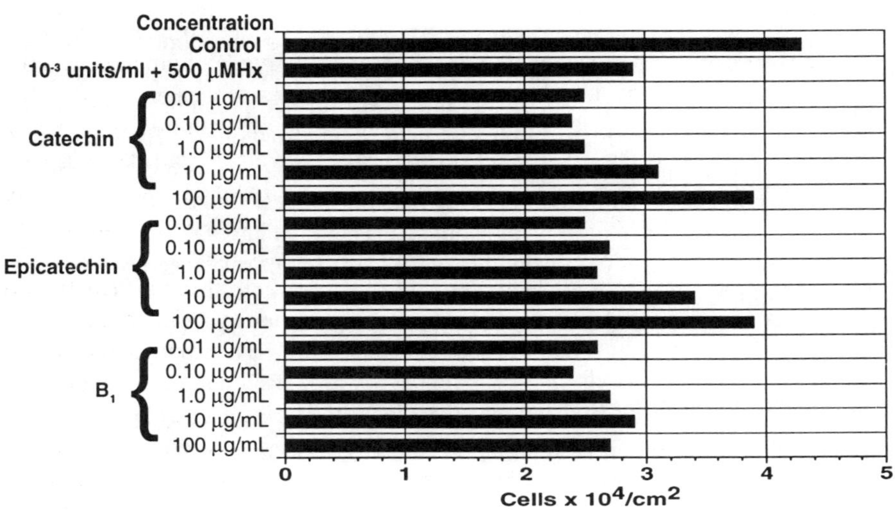

Fig. 9.19. Oxidative stress study with xanthine/xanthine oxidase (X/XO) and different concentrations of proanthocyanadins.

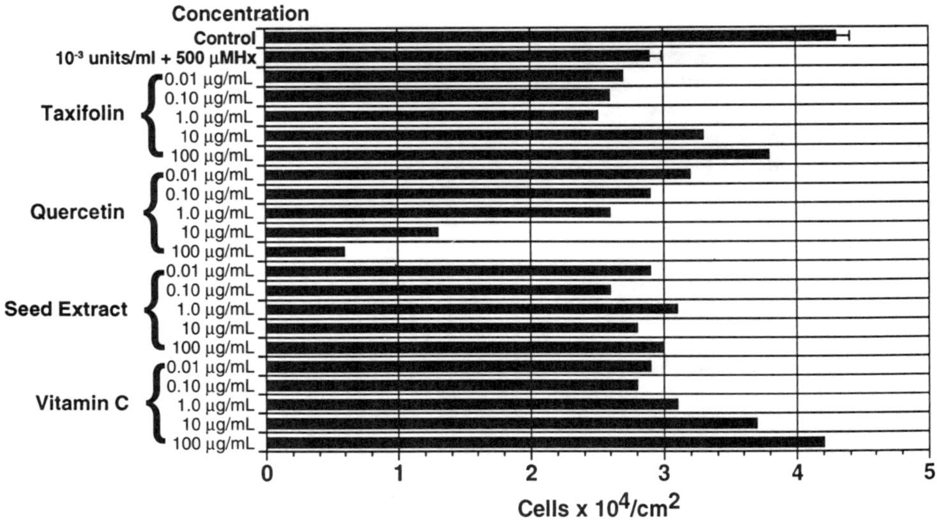

Fig. 9.20. Oxidative stress study with xanthine/xanthine oxidase (X/XO) and different concentrations of proanthocyanadins.

only other bioflavonoid that appears to provide any protective influence, and only at relatively high concentrations (100 µg/mL). Once again, quercetin appears to produce considerable cytotoxicity even at 10 µg/mL.

From these studies, we would suggest that some of the more complex proanthocyanidins may exhibit a synergistic effect with regard to free radical-induced cell damage and cell growth. In view of the potential for the dimeric proanthocyanidins to scavenge free radicals and their capacity to accommodate up to eight free radical species, it may well be that the newly formed proanthrocyanidin free radicals exhibit greater oxidative potential than originally thought. The interaction or complexation of these species with carbohydrates and proteins and their subsequent conversion to proanthocyanidin free radicals suggest that their potential for cellular damage may have been underestimated. These oxidative stress studies with human fibroblast cells in culture will be repeated to confirm these observations, but the preliminary data indicate the need to stop and think about the role of proanthocyanidins as free radical scavengers at these relatively high concentrations.

Proanthocyanidins and Potential Estrogenic Activity

Dietary phytoestrogens can be found in a variety of food sources including wholegrain products, seeds, fruits, berries, and soy products (59). The ingestion of these phytoestrogens as part of the regular diet has been tentatively linked to low levels of various diseases including breast cancer (60) and prostatic cancer (61). The mechanism associated with the protective influence from these phytoestrogens has only recently begun to be illuminated. Markaverich *et al.* (62,63) were perhaps the first to identify and speculate on the presence of a second estrogen receptor in a variety of cell types. This receptor is now referred to as the Type II estrogen binding site in contrast to the estrogen Type I receptor for which estradiol is a well-known agonist. Subsequently, these same researchers have identified the endogenous agonist for this Type II receptor as methyl para-hydroxyphenyllactate or MeHPLA (64,65). The biogenic source of this intriguing molecule has been associated with the metabolism of tyrosine (66) or the degradation of the bioflavonoid pelargonin (67). MeHPLA has been described as an inhibitor of cell growth and proliferation as a result of its action as a endogenous ligand for the nuclear Type II estrogen binding site.

These studies have now been joined by the work of Scambia *et al.*, who have demonstrated the growth inhibitory effects of quercetin and other flavonoids as potent anti-estrogenic agents operating at the Type II estrogen binding site in human MCF-7 breast cancer cells in culture (68). The structural and functional similarity of MeHPLA and quercetin to the proanthocyanidins is obvious (Fig. 9.21), and we have recently begun a study of the potential estrogenic activity of these grape seed and wine components in human MCF-7 breast cancer cells.

MCF-7 cells were established in a medium free of phenol red and supplemented with charcoal-stripped fetal calf serum. These conditions yielded a growth medium that was substantially estrogen free. Various individual polyphenolic agents isolated from grape seeds as well as the crude seed extract were exposed to these cell cultures at concentrations ranging from 1 ng/mL to 1 μg/mL for 1–4 h. The cells were then incubated for 1 h with ^{3}H-estradiol and analyzed for their ability to bind ^{3}H-estradiol to the protein fraction of the cell. All of the polyphenolic compounds tested, including the crude seed extract, blocked the binding of ^{3}H-estradiol to both estrogen type I and type II receptors. (+)-Catechin, (–)-epicatechin, quercetin, B_1, and *para*-hydroxyphenyllactic acid (HPLA) appeared to inhibit estrogen binding to both receptors with varying effectiveness. MeHPLA interfered only with ^{3}H-estradiol binding to the type II receptor as previously reported, and diethylstilbestrol (DES) interfered only with binding of estrogen to type I receptors

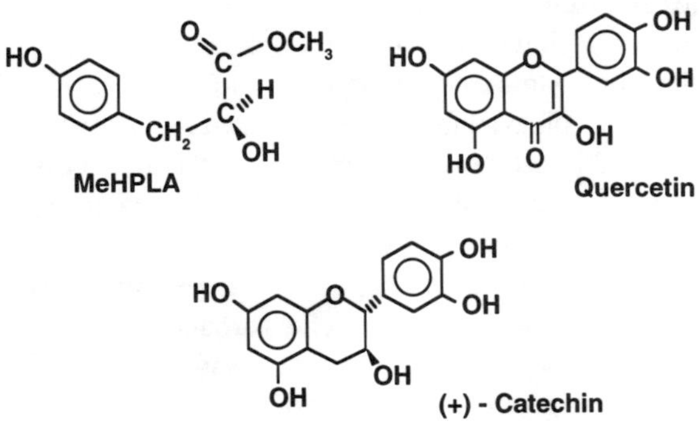

Fig. 9.21. Structural features of MeHPLA, quercetin, and proanthocyandins.

(1 ng/mL DES). On at least one occasion, quercetin appeared to stimulate the binding of ^{3}H-estradiol to both type I and type II receptors (29).

MCF-7 cells are reported to secrete proteins from estrogen-specific gene expression. However, studies examining the extracellular protein composition secreted from the MCF-7 cells treated with these same polyphenolics demonstrated no changes in extracellular-protein profiles as observed in SDS-polyacrylamide gel electrophoresis (unpublished data). Therefore, it is difficult at this time to assess the estrogen-binding capabilities of these polyphenolics as either pro- or anti-estrogen activities. These preliminary studies are continuing to more clearly define the estrogenic potential of the polyphenolic compounds isolated from grape seeds.

Conclusions

Research in the field of wine and health as it relates to the presence of proanthocyanidins has progressed in the last ten years. The antioxidant, free radical scavenging capacity of many of the proanthocyanidins has been demonstrated *in vitro* and *in vivo*, and the role of proanthocyanidins in a variety of protective mechanisms has been established. There are a number of unanswered questions, however, regarding the stability and bioavailability of these materials as well as the structure-activity-relationships (SAR) that have appeared in the literature.

One of the most important questions to be answered in the future concerns the proper dosage or exposure level required to achieve the protective influence attributed to these compounds. Analytical techniques have to be developed which can accurately detect the levels of these proanthocyanidins *in vivo* after moderate wine consumption or ingestion of grape seed extract products. There is further concern about the improper use of the grape seed products that are now appearing on the market as over-the-counter antioxidants. Our data would suggest that very high plasma concentrations of some of these agents might be counterproductive in some ways. Further study is required to evaluate the effects of these higher levels of proanthocyanidins on cell growth and antioxidant activity.

There is also the question of bioavailability or the ability of the proanthocyanidins to reach their target sites within the living system. Quercetin, which is a flavonoid found in many vegetables and fruits as well as wine, has been described as an anticancer agent *in vivo* (69). Our research with human fibroblast cells would suggest that this compound has considerable cytotoxicity even at very low dose levels. What is even more intriguing is the lack of bioavailability demonstrated by quercetin, because most of the quercetin is excreted intact. How can one explain the activity of this compound if indeed it has limited accessibility to the cells? What is the bioavailability of the other proanthocyanidins in this regard and what amounts of these compounds are metabolized before reaching their respective target sites? These questions and many more will continue to fuel the imagination of researchers around the world, and the importance of natural antioxidants and natural phytoestrogens in our diet will continue to be a very exciting area of investigation for years to come.

Acknowledgments

The authors wish to acknowledge the financial support of the Virginia Agricultural Council of the State of Virginia, the Virginia Wine Advisory Board, and the Department of Chemistry/Biochemistry, Old Dominion University. We are also indebted to the Virginia wine industry for their support and for the production of the experimental wines.

References

1. Weinges, K., Marx, W., Nader, E., Perner, and Seiler, D. (1968) *Liebigs Ann. 711*, 184.
2. Porter, L. (1988) *The Flavanoids. Advances in Research Since 1980*, Chapman and Hall, London.
3. Stafford, H.A., Lester, H.H., and Porter, L.J. (1985) *Phytochemistry 24*, 333.
4. Hemingway, R.W., and Laks, P.E. (1985) *J. Chem. Soc. Chem. Commun.*, 746.
5. Hergert, H.L. (1989) *Chemistry and Significance of Condensed Tannins* (Hemingway, R., ed.), Plenum Press, London, p.71.
6. Bourzeix, M. (1986) *Bulletin De L'O.I.V. 669–670*, 1171.
7. Lee, C.Y., and Jaworski, A. (1987) *Am. J. Enol. Vitic. 38*, 277.
8. Kantz, K., and Singleton, V. (1991) *Am. J. Enol. Vitic. 42*, 309.
9. Ricardo-Da-Silva, J., Rosec, J., Bourzeix, M., Mourgues, J., and Moutounet, M. (1992) *Vitis 31*, 55.
10. Kantz, K., and Singleton, V. (1990) *Am. J. Enol. Vitic. 41*, 223.
11. Kovac, P., Bourzeix, M., Heredia, M., and Ramos, T. (1990) *Cahier Scientifique 125*, 7.
12. Ricardo-Da-Silva, J., Belchior, A., Spanger, M., and Bourzeix, M. (1992) *Sciences Des Aliments 12*, 223.
13. Ricardo-Da-Silva, J., Rigaud, J., Cheynier, V., Cheminat, A., and Moutounet, M. (1991) *Phytochemistry 30*, 1259.
14. Oszmianski, J., and Lee, C. (1990) *Am. J. Enol. Vitic. 41*, 204.
15. Oszmianski, J., Romeyer, F., Sapis, J., and Macheix, J. (1986) *Am. J. Enol. Vitic. 37*, 7.
16. Singleton, V., and Trousdale, E. (1983) *Am. J. Enol. Vitic. 34*, 27.
17. Duvernay, J.M., Williams, R., and Recht, J. (1995) *Fourth International Symposium on Innovations in Wine Technology*, Vol. 1, Stuttgart, p. 233.
18. Singleton, V., and Draper, D. (1964) *Am. J. Enol. Vitic. 15*, 34.
19. Singleton, V., and Trousdale, E. (1992) *Am. J. Enol. Vitic. 43*, 63.
20. Delcour, J., Vandenberghe, M., Corten, P., and Dondeyne, P. (1984) *Am. J. Enol. Vitic. 35*, 134.
21. Delcour, J., Ferreira, D., and Roux, D. (1983) *J. Chem. Soc. Perkin Trans. I*, 1711.
22. Delcour, J., Serneels, E., Ferreira, D., and Roux, D. (1985) *J. Chem. Soc. Perkin Trans. I*, 669.
23. Botha, J., Ferreira, D., and Roux, D. (1981) *J. Chem. Soc. Perkin Trans. I*, 1235.
24. Thompson, R., Jacques, D., Haslam, E., and Tanner, R. (1972) *J. Chem. Soc. Perkin Trans. I*, 1387.
25. Karchesy, J., Bae, Y., Chalker-Scott, L., Helm, R., and Foo, L. (1989) *Chemistry and Significance of Condensed Tannins* (Hemingway, R., ed.), Plenum Press, London, p.139.
26. Oszmianski, J., Ramos, T., and Bourzeix, M. (1988) *Am. J. Enol. Vitic. 39*, 259.

27. Ricardo-Da-Silva, J. (1990) *J. Sci. Food Agric. 53*, 85.
28. Alonso, E., Revilla, E., Bourzeix, M., and Heredia, N. (1989) *Proceedings of the Fifth European Conference on Food Chemistry*, Vol. 2, Paris, 684.
29. Williams, R., Duvernay, J.M., and Recht, J. (1994) *Proceedings of the XVII International Conference of the Group Polyphenols*, Palma de Mallorca.
30. Michaud, J., LaCraze, P., and Masquelier, J. (1971) *J. Bull. Soc. Pharm. Bordeaux 110*, 111.
31. Reddy, J. (1993) M.S. Thesis, Old Dominion University, Norfolk, VA.
32. Haslam, E., Lilley, T., Warminski, E., Liao, H., Cai, Y., Martin, R., Gaffney, H., Goulding, P., and Luck, G. (1992) *Phenolic Compounds in Food and Their Effects on Health* (Ho, C.T., Lee, C., and Huang, M., eds.), Vol. 1, ACS Symposium Series 506, p. 8.
33. Hagerman, A. (1989) *Chemistry and Significance of Condensed Tannins* (Hemingway, R., ed.), Plenum Press, London, p. 323.
34. Masquelier, J., Michaud, J., Lappara, J., and Dumon, M. (1979) *Bull. Soc. Pharm. Bordeaux 118*, 95.
35. Masquelier, J. (1988) *Bull. De L'O.I.V. 689–690*, 554.
36. Masquelier, J. (1992) *Bull. De L'O.I.V. 733–734*, 177.
37. St. Leger, A., Cochrane, A., and Moore, F. (1979) *The Lancet i*, 1184.
38. Renaud, S., and Lorgeril, M. (1992) *The Lancet 339*, 1523.
39. Pratt, D. (1992) *Phenolic Compounds in Food and Their Effects on Health* (Huang, M., Ho, C., and Lee, C. eds.), Vol. 2, ACS Symposium Series 507, p. 54.
40. Kinsella, J., Kanner, E., Frankel, E., and German, B. (1992) *Proceedings, Potential Health Effects of Components of Plant Foods and Beverages in the Diet*, University of California, Davis, 107.
41. Hughes, L., Burton, G., Ingold, K., Slaby, M., and Foster, D. (1992) *Phenolic Compounds in Food and Their Effects on Health* (Huang, M., Ho, C., and Lee, C. eds.), Vol. 2, ACS Symposium Series 507, p. 184.
42. Ricardo-Da-Silva, J., Darmon, N., Fernandez, Y., and Mitjavila, S. (1991) *J. Agric. and Food Chem. 39*, 1549.
43. Ariga, T., Koshiyama, I., and Fukusima, D. (1988) *Agric. Biol. Chem. 52*, 2717.
44. Ariga, T., and Hamano, M. (1990) *Agric. Biol. Chem. 54*, 2499.
45. Ariga, T. (1989) U.S. Patent No. 4,797,421.
46. Hu, J., Calomme, M., Lasure, A., De Bruyne, T., Pieters, L., Vlietinck, A., and Vanden Berghe, D. (1995) *Biological Trace Element Res. 47*, 327.
47. Sichel, G., Corsaro, C., Scalla, M., Di Bilo, A., and Bonomo, R. (1991) *Free Radical Biol. Med. 11*, 1.
48. Cheynier, V., Rigaud, J., and Ricardo-Da-Silva J. (1992) *Plant Polyphenols* (Hemingway, R., and Laks, eds.), Plenum Press, New York, p. 281.
49. Frankel, E., Kanner, J., German, J., Parks, E., and Kinsella, J. (1993) *The Lancet 341*, 454.
50. Whitehead, T., Robinson, D., Allaway, S., Syms, J., and Hale, A. (1995) *Clin. Chem. 41*, 32.
51. Waterhouse, A. (1995) *Fourth International Symposium on Innovations in Wine Technology*, Vol. 1, Stuttgart, 240.
52. Demrow, H., Slane, P., and Folts, J. (1995) *Circulation 91*, 1182.
53. Duvernay, J.M., Recht, J., and Williams, R. (1993) *Proceedings of the Third International Conference on Wine and Health*, Coursan-Aude, France, p. 38.

54. Williams, R., Elliott, M., Reddy, J., and Recht, J. (1994) *Polyphenols Actualities 10*, 25.
55. Norwood, T., Smith, J., and Stein, G. (1990) *Handbook of the Biology of Aging* (Schneider, E., and Rowe, J., eds.), Academic Press, London, p. 131.
56. Richard, M., Guiraud, P., Monjo, A., and Favier, A. (1992) *Free Radical Res. Commun. 16*, 303.
57. Darmon, N., Fernadez, Y., Cambon-Gros, C., and Mitiavila, S. (1990) *Food Addit. Contam. 7*, S60.
58. Williams, R., and Elliott, M. (1994) *Proceedings of the 86th AOCS Meeting, Natural Antioxidants, Science and Applications*, May, in press.
59. Aldercreutz, H., Mousavi, Y., Clark, J., Hockerstedt, K., Hamalainen, E., Wahala, K., Makela, T., and Hase, T. (1992) *J. Steroid Biochem. Mol. Biol. 41*, 331.
60. Aldercreutz, H., Mousavi, Y., and Hockerstedt, K. (1992) *Acta. Oncologica. 31*, 175.
61. Aldercreutz, H., Markkanen, H., and Watanabe, S. (1993) *The Lancet 342*, 1209.
62. Markaverich, B., Williams, M., Upchurch, S., and Clark, J. (1981) *Endocrinology 109*, 62.
63. Markaverich, B., Roberts, R., Finney, R., and Clark, J. (1983) *J. Biol. Chem. 258*, 11663.
64. Markaverich, B., Gregory, R., Alejandro, M., Clark, J., Johnson, G., and Middleditch, B. (1988) *J. Biol. Chem. 263*, 7203.
65. Markaverich, B., Gregory, R., Alejandro, M., Kittrell, F., Medina, D., Clark, J., Varma, M., and Varma, R. (1990) *Cancer Res. 50*, 1470.
66. Karoum, F. (1985) *Biogenic Amines 2*, 269.
67. Griffiths, L., and Smith, G. (1972) *Biochem. J. 128*, 901.
68. Scambia, G., Ranelletti, F., Benedetti, P., Piantelli, M., De Vincenzo, R., Ferrandina, G., and Bonanno, G. (1993) *Int. J. Cancer 54*, 462.
69. Wiltrout, R., and Hornung, R. (1988) *J. Nat. Cancer Inst. 80*, 220.

Chapter 10

Flavonoids as Antioxidants

C. Kandaswami and E. Middleton, Jr.

Department of Medicine, Division of Allergy and Immunology, School of Medicine and Biomedical Sciences, State University of New York at Buffalo, Buffalo General Hospital, Buffalo, New York 14203.

Flavonoids and Their Biological Effects

The flavonoids (phenylchromones) are an unusually large group of naturally occurring phenolic compounds ubiquitously distributed in the plant kingdom (1–5). These aromatic compounds are formed in plants from the aromatic amino acids, phenylalanine and tyrosine, and acetate units (6,7). Phenylalanine and tyrosine are converted to cinnamic acid and *p*-coumaric acid which condense with acetate units to form the cinnamoyl structure (cinnamoyl fragment) of the flavonoids. A variety of phenolic acids such as caffeic acid, ferulic acid, and chlorogenic acid are cinnamic acid derivatives. Biotransformation of flavonoids in the gut can release these cinnamic acid derivatives (phenolic acids) (8). The flavonoids are phenylchromones (benzo-γ-pyrones) (Fig. 10.1). A phenyl group is usually substituted at the 2-position of the pyrone ring. In isoflavonoids, the substitution is at the 3-position. Flavonoids are complex and highly evolved molecules with intricate chemical variation. In plants, they generally occur as glycosylated derivatives. Conjugation with inorganic sulfate or organic acid is also known. Another known type of conjugation is malonylation. Flavonoids are categorized according to the structural class, and within each class, according to the hydroxylation pattern, other substitutions (e.g., isoprenylation), and molecular size. The different structural classes of flavonoids are shown in Table 10.1. Flavonoids and tocopherols (vitamin E) share a common structure, namely, the chromane ring. As of 1985, over 4000 chemically unique flavonoids have been identified in plants. This is only a fraction of the total number that are likely to be present in nature, because only a small percentage of plant species have been systematically examined for their flavonoid constituents (5). Unlike the alkaloids, which are restricted to about 20% of the flowering plant species, flavonoids occur universally in vascular plants (5).

The flavonoids are generally known to be present in plant, flower, leaf, and fruit as pigments (9). They are primarily responsible for plant colors, i.e., the brilliant shades of blue, scarlet, orange, and other colors present in flowers, fruits, and leaves. They are found in various fruits, vegetables, nuts, seeds, grains, spices and herbs, as well as in beverages such as tea, cocoa, and wine (10–12). Dietary exposure to flavonoids is significant. The average diet in the U.K. and the U.S. may contain up to 1 g of mixed flavonoids per day (11,13). This dietary intake far exceeds that of vitamin E, a monophenolic antioxidant, and of β-carotene (14).

A

Flavone

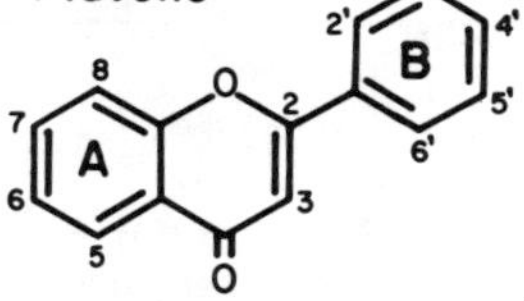

	5	6	7	8	3'	4'
Luteolin	OH	—	OH	—	OH	OH
Tangeretin	OCH_3	OCH_3	OCH_3	OCH_3	–	OCH_3
Apigenin	OH	–	OH	–	–	OH
Cirsiliol	OH	OCH_3	OCH_3	–	OH	OH

B

Flavonol

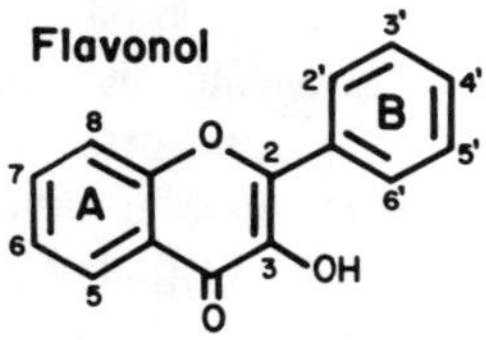

	5	7	2'	3'	4'	5'
Quercetin	OH	OH	–	OH	OH	–
Fisetin	–	OH	–	OH	OH	–
Kaempferol	OH	OH	–	–	OH	–
Myricetin	OH	OH	–	OH	OH	OH
Morin	OH	OH	OH	–	OH	–

C

Flavonol Glycosides

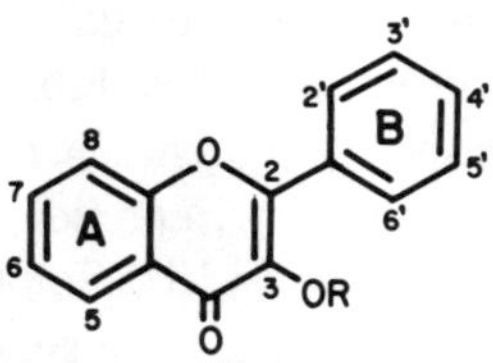

	3	5	7	3'	4'	5'
Rutin	R^1	OH	OH	OH	OH	–
Myricitrin	R^2	OH	OH	OH	OH	OH

R^1 = Rhamnosylglucoside

R^2 = Rhamnoside

D

Flavan-3-ol

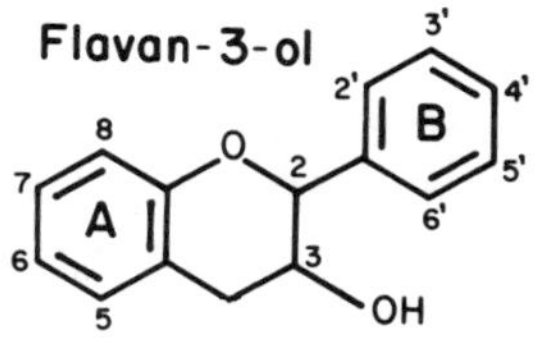

	5	7	3'	4'
Catechin	OH	OH	OH	OH

E

Isoflavone

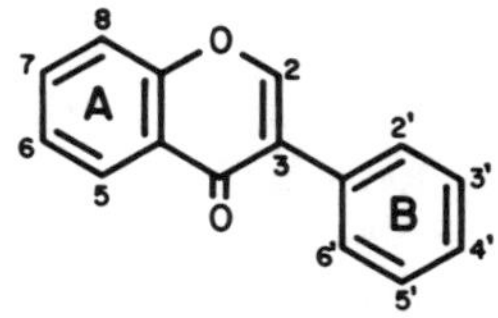

	5	6	7	4'	5'
Genistein	OH	–	OH	OH	–
Orobol	OH	–	OH	OH	OH
Tectorigenin	OH	OCH_3	OH	OH	–
Biochanin A	OH	–	OH	OCH_3	–
Formononetin	–	–	OH	OCH_3	–

F

Flavanone

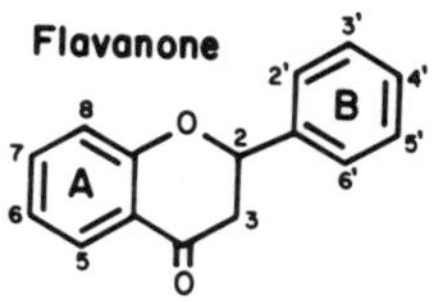

	5	7	3'	4'
Hesperetin	OH	OH	OH	OCH_3

Flavanonol

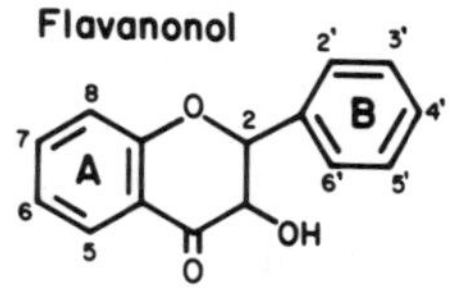

	5	7	3'	4'
Taxifolin	OH	OH	OH	OH

Silymarin

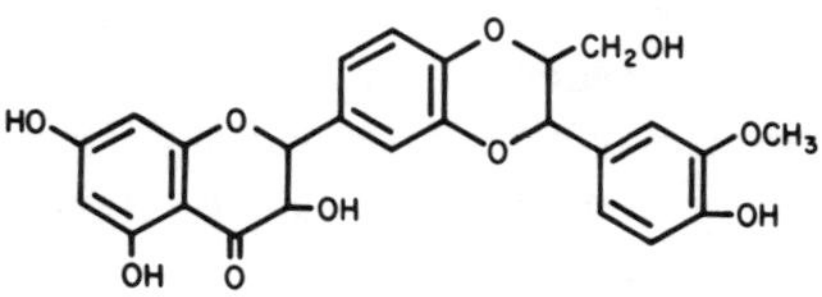

Fig. 10.1. Structures of flavonoids.

TABLE 10.1
Structural Classes of Flavonoids

Flavones	Flavanones
Flavanols	Flavananoles
Flavans, flavanols and proanthocyanidins	Biflavonoids
Isoflavonoids	Chalcones and aurones
Anthocyanins	Neoflavones (coumarins)

The past two decades have witnessed a renewed interest in the study of flavonoids and of their biological interactions with mammalian cells and tissues. Flavonoids are known to display a bewildering array of pharmacological and biochemical actions (15,16). They have long been recognized as possessing anti-inflammatory, antiallergic, antimicrobial, anthelminthic, hepatoprotective, antihormonal, antithrombotic, antiviral, antimutagenic/anticarcinogenic, and antineoplastic activities. The pleiotropic and potentially health-promoting effects of several flavonoids have come to be appreciated in many experimental situations. The flavonoids are typical phenolic compounds and therefore act as potent metal chelators and free radical scavengers (12,17–20). They are powerful chain-breaking antioxidants. The biological advantages of the ability of flavonoids to safely sequester and thus reduce the activity of the deleterious oxidant-inducing metals such as iron and copper cannot be overemphasized. Interestingly, flavonoids are known to possess vitamin C stabilizing and antioxidant-dependent vitamin C-sparing activities (12,18,21–23). They are also known to increase the absorption of vitamin C.

Flavonoids are known to modify the activities of a host of enzyme systems including protein kinase C and various other kinases, protein tyrosine kinase, aldose reductase, myeloperoxidase, NADPH oxidase, xanthine oxidase, phospholipase A_2, phospholipase C, reverse transcriptases, ornithine decarboxylase, sialidase, several ATPases, nucleotide phosphodiesterases, lipoxygenases, cyclooxygenase, cytochrome P450-dependent mixed-function oxidases, epoxide hydrolase, glutathione-*S*-transferase, and aromatase, among others (15). Some of these enzyme systems are critically involved in immune function, carcinogenesis, cellular transformation, and tumor growth and metastasis. Studies with mammalian cell systems indicate that different flavonoids can alter the function of mast cells, basophils, neutrophils, eosinophils, macrophages/monocytes, B and T lymphocytes, platelets, nerve, smooth muscle, and various cancer cells. The physiologic and pathologic processes affected by flavonoids are diverse and numerous, and include secretion, mitogenesis, platelet aggregation and adhesion to endothelial surfaces, cell motility and malignant cell proliferation, cancer metastasis and, the function/expression of adhesion molecules in various mammalian cell types (15). The antioxidant function and enzyme-modifying actions of flavonoids could account for many of their pharmacological activities.

With this general background, the antioxidant activity of flavonoids will be discussed. Reactive oxygen species (ROS) that can be scavenged or whose formation can be inhibited by flavonoids are shown in Table 10.2. Plant flavonoids are, in general, lipid soluble, and as antioxidants they can be recycled.

Influence of Flavonoids on ROS Production by Phagocytic Cells

Phagocytosis is an important physiological process which accompanies the functional production of $O_2^{\bullet-}$. Activated phagocytic cells such as monocytes, neutrophils, eosinophils and macrophages generate $O_2^{\bullet-}$ (24,25). Radical production by phagocytes is extremely important for their bacteriocidal and tumoricidal functions. Phagocytosis is accompanied by a dramatic increase in oxygen consumption (respiratory burst) with the attendant production of $O_2^{\bullet-}$, catalyzed by a membrane-bound NADPH oxidase system (24,25).

$O_2^{\bullet-}$ is generated by phagocytes dismutates to H_2O_2, a fairly unreactive molecule, which in turn gives rise to •OH by reaction with transition metal ions (26,27). This radical is extremely reactive and is one of the strongest oxidizing agents. The enzyme myeloperoxidase (MPO) provides another bacterial killing mechanism in neutrophils (28). This enzyme catalyzes the oxidation of chloride ions by H_2O_2 resulting in the formation of HOCl, a powerful bacteriocidal agent.

Even though $O_2^{\bullet-}$ is far less reactive than •OH, it can attack a number of biological targets. It can react with nitric oxide (NO•), a reactive free radical produced

TABLE 10.2
Reactive Oxygen Species That Can Be Scavenged or Whose Formation Can Be Inhibited by Flavonoids

$O_2^{\bullet-}$, superoxide anion	One electron reduction product of O_2. Produced by phagocytes. Formed in autoxidation reaction (flavoproteins, redox cycling. Generated by oxidases (heme proteins).
H_2O_2, hydrogen peroxide	Two-electron reduction product of O_2. Formed from $O_2^{\bullet-}(HO_2^{\bullet})$ by dismutation or directly from O_2. Reactivity of $O_2^{\bullet-}$ and H_2O_2 amplified in the presence of heme protein.
$^{\bullet}$OH, hydroxyl radical	Three-electron reduction product of O_2. Generated by Fenton reaction, transition metal (iron, copper)-catalyzed Heber-Weiss reaction. Formed by decomposition of peroxynitrite produced by the reaction of $O_2^{\bullet-}$ with NO (nitric oxide radical).
$RO^{\bullet}$, alkoxyl radical	Example: lipid radical ($LO^{\bullet}$)
$ROO^{\bullet}$ peroxyl radical	Example: lipid peroxy radical ($LOO^{\bullet}$). Produced from organic hydroperoxide (e.g., lipid hydroperoxide, LOOH), ROOH by hydrogen abstraction.
$^1\Delta gO_2$(also$^1O_2$)	Singlet molecular oxygen.

by cells such as phagocytes and vascular endothelial cells, to yield an even more reactive species, peroxynitrite, (29) which can decompose to form •OH in a reaction independent of transition metal ions (30). NO• is considered to be a smooth muscle relaxing factor. Endothelium-derived relaxing factor (EDRF), an important mediator of vasodilator responses, has been identified to be NO• (31,32). $O_2^{\bullet-}$ has been reported to react with NO• and inhibit its action (33). By impairing the physiological function of NO•, $O_2^{\bullet-}$ can act as a vasoconstrictor which could have deleterious consequences in some clinical situations (34).

While ROS generated by phagocytes play an important physiological function, they can also cause cellular damage. They are generated sequentially starting with $O_2^{\bullet-}$ production by a membrane-bound NADPH oxidase (24,25). The highly reactive oxygen metabolites along with other mediators elaborated by neutrophils and macrophages can promote inflammation and cause tissue damage (35). Busse *et al.* (36) showed that flavonoids inhibited ROS release (as assayed by the production of luminol-dependent chemiluminescence) by human neutrophils. Quercetin and other flavonoids were quite effective inhibitors of $O_2^{\bullet-}$ production by the cells. 'T. Hart *et al.* (37) recently reported a similar inhibitory effect of different flavonoids on ROS production by activated human neutrophils using the chemiluminescence method. Four selected flavonoids inhibited MPO release, while two of these strongly inhibited this activity. Considering luminol-dependent chemiluminescence production by neutrophils to be an MPO-dependent process, these authors contend that these effects might mask the effects of flavonoids on ROS production. Using the luminescent probe lucigenin for the exclusive detection of $O_2^{\bullet-}$ release, 'T. Hart *et al.* (37) showed that the release of this species by human neutrophils was inhibited by flavonoids. Essential determinants for inhibition of $O_2^{\bullet-}$ release appear to be the OH groups located in the B-ring of the flavonoid molecule. The formation of $O_2^{\bullet-}$ is dependent on the activation of NADPH oxidase localized in the plasma membrane, which is subject to flavonoid inhibition (38). The inhibition of protein kinase C by flavonoids can also be implicated in the impairment of the NADPH oxidase activation (39).

In addition to inhibiting the activity of a purified human neutrophil MPO, quercetin was also found to depress this activity in a system employing intact human neutrophils (40). In this case, in inhibiting the activity of the purified MPO, quercetin was significantly more potent than methimazole, a specific inhibitor of MPO (41). In addition, quercetin was found to have an ability to directly scavenge HOCl, a highly reactive chlorinated species generated by the MPO-H_2O_2-Cl system (40). Flavonoids can inhibit the formation of $O_2^{\bullet-}$ and the generation of $^{\bullet}OH$ radicals, in addition to their radical-scavenging effects. The inhibition of neutrophil MPO activity by flavonoids can result in the impairment of ROS production. Such impairment could diminish the formation of highly toxic HOCl and the hypochlorite ion (OCl^-). A consequence of this would be a decrease in the inactivation of α-1-antitrypsin, which could result in turn in the enhanced inactivation of neutrophil-derived and other tissue-damaging enzymes (42). Quercetin was found to be a potent inhibitor of human neutrophil degranulation and $O_2^{\bullet -}$ production induced by different secretogogues (43). Quercetin also inhibited the phosphorylation of neutrophil proteins accompanying neutrophil activation by phorbol myristic acetate. Phosphorylation of a specific neutrophil protein (MW 67,000) was reported to be particularly sensitive to quercetin at concentrations that also diminished neutrophil degranulation and $O_2^{\bullet -}$ production, thus suggesting that the phosphorylation of this particular protein is an important intracellular event associated with neutrophil activation (43).

Ogasawara *et al.* (44) described inhibition of anti-IgE-induced H_2O_2 generation and of human basophil histamine release by quercetin, apigenin, and taxifolin. All three flavonoids inhibited the generation of H_2O_2, but only quercetin and apigenin inhibited anti-IgE-induced histamine release. The results suggest that quercetin and apigenin possess the structural features necessary for inhibition of histamine secretion, whereas all three compounds possess structural features required for inhibition of H_2O_2 generation, suggesting a scavenging activity of the flavonoids.

Effect of Flavonoids on Lipid Peroxidation and Oxy-Radical Production

Oxidative stress can damage many biological molecules. Proteins and DNA appear to be some significant targets of cellular injury. Another target of free radical attack in biological systems is the lipids of cell membranes (26,45). Highly reactive radicals such as $^{\bullet}OH$ have the propensity to attack biological molecules by abstracting hydrogen. The most widely studied oxidative damage caused by $^{\bullet}OH$ is its capacity to initiate the free radical chain reaction, lipid peroxidation. This damage readily ensues when $^{\bullet}OH$ radicals abstract a hydrogen atom from a methylene carbon of a fatty acid or fatty acid side chain of a lipid, for instance. The lipids initially attacked by free radicals consequently become oxidized to lipid peroxides. Lipid peroxides are potentially toxic and possess the capacity to damage most cells (26,27,45,46). Accumulation of lipid peroxides has been reported in atherosclerotic plaques, in brain tissues damaged by trauma or oxygen deprivation, and in tissues poisoned by toxins. The idea that lipid peroxidation is often a secondary event consequent to primary cell damage induced by oxidative stress has been discussed (45). Rises in intracellular "free" Ca^{2+}, protein and DNA damage, and abnormalities in cellular metabolism produced by oxidative stress have been considered to be more important in causing cellular injury than is the peroxidation of membrane lipids (45).

Whether lipid peroxidation is a primary event produced by oxidative stress or a consequence of tissue damage, it can still be biologically important in exacerbating tissue injury, in view of the potential cytotoxicity and genotoxicity of the end products of lipid peroxidation (47). Lipid peroxidation products originating from dying cells could exert a cancer promotional effect (48). Great emphasis has recently been placed on the significant contribution of lipid peroxidation to the development of atherosclerosis, stroke and myocardial infarction, and to the deterioration of the brain or spinal cord that occurs following trauma or ischemia (46). Lipid peroxidation has also been implicated in several pathologic conditions including aging, hepatotoxicity, hemolysis, cancer, tumor promotion, inflammation, and iron toxicity (49–52).

Several flavonoids have been reported to inhibit either enzymic or nonenzymic lipid peroxidation. Flavonoids such as quercetin (flavonols) can suppress lipid peroxidation in model systems (53) as well as in several biological systems, such as mitochondria and microsomes (54,55), chloroplasts (56), and erythrocytes (57,58). Several studies have reported the inhibitory effects of (+) catechin, quercetin and other flavonoids on *in vitro* lipid peroxidation (59–63), generally assessed by measuring colorimetrically the formation of thiobarbituric acid-reactive substances.

Bindoli *et al.* (54) demonstrated that silymarin, a 3-OH flavanone present in *Silybum marianum* (the European milk thistle), protected rat liver mitochondria and microsomes from lipid peroxide formation induced by Fe^{2+}-ascorbate and NADPH-Fe^{3+}-ADP systems. Its antiperoxidative action was 10-fold greater than that of β-tocopherol at micromolar concentrations. While the impairment of enzymic lipid peroxidation by the flavone might involve its effect on the cytochrome P450 system, inhibition of non-enzymic lipid peroxidation has been considered to involve interaction of silymarin with free radical species responsible for lipid peroxidation (54). Silymarin and silybin are flavonoid compounds isolated from the European milk thistle. Cavallini *et al.* (55) reported that the inhibitory activity of silybin was superior to that of flavonoids even with *o*-dihydroxy or trihydroxy substitution patterns. Soybean isoflavones have been examined for their antioxidative potency by measuring the extent of inhibition of soybean lipoxygenase action and their ability to prevent peroxidative hemolysis of sheep, rat and rabbit erythrocytes (64). The extent of inhibition of the enzyme activity was positively correlated with the number of hydroxyl groups in the isoflavone nucleus. A number of isoflavones and their reduced derivatives (isoflavanones and isoflavans) were examined for inhibitory effects on lipid peroxidation in rat liver microsomes (65). The parent isoflavones and the isoflavans were by far the most potent inhibitors. Some isoflavans (6,7,4′-trihydroxy- and 6,7-dihydroxy-4-methoxyisoflavones) exceeded α-tocopherol and butylated hydroxyanisole (a synthetic antioxidant) in terms of inhibitory effect. The 6,7-dihydroxylated isoflavans were 80 times stronger than α-tocopherol in inhibiting lipid peroxidation. Methylation of the C_7-OH of the isoflavones did not reduce the inhibitory effect, whereas methylation of the C_6-OH group or both hydroxyl groups (C_6 and C_7) resulted in lowered inhibition. The position of the single phenolic group (OH) in the chromane ring of α-tocopherol corresponds to the 6-OH group of the isoflavonoids. A common feature of the active isoflavonoids is an *ortho*-dihydroxybenzene or catechol structure, which is considered to be important for antioxidative effectiveness of flavonoids (66–69).

Kimura *et al.* (70) reported that flavonoids such as wogonin, orxylin A, chrysin, skull capflavone II, baicalein and baicalin isolated from the roots of *Scutellaria baicalensis* Georgi, inhibited lipid peroxidation induced by ADP-NADP and Fe^{2+}-ascorbate in rat liver homogenates. The dried roots of *S. baicalensis* have been used for the treatment of suppurative dermatitis, diarrhea, inflammatory diseases, hyperlipidemia, and atherosclerosis in Chinese and Japanese traditional medicine. Another flavonoid isolated from these roots, 2′,5,5′,7′-tetrahydroxy-6′, 8-dimethoxyflavone, was found to be a very potent inhibitor of lipid peroxidation (71). It exhibited over 90% inhibition toward lipid peroxidation induced by both ADP plus ascorbate and ADP plus NADPH in rat liver mitochondria and microsomes at a concentration of 100 μM. Wogonin, at the same concentration, inhibited the ADP plus NADPH-induced lipid peroxidation of rat liver microsomes by 90%, whereas it inhibited the ADP plus ascorbate-induced lipid peroxidation of rat liver mitochondria by only 19%. It is worth noting that wogonin does not possess any hydroxyl substitution in its B-ring.

It was reported that lipid peroxidation can be inhibited by flavonoids possibly acting as strong $O_2^{\bullet-}$ scavengers (72) and $^1O_2$ quenchers (57). Although $O_2^{\bullet-}$ itself does not appear to be capable of initiating lipid peroxidation $HO_2^{\bullet}$ (protonated form of $O_2^{\bullet-}$) appears to do so in isolated polyunsaturated fatty acids (PUFA) (46). The role of $^1O_2$ in lipid peroxidation appears to be minor. The initiation of lipid peroxidation can be induced by $^{\bullet}OH$ and metal-ion-free radical complexes (such as perferryl and ferryl) (46). The scavenging of $^{\bullet}OH$ by flavonoids can impair lipid peroxidation. The induction of lipid peroxidation is shown below.

Initiation:	$LH + {}^{\bullet}OH \longrightarrow$	$H_2O + L^{\bullet}$
Propagation:	$L^{\bullet} + O_2 \longrightarrow$	$LOO^{\bullet}$
	$LOO^{\bullet} + LH \longrightarrow$	$LOOH + L^{\bullet}$
Termination:	$LOO^{\bullet} + LOO^{\bullet} \longrightarrow$	Inert Product
	$L^{\bullet} + L^{\bullet} \longrightarrow$	Inert Product
	$LOO^{\bullet} + L^{\bullet} \longrightarrow$	Inert Product

Lipid peroxidation may be prevented at the initiation stage by free radical scavengers, while the chain propagation reaction can be intercepted by peroxy-radical scavengers such as phenolic antioxidants (73). The chain-breaking antioxidant action of the flavonoids can be represented as shown below:

$$LOO^{\bullet} + FL\text{-}OH \longrightarrow LOOH + FL\text{-}O^{\bullet}$$

FL-OH, Flavonoid

Termination of lipid ($L^{\bullet}$) radical, lipid peroxyl radical ($LOO^{\bullet}$), and alkoxyl ($LO^{\bullet}$) radical (formed by reinitiation of lipid peroxidation induced by metal ions) by phenolic antioxidants is shown:

$$LOO^\bullet/L^\bullet/LO^\bullet + A\text{-}OH \longrightarrow LOOH/LH/LOH + AO^\bullet$$

A-OH, Phenol [e.g., α-tocopherol, flavonoids]

$AO^\bullet$, Phenoxy radical

It has also been proposed that flavonoids react with lipid peroxyl radicals ($LOO^\bullet$), leading to the termination of radical chain reactions. The oxidation of quercetin and rutin by lauroyl peroxide radicals is suggestive of such a mechanism (56). The autoxidation of linoleic acid and methyl linoleate was inhibited by flavonoids such as fustin, catechin, quercetin, rutin, luteolin, kaempferol, and morin (20). Morin and kaempferol were the most inhibitory for the autoxidation of linoleic acid. From the inhibition of the formation of *trans*, *trans* hydroperoxide isomers of linoleic acid by flavonoids, inhibition of the autoxidation of fatty acids by radical chain reaction termination was discerned (20).

Ratty and Das (74) showed that a number of flavonoids inhibited both ascorbic acid- and ferrous sulfate-induced lipid peroxidation in rat brain mitochondria. The concentrations of the flavonoids tested were rather high (0.1–4.0 mM). Structural requirements for antiperoxidative activity included a 3-OH substitution, a 4-keto group, a 2-3 double bond, and OH substitutions on rings A and B. Vicinal OH groups in the B-ring (3′,4′-OH) had no particular effect in increasing the inhibitory potency.

The mechanism of antiradical action of quercetin and its glycoside, rutin, has been evaluated by Afanas'ev *et al.* (75) sing NADPH- and carbon tetrachloride (CCl_4)-dependent lipid peroxidation of rat liver microsomes and iron ion-induced peroxidation of lecithin liposomes. Both flavonoids were significantly more effective inhibitors of the iron-ion-dependent lipid peroxidation system due to their chelation of iron ions. The chelating mechanism of inhibition was more important for rutin than for quercetin. Neither flavonoid impaired the activity of cytochrome P450 as assessed by their influence on microsomal aminopyrine demethylase. It is surprising that no effect of quercetin was found on this mixed-function oxidase activity. The inhibitory action of rutin and quercetin was demonstrated in all of the peroxidation (iron ion-dependent and non-dependent) systems studied. This action was explained by both chelating and antioxidative properties of the flavonoids. The inhibitory effects of both quercetin and rutin were more pronounced on NADPH-dependent than on CCl_4-dependent lipid peroxidation in rat liver microsomes. Microsomal NADPH-dependent lipid peroxidation is known to be catalyzed by NADPH cytochrome P450 reductase and proceeds in the presence of iron ions (76). On the other hand, the activation of CCl_4 involves cytochrome P450 and does not require iron ions (77). A much stronger inhibitory effect of the flavonoids on NADPH-dependent peroxidation was ascribed to their metal chelating properties. The flavonoids were reported to chelate iron ions and to form inert complexes unable to initiate lipid peroxidation, yet retaining their free radical-scavenging properties. At this juncture, it may be recalled that ascorbate can exhibit antioxidant activity only in the absence of transition metal ions (27). A stronger total inhibitory effect of quercetin in both peroxidation systems was thought to be due to its additional phenolic group (3-OH). Quercetin was also found to be oxidized by radicals generated in the decomposition of linoleic acid hydroperoxide in the presence of cytochrome C. The authors surmised that quercetin and rutin were able to suppress free radical processes by inhibiting the formation of $O_2^{\bullet -}$, $^{\bullet}OH$, and lipid peroxyl radicals.

In a recent study, baicalein was found to be a strong inhibitor of lipid peroxidation in rat forebrain homogenates (78). Its IC_{50} (0.42 μM) was much lower than that of quercetin (1.2 μM). Flavone was found to be inactive. Baicalein also showed free radical-scavenging action against 1,1-diphenyl-2-picrylhydrazyl (DPPH). This flavone also inhibited phorbol ester-induced ear edema in mice. Lipid peroxidation was considered to play an important role in the pathogenesis of phorbol ester-induced ear edema in mice.

Polymethoxylated flavones and C-glycosyl derivatives of flavones isolated from medicinal plants were studied for their influence on lipid peroxidation induced by $FeSO_4$ + cysteine in rat liver microsomes (79). Several hydroxylated flavones, C-glycosyl flavones, methoxyflavones, and flavonols, as well as the flavanol, leucocyanidol, and the biflavone, amentoflavone, showed inhibitory activity at a concentration of 100 μM. Some hydroxyflavones were as effective as hydroxylated flavonols in inhibiting lipid peroxidation. The same was the case with C-glycosylflavonols (e.g., rutin) and C-glycosylflavones (e.g., orientin and isoorientin). Some methoxyflavones were also quite potent in inhibiting lipid peroxidation, although their IC_{50} values were much higher than those of hydroxyflavones. The flavanone, naringin, displayed no inhibition at the stated concentration (100 μM). However, the corresponding flavone apigenin (with a 2-3 double bond) was a potent inhibitor. Galangin, a flavonol possessing no B-ring hydroxyl groups, was as effective as quercetin in inhibiting lipid peroxidation. Cirsiliol and sideritoflavone, potent lipoxygenase inhibitors (80), showed no inhibitory activity, indicating that the inhibition of arachidonic acid metabolism by these compounds is dependent on flavonoid-enzyme interactions and not related to possible antioxidant properties. A similar conclusion was also reached by Laughton *et al.* (81) who investigated the ability of various flavonoids to inhibit 5-lipoxygenase and cyclooxygenase activities of rat peritoneal leukocytes, and lipid peroxidation induced by $FeCl_3$ + ascorbate in rat liver microsomes. Several flavonols were potent inhibitors of lipid peroxidation in this system. Rutin was far less potent than quercetin. The lipid peroxidation inhibitory capacity of the flavonoids was not significantly correlated with their ability to inhibit lipoxygenase or cyclooxygenase activity, suggesting that their mode of inhibition of 5-lipoxygenase/cyclooxygenase is not simply due to scavenging of peroxyl radicals generated at the active site of the enzymes. Robak *et al.* (82) examined a series of flavonoids, isolated from plants, for their influence on soybean lipoxygenase activity, cyclooxygenase activity, and inhibition of ascorbate-stimulated lipid peroxidation in rat liver microsomes. Most of the tested flavonoids stimulated cyclooxygenase when arachidonic acid was used as a substrate at 100 μM. A number of flavonoids were inhibitors of soybean lipoxygenase activity and of lipid peroxidation. The most active inhibitors possessed vicinal hydroxyl groups in their B-ring.

An isoflavonoid glycoside containing OH groups at positions 3 and 4 of the B-ring, isolated from the roots of *Pueraria labata*, was found to inhibit enzymic (NADPH-induced) and non-enzymic (ascorbate or H_2O_2 + Fe^{2+}-induced) lipid peroxidation in rat liver microsomes (83). On the other hand, wogonin, a flavone with no OH substitution in the B-ring, inhibited only the enzymically-induced lipid peroxidation (83). Formation of Fe^{2+} by NADPH-dependent cytochrome P450 reductase was inhibited by wogonin, but not by the isoflavonoid glycoside. The glycoside had no effect on terminating radical chain reaction during lipid peroxidation in the enzymatic system or in the linoleic acid hydroperoxide-induced peroxidation system, suggesting that its antioxidant activity was probably due to its ability to scavenge free radicals involved in the initiation of lipid peroxidation.

Laughton *et al.* (84) found that both quercetin and myricetin were powerful inhibitors of iron-induced lipid peroxidation in rat liver microsomes. In these studies, peroxidation was induced by adding Fe^{2+} (as ferrous ammonium sulfate), Fe^{3+} (as ferric chloride), Fe^{3+}-ascorbic acid, Fe^{3+}-EDTA or Fe^{3+}-ADP/NADPH. Myricetin possesses *o*-trihydroxy substitution (pyrogallol structure) in its B-ring. The inhibitory effect was particularly pronounced when lipid peroxidation was stimulated by adding Fe^{3+}/ascorbate. At low concentration, the phenols caused a "lag period" during the course of lipid peroxidation. This effect was attributed to their action as lipid-soluble chain-breaking inhibitors of the peroxidative process, scavenging intermediate peroxyl and alkoxyl radicals. At 100 μM, both quercetin and myricetin accelerated the generation of $^{\bullet}OH$ radicals from H_2O_2 in the presence of Fe^{3+}-EDTA. $^{\bullet}OH$ production was inhibited by catalase and SOD which prompted the authors to suggest a mechanism in which the phenols oxidize to produce $O_2^{\bullet-}$, which then induces $^{\bullet}OH$ generation from H_2O_2 in the presence of Fe^{3+}-EDTA. At concentrations up to 75 μM, quercetin and myricetin also accelerated bleomycin-dependent DNA damage in the presence of Fe^{3+}, which was suggested to be due to the reduction of the Fe^{3+}-bleomycin-DNA complex to the Fe^{2+} form. These phenols, however, caused no acceleration of microsomal lipid peroxidation in the presence of Fe^{3+} or other iron complexes. The authors contend that the chain-breaking antioxidant activity of the phenolics outweighs any iron-reducing activity. In view of their observed prooxidant effects, the authors remark that these phenolics cannot be classified simplistically as "antioxidants." At this juncture, it may be recalled that both α-tocopherol and ascorbate have similar prooxidant effects (85–87).

Semisynthetic hydroxyethyl derivatives of flavonols have also been shown to display antioxidant action (88). These derivatives are water soluble. Several hydroxyethyl rutosides and 7,3′,4′-trihydroxyethyl quercetin exhibited considerable inhibition of rat liver microsomal lipid peroxidation induced by $FeSO_4$ and ascorbate. They were less active than quercetin. They were also shown to be potent •OH scavengers and interacted with the DPPH stable free radical. Increasing substitution on the phenolic groups resulted in a concomitant diminution in the observed inhibition of lipid peroxidation.

The antioxidant action of the flavonoids, silybin and (+)-cyanidanol-3 [(+)-catechin] was assessed in a peroxidation system consisting of linoleate and Fe^{2+} (89). At a concentration of 2 mM, silybin (a water-soluble preparation of silybin as dihemisuccinate disodium salt) inhibited Fe^{2+}-induced linoleate peroxidation. The antioxidant effect exerted by (+)-cyanidanol-3 was far greater than that of silybin at concentrations ranging from 250 μM to 2.0 mM. At a concentration of 2 mM, the inhibitory action of silybin was comparable to that of butylated hydroxyanisole, while the antioxidant effect of (+)-cyanidanol-3 was similar to that obtained with butylated hydroxytoluene, one of the most powerful synthetic antioxidants. (+)-Cyanidanol-3 has been shown to have a powerful free radical scavenging activity and to inhibit lipid peroxidation in different experimental systems (60,90–92). These include the inhibition of ethanol-induced enhancement of liver conjugated dienes (60) and of the chemiluminescence of rat liver *in situ* (92).

Fraga *et al.* (93) reported that (+)-catechin, eriodictoyl and myricetin, at low concentrations (IC50 3–15 μM) inhibited the tert-butyl hydroperoxide-initiated chemiluminescence of mouse liver homogenates that is associated with lipid peroxidation resulting from the formation of hemoprotein-catalyzed radicals following rupture of the hydroperoxide (94). Administration of eriodictyon and (+)-catechin to mice also depressed the enhancement of *in situ* liver chemiluminescence produced by CCl_4 (93). CCl_4 reacts with cytochrome P450 to initiate *in vivo* lipid peroxidation (95). Both carbon- and oxygen-centered radicals (96) and excited species (97) are formed during this process. The observed inhibition of chemiluminescence was proposed to involve free radical-scavenging as well as excited species quenching.

Sorata and co-workers (57) demonstrated that quercetin and rutin inhibited human erythrocyte lipid peroxidation accompanying photohemolysis. A number of flavonoids were observed to inhibit *N*-ethyl maleimide-induced lipid peroxidation in human platelets (98). Very low IC_{50} values were observed, and silymarin appeared to be particularly active. Utilizing phenazine methosulfate as an intracellular generator of oxygen free radicals, Maridonneau-Parini *et al.* (58). reported a heterogenous effect of flavonoids on K^+ loss and lipid peroxidation induced by oxygen radicals in human erythrocytes. These authors suggested that the flavonoids could be classified according to the activity applied, for the most part, to both K^+ permeability and to membrane lipid peroxidation. This activity would include protective, toxic, biphasic, and inactive responses. Kappus *et al.* (99) showed the inhibition of lipid peroxidation in isolated rat hepatocytes by (+)-cyanidanol-3.

Cholbi and Alcaraz (100) described the activity of apigenin, luteolin, gardenin D, galangin, datiscetin and morin as well as catechin as inhibitors of CCl_4-induced rat liver NADPH-dependent microsomal lipid peroxidation. The polymethoxylated flavone, gardenin D, possesses OH groups at the 5- and 3′-positions, and OCH_3 groups at the 6-,7-,8-, and 4′-positions. Its potency was reported to be comparable to that of (+)-catechin, showing its strong inhibitory effect on cytochrome P450.

The flavonols, quercetin, rutin, and morin and flavanones, naringin and hesperidin, were studied as chain-breaking antioxidants for the autoxidation of linoleic acid in cetyl trimethylammonium bromide micelles (101). All three flavonols exhibited antioxidant activities, whereas the two flavanones, naringin and hesperidin, did not suppress the oxidation appreciably. The 7-hydroxy group of the flavonoids is considered to be the first to dissociate and is thus the most likely site of attack by peroxy radical (102,103). The 7-hydroxy group is free for quercetin, rutin and morin, but in naringin and hesperidin, this phenolic site is blocked with a glycoside. Therefore, it was suggested that the former compounds exhibited potent antioxidant activity, whereas the latter were inactive.

Middleton, Drzewiecki, and Kandaswami (unpublished results) examined the scavenging action of a wide range of flavonoids against the DPPH radical. A number of flavonols, flavones and flavan-3-ols were active, although flavone, apigenin, naringin, naringenin, chrysin, and others showed no activity. The 2,3-double bond and the 3-OH group appeared to intensify the radical scavenging potency at lower concentrations.

Bors and Saran (104) studied the radical scavenging efficiencies of different classes of flavonoids by employing the method of pulse radiolysis. Aroxyl radicals were generated by univalent oxidation of a number of flavonoids by azide (N_3) radicals at pH 11.5. Compounds with a saturated ring were predominantly attacked at the *o*-dihydroxy site at the B-ring, and the semiquinones formed were quite stable. For a substance to act as an antioxidant, the stability of the radicals formed from it is of prime importance. Radicals derived from flavonoids with a 2,3-double bond and both 3- and 5-OH substituents (flavonols) apparently did not seem to possess a higher stability. The very high rate constant of formation and the relative stability of some of the aroxyl radicals led to the supposition that the biological function of flavonoids might be the scavenging of radicals. In a study dealing with the reaction of fatty acid peroxyl radicals, both kaempferol and quercetin turned out to be exceptionally good scavengers of linoleic acid peroxyl radicals (105).

Bors *et al.* (102) examined the radical scavenging and antioxidant potential of different classes of flavonoids, using the method of pulse radiolysis. Their studies demonstrated the effective radical scavenging capabilities of most flavonoids and indicated the existence of multiple mesomeric structures for aroxyl radical species of flavonoids. Three structural groups were important determinants for radical scavenging and for antioxidant potential: (i) the *o*-dihydroxy (catechol) structure in the B-ring, the obvious radical target site for all flavonoids with a saturated 2,3-double bond (flavan-3-ols, flavanones, cyanidin chloride); (ii) the 2, 3-double bond in conjunction with a 4-oxo function; and (iii) the additional presence of both 3- and 5-OH groups for maximal radical-scavenging potential. The capacity of flavonoids to scavenge $O_2^{\bullet -}$, $^{\bullet}OH$, and lipid radicals has been frequently reported

(20, 106–111). Flavonoids do react rapidly with $^{\bullet}OH$ because of the generally high reactivity of this radical with aromatic compounds (102). In contrast, for $O_2^{\bullet-}$, even for the very efficient flavonol radical scavengers kaempferol and quercetin, only very low rate constants were found (102), even though flavonoids have been considered as scavengers of this radical (110,111). Bors *et al.* (102) have questioned reports on the specific scavenging of different radicals by flavonoids. Sichel *et al.* (112) have recently reported the scavenger activity of some flavonoids against $O_2^{\bullet-}$ using electron spin resonance (ESR) spectrometry. These authors suggest that the presence of hydroxyl groups in the B-ring of flavonoids is essential for this scavenging activity. Cotelle *et al.* (113) showed the formation of stable radicals from synthetic flavonoids by ESR spectroscopy.

Certain flavonoids have been shown to inhibit mitochondrial succinoxidase NADH oxidase, as well as other oxidase activities (114–116). In a structure-activity investigation of 14 different flavonoids, four flavonoids, quercetagetin, quercetin, myricetin, and delphinidin chloride, were shown to generate a cyanide-insensitive respiratory burst in the presence of isolated beef heart mitochondria and to autoxidize in buffer alone (114). Subsequently, the same flavonoids were shown to autoxidize with the concomitant production of semiquinone radicals, $O_2^{\bullet-}$, $^{\bullet}OH$, and H_2O_2 (117). The inhibition of the above mitochondrial enzymes by flavonoid compounds was suggested to contribute to their antineoplastic activities. The inhibition of enzymes that catalyze oxidation-reduction reactions by flavonoids may involve flavonoid-generated ROS (114–116).

The autoxidation of flavonoids such as quercetin and myricetin (having catechol and pyrogallol configuration in the B-ring, respectively) in aqueous media at pH 7.5 has been described (118). This autoxidation resulted in the generation of $O_2^{\bullet}$, H_2O_2, and $^{\bullet}OH$. The autoxidation, however, was quite slow at pH 7.5 for quercetin. Such prooxidant effects are of interest in the context of tumor cell cytotoxicity, although not considered to have toxicological consequences *in vivo*.

Antitoxic Effects of Flavonoids

Silymarin has been shown to have hepatoprotective effects *in vivo*. Both silymarin and silybin dihemisuccinate have been shown to be effective protective agents against the hepatotoxicity of CCl_4, phalloidin, and α-amanitin (119). With regard to its protective mechanism, it is considered that the flavonoid exerts a membrane-stabilizing action, thus preventing or inhibiting lipid peroxidation (120). Silymarin has been widely used in Europe in the treatment of alcoholic liver disease and diseases associated with increased vascular permeability and capillary fragility (121).

It was reported that *in vivo* treatment with silymarin protected against lipid peroxidation and hemolysis induced in rat erythrocytes, when incubated with phenylhydrazine (122). In addition, *in vivo* treatment with silybin dihemisuccinate was shown to inhibit the release of malondialdehyde induced by phenylhydrazine in the perfused rat liver (123). Silymarin also prevented liver glutathione depletion and lipid peroxidation induced by an acute intoxication with ethanol in the rat (124). These effects attest to the suggested action of the flavonoid as a cytoprotective agent. Intraperitoneal administration (50 mg/kg) of silybin dihemisuccinate to rats inhibited lipid peroxidation, methemoglobin formation, and osmotic fragility induced *in vitro* by phenylhydrazine in erythrocytes (125). Effects on osmotic fragility was suggested to be due to a consequence of the membrane-stabilizing properties of the flavonoid. These effects were also ascribed to the antioxidant properties of the flavonoid, because spontaneous or induced oxidative stress may labilize cell membranes. The observed novel pharmacological action of silybin dihemisuccinate, primarily used in the treatment of hepatic diseases, could have other therapeutic implications. Several drugs are metabolized to hydrazine derivatives producing not only liver damage, against which silybin has been shown to have a protective effect (123), but also hematological disorders. Prophylactic or therapeutic treatment with the above flavonoids has been suggested to confer protection against these deleterious effects (125).

Elucidation of the mechanism for the protective effect of silymarin against the hepatotoxicity of CCl_4 has received considerable interest. A short report showed decreased amounts of diene conjugates in rats pretreated with silymarin prior to the administration of CCl_4 (126). The possible mechanisms for the protective effect of silymarin against the hepatotoxicity of CCl_4 have recently been elucidated by Letteron *et al.* (127). Intraperitoneal administration (800 mg/kg) of silymarin to mice protected the liver from CCl_4-induced lipid peroxidation and hepatotoxicity. Silymarin inhibited the metabolic activation of CCl_4 *in vivo*, as suggested by a decreased covalent binding of CCl_4 metabolites to hepatic lipids *in vivo*. Decreased metabolic activation of CCl_4 by cytochrome P450 will depress the initial formation of the trichloromethyl free radical and therefore diminish the initiation of lipid peroxidation. Silymarin (800 μg/mL) impaired the irreversible binding of CCl_4 metabolites to hepatic microsomal protein by only 21%, although it decreased by 72% the *in vivo* lipid peroxidation mediated by CCl_4 metabolites. Silymarin treatment *in vivo* diminished the irreversible binding of CCl_4 metabolites to hepatic lipids by only 39%, although it depressed by 60% the exhalation of ethane during the first hour after the administration of CCl_4. Silymarin (800 μg/mL) decreased by 70% *in vitro* lipid peroxidation mediated by CCl_4 metabolites, and decreased by 90% lipid peroxidation mediated by NADPH alone. In this system, lipid peroxidation is thought to be mediated by the reduction of iron to the ferrous state (128). It was reported earlier that silymarin can prevent lipid peroxidation mediated by the addition of Fe^{2+}-ascorbate, cumene hydroperoxide, or tert-butylhydroperoxide, suggesting that they can act as chain-breaking antioxidants (54,63,89,98). Letteron *et al.* (127) concluded that silymarin prevented CCl_4-induced lipid peroxidation and hepatotoxicity in mice by a dual mechanism, i.e., by decreasing the metabolic activation of CCl_4 into free radicals and by scavenging free radicals. Fehrer et al. (129) showed that silymarin treatment corrected the decreased SOD activity of erythrocytes and lymphocytes in patients with alcoholic cirrhoses, thus exemplifying the therapeutic utility of the flavonoid.

The activity of intravenous S 5682, a purified fraction containing 90% diosmin (a flavone derivative) and 10% hesperidin (a flavanone derivative) was evaluated in the rat by measuring the degree of hyperglycemia provoked by an intravenous injection of alloxan, whose metabolism produces ROS which are toxic to B cells of the pancreas. S 5682 produced a decrease in hyperglycemia in a dose-dependent manner (25 and 50 mg/kg) (129). The authors suggest that the radical scavenging properties of S 5682 might explain its diverse pharmacological effects such as (i) the reduction in capillary permeability induced in the rat and rabbit by the injection of antigenic particles, the application of chloroform swabs, or by irradiation, and (ii) the anti-inflammatory and antiedematous effects seen in inflammatory granulomas in the rat (130).

The flavonoids quercetin, kaempferol, catechin, and taxifolin suppressed the cytotoxicity of $O_2^{\bullet -}$ and H_2O_2 on Chinese hamster V79 cells, as assessed with a colony formation assay (131). Quercetin and kaempferol showed protective effects at 5–10 μM concentrations, whereas much higher concentrations of catechin and taxifolin were necessary for the prevention of cytotoxicity. The protective activity was ascribed to the *o*-dihydroxy structure in the B-ring, or 3- and 5-OH groups with the 4-oxo function or the 2,3-double bond in conjunction with the 4-oxo function. The authors earlier suggested that the *o*-dihydroxy structure of polyphenols was essential for protection against H_2O_2-induced cytotoxicity in V79 cells, because antioxidants bearing only one phenolic OH, such as ferulic acid methyl ester and α-tocopherol, exhibited no protective effects (132). The observation that kaempferol, lacking the above structure, showed protective effect seems to be an exception. The conversion of kaempferol to quercetin by *o*-hydroxylation under the experimental conditions might explain this effect. The mutagenic effect of chrysotile asbestos fibers, and zeolite and latex particles on human lymphocytes in whole blood was inhibited by antioxidant enzymes, SOD and catalase, and radical scavengers such as rutin, ascorbic acid, and bemitil, indicating that the mutagenic effects of the particles was mediated by oxygen radicals (133). Of the radical scavengers studied, rutin was the most effective inhibitor of the mutagenic effect of mineral fibers and dusts. The study of lucigenin- and luminol-amplified chemiluminescence of peritoneal macrophages stimulated by the above fibers and particles showed that their mutagenic action was probably mediated by different oxygen species. Rutin was more potent than ascorbate in inhibiting luminol-dependent chemiluminescence of peritoneal macrophages activated by chrysotile fibers or zeolite particles (133).

Kantengwa and Polla (134) reported that erythrophagocytosis in human monocytes-macrophages induced the synthesis of stress proteins including the classical heat shock proteins and heme oxygenase. Quercetin and kaempferol inhibited this induction. The results suggest that (i) erythrophagocytosis-related oxygen radicals are involved in the induction of the stress response in phagocytic cells; (ii) the induction of classical heat shock proteins appears, at least in part, to be dependent on protein kinase C; whereas heme oxygenase appears to be strictly dependent on reactive oxygen species; and (iii) the effects of the flavonoids on heme oxygenase are linked to their scavenging activity rather than to protein kinase C modulation. Antioxidant catechins (flavans) isolated from Chinese green tea showed scavenging activity against H_2O_2 and $O_2^{\bullet -}$ (generated by the xanthine-xanthine oxidase system (135). The flavans also prevented oxygen radical-induced cytotoxicity and inhibition of intercellular communication in cultured B6C3F1 mouse hepatocytes and keratinocytes (NHEK cells). Cytotoxicity and inhibition of intercellular communication represent two possible mechanisms by which tumor promoters produce their promoting effects (136). The prevention of these two effects of prooxidants by tea flavans may suggest a mechanism by which these catechins inhibit tumor promotion *in vivo*.

The cytoprotective effect of three flavonoids, catechin, quercetin, and diosmetin, was recently investigated on iron-loaded rat hepatocyte cultures, considering two parameters, namely, the prevention of iron-induced increase in lipid peroxidation and the inhibition of intracellular lactate dehydrogenase release (137). The potency of these flavonoids for the above two aspects of cytoprotection was classified as follows: catechin > quercetin > diosmetin. The investigation of the capacity of these above flavonoids to remove iron from iron-loaded hepatocytes revealed that the iron-chelating capacity of the three compounds followed the same order as did the cytoprotective effect (catechin > quercetin > diosmetin). The authors suggest that this relationship has to be taken into consideration in further development of these protective flavonoids which could have important applications in human diseases, such as the widely known silymarin used in liver dysfunction, and diosmin acting as vascular protectant. Some flavonoids have been reported to be able to mobilize iron from ferritin (138) and to be capable of reducing Fe^{3+} to Fe^{2+} ions (139). These considerations were thought to be of importance, although some authors ruled out the possibility that the antiperoxidative action was related to an interaction of the flavonoids with iron ions (54,140).

Flavonoid Action in Relation to Coronary Artery Disease and Ischemia Reperfusion

De Whalley *et al.* (141) showed that certain flavonoids were potent inhibitors of the modification of low density lipoproteins (LDL) by mouse macrophages with IC_{50} values in the micromolar range (e.g., 1–2 μM for fisetin, morin, and quercetin). Flavonoids also inhibited the cell-free oxidation of LDL mediated by $CuSO_4$. The flavonoids appeared to act by protecting LDL against oxidation caused by the macrophages, because they inhibit the generation of lipid hydroperoxides and protect α-tocopherol, a major lipophilic antioxidant carried in lipoproteins, from being consumed by oxidation in the LDL. The flavonoids protect the α-tocopherol (and possibly other endogenous antioxidants) in LDL from oxidation, maintain their levels for longer periods of time and delay the onset of lipid peroxidation. While the mechanisms by which flavonoids inhibit LDL oxidation are not certain, the following possibilities have been advanced. They may reduce the generation or release of free radicals in the macrophages or may protect the α-tocopherol in LDL from oxidation, by being oxidized by free radicals themselves in preference to it. Another possible mechanism is that the flavonoids could have regenerated active α-tocopherol by donating a hydrogen atom to the α-tocopheryl radical, which is formed when it transfers its own OH hydrogen atom to a lipid peroxy radical to terminate the chain reaction of lipid peroxidation. Another possibility is the sequestration of metal ions such as iron and copper by flavonoids, thereby diminishing the engendered free radicals in the medium. Because some flavonoids at a concentration of only 10 μM completely inhibited the modification of LDL by 100 μM Cu^{2+}, doubt was raised whether metal complexation by flavonoids could explain all their effects. Macrophage-associated free radicals could be derived from a number of sources, two of which are as by-products of the action of 5-lipoxygenase and cyclooxygenase. No obvious correlations were apparent, however, between the known potencies of individual flavonoids in inhibiting these two enzymes and their potencies in inhibiting LDL modification. Flavone itself was not a good inhibitor of LDL modification by macrophages, whereas the polyhydroxylated aglycone flavonoids were potent inhibitors. The importance of OH groups of the flavone nucleus could thus be discerned.

Negre-Salvayre *et al.* (142) reported the protection of lymphoid cell lines against peroxidative stress induced by oxidized LDL utilizing a combination of α-tocopherol, ascorbic acid, and the quercetin glycoside, rutin. These investigators have also shown that the cytotoxicity of oxidized LDL can be prevented by flavonoids in two ways, either by inhibiting the lipid peroxidation of LDL [induced by ultraviolet (UV) irradiation] or by blocking at the cellular level the cytotoxicity of previously oxidized LDL (143). Their studies showed that (i) probucol (25 μM), a synthetic antioxidant, was very effective in preventing UV-induced lipid peroxidation of LDL and their subsequent cytotoxicity on lymphoid cell lines (EBV-transformed cell lines), but it could not protect cells against the cytotoxicity of previously oxidized LDL; (ii) vitamin E (100 μM) prevented the lipid peroxidation of LDL poorly, but it was able to abrogate the cellular oxidative stress and cytotoxicity induced by previously oxidized LDL; and (iii) catechin (10 μM) exhibited two types of protective effects, namely, it inhibited the peroxidation of LDL and their subsequent cytotoxicity and very effectively protected the cells against the toxicity of previously oxidized LDL. In subsequent studies, the above investigators showed that both quercetin and rutin exhibited effects similar to those of catechin, *viz.*, inhibiting the lipid peroxidation of LDL and blocking at the cellular level the cytotoxicity of previously oxidized LDL (144). Flavone was completely inefficient in exerting any of these effects. The oxidation of LDL induced by UV-radiation attacks mainly the lipid core of the LDL, in contrast to the cell- or copper-mediated oxidation which attacks primarily the LDL surface components (145). The inhibition of LDL lipid peroxidation by the flavonoids was well correlated with the prevention of the cytotoxicity of oxidized LDL.

In the protection of the cells by polyphenolic flavonoids, two lines of defense were inferred: (i) at high concentrations (IC_{50}, 10–20 μM for quercetin or rutin), an antioxidant effect inhibiting the lipoprotein oxidation and subsequent cytotoxicity; (ii) at low concentrations (IC50, 0.1 and 3 μM for quercetin or rutin), direct protection of cells against the cytotoxic effect of oxidized LDL. The intracellular mechanisms for this direct prevention of the cytotoxic effect of oxidized LDL are unknown. The authors suggest that quercetin acts at the cellular level by blocking the intracellular "transduction" of the cytotoxic "signal" contained in oxidized LDL. The authors suggest that the cellular mechanisms underlying the protective effect could be related to the various biological actions of quercetin such as (i) antioxidant properties preventing oxidative attack of membrane lipids by sparing vitamin E or regenerating it as does ascorbic acid in the maintenance of α-tocopherol levels; (ii) inhibition of lipoxygenases which are known to be stimulated by lipid peroxides and which can be involved in oxidative stress, as suggested by their role in LDL oxidation in cells; and (iii) inhibition of cellular enzymes involved in signal transduction. The above results suggest that dietary flavonoids or related compounds could be involved in the prevention of atherosclerosis not only by inhibiting LDL oxidation but also by increasing the cellular resistance to the deleterious effects of oxidized LDL. Recruitment of different flavonoids effective in directly protecting cells represents a novel approach in the prevention of atherosclerosis by nutritional intervention.

A recent study from the Netherlands showed an inverse correlation between dietary flavonoid intake and the incidence of coronary artery disease (146). The individuals with the lowest dietary intake of flavonoids had the highest incidence of heart disease. Interestingly, the relative incidence of heart disease among men who had the highest intake of flavonoids was only a third of those who had the lowest intake of flavonoids. The results were the same even after adjustment for age, body fat, smoking, cholesterol, blood pressure, physical activity, coffee consumption, and the intake of calories, vitamin C, vitamin E, β-carotene and dietary fibers. The main sources of dietary flavonoids for the above individuals were apples, onions, and tea.

Consumption of diets high in saturated fat and cholesterol is associated with increased risk of coronary artery disease. However, epidemiological evidence indicates that the incidence of heart disease is lower in the French than expected, based on saturated fat intake and cholesterol levels. This unusual effect, known as the "French Paradox," has been attributed to the drinking of red wine. A recent study indicates that polyphenolic compounds (e.g., anthocyanin flavonoids and related compounds) present in wine could exert a protective effect (147). Quercetin and phenolic compounds isolated from red wine effectively impaired copper ion-catalyzed oxidation of LDL. The antioxidant activity of the extracts from red wine, even after 1000-fold dilution, far exceeded that of vitamin E. α-Tocopherol exhibited only 60% of the potency of wine phenolics or quercetin (147).

Two flavonoids, quercetin and silybin, were reported to exert a protective effect by preventing the decrease in the xanthine dehydrogenase/oxidase ratio observed during ischemia-reperfusion in the rat (148). The results indicated the conversion of xanthine dehydrogenase to xanthine oxidase during the early stages of kidney ischemia. The enzyme xanthine oxidase, implicated in tissue oxidative injury after ischemia-reperfusion, is a source of ROS and is formed from a dehydrogenase during ischemia (149). The protective effect of quercetin and silybin on the xanthine dehydrogenase/oxidase ratio, observed in the above study, was postulated to be due to the inhibition of the dehydrogenase to oxidase transformation by the flavonoids. The inhibition of xanthine oxidase activity by flavonoids has been described earlier (150). Ning *et al.* (151) reported that flavone administration markedly improved functional recovery in the reperfused rabbit heart after a bout of global ischemia. The effects of the compound on postischemic recovery were proposed to be due to its stimulation of the cytochrome P450 system. Cytochrome P450 reductase, which transfers electrons from NADPH to cytochrome P450 during P450-dependent catalysis, is capable of reducing oxygen to yield $O_2^{\bullet -}$, and the oxygenated intermediates of P450 themselves decompose in a side reaction to release $O_2^{\bullet -}$ (152,153). It was advanced that flavone might be acting as an allosteric effector that improves catalytic efficiency, thereby diminishing detrimental ROS production (151). Ning *et al.* (151) have highlighted the potential utility of flavonoids as a means of enhancing myocardial ischemic tolerance or resistance to reperfusion injury, or both. They also point out the recent identification of an interesting flavonoid compound, puerarin (8-C-C-glycopyranosyl-1-4′-7-dihydroxyisoflavone), as an active ingredient of *Radix puerariae*, a traditional Chinese medicinal herb that has been used for decades for the treatment of hypertension and angina pectoris in China (154).

The vascular endothelium is extremely sensitive to oxidative damage mediated by ROS released from inflammatory cells (155,156). Of these metabolites, H_2O_2 appears to be an important mediator of acute cellular injury in a variety of settings (156). Such oxidative damage may play a role in the pathogenesis of atherosclerosis (157). The flavan-3-ol compounds, gallocatechin-3-*O*-gallate and epicatechin-3-*O*-gallate, isolated from tea, were effective in preventing H_2O_2-induced injury to bovine endothelial cells in culture (158). These observations suggest a possible role for these catechins in maintaining vascular homeostasis.

Gryglewski and coworkers studied the mechanism of the antithrombotic action of flavonoids (159). Four flavonoids (quercetin, rutin, cianidanol, and meciadonol) inhibited platelet lipoxygenase activity and ascorbate-induced rat liver microsomal lipid peroxidation, whereas only quercetin and rutin stimulated cyclooxygenase and bound to platelet membranes. Quercetin and rutin were capable of dispersing platelet thrombi adhering to rabbit aortic endothelium *in vitro* and prevented platelets from aggregating over a blood-superfused collagen strip (adhesion-related phenomena). The *in vivo* counterpart of these experiments involved the infusion of quercetin and rutin into an extracorporeal stream of blood. Quercetin and rutin inhibited the deposition of platelet thrombi on the blood-superfused collagen strip at calculated plasma concentrations of 0.05 and 0.03 μM, respectively. Analogously, in the model for studying platelet-endothelium interactions, quercetin and rutin, when infused into the stream of blood which superfused a rabbit aortic endothelial surface, caused the disaggregation of preformed platelet thrombi, again at low concentrations. Clearly, the expression and/or activity of platelet/endothelium adhesion molecules is affected by the flavonoids. The authors concluded that flavonols are antithrombotic because they are bound selectively to mural platelet thrombi and, because of their free radical-scavenging properties, modify damaged endothelial cells and permit normal prostacyclin and EDRF (159).

Flavonoids and Ascorbic Acid Interactions

Ascorbic acid is a universal component of plant cells. Ascorbic acid and flavonoids coexist in plants and thus the two are consumed together in the diet (18,21). A large literature has accumulated concerning the interactions of flavonoids with ascorbic acid in biological systems (12,18,22). Several flavonoids serve as antioxidants for ascorbic acid. One of the mechanisms for this effect is thought to be by chelating metals, even though the free radical accepting action may be more important. The sparing effect of flavonoids on ascorbate oxidation may explain many of the interactions of flavonoids with ascorbic acid described in the voluminous literature on these compounds. Of historical importance is the observation that a mixture of two flavonoids called citrin (eriodictoyl and hesperidin) was considered to possess vitamin-like activity (12,18). The term vitamin P was coined to indicate that this material had the property of decreasing capillary permeability (and fragility), prolonging the life of marginally scorbutic guinea pigs, and reducing the signs of hypovitaminosis C in experimental animals. The term vitamin P was subsequently abandoned, because citrin was not found to fulfill the classical function of a vitamin. Nevertheless, subsequent studies have shown that flavonoids have potent antioxidant-dependent vitamin C-sparing activity (12,18). Human studies showed increased tissue concentration of ascorbic acid as well as increased urinary output of the vitamin (18,23). Considerable evidence indicates that flavonoids may influence the metabolism of ascorbic acid although the basis of this impact is not understood (18,23).

In vitro studies indicated that flavonoids had a considerable capacity for retarding the breakdown of ascorbate to dehydroascorbate (160). One mechanism for this protection might involve the chelation of copper and other trace metals by flavonoids, resulting in the retardation of metal-catalyzed oxidation of ascorbic acid. Another protective mechanism is based on the ability of flavonoids to act as free radical acceptors. Free radical formation is considered to be an all-important phase of ascorbate oxidation. Clemtson and Anderson related ascorbate-protective capacity to the structure of the flavonoids (22). They examined the effect of some 34 different flavonoids on the oxidation of ascorbic acid at physiological pH and concluded that significant antioxidant activity was confined to compounds possessing (i) 3′,4′-OH groups (couplet) of the B-ring, and (ii) the 3-hydroxy-4-carbonyl group (couplet) of the γ-pyrone ring. In agreement with this, quercetin and rutin were found to have a greater ascorbic acid-protective capacity than the other flavonoids examined (18). An apparent exception to the above generalization is hesperidin which did not conform to the prescribed pattern and yet had *in vitro* protective capacity and increased the tissue ascorbic acid concentrations *in vivo* (161,162). It was reported that commercial samples of hesperidin contained other flavonoids as impurities (22).

Thiol compounds such as glutathione are potential hydrogen donors for the reduction of dehydroascorbic acid to ascorbic acid (18,163). Flavonoids such as quercetin and hesperidin were shown to enhance the reduction of dehydroascorbic acid by glutathione. Parrot and Gazave (163) reported that (+)-catechin potentiated the reduction of dehydroascorbic acid by glutathione. It has been suggested that certain flavonoids [flavan-3-ols (e.g., catechin)] designated as vitamin C_2 (or C_2 factor) and regarded as a second antiscorbutic factor, can potentiate the chemical reduction of dehydroascorbic acid (18). While studying the reduction of dehydroascorbic acid to ascorbic acid by thiols in an aerobic environment, Regnault-Roger *et al.* (164) reported that the flavan-3-ol configuration of C_2 factor compounds such as epicatechin plays a specific role as a catalyst in this reaction, which might not be dependent on the redox potential alone. The possibility that flavonoids might stimulate the tissue reduction of dehydroascorbic acid was examined by Zloch (165). In Guinea pigs given a standard diet of dehydroascorbic acid with and without flavonoids (rutin, epicatechin), the tissue ascorbic acid content was 30–100% greater in the case of the flavonoid-treated group.

Several physiological interactions of ascorbic acid with plant flavonoids have been considered (18) such as (i) increase in ascorbic acid absorption, (ii) stabilization of ascorbic acid, (iii) reduction of dehydroascorbate to ascorbate, and (iv) metabolic sparing of ascorbic acid by flavonoids. Flavonoids have been considered to function as antioxidants and UV light filters in higher plants (21). This antioxidant activity has been related to their protection against ascorbic acid oxidation. The oxidation of ascorbic acid by metal ions such as Cu^{2+} and copper-containing enzymes is well known (166). The inhibitory effect of flavonoids on ascorbic acid oxidation is considered to be due to metal-flavonoid complexation and/or free-radical trapping by the flavonoids (18). The protection of ascorbic acid by flavonoids could have important biological implications as emphasized by Hughes and Wilson (18). Ascorbic acid metabolites can be mutagenic for mammalian cells (167). An increased production of these metabolites could be a key factor in aging, according to the intrinsic mutagenesis theory of aging (168). Flavonoids and other factors which suppress the breakdown of ascorbic acid could, therefore, function as anti-aging factors. Ascorbate may also protect flavonoids from oxidation. Purified cyanidin 3-gentiobioside, cyanidin 3-rhamnoside, and pelargonidin 3-glucoside were decolorized by low levels of H_2O_2 and horseradish peroxidase. Ascorbate added to this system inhibited the decolorization of the anthocyanins to one tenth the rate of the control, apparently by reducing an early oxidation product of anthocyanin breakdown (21). This scheme has implications in flavonoid metabolism.

Sorata *et al.* (169) studied the promoting effect of ascorbate on quercetin-induced suppression of photohemolysis in human erythrocytes. These authors suggested that the cooperation of quercetin with ascorbate in photohemolysis was due to the reduction of oxidized quercetin by ascorbate, resulting in the regeneration of the flavonol. Takahama's studies also suggested the reduction of oxidized quercetin to quercetin by ascorbate (107). This author reported the suppression of photooxidation of quercetin by ascorbate; during this suppression, ascorbate was oxidized. Jan *et al.* (170) reported that the antioxidative function of quercetin in inhibiting the photooxidation of α-tocopherol was enhanced by ascorbate. The enhancement was attributed to the reduction of oxidized quercetin by ascorbate. Takahama showed that the intermediates formed during the oxidation of flavonoids by the horseradish peroxidase-H_2O_2 system might be reduced by ascorbate; the oxidized product which could be reduced by ascorbate appeared to be an ortho-quinone derivative (171).

An example with potential clinical relevance is the preservation of antiviral activity of quercetin in the presence of ascorbate which inhibits the oxidative degradation of the quercetin (172). Maintenance of biological activity of other flavonoids by ascorbate is also suggested by the experiments of Kandaswami *et al.* (173) who found that ascorbic acid augmented by about twofold the antiproliferative effect of fisetin and quercetin on proliferation of HTB43 squamous cell carcinoma in tissue culture. Flavone had no effect, indicating the requirement for hydroxylation; most likely, the ascorbic acid had flavonoid protective activity. In other experiments (Middleton, Drzewiecki, and Kandaswami, unpublished observations), it was demonstrated that low concentrations of ascorbic acid completely blocked the oxidation of quercetin in aqueous media at pH 7.5 as determined spectrophotometrically over a 24-h period. Considering the redox potentials for the reduction of ascorbic and metal ions (166), ascorbic acid can itself reduce cupric and ferric ions. Metal ions such as Cu^{2+} are known to oxidize flavonols such as quercetin in aqueous media (174). Chelation of the vicinal hydroxyl groups of quercetin by Cu^{2+} would result in its conversion to quinone. The reduction by ascorbic acid of the quinone to the flavonol could have enhanced its biological activity in the above instances.

Conclusions

A large number of studies have emphasized the potential health-promoting and disease-preventive effects of fruits and vegetables. The beneficial effects of fruits and vegetables have frequently been attributed to ascorbic acid and the carotenoids present in these foods. However, as stated elsewhere, fruits and vegetables contain a multitude of flavonoids and related phenolic compounds. The importance of flavonoids in disease prevention is being increasingly realized. The significance of these protective phytochemicals is emerging as an important issue. The natural antioxidants from plants are phenolic compounds. Flavonoids and related cinnamic acid derivatives, coumarins, tocopherols, and phenolic acids constitute the most common antioxidants. Flavonoids can function as (i) metal chelators and reducing agents,

(ii) scavengers of ROS, (iii) chain-breaking antioxidants, and (iv) quenchers of the formation of singlet oxygen. Protection of ascorbic acid appears to be one of their important functions. They form complexes with metals. However, their primary antioxidant activity could be of greater value. In many of the studies reported, it is not certain whether flavonoids inhibit the formation of ROS or scavenge them. It is obvious that flavonoids react with $^{\bullet}OH$ and, therefore, can be very important chain-breaking antioxidants. They could play an important role in conserving tocopherols in biological membranes. Flavonoids could also be important in protecting LDL from oxidation, thus reducing their atherogenicity. In general, flavonoids could potentially influence disease states in which lipid peroxidation products are intricately involved. Flavonoids can be important for protection against liver diseases, vascular disorders, and heart diseases. Recent studies emphasize the importance of olive oil, red grapes, and red wine in the protection against coronary artery disease. The flavonoid constituents of those food substances appear to be responsible for disease prevention. Studies of blood lipids and recent evidence concerning the susceptibility of LDL to oxidation suggest that consumption of olive oil as a primary fat is responsible in part for the decreased incidence of cardiovascular disease reported in the Mediterranean countries (175). Flavonoids and related phenolics found in olive oil could account for the potent antioxidant activity of olive oil (176,177) and could also be responsible in part for the salutary effects of olive oil. Recent studies have identified isoflavonoids as constituents of plasma in healthy human subjects. No information is available as yet on the plasma concentrations of other flavonoids. Obtaining such information is of crucial importance, because dietary exposure to flavonoids is substantial. Antioxidant flavonoids have been shown to have cancer-preventive effects in experimental animals. They could have a marked influence on the metabolic activation of chemical carcinogens by virtue of their modulating effects on carcinogen-metabolizing enzymes. Flavonoid inhibition of enzymes such as lipoxygenase and phagocyte NADPH oxidase involved in oxidative stress could play a role in the inhibition of tumor promotion. Plant flavonoids are a relatively unexplored group of potentially important nontoxic dietary antioxidants that warrant further intensive investigation.

Acknowledgments

The financial assistance from the Cancer Research Foundation of America, the Department of Citrus, State of Florida, and Margaret Duffy and Robert Cameron Troup Memorial Fund is gratefully acknowledged.

References

1. Harborne, J.B., Mabry, T.J., and Mabry, M. (1975) *The Flavonoids*, Academic Press, New York.
2. Harborne, J.B., and Mabry, T.J. (1982) *The Flavonoids: Advances in Research*, Chapman and Hall, London.
3. Harborne, J.B. (1988) *The Flavonoids: Advances in Research Since 1980*, Chapman and Hall, London.

4. Harborne, J.B. (1993) *The Flavonoids: Advances in Research Since 1986,* Chapman and Hall, London.
5. Harborne, J.B. (1986) in *Plant Flavonoids in Biology and Medicine: Biochemical Pharmacological and Structure-Activity Relationships* (Cody, V., Middleton, E., and Harborne, J.B., eds.), Alan R. Liss, New York, p. 15.
6. Harborne, J.B. (1988) in *Plant Flavonoids in Biology and Medicine: Biochemical, Cellular and Medicinal Properties* (Cody, V., Middleton, E., and Harborne, J.B., eds.), Alan R. Liss, New York, p. 17.
7. Ebel, J., and Hahlbrock, K. (1982) in *The Flavonoids: Advances in Research* (Harborne, J.B., and Marby, T.J., eds.), Chapman and Hall, London, p. 641.
8. Scheline, R.R. (1991) *Handbook of Mammalian Metabolism of Plant Compounds*, CRC Press, Boca Raton.
9. Brouillard, R., and Cheminant, A. (1988) in *Plant Flavonoids in Biology and Medicine: Biochemical, Cellular and Medicinal Properties* (Cody, V., Middleton, E., and Harborne, J.B., eds.), Alan R. Liss, New York, p. 93.
10. Hermann, K. (1976) *J. Food Technol. 11*, 433.
11. Kuhnau, J. (1976) *World Rev. Nutr. Diet 24*, 117.
12. Clemetson, C.A.B. (1989) *Vitamin C*, CRC Press, Boca Raton.
13. Pierpoint, W.S. (1986) in *Plant Flavonoids in Biology and Medicine: Biochemical, Pharmacological and Structure-Activity Relationships* (Cody, V., Middleton, E., and Harborne, J.B., eds.), Alan R. Liss, New York, p. 125.
14. Hertog, M.G.L., Hollman, P.C.H., Katan, M.B., and Kromhout, D. (1993) *Nutr. Cancer 20*, 21.
15. E. Middleton, Jr., and Kandaswami, C. (1993) in *The Flavonoids: Advances in Research Since 1986* (Harborne, J.B., ed.), Chapman and Hall, London, p. 619.
16. Middleton, E. Jr., and Kandaswami, C. (1992) *Biochem. Pharmacol. 43*, 1167.
17. Pratt, D.E. (1992) in *Phenolic Compounds in Food and Their Effects on Health II* (Huang, M.-T., Ho, C.-H., and Lee, C.Y., eds.), American Chemical Society, Washington, p. 54.
18. Hughes, R.E., and Wilson, H.K. (1977) in *Progress in Medicinal Chemistry* (Ellis, G.P., and West, G.B., ed.), Vol. 14, Elsevier, Amsterdam, p. 285.
19. Lea, C.H., and Swoboda, P.A.T. (1956) *Chem. Ind.*, 1426.
20. Torel, J., Cillard, J., and Cillard, P. (1986) *Phytochemistry 25*, 383.
21. McClure, J.W. (1975) in *The Flavonoids* (Harborne, J.B., Mabry, T.J., and Mabry, H., eds.), Academic Press, New York, p. 970.
22. Clemetson, C.A.B., and Anderson, L. (1966) *Ann. N.Y. Acad. Sci. 136*, 341.
23. Jones, E., and Hughes, R.E. (1984) *IRCS Med. Sci. 12*, 320.
24. Babior, B.M., and Woodman, R.C. (1990) *Semin. Hematol. 27*, 24.
25. Curnutte, J.T., and Babior, B.M. (1987) *Adv. Hum. Genet. 16*, 229.
26. Halliwell, B., Gutteridge, J.M.C., and Cross, C.E. (1992) *J. Lab Clin. Med. 119*, 598.
27. Halliwell, B. (1991) *Am. J. Med. 91*, 3C–14S.
28. Weiss, S.S. (1989) *N. Engl. J. Med. 320*, 365.
29. Michel, S.M., and Bors, C. (1991) *Free Radical Res. Commun. 10*, 221.
30. Beckman, J.S., Beckman, T.W., Chen, J., Marshall, P.A., and Freeman, B.A. (1990) *Proc. Natl. Acad. Sci. USA 87*, 1620.
31. Marletta, M.A. (1989) *Trends Biochem. Sci. 14*, 488.
32. Moncada, S., Plamer, R.M.J., and Higgs, E.A. (1989) *Biochem. Pharmacol. 38*, 1709.

33. Gryglewski, R.J., Palmer, R.M.J., and Moncada, S. (1986) *Nature (London) 320*, 454.
34. Laurindo, F.R.M., daLuz, P.L., Uint, L., Rocha, T.F., Jaegar, R.G., and Lopes, E.A. (1991) *Circulation 83*, 1705.
35. Fantone, J.C., and Ward, P.A. (1982) *Am. J. Pathol. 107*, 397.
36. Busse, W.W., Kopp, D.E., and Middleton, E. (1984) *J. Allergy Clin. Immunol.* 73, 801.
37. 'T Hart, B.A., Ram, T., Vai Ching, I.P., Van Di, H., and Labadie, R.P. (1990) *Chem. Biol. Interactions 73*, 323.
38. Tauber, A.I., Fay, J.R., and Marletta, M.A. (1984) *Biochem. Pharmacol.* 33, 1367.
39. Ferriola, P.C., Cody, V., and Middleton, E. (1989) *Biochem. Pharmacol. 38*, 1617.
40. Pincemail, J., Deby, C., Thirion, A., de Bruyn-Dister, M., and Goutier, R. (1988) *Experientia 44*, 450.
41. Winterbourn, C.C. (1985) *Biochim. Biophys. Acta 840*, 204.
42. Stolc, V. (1979) *J. Biol. Chem. 254*, 1273.
43. Blackburn, W.D., Heck, L.W., and Wallace, R.W. (1987) *Biochem. Biophys. Res. Commun. 144*, 1229.
44. Ogasawara, H., Fujitani, T., Drzewiecki, G., and Middleton, E., Jr., (1986) *J. Allergy Clin. Immunol. 78*, 321.
45. Halliwell, B., and Chirico, S. (1993) *Am. J. Clin. Nutr. 57*, 715S.
46. Halliwell, B., and Gutteridge, J.M.C. (1990) in *Methods in Enzymology* (Packer, L., and Glazer, A.N., eds.), Vol. 186, Academic Press, San Diego, p. 1.
47. Esterbauer, H., Zollner, H., and Schaur, R.J. (1988) *ISI Atlas Sci. Biochem. 1*, 311.
48. Cerutti, P.A. (1985) *Science 227*, 375.
49. Bus, J.S., and Gibson, J.E. (1979) *Rev. Biochem. Toxicol. 1*, 125.
50. Plaa, G.L., and Witschi, H. (1976) *Ann. Rev. Pharmacol. Toxicol. 16*, 125.
51. Recknagel, R.G., and Glende, E.A. (1979) *Handbook of Physiol. 9*, 591.
52. Tappel, A.L. (1978) *Exp. Med. Biol. 97*, 111.
53. Letan, A. (1966) *J. Food Sci. 31*, 518.
54. Bindoli, A., Cavallini, L., and Siliprandi, N. (1977) *Biochem. Pharmacol. 26*, 2405.
55. Cavallini, L., Bindoli, A., and Siliprandi, N. (1978) *Pharmacol. Res. Commun. 10*, 133.
56. Takahama, U. (1983) *Photochem. Photobiol. 38*, 363.
57. Sorata, Y., Takahama, U., and Kimura, M. (1984) *Biochim. Biophys. Acta 799*, 313.
58. Maridonneau-Parini, I., Braquet, P., and Garay, R.P. (1986) *Pharmacol. Res. Commun. 18*, 61.
59. Young, M., and Sieger, C.P. (1981) *Planta Med. 43*, 240.
60. Videla, L.A., Fernandez, V., Valenzuela, A., and Ugarte, G. (1981) *Pharmacology 22*, 343.
61. Muller, A., and Sies, H. (1981) *Biochem. J. 206*, 153.
62. Videla, L.A., Valenzuela, A., Fernandez, V., and Kriz, A. (1985) *Biochem. Int. 10*, 425.
63. Valenzuela, A., and Guerra, R. (1986) *Experientia 42,* 139.
64. Naim, M., Gestetner, B., Bondi, A., and Birk, Y. (1975) *J. Agric. Food Chem. 24*, 1174.
65. Jha, H.C., von Recklinghausen, G., and Zilliken, F. (1985) *Biochem. Pharmacol. 34*, 1367.
66. Hudson, B.J.F., and Lewis, J.I. (1965) *Food Chem. 10*, 47.
67. Simpson, T.H., and Uri, N. (1956) *Chem. Ind.*, 956.
68. Mehta, A.C., and Seshadri, T.R. (1959) *J. Sci. Ind. Res. 18B*, 24.
69. Heimann, A., Heimann, W., Gremminger, M., and Holman, H.H. (1953) *Fette u. Soifen 55*, 394.

70. Kimura, Y., Kubo, M., Tani, T., Arichi, S., and Okuda, H. (1981) *Chem. Pharm. Bull. (Tokyo) 29*, 2610.
71. Kimura, Y., Okuda, H., Taira, Z., Shoji, N., Takemoto, T., and Arichi, S. (1984) *Planta Med. 50*, 290.
72. Baumann, J., Wurm, G., and Bruchhausen, F.V. (1980) *Arch. Pharm. 313*, 330.
73. Burton, G.W., and Ingold, K.U. (1981) *J. Am. Chem. Soc. 103* 6472.
74. Ratty, A.K., and Das, N.P. (1988) *Biochem. Med. Metab. Biol. 39*, 69.
75. Afanas'ev, I.B., Dorozhko, A.I., Brodskii, A.V., Kostyuk, V.A., and Potapovitch, A.I. (1989) *Biochem. Pharmocol. 38*, 1763.
76. Svingen, B.A., Buege, J.A., O'Neal, F.O., and Augst, S.D. (1979) *J. Biol. Chem. 254*, 5892.
77. Albano, E., Lott, K.A.K., Slater, T.F., Stier, A., Symons, M.S.R., and Tomasi, P. (1982) *Biochem. J. 204*, 593.
78. Hara, H., Sukamoto, T., Ohtaka, H., Abe, K., Tatumi, Y., Saito, Y., Suzuki, A., and Tsukamoto, G. (1992) *Eur. J. Pharmacol. 221*, 193.
79. Mora, A., Paya, M., Rios, J.L., and Alcaraz, M.J. (1990) *Biochem. Pharmacol. 40*, 793.
80. Alcaraz, M.J., and Ferrandiz, M.L. (1987) *J. Ethnopharmacol. 21*, 209.
81. Laughton, M.J., Evans, P.J., Moroney, M.A., Hoult, J.R.S., and Halliwell, B. (1991) *Biochem. Pharmacol. 42*, 1673.
82. Robak, J., Shridi, F., Wolbis, M., and Krolikowska, M. (1988) *Pol. J. Pharmacol. Pharm. 40*, 451.
83. Sato, T., Kawamoto, A., Tamuro, A., Tatsumi, Y., and Fugii, T. (1992) *Chem. Pharm. Bull. 40*, 721.
84. Laughton, M.J., Halliwell, B., Evans, P.J., and Hoult, J.R.S. (1989) *Biochem. Pharmacol. 38*, 2859.
85. Husain, S.R., Cillard, J., and Cillard, P. (1987) *J. Am. Oil Chem. Soc. 64*, 109.
86. Yamamoto, K., and Niki, E. (1988) *Biochim. Biophys. Acta 958*, 19.
87. Girotti, A.W., Thomas, J.P., and Jordan, J.E. (1985) *Photochem. Photobiol. 41*, 267.
88. Rekka, E., and Kourounakis, P.N. (1991) *J. Pham. Pharmacol. 43*, 486.
89. Valenzuela, A., Guerria, R., and Videla, L.A. (1986) *Planta Med. 52*, 438.
90. Slater, T.F., and Eakins, M.N. (1975) in *New Trends in the Therapy of Liver Disease* (Bertelli, A., ed.), Karger, Basel, p. 84.
91. Videla, L.A. (1983) *Experientia 34*, 500.
92. Videla, L.A., Fraga, C., Koch, O., and Boveris, A. (1983) *Biochem. Pharmacol. 32*, 2822.
93. Fraga, C.G., Martino, V.S., Ferraro, G.E., Coussio, J.D., and Boveris, A. (1987) *Biochem. Pharmacol. 36*, 717.
94. Boveris, A., Llesuy, S.F., and Fraga, C.G. (1985) *Free Radical Biol. Med. 1*, 131.
95. Slater, T.F. (1984) *Biochem. J. 221*(1), 100.
96. McCay, P.B., Lai, E.K., Poyer, J.L., DuBoise, C.M., and Janzen, E.G. (1984) *J. Biol. Chem. 259*, 2135.
97. Chance, B., Sies, H., and Boveris, A. (1979) *Physiol. Rev. 59*, 527.
98. Koch, H.P., and Loffler, E. (1985) *Methods Fund. Exp. Clin. Pharmacol. 7*, 13.
99. Kappus, H., Koster-Albrecht, D., and Remmer, H. (1979) *Arch. Toxicol. 2*, 321.
100. Cholbi, M.R., and Alcaraz, M.J. (1991) *Experientia 47*, 195.
101. Wang, P.-F., and Zheng, R.-L. (1992) *Chem. Phy. Lipids 63*, 37.

102. Bors, W., Heller, W., Michel, C., and Saran, M. (1990) in *Methods in Enzymology* (Packer, L., and Glazer, A.M., ed.), Academic Press, New York, p. 343.
103. Mabry, T.J., Markham, K.R., and Thomas, M.B. (1970) *The Systematic Identification of Flavonoids Part 2*, Spring-Verlag, Berlin.
104. Bors, W., and Saran, M. (1987) *Free Radical Res. Commun. 2*, 289.
105. Erben-Russ, M., Bors, W., and Saran, M. (1987) *Int. J. Radiat. Biol. 52*, 393.
106. Ueno, I., Kohno, M., Haraikawa, K., and Hirono, I. (1984) *J. Pharmacobio-Dyn. 7*, 798.
107. Takahama, U. (1985) *Photochem. Photobiol. 42*, 89.
108. Husain, S.R., Cillard, J., and Cillard, P. (1987) *Phytochemistry 26*, 2489.
109. Takahama, U. (1987) *Plant Cell Physiol. 28*, 953.
110. Robak, J., and Gryglewski, R.J. (1988) *Biochem. Pharmacol. 37*, 837.
111. Huguet, A.I., Manez, S., and Alcaraz, M.J. (1990) *Z. Naturforsch 45C*, 19.
112. Sichel, G., Corsaro, C., Scalia, M., Bilio, A.J., and Bonomo, R.P. (1991) *Free Rad. Biol. Med. 11*, 1.
113. Cotelle, N., Bernier, J.L., Henichart, J.P., Catteau, J.P.C., Gaydou, E., and Wallet, J.C. (1992) *Free Radical Biol. and Med. 13*, 211.
114. Hodnick, W.F., Kung, F.S., Roettger, W.J., Bohmont, C.W., and Pardini, R.S. (1986) *Biochem. Pharmacol. 35*, 2345.
115. Hodnick, W.F., Bohmont, C.W., Capps, C., and Pardini, R.S. (1986) *Biochem. Pharmacol. 36,* 2873.
116. Elliott, A.J., Schreiber, S.A., Thomas, C., and Pardini, R.S. (1992) *Biochem. Pharmacol. 44,* 1603.
117. Hodnick, W.F., Kalyanaraman, B., Fritsos, C.A., and Pardini, R.S. (1988) in *Oxygen Radicals in Biology and Medicine* (Simic, M.G., Taylor, K.A., Ward, J.F., and VonSonntag, C., eds.), Plenum Press, New York, p. 149.
118. Canada, A.T., Gianella, E., Nguyen, T.D., and Mason, R.P. (1990) *Free Radical Biol. Med. 9*, 441.
119. Hahn, G., Lehmann, H.D., Kurten, M., Uebel, H., and Vogel, G. (1968) *Arzneim.-Forsh. (Drug Res.) 18*, 698.
120. Greimel, A., and Koch, H. (1977) *Experientia 33,* 1417.
121. Perrissoud, D. (1986) in *Plant Flavonoids in Biology and Medicine: Biochemical, Pharmacological and Structure-Activity Relationships* (Cody, V., Middleton, E., and Harborne, J.B., eds.), Alan R. Liss, New York, p. 559.
122. Valenzuela, A., Barria, T., Guerra, T., and Garrido, A. (1985) *Biochem. Biophys. Res. Commun. 126*, 712.
123. Valenzuela, A., and Guerra, R. (1985) *FEBS Lett. 181*, 271.
124. Velenzuela, A., Lagos, C., Schmidt, K., and Videla, L.A. (1985) *Biochem. Pharmacol. 39*, 2209.
125. Valenzuela, A., Guerra, R., and Garrido, A. (1987) *Planta Medica 53*, 402.
126. Rauen, H.M., Schriewer, H., Tegtbauer, U., and Lasana, J.E. (1973) *Experientia 29*, 1372.
127. Letteron, P., Labre, G., Degott, C., Berson, A., Fromenty, B., Delaforge, M., Larrey, D., and Pessayre, D. (1990) *Biochem. Pharmacol. 39*, 2027.
128. Labbe, G., Descatoire, V., Letteron, P., Degott, C., Tinel, M., Larrey, D., Carrion-Pavlor, Y., Amouyal, G., and Pessayre, D. (1987) *Biochem. Pharmacol. 36*, 907.
129. Feher, J., Cornides, A., Pal, J., Lang, I., and Csomos, G. (1989) *Acta Physiol. Hungarica 73*, 285.

130. Lonchampt, M., Guardiola, B., Sicot, N., Bertrand, M., Perdix, L., and Duhault, J. (1989) *Arzneim.-Forsch (Drug Res.) 39*, 882.
131. Nakayama, T., Yamada, M., Osawa, T., and Kawakishi, S. (1993) *Biochem. Pharmacol. 45*, 265.
132. Nakayama, T., Niimi, T., Osawa, T., and Kawakishi, S. (1992) *Mutat. Res. 281*, 77.
133. Korkina, L.G., Durnev, A.D., Suslova, T.B., Cheremisina, Z.P., Daugel-Dauge, N.O., and Afanas'ev, I.B. (1992) *Mutat. Res. 265*, 245.
134. Kantengwa, S., and Polla, B.S. (1991) *Biochem Biophys. Res. Commun. 180*, 308.
135. Ruch, R.J., Cheng, S.-J., and Klaunig, J.E. (1989) *Carcinogenesis 10*, 1003.
136. Trosko, J.E., and Chang, C.C. (1984) in *Mechanisms of Tumor Promotion: Cellular Responses to Tumor Promoters* (Slaga, T.J., ed.), Vol. 4, CRC Press, Boca Raton, p. 119.
137. Morel, I., Lescoat, G., Cogrel, P., Sergent, O., Pasdeloup, N., Brissot, P., Cillard, P., and Cillard, J. (1993) *Biochem. Pharmcol. 43*, 13.
138. Boyer, R.F., Clark, H.M., and LaRoche, A.P. (1988) *J. Inorg. Biochem. 32*, 171.
139. Aruoma, O.I. (1991) in *Free Radicals and Food Additives* (Aruoma, O.I., and Halliwell, B., ed.), Taylor and Francis, London, p. 173.
140. Kapus, A., and Lukacs, G.L. (1986) *Biochem. Pharmacol. 35*, 2119.
141. de Whalley, C.V., Rankin, S.M., Hoult, R.S., Jessup, W., and Leake, D.S. (1990) *Biochem. Pharmacol. 39*, 1743.
142. Negra-Salvayre, A., Reaud, V., Hariton, C., and Salvayre, R. (1991) *Biochem. Pharmacol. 2*, 450.
143. Negra-Salvayre, A., Alomar, Y., Troly, M., and Salvayre, R. (1991) *Biochim. Biophys. Acta 1096*, 291.
144. Negre-Salvayre, A., and Salvayre, R. (1992) *Free Radical Biol. Med. 12*, 101.
145. Negra-Salvayre, A., Lopez, M., Levade, T., Pierraggi, M.T., Dousset, N., Douste-Blazy, L., and Salvayre, R. (1990) *Biochim. Biophys. Acta 1045*, 224.
146. Hertog, M.G.L., Feskens, E.J.M., Hollman, P.C.H., Katan, M.B., and Kromhout, D. (1993) *Lancet 342*, 1007.
147. Frankel, E.N., Kanner, J., German, J.B., Parks, E., and Kinsella, J.E. (1993) *Lancet 341*, 454.
148. Sanhueza, J., Valdes, J., Campos, R., Garrido, A., and Valenzuela, A. (1992) *Res. Commun. Chem. Pathol. Pharmcol. 78*, 211.
149. McCord, J.M. (1986) *N. Engl. J. Med. 312*, 159.
150. Iio, M., Ono, Y., Kai, S., and Fukumoto, M. (1986) *J. Nutr. Sci. Vitaminol. 32*, 635.
151. Ning, X.-H., Ding, X., Childs, K.F., Bolling, S.F., and Gallagher, K.P. (1993) *J. Thorac. Cardiovasc. Surg. 105*, 541.
152. White, R.E., and Coon, M.J. (1980) *Ann. Rev. Biochem. 49*, 315.
153. Halliwell, B., and Gutteridge, J.M.C. (1985) *Free Radicals in Biology and Medicine*, Oxford, New York.
154. Fan, L.L., O'Keefe, D.D., and Powell, W.J. (1985) *J. Chin. Med. (England) 98*, 821.
155. Sacks, T., Moldow, C.F., Craddock, P.R., Bowers, T.K., and Jacobs, H.S. (1978) *J. Clin. Invest. 61*, 1161.
156. Weiss, S.J., Young, J., LoBuglio, A.F., Slivka, A., and Nimch, N.G. (1981) *J. Clin. Invest. 68*, 714.
157. Mazzone, T., Jensen, M., and Chait, A. (1983) *Proc. Natl. Acad. Sci. USA 80*, 5094.
158. Chang, W.-C., and Hsu, F.-L. (1991) *Prostaglandins Leukotr. Essen. Fatty Acids 44*, 51.

159. Gryglewski, R.J., Korbut, R., Robak, J., and Swies, J. (1987) *Biochem. Pharmacol. 36*, 317.
160. Harper, K.A., Morton, A.D., and Rolfe, F.J. (1969) *J. Food Technol. 4*, 255.
161. Bhagvat, K. (1946) *Ind. J. Med. Res. 34*, 87.
162. Wilson, H.K., and Price-Jones, C. (1971) *J. Sci. Food Agr. 22*, 551.
163. Parrot, J.L., and Gazave, J.M. (1951) *C.R. Soc. Biol. 145*, 821.
164. Regnault-Roger, C., Gazave, J.M., and Devynck, J. (1982) *Int. J. Vitamin. Nutr. Res. 52*, 158.
165. Zloch, Z. (1973) *Int. J. Vitamin. Nutr. Res. 43*, 378.
166. Basu, T.K., and Schorah, C.J. (1982) *Vitamin C in Health and Disease*, AVI Publishing, Westport.
167. Stich, H.G., Karim, J., Moropatnick, J., and Lo, L. (1976) *Nature (London) 260*, 722.
168. Burnet, M. (1974) *Intrinsic Mutagenesis: A Genetic Approach to Aging*, MTP, Lancaster.
169. Sorata, Y., Takahama, U., and Kimura, M. (1988) *Photochem. Photobiol. 48*, 195.
170. Jan, C.-Y., Takahama, U., and Kimura, M. (1991) *Biochim. Biophys. Acta 1086*, 7.
171. Takahama, U. (1986) *Biochim. Biophys. Acta 882*, 445.
172. Vrijsen, R., Everaert, L., and Boeye, A. (1988) *Gen. Virol. 69*, 1749.
173. Kandaswami, C., Perkins, E., Soloniuk, D.S., Drzewiecki, G., and Middleton, E. Jr. (1993) *Anti-Cancer Drugs 4*, 91.
174. Kochi, J.K. (1978) *Organometallic Mechanisms and Catalysis*, Academic Press, New York.
175. Kushi, L.H., Lenart, E.B., and Willett, W.C. (1995) *Am. J. Clin. Nutr. 61*, 1416.
176. Ferro-Luzzi, A., and Ghiselli, A. (1993) *Adv. in Exp. Med. Biol. 348*, 137.
177. Ferro-Luzzi, A., and Branca, F. (1995) *J. Clin. Nutr.*, 1338S.

Chapter 11

Antioxidative Activity of Condensed Tannins

A.D. Muir

Agriculture and Agri-Food Canada, Saskatoon, Saskatchewan, Canada.

Introduction

Over the past decade or so, there has been growing public skepticism of the safety of the synthetic antioxidants (e.g., BHA, BHT, and TBHQ) widely used in food processing and preservation. Accompanying this safety concern has been a steady increase in the demand for "natural" antioxidants, based on the premise that these compounds are inherently safe. It is not my intention to debate the validity of this assumption, but rather to review the antioxidative properties of a group of compounds, known as condensed tannins, that is widespread in our food.

Condensed tannins are small-to-medium-sized polymers composed principally of 4–8 linked flavan-3-ols (I, II); other branching patterns also exist, including 4–6 (III) and 2-O-7,4-6 linked flavan-3-ols (IV) (Scheme 11.1). These compounds exist naturally in a wide range of forms ranging from the monomer to polymers composed of 30 or more flavan-3-ol units. There are at least 13 different flavan-3-ols found in condensed tannins (1). Each flavan-3-ol has two chiral centers at positions 2 and 3, and when dimers or higher oligomers are formed with 4-6 or 4-8 linkages, a third chiral center at position 4 is created, thus creating a very large number of possible combinations. The 3-OH and occasionally the B-ring hydroxyl groups can also be esterified with gallic acid to add a third level of variation, although it is unusual to find gallic acid esters of molecules larger that trimers.

The antioxidant activity of condensed tannins and related compounds can be grouped into three classes based on their chemistry; monomers, dimers and trimers, and higher oligomers. Antioxidant activity can also be divided into three classes based upon the origin of the condensed tannin material; grape tannins, tea tannins, and other sources. The last-mentioned classification reflects the fact that most of the published research has centered around grape and tea tannins, while a number of published reports have used mixed preparations in which the chemistry of the tannins is not defined.

Antioxidant Assays

A large number of different antioxidant assays have been used to assess antioxidant activity, and it is not the intent of this paper to review all of the assays available but rather to concentrate on those assays that have been used to assess flavan-3-ols and oligomers of flavan-3-ols. The two most commonly used assays are the

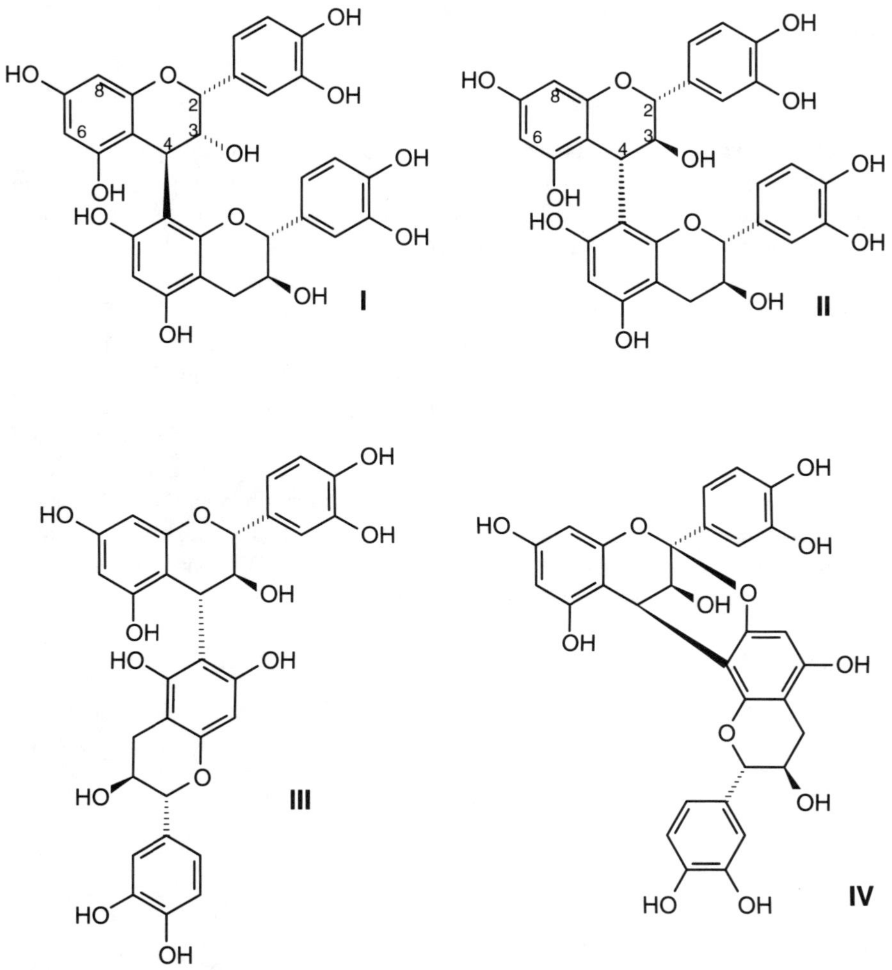

Scheme 11.1. Chemical structures of monomers of condensed tannins.

DPPH radical scavenging assay (2–7) and the scavenging of hydroxyl radicals generated by Fenton's reaction (2,8,9).

The scavenging of superoxide anions generated by the xanthine oxidase enzyme is also used frequently (2,5,9). However, these results must be viewed with caution when dimers and higher oligomers are tested, because there does not appear to have been any assessment of the ability of these compounds to precipitate the xanthine oxidase enzyme. This is of particular concern because protein precipitation is the key biological property that defines a condensed tannin.

Other assays reported include electron spin resonance (ESR) (9,10), an ultrasound-induced lipid peroxidation assay (9), inhibition of the oxidation of lard in a

Rancimat (11), a β-carotene-linoleic acid assay (3), and a rat heart mitochondria lipid oxidation assay (6).

Occurrence in Edible Plants

Condensed tannins and their precursors occur in a number of edible plants that may constitute a significant proportion of the human diet. For example, people who consume green tea may ingest up to 2 g/d of monomeric flavan-3-ols composed principally of (-)-epigallocatechin gallate (EGCG) (IX) (Scheme 11.2) (12,13), while people who drink black tea may ingest up to 1 g/d of monomeric flavan-3-ols (14). Condensed tannins occur in a number of seeds including peanuts (15), faba beans (16), millet (17), kidney beans (18), red sorghum (18,19), azuki beans (20), lentil (21), with traces in wheat bran (22). They also can occur in high concentrations in persimmons (23) and in condiments including turmeric (18). Monomeric flavan-3-ols, particularly epicatechin (VI) (Scheme 11.2), occur widely in pome and stone fruits including apples, pears, cherries, apricots (24), and peaches (25), while polymeric forms occur in kiwi fruit, black and red currants, bananas and cranberries (26). Monomeric and dimeric flavan-3-ols are also found in beer (27,28) and wine (29,30), while higher oligomers are sometimes found in wines and ciders (29,31,32). Monomers and dimers have also been found in yams (33) and cassava (34).

Condensed Tannin Monomers

In common with a number of other flavonoids (35-39), flavan-3-ols such as catechin and epicatechin have been shown to possess significant antioxidant activity.

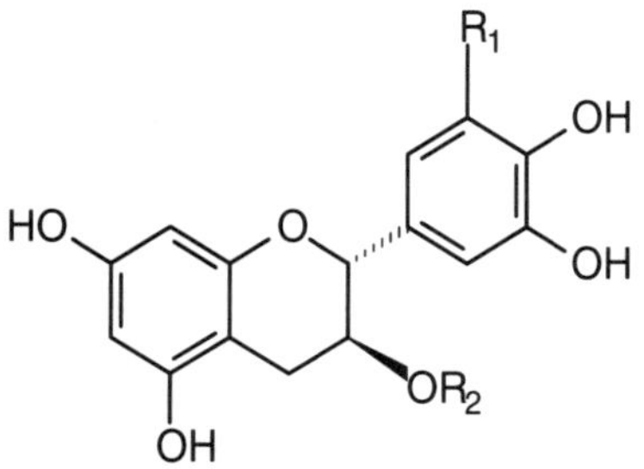

V $R_1=R_2=H$

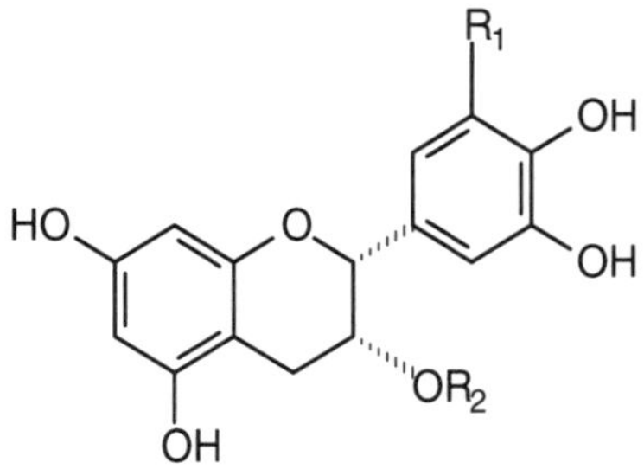

VI $R_1=R_2=H$

VII $R_1=H$, $R_2=$Galloyl

VIII $R_1=OH$, $R_2=H$

IX $R_1=OH$, $R_2=$Galloyl

Scheme 11.2. Chemical structures of selected catechins.

Epigallocatechin (VIII), epicatechin (VI), their corresponding gallates (VII, IX) and catechin (V) were all more effective scavengers of the DPPH radical than ascorbic acid and α-tocopherol (2,4,5), with epicatechin gallate (ECG) (VII) and EGCG (IX), the most effective compounds (Scheme 11.2). In studies of green, semifermented, and black tea, the principal flavan-3-ols and their corresponding gallates were shown to inhibit both oxidation of lard in Rancimat studies and lipoxygenase activity (11). In these studies, epigallocatechin gallate and epigallocatechin were the most effective inhibitors of lard oxidation and, together with epicatechin gallate, were the most effective lipoxygenase inhibitors. In both model systems, epicatechin was the least effective compound. In a study of rat heart mitochondria lipid peroxidation (6), flavan-3-ol 3-O-gallates were the most effective inhibitors, and all flavan-3-ols were more effective that Trolox (a water-soluble analogue of Vitamin E).

Condensed Tannin Dimers

The dimers procyanidin B-1(I) and B-3 (II) (Scheme 11.1), isolated from Azuki beans, have been shown to possess significant antioxidative (3) and radical scavenging activity (10). In the β-carotene assay, procyanidin B-3 (II) was significantly more effective at inhibiting the oxidation of β-carotene than α-tocopherol. In the DPPH assay, both dimers were more effective at donating H^+ to DPPH than (+) catechin, ascorbic acid, BHA, or α-tocopherol. In another experiment (2), the trigallate of procyanidin C-1 was found to be a more effective DPPH radical scavenger that the corresponding procyanidin B-2 and B-5 digallates which in turn were more effective than ECG and EGCG on a molar basis. This same group of compounds was also observed to be effective hydroxyl radical (Fenton's reaction) scavengers with the same order of activity. In these latter experiments (2), nongallated monomers and dimers were not included. A series of dimers and trimers isolated from grape seeds were also shown to be effective superoxide radical (xanthine oxidase) and hydroxyl radical (Fenton's reaction) scavengers (8). In these model systems, galloyl esters were more effective, with the most activity associated with the 3′-galloyl esters.

Condensed Tannin Oligomers and Polymers

In many plants, a significant proportion of the flavan-3-ols occur as higher oligomers or polymers with molecular weights ranging from 1000 to over 30,000. These compounds may have different solubilities from the monomers and dimers, but still retain many of the same chemical properties. The one property which is significantly different in the higher molecular weight polymers is the ability to precipitate proteins which increases with increasing molecular weight. In spite of their abundance, little attention has been paid to their potential antioxidant activity. Bahorun *et al.* (40) observed antioxidant activity in monomeric and dimeric fractions but found no significant antioxidant activity in the polymeric fractions obtained from hawthorn (*Crataegus monogyna*) (40). Maffei Facino *et al.* (9) investigated the antioxidant activity of a grape seed condensed tannin preparation (mean MW 1800) in two antioxidant assays and determined that the grape seed preparation was significantly more effective than catechin. However, catechin has previously been reported to be the least effective antioxidant of the flavan-3-ol monomers (4), suggesting that the activity observed was more likely due to the abundant monomers and dimers in this material rather than the higher oligomers. Uchida *et al.* (2) also observed that a crude persimmon tannin preparation could effectively scavenge the DPPH radical and hydroxy radicals generated by Fenton's reaction.

In the course of investigating the effects of condensed tannins found in forage legumes on rumen function (41,42), we isolated condensed tannin polymers from a number of plants by conventional isolation procedures (43). The antioxidant activity of nine polymers (Table 11.1) was assessed using three antioxidant assays: a thiocyanate assay (44,45), a thin-layer chromatographic (TLC) linolenic acid oxidation assay (45), and a DPPH radical scavenging assay (5,7).

Of the polymeric tannins tested, all were less effective antioxidants than vitamin E in the thiocyanate assay (Fig. 11.1), which in turn was significantly less effective than either BHA or BHT in this antioxidant assay. However, in the TLC linolenic acid oxidation assay, three of the polymer preparations offered antioxidant protection equal to or greater than that of BHT (Fig. 11.2), while one of the polymer preparations exhibited equivalent antioxidant protection to Vitamin E. In this assay, BHA was the most effective antioxidant.

In the third assay, the DPPH radical scavenging assay, all of the tannin preparations exhibited significant radical scavenging ability (Fig. 11.3). All polymer preparations exhibited greater radical scavenging activity than BHT. Eight of the nine polymers tested exhibited radical scavenging activity equivalent to BHA and Vitamin E. The only exception was the polymer isolated from alfalfa seed. As has been previously reported, flavan-3-ol monomers are also effective radical scav-

TABLE 11.1
Condensed Tannin Polymers

Common name	Plant part	Latin name
Lotus uliginosus var. glab.	leaf	*Lotus uliginosus* L. var. *glabriusculus*
Big trefoil	whole plant	*Lotus uliginosus* L.
Alfalfa	seed	*Medicago sativa* L.
Sainfoin	leaf	*Onobrychis viciifolia* Scop.
Crown vetch	leaf	*Coronilla varia* L.
Hedysarum	stems	*Hedysarum alpinum* L. var. *Americanum*
Big trefoil	leaf	*Lotus uliginosus* L.
Birdsfoot trefoil	leaf	*Lotus corniculatus* L.
Lespedeza	leaf	*Lespedeza cuneata* Don.

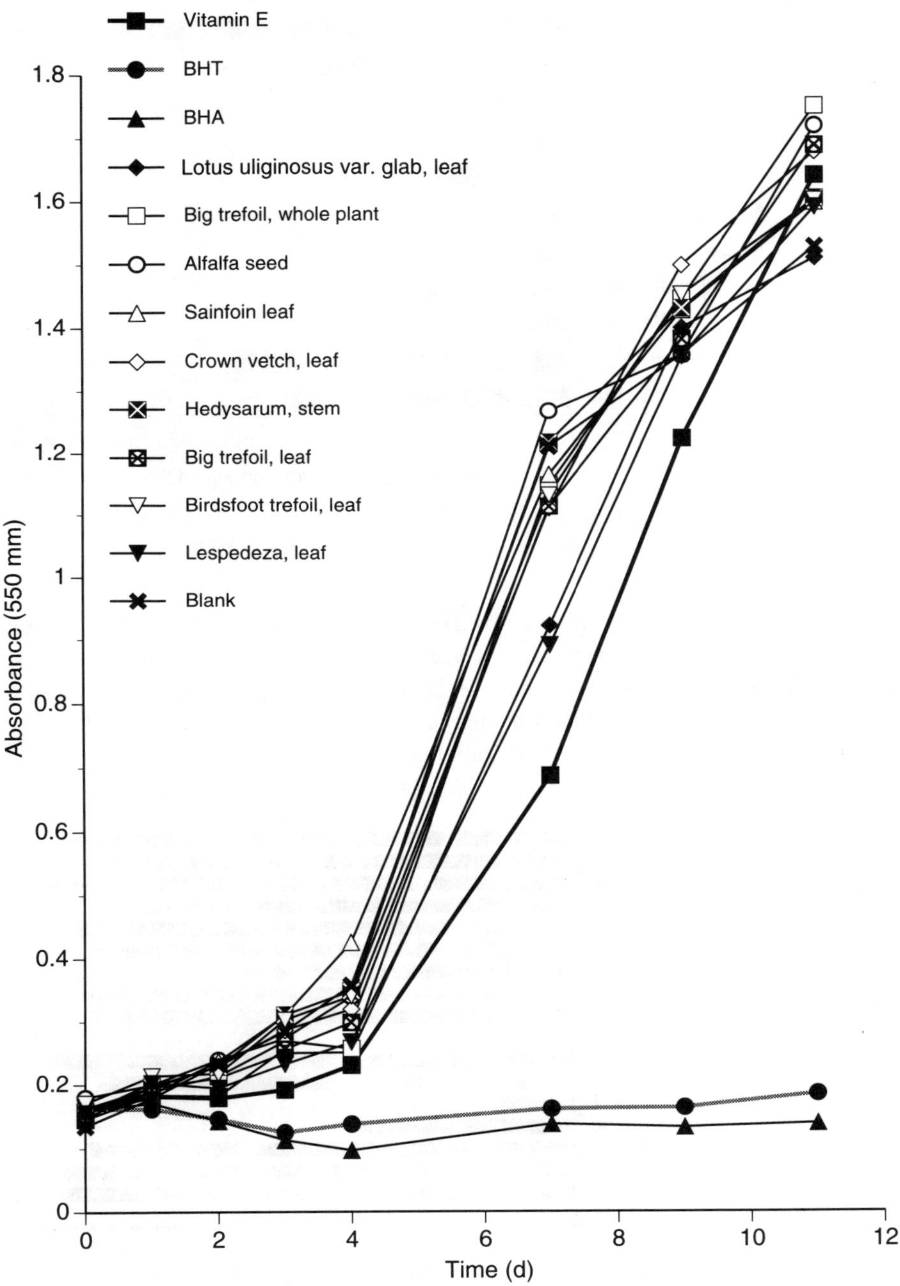

Fig. 11.1. The effects of condensed tannin polymers on the oxidation of linolenic acid as measured by the thiocyanante assay.

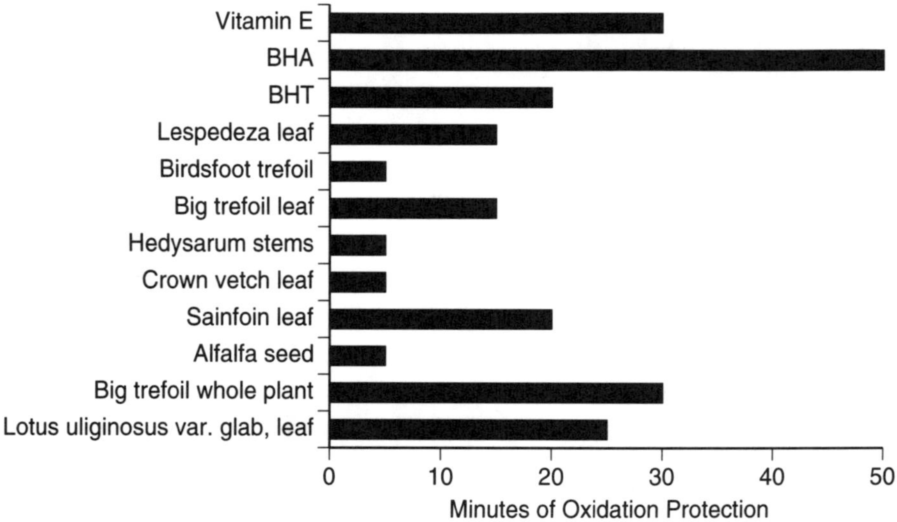

Fig. 11.2. Effect of condensed tannin polymers on the oxidation of linoleic acid as determined by the thin-layer chromatographic (TLC) method.

engers and on a weight for weight basis, most of the polymer preparations exhibit equivalent radical scavenging activity. We also examined the possibility that the radical scavenging activity might be correlated with other properties of these polymers and found that the radical scavenging activity was not correlated with polymer molecular weight or protein precipitating ability.

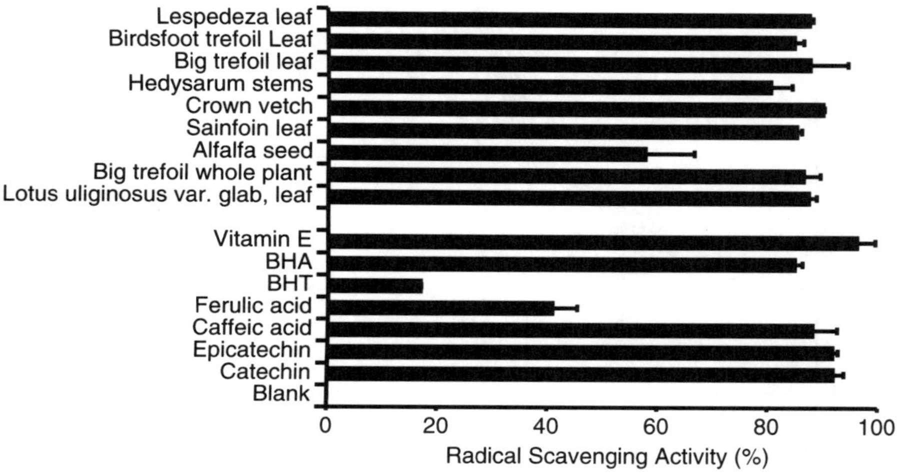

Fig. 11.3. Radical scavenging activity of condensed tannin polymers as determined by the DPPH assay (SE, $n = 3$).

Conclusions

These results are consistent with the observation that condensed tannin polymers are readily oxidized to amorphous brown polymeric materials. The ability of these oligomeric flavan-3-ols to act as radical scavengers suggests another possible role for these compounds in the plant while at the same time offering the possibility that plant material rich in condensed tannins may have applications in food preservation and contribute to the maintenance of the antioxidant balance in the digestive tract. Because oligomeric flavan-3-ols, unlike monomers, are not thought to be transported across the intestine wall (46), it is unlikely that the intact polymer could have physiological effects other than in the digestive tract.

Acknowledgements

The author wishes to thank Krista Ballantyne and Andrew Aubin for their contributions to this work. Saskatoon Research Centre, Agriculture and Agri-Food Canada Publication #1165.

References

1. Porter, L.J. (1988) in *The Flavonoids* (Harborne, J.B., ed.), Chapman and Hall Ltd., London. p. 21–62.
2. Uchida, S., Edamatsu, R., Hiramatsu, M., Mori, A., Nonaka, G.-I., Nishioka, I., Niwa, M., and Ozaki, M. (1987) *Med. Sci. Res. 15*, 831.
3. Ariga, T., Koshiyama, I., and Fukushima, D. (1988) *Agric. Biol. Chem. 52*, 2717.
4. Yoshida, T., Mori, K., Hatano, T., Okumura, T., Uehara, I., Komagoe, K., Fujita, Y., and Okuda, T. (1989) *Chem. Pharm. Bull. 37*, 1919.
5. Hatano, T., Edamatsu, R., Hiramatsu, M., Mori, A., Fujita, Y., Yasuhara, T., Yoshida, T., and Okuda, T. (1989) *Chem. Pharm. Bull. 37,* 2016.
6. Hong, C.Y., Wang, C.P., Lo, Y.C., and Hsu, F.L. (1994) *Am. J. Chinese Med. 22*, 285.
7. Brand-Williams, W., Cuvelier, M.E., and Berset, C. (1995) *Lebensmittel-Wissenschaft & Technologie 28*, 25.
8. Ricardo-Da-Silva, J.M., Darmon, N., Fernandez, Y., and Mitjavila, S. (1991) *J. Agric. Food Chem. 39*, 1549.
9. Maffei Facino, R., Carini, M., Aldini, G., Bombardelli, E., Morazzoni, P., and Morelli, R. (1994) *Arzneimittel-Forschung 44*, 592.
10. Ariga, T., and Hamano, M. (1990) *Agric. Biol. Chem. 54*, 2499.
11. Ho, C.-T., Chen, Q., Shi, H., Zhang, K.-Q., and R.T. Rosen (1992) *Preventive Med. 21*, 520.
12. Bradfield, A.E., Penney, M., and Wright, W.B. (1947) *J. Chem. Soc., 32*.
13. Fujita, Y., Yamane, T., Tanaka, M., Kuwata, K., Okuzumi, J., Takahashi, T., Fujiki, H., and Okuda, T. (1989) *Japan J. Cancer Res. 82*, 503.
14. WHO (1991) International Agency of Research on Cancer. *IARC Monogr. Carcinog. Risks Hum. 51*, pp. 207–271.
15. Bate-Smith, E.C., and Ribereau-Gayon, P. (1959) *Qualitas Plantarum et Materiae Vegetabiles 5*, 189.
16. Cansfield, P.E., Marquardt, R.R., and Campbell, L.D. (1980) *J. Sci. Food. Agric. 31*, 802.

17. Odumodu, C.U. (1992) *Tropical and Geographical Medicine 44*, 260.
18. Narasinga Rao, B.S., and Prabhavathi, T. (1982) *J. Sci. Food. Agric. 33*, 89.
19. Bate-Smith, E.C., and Rasper, V. (1969) *J. Food Sci. 34*, 203.
20. Price, M.L., Hagerman, A.E., and Butler, L.G. (1980) *J. Agric. Food Chem. 28*, 459.
21. Vaillancourt, R., Slinkard, A.E., and Reichert, R.D. (1986) *Can. J. Plant Sci. 66,* 241.
22. McCallum, J.A., and Walker, J.R.L. (1990) *Cereal Chem. 67*, 282.
23. Ito, S. (1980) in *Tropical and Subtropical Fruits, Composition, Properties and Uses* (Nagy, S., and Shaw, P.E., eds.), AVI Publishing, Westport, CT, pp. 442–468.
24. Mosel, H.-D., and Herrmann, K. (1974) *Z. Lebensm Unters Forsch. 154*, 6.
25. Senter, S.D., and Callahan, A. (1990) *J. Food Sci. 55*, 1585.
26. Foo, L.Y., and Porter, L.J. (1981) *J. Sci. Food Agric. 32*, 711.
27. Eastmond, R. (1974) *J. Inst. Brew. 80*, 188.
28. McGuinness, J.D., Laws, D.R.J., Eastmond, R., and Gardner, R.J. (1975) *J. Inst. Brew. 81*, 237.
29. Lea, A.G.H., Bridle, P., Timberlake, C.F., and Singleton, V.L. (1979) *Am. J. Enol. Vitic. 30*, 289.
30. Ricardo-Da-Silva, J.M., Belchior, A.P., Spranger, M.I., and Bourzeix, M. (1992) *Science des Aliments 12*, 223.
31. Lea, A.G.H., and Arnold, G.M. (1978) *J. Sci. Food Agric. 29*, 478.
32. Oszmianski, J., and Lee, C.Y. (1990) *Am. J. Enol. Vitic. 41*, 204.
33. Ozo, O.N., Caygill, J.C., and Coursey, D.G. (1984) *Phytochemistry 23*, 329.
34. Rickard, J.E. (1986) *J. Sci. Food. Agric. 37*, 37.
35. Lea, C.H., and Swoboda, P.A.T. (1956) *Chemistry & Industry*, 1426.
36. Pratt, D.E. (1992) in *Phenolic Compounds in Food and Their Effect on Health II. Antioxidants and Cancer Prevention* (Huang, M.Y., Ho, C.T., and Lee, C.Y., eds.), ACS, Washington, D.C., pp. 54–71.
37. Okamura, H., Mimura, A., Yakou, Y., Niwano, M., and Takahara, Y. (1993) *Phytochemistry 33*, 557.
38. Nieto, S., Garrido, A., Sanhueza, J., Loyola, L.A., Morales, G., Leighton, F., and Valenzuela, A. (1993) *J. Am. Oil Chem. Soc. 70,* 773.
39. Igile, G.O., Oleszek, W., Jurzysta, M., Burda, S., Fafunso, M., and Fasanmade, A.A. (1994) *J. Agric. Food Chem. 42*, 2445.
40. Bahorun, T., Trotin, F., Pommery, J., Vasseur, J., and Pinkas, M. (1994) *Planta Med. 60*, 323.
41. Bae, H.D., McAllister, T.A., Yanke, J., Cheng, K.-J., and Muir, A.D. (1993) *Appl. Environ. Microbiol. 59,* 2132.
42. Jones, G.A., McAllister, T.A., Cheng, K.-J., and Muir, A.D. (1994) *Appl. Environ. Microbiol. 60*, 1374.
43. Bae, H.D., McAllister, T.A., Muir, A.D., Yanke, J., Bassendowski, K.A., and Cheng, K.-J. (1993) *J. Agric. Food Chem. 41*, 1256.
44. Masuda, T., Isobe, J., Jitoe, A., and Nakatani, N. (1992) *Phytochemistry 31*, 3645.
45. Masuda, T., and Jitoe, A. (1994) *J. Agric. Food Chem. 42*, 1850.
46. Jimenez-Ramsey, L.M., Rogler, J.C., Housley, T.L., Butler, L.G., and Elkin, R.G. (1994) *J. Agric. Food Chem. 42*, 963.

Chapter 12

Natural Antioxidants from Tea

C.-T. Ho[a], C.-W. Chen[a], U.N. Wanasundara[b], and F. Shahidi[b]

[a]Department of Food Science, Rutgers University, New Brunswick, New Jersey; and [b]Department of Biochemistry, Memorial University of Newfoundland, St. John's, Newfoundland, Canada.

Introduction

Tea, a beverage originating from a single species of plant, *Camellia sinensis*, is widely cultivated around the world in both tropical and subtropical regions (annual production of about 2.5 million tons) and has become the second most popular drink after water. There are three major forms of manufactured teas: green tea, Oolong tea, and black tea. Green tea is prepared in such a way as to preclude the oxidation of green leaf polyphenols. The manufacture of black tea is carried out so that a high degree of oxidation of the tea leaf polyphenols is ensured, and Oolong tea is a partially oxidized product. There are three major polyphenols in teas: catechins, theaflavins, and thearubigins. Catechins are major constituents of green tea leaves and are also present in Oolong and black teas, whereas thearubigins and theaflavins are found only in black and Oolong teas. The chemical structures of catechins and theaflavins have been identified as shown in Fig. 12.1, but the structure and chemistry of thearubigens have not been well defined or characterized.

Green tea polyphenols are known to inhibit mutagenicity induced by benzo(a)pyrene, aflatoxin B1, 2-aminofluorene, 4-nitroquinoline-*N*-oxide, 2-amino-3,4-dimethyl-imidoazo[4,5f]-quinoline, cigarette smoke condensate, and extracts of fried fish in *Salmonella typhimurium* TA 100 and/or TA 98 and/or V79 cells (1,2). Infusions or water extracts of green tea inhibited forestomach and lung tumorigenesis of mice induced by *N*-nitrosodiethylamine (3). Not only green tea, but also Oolong and black teas exhibited an antitumorigenesis effect on rat esophagus tumors induced by sodium nitrite and methylbenzylamine (4). The most abundant polyphenol in green tea, (-)-epigallocatechin gallate (EGCG), was the most potent of the inhibitory tea polyphenols against 12-*O*-tetradecanoylphorbol-13-acetate(TPA)-induced mouse ear skin inflammation (5,6) and also inhibited tumor promotion in the gastrointestinal tract of mouse duodenal carcinogenesis induced by *N*-ethyl-*N*′-nitro-*N*-nitrosoguanidine (7). In addition to the above properties, green tea polyphenols showed a strong inhibitory effect on TPA-induced biochemical and morphological changes in mouse skin (8,9), on mouse skin tumor initiation, promotion and progression (9–12), and on ultraviolet (UV) light-induced sun-

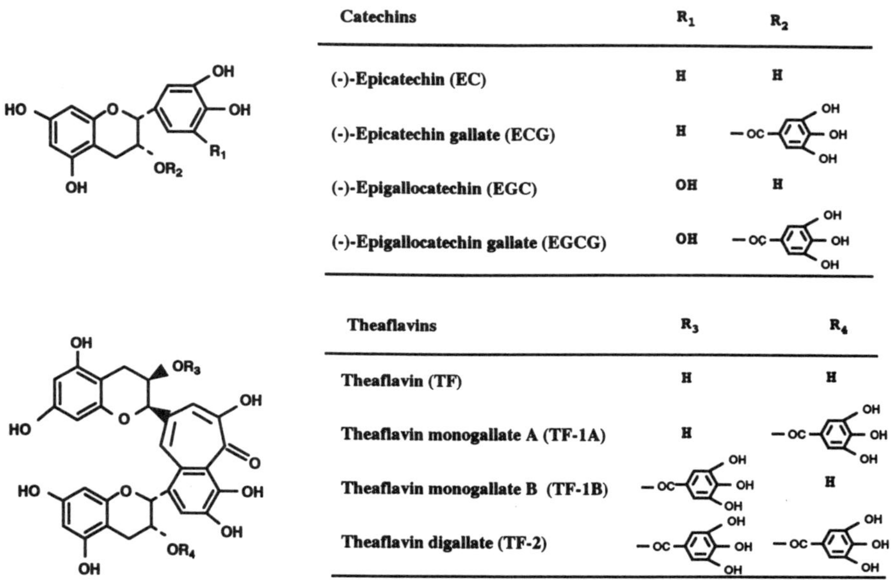

Fig. 12.1. The structures of catechins and theaflavins.

burn lesions and carcinogenesis in mouse skin as summarized in Table 12.1 (13–15). The mechanisms of antimutagenicity and anticarcinogenicity of tea polyphenols have been summarized by Cheng *et al.* (16) as given below:

1. Tea polyphenols induce detoxification activity of enzymes such as glutathione-*S*-transferase.
2. They reduce the TPA-induced ornithine decarboxylase activity and inhibit tumor promotion.
3. They block certain carcinogens from binding to DNA.
4. They act as a free radical trap and prevent *in vivo* lipid oxidation.

In addition to anticarcinogenic and antimutagenic activities, green tea extracts exhibited good hydrogen peroxide and superoxide radical-scavenging activities (17). Individual catechins and theaflavins, which were purified from green tea and black tea, respectively, showed different abilities to scavenge superoxide or 1,1-diphenyl-2-picrylhydrazyl (DPPH) radicals and to inhibit lipoxygenase and lipid peroxidation (18–20). These data may be used to partially elucidate the mechanism of action of the antioxidative effect of tea polyphenols. Hara (21) has evaluated the antioxidative potency of crude extracts of green tea and individual catechins in lard by the Active Oxygen Method. Crude tea catechins reduced the formation of peroxides more effectively than α-tocopherol or butylated hydroxyanisole (BHA). The antioxidant potency of individual catechins, evaluated in the same manner,

TABLE 12.1
Inhibitory Effects of Green Tea Polyphenol Fraction on Biochemical and Morphological Changes, Skin Tumor Initiation, Promotion and Progression, and Ultraviolet Light-Induced Sunburn Lesions and Carcinogenesis in Mouse Skin[a]

Inhibitory effects of green tea	Reference
TPA-induced biochemical changes	
Skin inflammation (edema of mouse ears)	(5,6,9)
Ornithine decarboxylase activity	(8,9)
Production of hydrogen peroxide	(9)
Myeloperoxide activity	(9)
TPA-induced morphological changes	
Epidermal thickening	(5,6)
Increased epidermal cell layers	(5,6)
Leukocyte infiltration	(5,6)
Intercellular edema	(5,6)
Increased keratin layer thickness	(5,6)
Initiation	
[^{3}H]B[a]P-DNA, [^{3}H]DMBA-DNA adduct formation	(10,11)
B[a]P or DMBA initiation	(9)
Promotion	
TPA promotion	(9–11)
Teleocidin promotion	(41)
Okadaic acid promotion	(12)
Progression	
Benzoylperoxide or 4-nitroquinoline-*N*-oxide progression	(5,6)
Sunburn lesions	(14,15)
UV-B initiation, TPA promotion	(14,15)
DMBA initiation, UV-B promotion	(14,15)
UV-B complete carcinogenesis	(13)

[a]Abbreviations: TPA, 12-*O*-tetradecanoylphorbol-13-acetate; DMBA, 7,12-dimethylbenz[a]anthracene; UV-B, ultraviolet-B.

was in the order of (-)-epigallocatechin gallate (EGCG) > (-)-epigallocatechin (EGC) > (-)-epicatechin gallate (ECG) > (-)-epicatechin (EC).

Composition of Tea Polyphenols

Tea composition varies with climate, season, tea variety, and the age of the leaf. In general, fresh green tea leaves contain 36% polyphenols (22). Catechins are the predominant polyphenols in green tea, and epigallocatechin gallate appears to be the predominant catechin present in green tea leaves. The composition of green tea polyphenols is shown in Table 12.2 (9).

During the manufacturing of Oolong tea or black tea, part of the catechins in green tea leaves undergoes condensation and polymerization to form theaflavins and thearubigins (23). The total content of theaflavins in Oolong tea and black tea is about 0.84 and 1.64%, respectively, and the total content of thearubigins in Oolong tea and black tea is 17.53 and 27.76%, respectively (20).

TABLE 12.2
Composition of Green Tea Polyphenol Fraction

Compound	Percentage of solids (%)
(-)-Epigallocatechin gallate (EGCC)	48–55
(-)-Epigallocatechin (EGC)	9–12
(-)-Epicatechin gallate (ECG)	9–12
Caffeine	7–9
(-)-Epicatechin (EC)	5–7
(-)-Catechin	0.3–0.6
Gallic acid	0.3–0.5

DPPH Radical-Scavenging Ability

One method of evaluating antioxidant activity of a compound is to assess its free radical inhibitory activity. The antioxidant is supposed to react with free radicals such as the hydroperoxy radical generated from lipid peroxidation and to terminate the propagation of chain reaction. The DPPH radical, which is a very stable radical, has been employed to determine the free radical inhibitory effect of some antioxidants (18,24,25). The mechanism of the reaction of antioxidants with the DPPH radical is shown below (24).

$$(DPPH)^{\bullet} + HO\text{-}R\text{-}OH \rightarrow (DPPH){:}H + HO\text{-}R\text{-}O^{\bullet}$$

$$HO\text{-}R\text{-}O^{\bullet} + (DPPH)^{\bullet} \rightarrow (DPPH){:}H + O{=}R{=}O$$

The DPPH radical with a deep violet color receives a proton from the antioxidant and becomes a colorless protonated DPPH species. Using this reagent, the free radical-scavenging ability of the antioxidant may be measured by spectrophotometric methods. As shown in Table 12.3, tea catechins and theaflavins show strong and different DPPH radical-scavenging abilities compared with butylated hydroxytoluene (BHT) (18). The DPPH radical-scavenging ability of catechins is in the order of EGCG > ECG > EGC > EC, and for the theaflavins, the order is theaflavin digallate (TF-2) > theaflavin monogallate (TF-1) > theaflavin (TF) (Table 12.1). This DPPH radical-scavenging ability of polyphenolic compounds is due to their hydrogen-donating ability (24–26). The number of hydroxyl groups in the structures of catechins or theaflavins may be related to their hydrogen-donating ability, and thus the presence of more hydroxyl groups in the catechin or theaflavin molecules enhances their free radical-scavenging ability (18).

Superoxide-Scavenging Ability

The superoxide radical ($O_2^{-\bullet}$) is produced by the addition of an electron onto the oxygen molecule. After $O_2^{-\bullet}$ is formed, other reactions will proceed (27):

$$O_2^{-\bullet} + H^+ \rightarrow HOO^{\bullet}$$

$$HOO^{\bullet} + HOO^{\bullet} \rightarrow O_2 + 2HO^{\bullet}$$

The hydroxyl radical ($HO^{\bullet}$) is much more reactive than the superoxide radical and is able to attack DNA, leading to *in vivo* mutagenicity (28).

Superoxide dismutase, which is present within the cells of the human body, is able to remove $O_2^{-\bullet}$ by catalyzing the following reaction (29):

$$O_2^{-\bullet} + O_2^{-\bullet} + 2H^+ \rightarrow H_2O_2 + O_2$$

Hydrogen peroxide (H_2O_2) is a sluggish molecule in terms of reactivity, but it may be converted to a more reactive $OH^{\bullet}$ radical via the Fenton reaction (28):

$$Fe^{2+} + H_2O_2 \rightarrow Fe^{2+} + OH^{\bullet} + OH^{-}$$

The hydroxyl radical ($OH^{\bullet}$) is so reactive that green tea polyphenols exhibited little scavenging effect on it in the Fenton reaction model system (30). However, green tea catechins exhibited excellent ability in scavenging H_2O_2 and $O_2^{-\bullet}$, the precursors of $OH^{\bullet}$ (17). In our study, the individual catechins and theaflavins which were isolated from green tea and black tea, respectively, effectively inhibited the production of superoxide generated by phenazine methosulfate (PMS) and NADH (Table 12.3) (18). The effectiveness of the three theaflavins in this work was similar in scavenging the superoxide radical, but the ability of catechins was in the order of EGCG > ECG > EGC > EC. This trend is the same as that found for DPPH radical-scavenging activity of catechins. The excellent superoxide-scavenging ability of catechins and theaflavins may be related to their potent antimutagenic and anticarcinogenic activities.

TABLE 12.3
The DPPH Radical-, Superoxide-, Lipoxygenase-, and Lipid Peroxidation-Inhibition Abilities of Catechins, Theaflavins, and Butylated Hydroxytoluene (BHT)

Compound[a]	DPPH radical[b] inhibition (%)	Superoxide[b] inhibition i(%)	Lipoxygenase inhibition[c] IC50 (μg/mL)[d]	Rancimat test[b] Induction time (h)
EGCG	74.8	69.4	4.6	55.30
ECG	59.3	39.9	7.7	53.30
EGC	36.1	23.9	6.1	19.15
EC	32.0	11.2	40.6	3.00
TF-2	58.2	70.5	0.2	2.75
TF-1	43.3	65.2	22.3 (0.4)[e]	3.43
TF	32.3	64.4	124.7	3.70
BHT	4.7	0.5	0.1	5.20
control	—	—	—	2.25

[a]The concentration of compounds for DPPH radical-scavenging test, superoxide-scavenging test, and Rancimat test were 10 μM, 50 μM, and 200 μM, respectively.
[b]*Source:* Ref. (18).
[c]*Source:* Ref. (20).
[d]IC50, compound concentration at which 50% of lipoxygenase activity is inhibited.
[e]The values of 22.3 and 0.4 μg/mL are the lipoxygenase inhibition IC50 of theaflavin monogallate A and theaflavin monogallate B, respectively.
Abbreviations: See Table 12.2.

Lipoxygenase-Inhibition Ability

The lipoxygenase pathways in the metabolism of arachidonic acid produce reactive oxygen species. These reactive species as well as other metabolites from arachidonic acid metabolism result in inflammation and tumor promotion (31). The inhibitors which could act on the lipoxygenase pathways of arachidonic acid metabolism are able to inhibit tumor promotion in animals (32). Experimentally, inhibition of soybean lipoxygenase has been used to replace the inhibition of mammalian lipoxygenase as an *in vitro* method for the screening of antitumor promotion activity of natural products due to the structural and mechanistic similarities between soybean and mammalian lipoxygenases (33–35).

Among theaflavins, theaflavin monogallate B and theaflavin digallate appeared to be most active in inhibiting soybean lipoxygenase, whereas theaflavin showed no inhibitory effect (Table 12.3). In catechins, EGCG, ECG, and EGC displayed good lipoxygenase-inhibition ability, whereas EC showed little effect. The lipoxygenase-inhibition activity of catechins and theaflavins may be related to good antioxidant activity (19,20).

Lipid Oxidation-Inhibition Ability

A good antioxidant provides not only health benefits but may also be used in foods to control lipid oxidation. BHA, BHT and *tert*-butylhydroquinone (TBHQ) are commonly used as food antioxidants. However, possible toxicity of synthetic antioxidants and consumer demands have led to decreased use of synthetic antioxidants (36). Therefore, research on natural antioxidants has gained momentum because they are considered to pose no health risk to consumers. Naturally occurring antioxidative compounds in foods include flavonoids, phenolic acids, lignans, terpenes, tocopherols, phospholipids, and polyfunctional organic acids (37,38). Recent studies have shown that phenolic compounds extracted from green tea (catechins) and black tea (theaflavins) had strong antioxidant activity in different lipids and lipid-containing foods (18,39).

Lard containing 200 ppm of individual catechins or theaflavins (except EC and TF-2) showed significantly longer induction periods as determined by the Rancimat method, than the control sample, with no additives (Table 12.3) (18). According to the induction time obtained, all theaflavins showed little effect on the inhibition of lipid peroxidation, but catechins (except EC) exhibited excellent lipid peroxidation-inhibition in the order of EGCG > ECG > EGC > EC, similar to that of their DPPH radical- and superoxide-scavenging abilities (Table 12.3). However, Amarowicz and Shahidi (40) have shown that, among the tea catechins, ECG possesses the strongest and EGC the weakest antioxidative effect in a β-carotene-linoleate model system.

Green tea catechins also showed strong antioxidant activity in prevention of oxidation of marine oils. The antioxidant activity of purified green tea catechins (EC, ECG, EGCG, and EGC at 200 ppm) was compared with that of commercial antioxidants (BHA, BHT, and TBHQ at 200 ppm and α-tocopherol at 500 ppm) in seal blubber (SBO) and menhaden (MHO) oils under Schaal oven test conditions at 65°C for 144 h. The formation of primary oxidation products (hydroperoxides or peroxides) was monitored by measuring peroxide values (PV) of oils. Catechin-treated oils exhibited significantly ($P < 0.05$) lower (at least by 60% even after 144 h) PV than those containing α-tocopherol, BHA and BHT (Fig. 12.2). Among tea catechins tested, ECG served best in lowering peroxide formation, even better than TBHQ which is the most effective antioxidant used by the food industry. ECG, the superior antioxidant used in this study, gave PV results of 4.62, 7.90, 27.57, and 46.96 meq/kg SBO after 24, 48, 84, and 144 h of storage, respectively; corresponding values of the control samples were 25.22, 49.26, 118.75 and 183.33 meq/kg oil. Similarly, MHO treated with ECG had PV of 7.62, 9.69, 75.94, and 101.0 (meq/kg oil) after 24, 48, 84, and 114 h storage, respectively. Corresponding values for untreated MHO were 38.07, 96.54, 282.90, and 347.50 meq/kg oil. However, in MHO, the TBHQ-treated samples maintained lower PV than ECG for up to 48 h of storage, after which the oil containing ECG had significantly ($P < 0.05$) lower PV than all other treatments. On the other hand, ECG was 5.6 and 6.8 times more potent than α-tocopherol and 6.8 and 7.4 times more effective than BHA in SBO and MHO, respectively, after 48 h of storage.

Addition of tea catechins, α-tocopherol, and other antioxidants to both SBO and MHO had a significant ($P < 0.05$) effect in lowering the formation of 2-thiobarbituric acid reactive substances (TBARS) compared with the control sample. The order of potency of these additives in inhibiting the formation of TBARS in both SBO and MHO was ECG > TBHQ > EGCG > EGC > EC > BHT > BHA > α–tocopherol (Fig. 12.3). Among the catechins tested, ECG and EGCG exhibited >50% inhibition of TBARS formation in treated SBO, whereas for MHO, only the ECG-treated sample showed a similar inhibition of oxidation. The TBHQ-treated samples also exhibited excellent stability because TBARS production was inhibited by 57.4 and 51.1% for SBO and MHO, respectively. However, TBHQ is not yet licensed for food use in Canada and the European countries. The most commonly used synthetic antioxidants, namely, BHA and BHT, were not as effective as tea catechins in inhibiting the formation of flavor-active secondary oxidation products. Among catechins tested, ECG was 2.6 and 1.7 times more potent in SBO and 2.1 and 1.7 times more effective in MHO in inhibiting TBARS formation compared with BHA and BHT, respectively.

The main purpose of using antioxidants in lipids is to delay the accumulation of free radicals (to lower the free radical burden) and thus to enhance their oxidative stability. Catechins with free hydroxyl groups may act as free-radical acceptors and could also delay the formation of free radicals. Catechins possessing multiple hydroxyl groups (Fig. 12.1) exhibited better antioxidant activity than BHA and BHT which have only one hydroxyl group in their chemical structures. When in *ortho* configuration, multiple hydroxyl groups may also participate in chelation of metal ions, in addition to their free-radical scavenging effects.

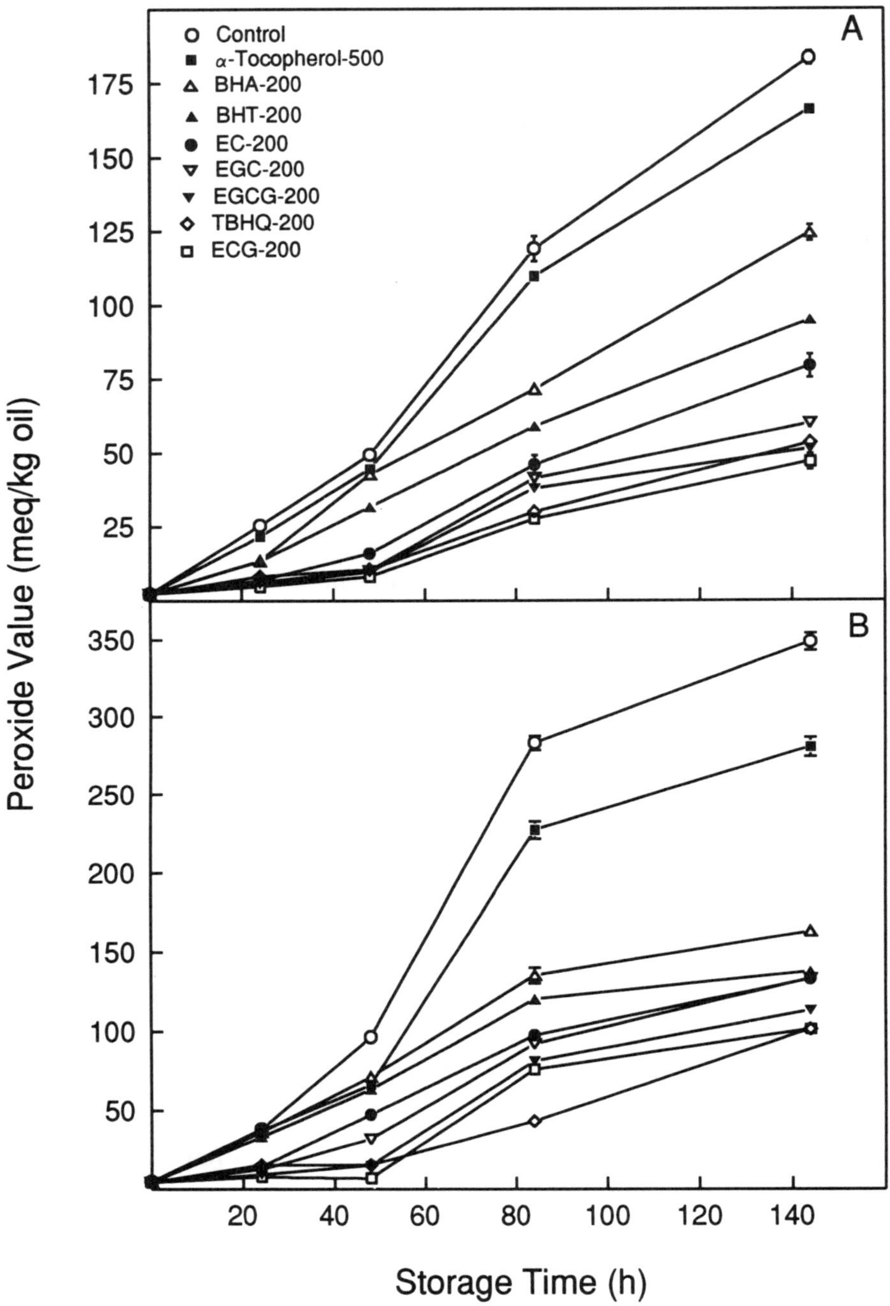

Fig. 12.2. Effect of tea catechins and conventional antioxidants on the peroxide formation of (A) RBD-seal blubber and (B) RBD-menhaden oils. *Abbreviations:* BHA, butylated hydroxyanisole; BHT, butylated hydroxytoluene; EC, (-)-epicatechin; EGC, (-)-epigallocatechin; EGCG, (-)-epigallocatechin gallate; TBHQ, *tert*-butylhydroquinone; ECG, (-)-epigallocatechin.

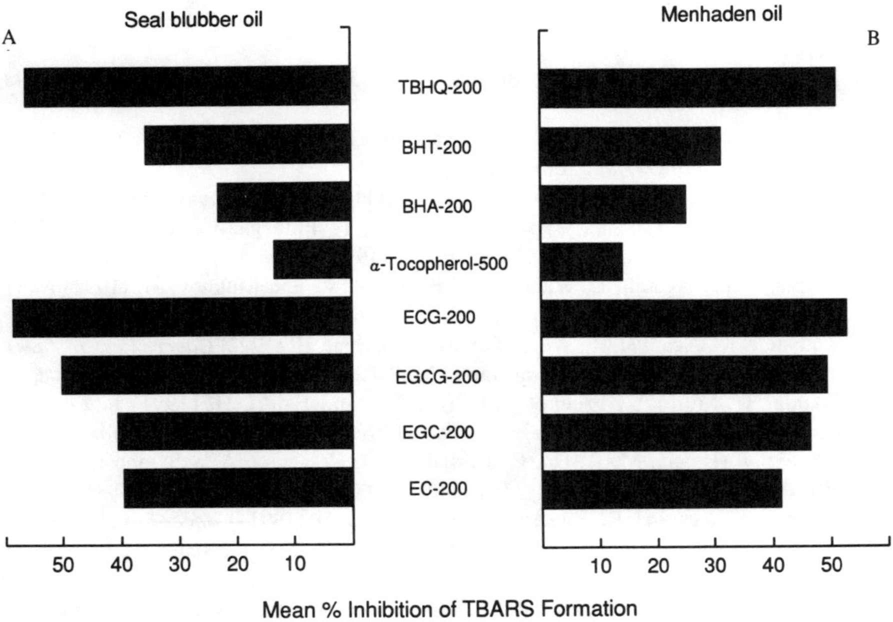

Fig. 12.3. Effect of tea catechins and conventional antioxidants on the 2-thiobarbituric acid reactive substances (TBARS) formation of (A) RBD-seal blubber and (B) RBD-menhaden oils. See Fig. 12.2 for abbreviations.

Conclusions

Green tea polyphenols namely, EGCG, ECG, EGC, and EC, exhibited good DPPH radical-, superoxide-, lipoxygenase-, as well as lipid oxidation-inhibition abilities in model systems and in marine oils. Tea catechins also showed high anticarcinogenic and antimutagenic abilities, and their use in foods, in addition to control of oxidation, may offer health benefits. Theaflavins, especially TF-2 and TF-1, exhibited the ability to inhibit the DPPH and superoxide radicals as well as lipoxygenase activity. Despite their good anticarcinogenic and antimutagenic activities, theaflavins are poor lipid peroxidation inhibitors and as such might not serve as good food antioxidants.

References

1. Cheng, S.J., Ho, C.-T., Lou, H.Z., Bao, Y.D., Jian, Y.Z., Li, M.H., Gao, Y.N., Zhu, G.F., Bai, J.F., Guo, S.P., and Li, X.Q. (1986) *Acta Biol. Exp. Sinica 19*, 427.
2. Wang, Z.Y., Cheng, S.J., Zhou, Z.C., Athar, M., Khan, W.A., Bickers, D.R., and Mukhtar, H. (1989) *Mutat. Res. 223*, 273.
3. Wang, Z.Y., Hong, J.Y., Huang, M.T., Renhl, K.R., Conney, A.H., and Yang, C.S. (1992) *Cancer Res. 52*, 1943.
4. Han, C., and Xu, Y. (1990) *Biomed. Environ. Sci. 3*, 35.

5. Katiyar, S.K., Agarwal, R., Ekker, S., Wood, G.S., and Mukhtar, H. (1993) *Carcinogenesis 14*, 361.
6. Katiyar, S.K., Agarwal, R., and Mukhtar, H. (1993) *Proc. Am. Associ. Cancer Res. 34*, 555.
7. Fujita, Y., Yamane, T., Tanaka, M., Kuwata, K., Okuzumi, J., Takahashi, T., Fujiki, H., and Okuda, T. (1989) *Jpn. J. Cancer Res. 80*, 503.
8. Agarwal, R., Katiyar, S.K., Zaidi, S.I.A., and Mukhtar, H. (1992) *Cancer Res. 52*, 3582.
9. Huang, M.-T., Ho, C.-T., Wang, Z.Y., Ferraro, T., Finnegan-Olive, T., Lou, Y.-R., Mitchell, J.M., Laskin, J.D., and Newmark, H. (1992) *Carcinogenesis 13*, 947.
10. Katiyar, S.K., Agaral, R., Wang, Z.Y., Bhatia, A.K., and Mukhtar, H. (1992) *Nutri. Cancer 18*, 73.
11. Katiyar, S.K., Agarwal, R., Wood, G.S., and Mukhtar, H. (1992) *Cancer Res. 52*, 6890.
12. Yoshizawa, S., Horiuchi, T., Suganuma, M., Nishiwaki, S., Yatsunami, J., Okabe, S., Okuda, T., Muto, Y., Frenkel, K., Troll, W., and Fujiki, H. (1991) in *Phenolic Compounds in Food and Their Effects on Health II—Antioxidants and Cancer Prevention* (Huang, M.-T., Ho, C.-T., and Lee, C.-Y., eds.), ACS Symposium Series 507, American Chemical Society, Washington, D.C., pp. 316–325.
13. Wang, Z.Y., Agarwal, R., Bickers, D., and Mukhtar, H. (1991) *Cancer Res. 12*, 1527.
14. Wang, Z.Y., Huang, M.-T., Ferraro, T., Wong, C.-Q., Lou, Y.-R., Reuhl, K., Iatropoulos, M., Yang, C.S., and Conney, A.H. (1992) *Cancer Res. 52*, 1162.
15. Conny, A.H., Wang, Z.Y., Huang, M.-T., Ho, C.-T., and Yang, C.S. (1992) *Preventive Medicine 52*, 361.
16. Cheng, S., Wang, Z., and Ho, C.-T. (1988) in *Current Medicine in China*, The People's Medical Publishing House, Beijing, pp. 165–172.
17. Randall, T.R., Cheng, S., and Klaunig, E. (1989) *Carcinogenesis 10*, 1003.
18. Chen, C.-W., and Ho, C.-T. (1995) *J. Food Lipids 2*, 35.
19. Ho. C.-T., Chen, Q., Shi, H., Zhang, K.-Q., and Rosen, R.T. (1992) *Preventive Medicine 21*, 520.
20. Xie, B., Shi, H., Chen, Q., and Ho, C.-T. (1993) *Proc. Nat. Sci. Counc. ROC Part B, Life Sci. 17*, 77.
21. Hara, Y. (1994) in *Food Phytochemicals for Cancer Prevention II—Tea, Spices and Herbs* (Ho, C.-T., Osawa, T., Huang, M.-T., and Rosen, R.T., eds.), ACS Symposium Series 547, American Chemical Society, Washington, D.C., pp. 34–50.
22. Lunder, T. (1989) *Farm. Tijdschr. Belg. 66*, 34.
23. Graham, H.N. (1992) *Preventive Medicine 21*, 334.
24. Blois, M.S. (1958) *Nature (London) 181*, 1199.
25. Yen, G.-C., and Duh, P.-D. (1994) *J. Agric. Food Chem. 42*, 629.
26. Shimada, K., Fujikawa, K., Yahara, K., and Nakamura, T. (1992) *J. Agric. Food Chem. 40*, 945.
27. Simic, M.G., and Jovanovic, S.V. (1990) in *Antimutagenesis and Anticarcinogenesis Mechanisms II* (Kuroda, Y., Shankel, D.M., and Waters, M.D., eds.), Plenum Press, New York, pp. 127–137.
28. Mason, R.P., Stolze, K., and Flitter, W.D. (1990) in *Antimutagenesis and Anticarcinogenesis Mechanisms II* (Kuroda, Y., Shankel, D.M., and Waters, M.D., eds.), Plenum Press, New York, pp. 119–125.
29. Halliwell, B. (1991) in *Free Radicals and Food Additives* (Aruoma, O.I., and Halliwell, B., eds.), Taylor, and Francis Ltd., London, pp. 37–57.

30. Zhao, B., Li, X., He, R., Cheng, S., and Wenjuan, X. (1989) *Cell Biophys. 14*, 175.
31. Huang, M.-T., Lysz, T., Ferraro, T., Abidi, T.F., Laskin, J.D., and Conney, A.H. (1991) *Cancer Res. 51*, 813.
32. Belman, S., Solomon, J., Segal, A., Block, E., and Barany, G. (1989) *J. Biochem. Toxicol. 4*, 151.
33. Block, E., Iyer, R., Griconi, S., Saha, C., Belman, S., and Lossing, F.P. (1988) *J. Am. Chem. Soc. 110*, 7813.
34. Hamberg. M., and Samuelsson, B. (1967) *J. Biol. Chem. 242*, 5329.
35. Percival, M.D. (1991) *J. Biol. Chem. 266*, 10058.
36. Namiki, M. (1990) *CRC Crit. Rev. Food Sci. Nutr. 29*, 273.
37. Shahidi, F., and Wanasundara, P.K.J.P.D. (1992) *CRC Crit. Rev. Food Sci. Nutr. 32*, 67.
38. Wanasundara, U.N., Amarowicz, R., and F. Shahidi, (1994) *J. Agric. Food Chem. 42*, 1285.
39. Wanasundara, U.N., and Shahidi, F. (1996) *J. Am. Oil Chem. Soc.,* in press.
40. Amarowicz, R., and Shahidi, F. (1995) *J. Food Lipids 2*, 47.
41. Yoshizawa, S., Horiuchi, T., Fujiki, H., Yoshida, T., Okuda, T., and Sugimura, T. (1987) *Phytotherapy 1*, 44.

Chapter 13

Optimizing Lipid Stability with Natural Inhibitors

R.J. Evans

KALSEC Inc., 1127 Buchelew Drive, Kingsport TN 37663.

Introduction

Antioxidant properties of naturally occurring substances have been evaluated extensively, often in model systems involving isolated lipids. The suggestions presented here on the substrate-specific nature of free radical interceptor (FRI) reactions and on a hypothesis to explain the mechanism of synergism observed in certain FRI combinations are based on published studies, hundreds of experiments, and on observed performance in commercially processed foods. Managing oxidation provides the benefit of extended shelf life for fats and oils. It also helps stabilize carotenoid pigments, muscle phospholipids, and proteins. The oxidation mechanisms involved vary. The relative superiority of any one inhibitor is dependent upon the substrate, environment, and test method.

Problems with oxidative rancidity have commanded special attention because they are encountered in many foods. The control of rancidity and of bacterial spoilage has been the subject of experimentation since man first attempted to store foods. Through the ages, these problems were managed with salt, cooking, dehydration, vinegar, wood smoke, freezing, and spices. The ethnic preferences for highly seasoned dishes often can be traced to the use of the available spices, primarily as oxidation inhibitors, over many centuries. Their use in preventing rancidity and as quasi-bacteriostats was restricted by their limited availability and the consequent high cost of spices. Rome was once ransomed for three thousand pounds of black pepper (1).

Newer options for inhibiting oxidation were not available until early in this century. Around 1910, the hydrogenation process made oils more stable and gave rise to the development of vegetable shortenings as alternatives to lard and tallow. In the late 1940s, the first synthetic antioxidant received clearance in the U.S. About the same time, the development of the molecular still made tocopherol concentrates practical. Improved extraction procedures yielded improved spice oleoresins. Spice extracts eliminated the sanitation problems associated with ground spices and also provided oil solubility. Another important property, good thermal stability, was provided by oleoresin rosemary. Higher initial costs associated with the use of these natural soy and spice extracts were responsible for their benefits often being overlooked in the U.S. In Japan and the EC, use of synthetic antioxidants is more restricted. In those areas, rosemary, sage, tea, and mixed tocopherols have frequently proven to be more effective in extending shelf life of formulated foods than when formulated with a synthetic FRI.

Research published over the last few decades, and subsequent publicity, has fostered significant consumer resistance to the use of synthetic antioxidants. Articles on dietary components that possibly predispose one to atherosclerosis have led to public aversion toward saturated fats and partial hydrogenation of oils. Other studies suggest that certain polyunsaturated fatty acids are essential, especially in prenatal and infant nutrition. Designed foods have achieved popularity. The result is more polyunsaturated oils in the diet. These oils are more susceptible to oxidation as shown in Table 13.1 (2). Higher polyunsaturate levels in the diet have resulted in increased oxidative stress. These stresses can be effectively managed by combinations of natural FRIs.

The restricted U.S. clearances for synthetic antioxidants are generally based on fat content. They are not permitted at practical levels in certain applications, such as further processed muscle foods. The stabilization of pigments and of protein against oxidation involves mechanisms different from those seen in lipid oxidation and are independent of the levels of the lipid in a food. These factors have also given impetus to evaluation of natural inhibitors. The natural extracts demonstrate specific benefits in a wide variety of substrates and in dealing the various oxidation reactions.

Basic Considerations

In today's environment, newly recognized market needs are justifying initial cost considerations. Natural inhibitors can protect the quality of many foods more effectively than synthetics. The economic benefits provided by improved keeping qualities are seen in reduced packaging cost, broader distribution, and consumer acceptance.

There is no evidence that a single food-grade synthetic antioxidant or natural inhibitor outperforms all others in all lipid substrates. Further, there is ample evidence that combinations of two or more FRIs offer improved performance. Effective formulations often include natural acids to combat prooxidants. Carotenoid pigments may also be added to minimize the damage from light. Formulating the best combination of the appropriate natural inhibitors involves a number of factors. These include: the specific oxidation mechanism to be suppressed; prooxidant factors in the substrate and

TABLE 13.1
Relative Speed of Oxidation of Fatty Acids Autoxidation at 20°C

C_{18} Fatty acid	Relative rate
18:0 (Stearic)	1
18:1 (Oleic)	100
18:2 (Linoleic)	1200
18:3 (Linolenic)	1500

in the process environment; solubility; flavor; color; thermal stability; cost; and the consumer's acceptance of the appropriate label statements. It is important to be aware that diverse oxidation reactions do take place in foods. Some are beneficial to performance such as the oxidation of protein to provide structural strength in bread. Other oxidation reactions often cause a loss in quality that may be effectively slowed by an appropriate inhibitor.

Identifying the specific reaction involved is fundamental to managing oxidation. It is equally important to realize that the prooxidant factors present in many foods have to be neutralized. Managing the prooxidant factors can be more productive than the use of FRI. The merit of this approach to managing oxidation is seen in the impressive shelf life of ultrarefined, additive-free, retail salad oils. Process conditions can be modified to minimize a host of factors including the catalytic effect of light, alkaline pH, metals, heat, and enzymes. When these factors are properly managed, packaging and use of formulated oxidation-inhibiting blends should be much more effective in protecting quality. Optimum performance from an inhibitor blend requires the earliest possible addition to the substrate. The adverse effects of delaying addition even a few hours are readily perceived, even in low-fat foods such as fish and poultry products.

There are several areas often overlooked by food processors that can influence stability. Specifications on purchased oils and fats can often be tightened at little or no cost. Moisture should be very close to zero. Free fatty acids and pigments can initiate oxidation and should be minimized. High Totox values indicate an abused oil even though it meets other specifications at the time of delivery. Trace metal content should be a specific concern. Process water can contain iron, copper, or other metals that, as shown in Table 13.2 (3), are oxidation catalysts. Copper gaskets and brass are not uncommon, nor is the wrong grade of steel in holding tanks and lines. Frequent evaluation of process water is suggested.

Proper storage is important. Sparging oils in bulk holding tanks with nitrogen has a positive benefit, as do stirrers in holding tanks. The use of chelating agents to complex and deactivate metals is helpful. Citric acid is one of many chelators used in fats and oils. Enzymes are a separate problem because they may initiate oxidation. Their presence in a variety of ingredients in processed foods complicates matters. Elevated temperatures can activate some enzymes, inactivate others.

TABLE 13.2
Concentration of Metal Required to Reduce the Keeping Time of Lard by 50% at 98°C

Metal	Concentration (ppm)
Copper	0.05
Manganese	0.06
Iron	0.06
Nickel	2.2
Aluminum	50

Selecting an Effective Oxidation Inhibitor

In the U.S., three synthetic antioxidants have been very popular, butylated hydroxyanisole (BHA), butylated hydroxytoluene (BHT) and tert-butylhydroquinone (TBHQ). (Propyl gallate's color reaction limits it use). The success each enjoys relates to its benefits in certain fats. Commercial recommendations suggest that the performance of each synthetic is highly specific and, because each is a distinctly different structure, this is not surprising (4). The effectiveness of an FRI is believed to relate to solubility, molecular configuration, concentration, and other factors which could affect its ability to react with specific types of free radicals. These free radicals differ with each of the unsaturated acids in the lipid substrate. This specificity has resulted in the need for the variety of different "antioxidant solutions" containing more than one FRI. Combinations can provide improved performance. No known combination of the three available synthetics totally arrests oxidation. The far greater number of functional FRI molecules in natural extracts of soybean, rosemary, sage, and tea suggests that their diversity offers a potential for significant improvements in stabilizing lipids.

A review of the basic oxidation reactions will help illustrate why a diversity of molecular structures in an FRI combination may outperform higher levels of a single molecule. The predominant form of oxygen present in the atmosphere is in the triplet state. It does not readily react with lipids (5). It reacts with unstable lipid-derived free radicals, created when a prooxidant abstracts a hydrogen from the lipid. The origins of the initial free radicals required to start the chain reaction of oxidation can be traced to prooxidants. The more common prooxidant initiators are often ignored when theorizing about oxidation management, and some may be inherent in the oil, even after refining (6).

The free radicals that develop in fats and oils are diverse in structure. Unchecked, they attack unsaturated fats, creating more and newer radical configurations. The chain reaction accelerates, leading to rancidity. As Table 13.1 illustrates, the more unsaturated the fat, the more rapid the onset of rancidity. Also, the more unsaturated the fat, the greater the diversity of free radical configurations. Grosch (7) lists some 70 breakdown products already identified that result from the unchecked oxidation of a linoleate ester. The variety of free radicals that may have been formed in this oxidation cascade illustrate the magnitude of the problem of intercepting all of the free radicals in a system with a single FRI. The structural component in most synthetics and natural inhibitors that facilitates free radical interception is phenolic. The hydroxyl group of the phenolic may readily donate an electron or the hydrogen to intercept free radicals. The intercepted radical is converted to a more stable compound.

Misconception #1

In some early texts, the FRI mechanism was depicted by Equation [1]. It is an accurate depiction only in those rare situations in which oxygen is present at extremely low levels. This concept leads to the erroneous assumption that an appropriate FRI, added at adequate levels, will stop oxidation.

$$R^{\bullet} + PH \rightarrow RH + P^{\bullet} \text{ (or P)} \quad [1]$$

In Equation 1, the $R^{\bullet}$ represents the reactive lipid free radical created by a prooxidant's abstraction of a hydrogen from a lipid. The lipid free radical can abstract a hydrogen from the appropriate FRI shown as PH. As a result, the free radical is now a stable RH and the FRI becomes a radical, $P^{\bullet}$, generally of low reactivity. $P^{\bullet}$ may also rearrange internally to become a stable molecule P. Because oxygen is commonly present in foods at levels adequate to negate Equation [1], it is not generally applicable.

The Probable Mechanism

Equations [2] and [3] illustrate the more probable reactions occurring in the presence of oxygen.

$$R^{\bullet} + O \rightarrow RO^{\bullet} \quad [2]$$

$$RO^{\bullet} + O \rightarrow ROO^{\bullet} \quad [3]$$

The radical $R^{\bullet}$ will preferentially react with oxygen by Equation [2] to form an alkoxyl radical, $RO^{\bullet}$, which then further reacts with oxygen by Equation [3] to form the peroxyl radical ROO°.

$$ROO^{\bullet} + LH \rightarrow L^{\bullet} + ROOH \quad [4]$$

The peroxyl radical can attack another lipid by Equation [4] creating a new lipid free radical and an unstable hydroperoxide. Hydroperoxide decomposition starts a second oxidation cascade, creating additional new free radicals capable of additional abstractions. Radical content increases exponentially and the "chain reaction" accelerates.

$$ROO^{\bullet} + PH \rightarrow ROOH + P^{\bullet} \text{ (or P)} \quad [5]$$

The peroxyl radical can preferentially react with an appropriate FRI by Equation [5]. This reaction does not yield the new lipid free radical generated by Equation [4] but does yield an unstable peroxide. The chain reaction is interrupted, but the hydroperoxide will propagate. Further oxidation reactions are slowed but not stopped.

The formation of peroxide intermediates provides compounds that are easily measured. The typical plot of peroxyl radicals and hydroperoxides levels in an accelerated aging of fat is shown in Fig. 13.1, line A.

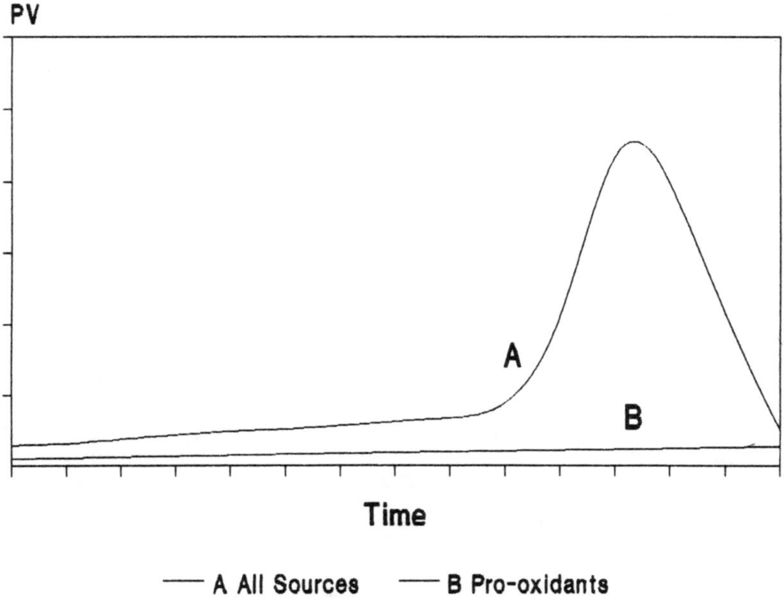

Fig. 13.1. The level of peroxides, expressed as peroxide value (PV), in a typical oxidizing lipid is illustrated by line A. Line B is an arbitrary illustrative plot of peroxide levels resulting solely from direct abstraction of a hydrogen from the lipid by a prooxidant such as iron. The peroxide content represented by the difference between lines B and A results from the propagating chain reaction of hydrogen abstraction by lipid free radicals initially induced by the action of the prooxidant.

Peroxides gradually increase during an initiation period to a critical concentration at which the rate of peroxide development accelerates exponentially, the propagation stage. Normally, it is after the sharp upward inflection of the curve that perceptible rancidity develops as determined by odor and taste. Eventually, in the termination phase, the peroxide content begins dropping. Only a small fraction of the susceptible fatty acids has been subjected to hydrogen abstraction. The high levels of unstable peroxides may accelerate their own decomposition, accounting for the fall-off in total peroxides in the termination stage. Figure 13.1, line B, is an arbitrary estimate included to reflect the linear increase in peroxides from the constant abstraction of hydrogen from lipids by prooxidants. The addition of an FRI retards peroxide development as shown in Fig. 13.2. Line A represents peroxide levels in the control. Line B shows the extension of the induction period by the added FRI.

Misconception #2

The peroxyl radicals are often presumed to combine with an FRI *via* Equation [5] as opposed to attacking another lipid as shown in Equation [4]. If this were true, it

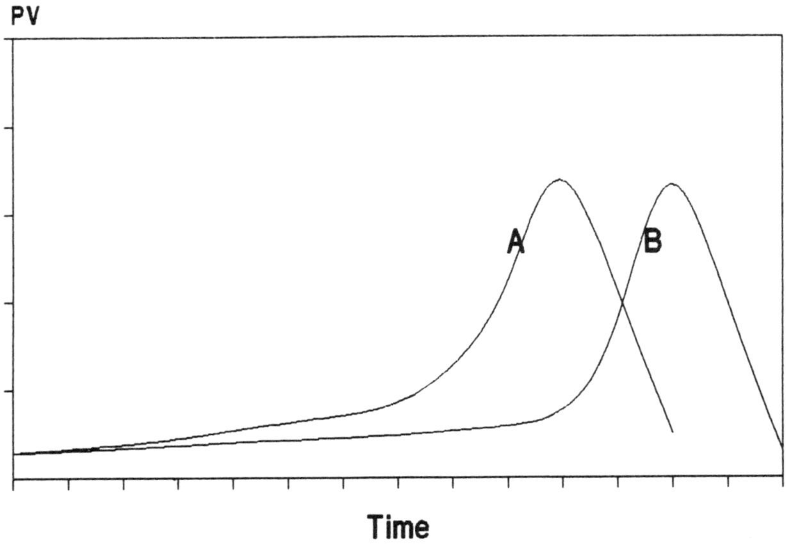

Fig. 13.2. Line A represents the typical peroxide levels observed in an oxidizing lipid (control). Line B illustrates the ability of a free radical interceptor (FRI) to delay the rapid increase in peroxides associated with rancidity.

is reasonable to expect that, if the FRI is present at a high enough concentration, the only increase in total peroxides would be the modest amount created by iron or other prooxidants. No peroxyl radicals would survive to attack other lipids. Yet, it appears that the chain-reaction effect of peroxyl radicals continues at a reduced rate in the presence of high levels of an FRI. Adequate levels do suppress the rate of peroxide build-up to varying degrees. Evidence of the total elimination of the chain-reaction effect of Equation [4] is rarely seen.

FRIs Are Substrate Specific

The common understanding of the lipid oxidation mechanism in Equation [5] may have to be modified. If the chosen FRI is able to react with only certain types of free radicals for steric, solubility, or other reasons, an FRI added to a lipid may not intercept all of the various radicals generated in that lipid. Some would be intercepted, some not. The effect of the added phenolic would increase the fat stability vs. a control fat because it has measurably suppressed induction by intercepting a certain type of radical. Other types of radicals are not intercepted and are free to react. The net result is that the overall stability of the fat is improved but it is not stable.

Schuler (8) cited unpublished data from Pongracz shown in Fig. 13.3. The effect of various levels of an added FRI on the stability of lard is shown. Carnosic

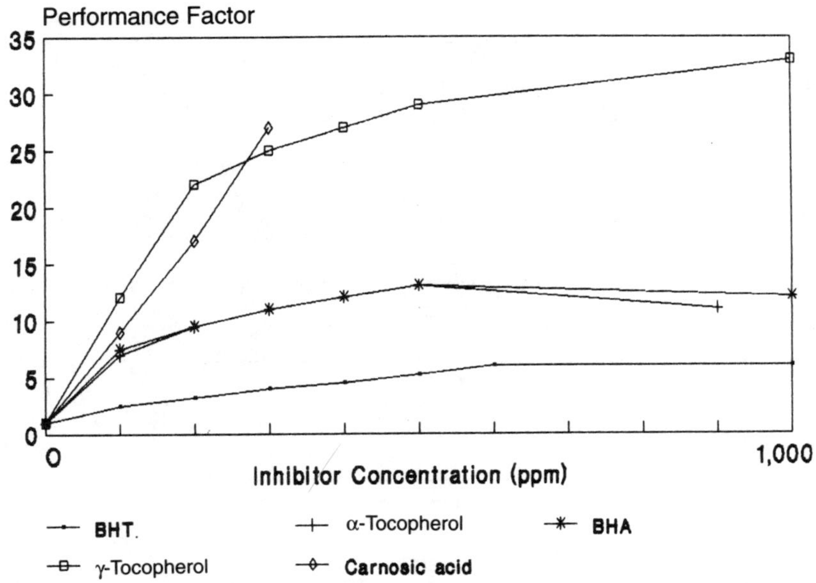

Fig. 13.3. The relative improvement (performance factor) in the oxidative stability of lard resulting from the addition of incremental levels of various free radical interceptors (FRI) is shown. Little or no increase in benefit is seen at higher levels of butylated hydroxyanisole (BHA), butylated hydroxytolune (BHT) or α-tocopherol, whereas γ-tocopherol continues to improve stability. Carnosic acid (from rosemary) provides a linear dose response at levels tested (Rancimat, 120°C).

acid (present in rosemary extracts) shows a linear dose response at levels tested. Others show diminishing utility at low levels. The data suggest that a specific free radical type, present at a high concentration in lard, is intercepted by carnosic acid. The rapidly diminishing increment in the benefit of the BHA and of BHT in Fig. 13.3 suggests that low levels of the radicals for which they were specific have been totally managed by interception. The slight decline in performance of α-tocopherol (*d* or *dl* not defined) may indicate the onset of a prooxidant effect. This prooxidant effect has been reported (9) when 0.02% of *dl*-α-tocopherol is added to vegetable oils. It may indicate the formation of prooxidant dimers resulting from the high concentration of spent tocopherol radicals (10).

When peroxides reach the inflection stage and start their exponential increase, the acceleration has often been attributed to exhaustion of the phenolic FRI. If this were true, adding excessive amounts of a phenolic to an incubating sample just prior to the time of inflection should significantly extend the induction beyond a single treated control. Figure 13.4 supports the data cited by Schuler and discounts FRI depletion.

If FRI are specific to certain radical configurations or solubilities, it would explain why mixtures of FRIs are frequently better than a single FRI, keeping total addition equal. It also explains why very high levels of a single phenolic normally

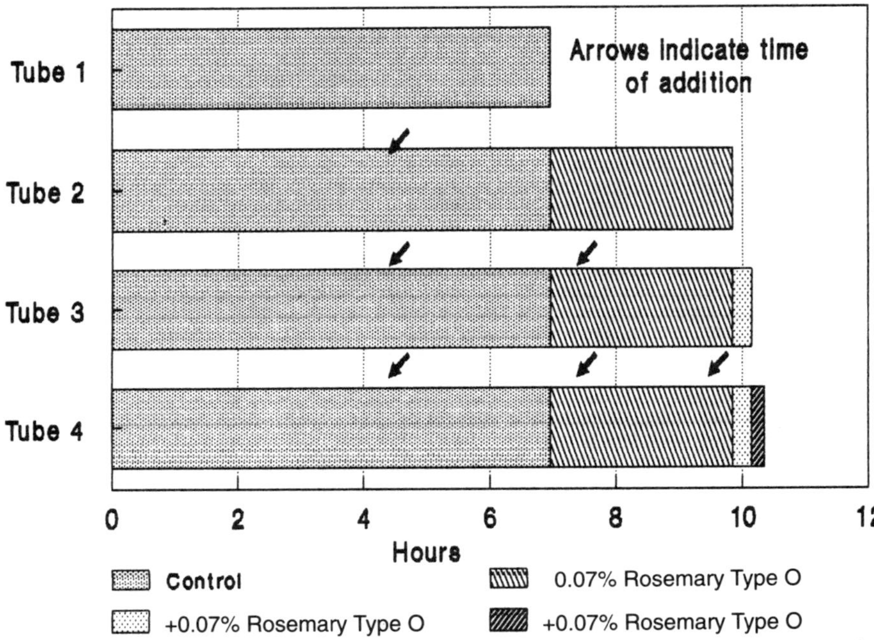

Fig. 13.4. The diminishing benefit of repeated supplementation of refined, bleached, and deodorized soy oil with 700 ppm of a rosemary extract is illustrated. Arrows show the time of initial fortification of tubes 2, 3, and 4 and of additional supplementation of tubes 3 and 4. Depletion should not have been a significant factor because later additions had little impact. Volatility loss with rosemary should be minimal. The onset of induction in the presence of excess free radical interceptor (FRI) suggests the free radical specific nature of FRI reactions (Rancimat, 120°C).

do not make a fat or oil extremely stable. The same theory helps to explain synergism. Figure 13.5 presents observed synergism, supporting the theory. The data are expressed as ratios of time to inflection using an Oxidograph. The control oil time is defined as 1, and the experimental time is compared with the control time to establish the recorded ratio. In the plot in Fig. 13.5, the temperature used with poultry fat was 120°C. Rosemary extract at 0.05% improved stability by 13%. Tocopherol at 0.10% provided a 226% improvement. By combining the two inhibitors, a 550% improvement resulted.

The rosemary used may have intercepted the free radicals emanating from fatty acids present at moderate levels in poultry. Other unintercepted radicals emanating from other groups of fatty acids continue the initiation process. Similarly, the tocopherol managed a different group of free radicals. Cort (4) reported BHT to be superior to tocopherol in stabilizing oleic acid, and BHT inferior with linoleic acid. Hussain (11) has suggested that α-tocopherol is a prooxidant with linoleic acid but is superior in stabilizing linoleic-derived hydroperoxides. FRIs are sub-

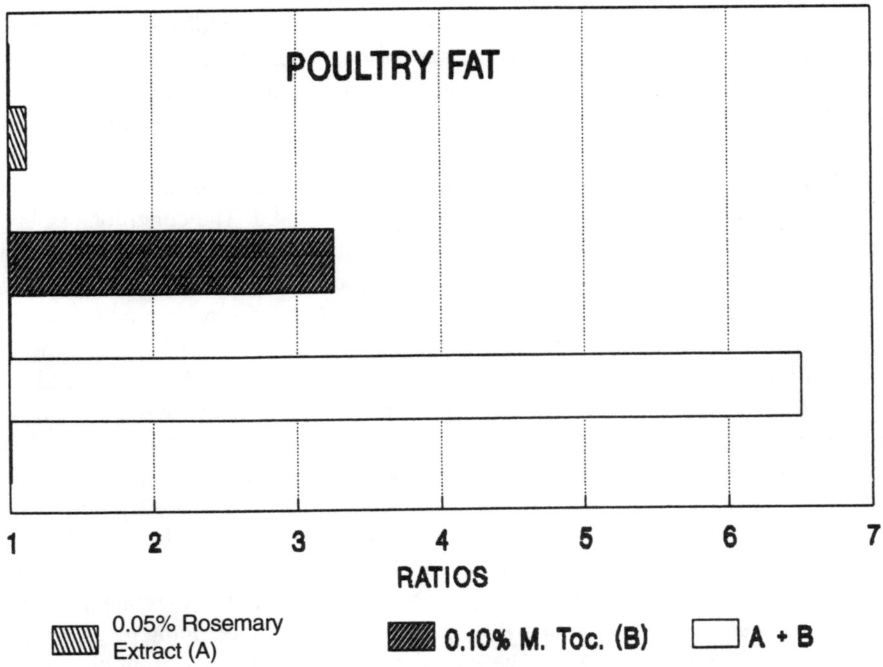

Fig. 13.5. The ratios of induction times observed in poultry fat stabilized with rosemary extract and tocopherol, alone and in combination, are compared with the control induction time. The benefit of the combination is synergistic (Rancimat, 120°C).

strate specific. If depletion of the FRI were responsible for inflection, the result of combining the two would be simply additive. In Fig. 13.5, the combination of the two extracts, each multiphenolic, allows for interception of more varieties of free radical configurations than either alone. FRI blends can be reasonably optimized for a freshly refined oil by trial and error. However, the level and type of radicals present will change rapidly if addition is delayed.

A Synergistic Mechanism?

One hypothesis may explain why results are sometimes synergistic rather than simply additive. In comparing the effect of FRIs, it is interesting to focus not on induction time but on the effect of the FRIs in reducing the unintercepted free radical concentration and its effect of the rate of propagation. The impact of this low concentration is important because the rate of propagation is probably related exponentially to the free radical content. As content is lowered, the concentration-dependent acceleration rate is lowered and the time required to reach a specific higher radical content, or critical stage, is significantly increased. The moderate decreases in free radical content have substantial benefits for stability.

An explanation for synergism can be derived from a theoretical lipid for which free radical configurations generated in the various steps in the cascade of oxidation can be grouped into three distinct types. Two theoretical FRIs, A and B are introduced, and each intercepts only one of the three groups of unique free radicals. Table 13.3 reflects the assumptions.

In Fig. 13.6, we have plotted the effect of accelerated conditions on the control, where 100% of the free radicals remain unintercepted. The conditions of this illustration involve heat and bubbled air which accelerate the reaction rate and account for the perceptible change early in the plotted rate of oxidation. Further, there seems to be a specific threshold concentration of reaction components responsible for the very rapid increase in the rate of peroxide formation resulting in propagation, the critical concentration. This critical level of free radical concentration is designated by an arbitrary line. Above the critical concentration, the rate of propagation accelerates more rapidly than below the line. In a 2nd sample, FRI A is added in excess to the oil and 20% of the radicals are intercepted. The induction period is extended about 25%. The important consideration is that 80% survive as free radicals. If only FRI B is added in a 3rd sample, 68% of the radicals are free to propagate. The induction time is extended 55%. This is a greater improvement than with A because more radicals are intercepted and the number of remaining free radical is lowered further. If A and B are added in a 4th sample, unintercepted radical content is reduced to 48%. The calculated improvement in induction time arrived at by adding the increases in induction times over the control time of both A (25%) and B (55%), represented by the broken line, is about 80%. The theoretical plot of the exponential benefit of reducing the initial radical content, shown in the plot labeled Observed Synergism (Fig. 13.6), improves performance by 170% over the control. This would explain the data reported in Fig. 13.5.

The effect of combining FRI A and FRI B in further reducing initial free radical content with a consequent reduction in the exponential rate of propagation can explain positive synergism.

The hypothesis also explains negative synergism. If A and B both have the ability to intercept only Type II radicals, then together they could reduce radical

TABLE 13.3
Interception of Free Radicals by FRI

Free radical type	% of total	Intercepted by
I	48	
II	20	A
III	32	B
Remaining unintercepted radical content		
Adding only FRI A	80%	
Adding only FRI B	68%	
Adding FRI A and B	48%	

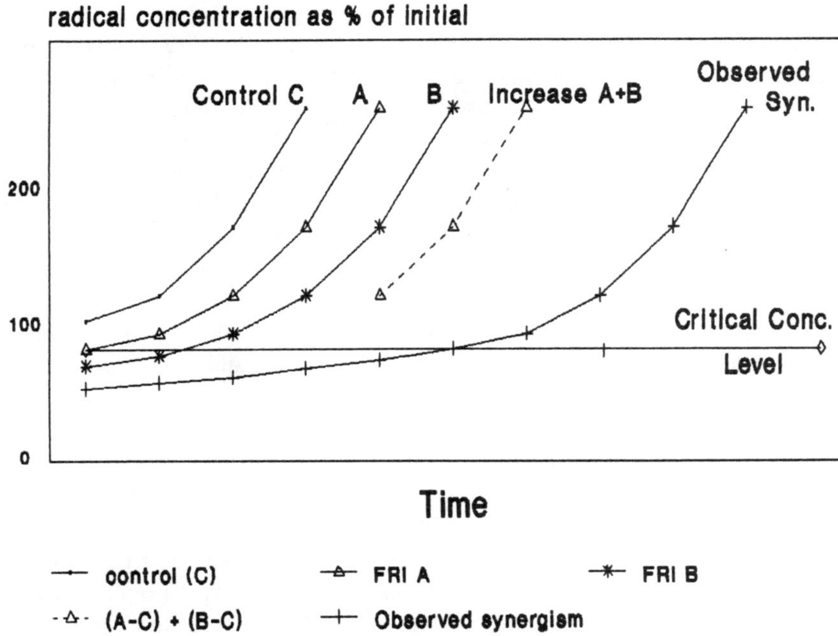

Fig. 13.6. A number of assumptions are made here to illustrate a concept. In theoretical oil, initial free radical content is 100%. A "critical concentration" for free radicals in this oil is defined at 75% of the zero-time radical concentration. Next, the rate of increase in acceleration of free radical propagation increases more rapidly above the critical concentration. Finally, the free radicals present are divided into three groups, each with different ability to react with a given free radical interceptor (FRI). FRI A is added and can react with only one group, present at 20% in the oil and can reduce free radical content to 80% of the original content. B reacts with a second group only, present at 32%. B would reduce free radical content to 68%. Adding A and B together reduces free radical content to 48%. The improvement in the oil stability, if simply additive, is plotted as Increase A + B. However, the exponential benefit of lower propagation rates below the critical free radical concentration provides more than an additive benefit. The plot of the curve "Observed Synergism" would explain synergistic results as derived from lower initial increases in acceleration rates.

content only down to 80%, because they eliminate only Type II radicals present at 20%. A alone would provide the plotted A response; B alone could not exceed A's performance due to the limited Type II radical content. Benefits would not be additive. The negative synergism sometimes seen with combinations is simply the result of overlapping capabilities of A and B and the low levels of the free radicals they are capable of intercepting.

This plot assumes some acceleration rates which are totally arbitrary but are consistent for all plots at the same levels of free radical concentration. Below the assigned critical radical concentration, the rates of increase in acceleration used for the various plots are low and are high above. Each rate allows a linear semi-log plot. While there is much in the literature defining reaction rates, data are on fatty acid esters. Cosgrove (12) observed that the rates for triglyceride oxidation do not conform. These assumptions help in understanding benefits and shortcomings of multi-FRI combinations. The validity of the general concept has been endorsed by years of work with natural FRI combinations in various substrates and has contributed to the design of proprietary blends of natural FRIs with predictable performance.

The preferential reaction of the peroxyl free radical with the FRI, Equation [5] rather than another lipid, Equation [4], holds only if the FRI has the right properties and is present in adequate concentration. Just as Equation [1] is the correct understanding only under certain conditions, a revision of Equation [5] to Equation [5a] may be appropriate. The mechanism is selective.

$$R^{\bullet} + \text{[a specific FRI, PH]} \rightarrow RH + P^{\bullet} \text{ (or P)} \qquad [5a]$$

The measurable differences in the effectiveness of the tocopherols illustrate how the molecular structure of a phenolic can affect its ability to intercept radicals. The inhibiting effects of α-, β-, δ- and γ-tocopherols have shown significant differences (13). These large hydroxyaromatic molecules differ slightly in the number and location of their methyl groups. Steric hindrance varies and performance vary. There is evidence that steric hindrance is a significant factor. The difference in the performance of the 2 vs. the 3 isomer of BHA is seen in numerous fats. Also, using a single BHA isomer, Fukuzuki and Naburo (14) found it more effective with the *cis* isomer of a C_{18} acid than with the *trans* isomer.

Which FRI Is Best?

Until recently, partial hydrogenation and the popular synthetics provided a practical, though imperfect, solution to the need for satisfactory oil stability. Now. there are other options. The determination of which FRI is best for the various fatty acid ratios in different oils is the tedious part of managing oxidation. Figure 13.7 illustrates the diverse structures in natural extracts. Pioneering work by Chang (15) with rosemary suggested more than 20 phenolics in rosemary, many of which have been identified. Mixed tocopherol concentrates provide α-, β-, δ- and γ-tocopherol. There are other identified free radical interceptors in minor concentrations in mixed tocopherol concentrates. Tea provides various catechins and theaflavin gallates. Tea also provides lipoxygenase-inhibiting activity (16). When compared with BHA in lard on an equimolar basis, the multiphenolic tea oleoresin provides superior performance (17). The numerous hydroxyl groups provided by tea catechins provide varied reaction sites. Other FRIs may remain to be identified in all three of these natural extracts.

The possible combination of any two or more of multiphenolic natural extracts provides a potpourri of FRIs. Theoretically, adding high levels of all the known natural inhibitors would optimize stability. A number of factors, including cost, limit

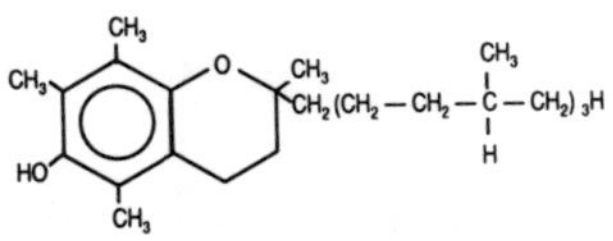

α-tocopherol

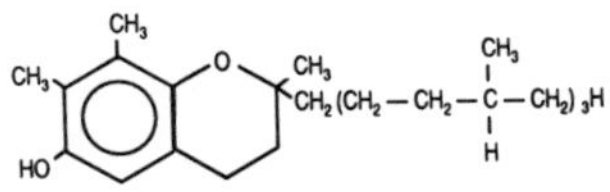

γ-tocopherol

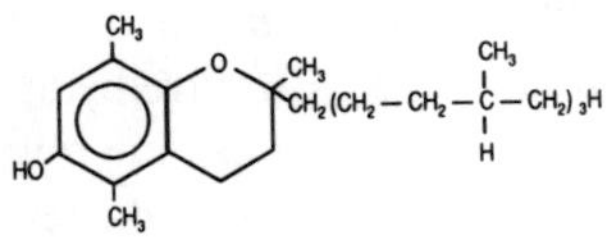

β-tocopherol

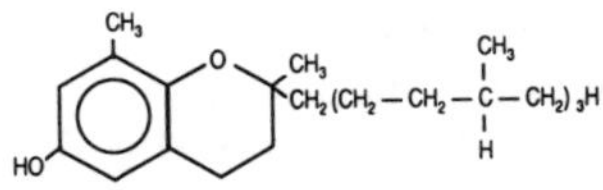

δ-tocopherol

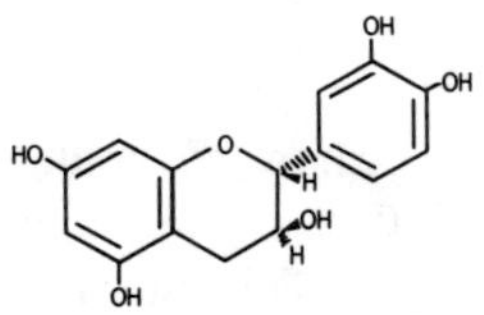

(-)-Catechin

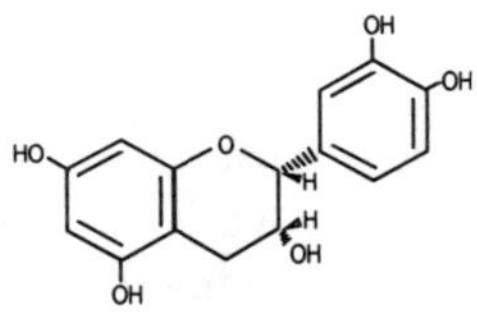

(-)-Epicatechin

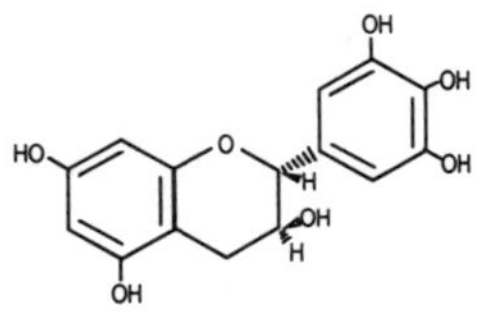

(+)-Gallocatechin

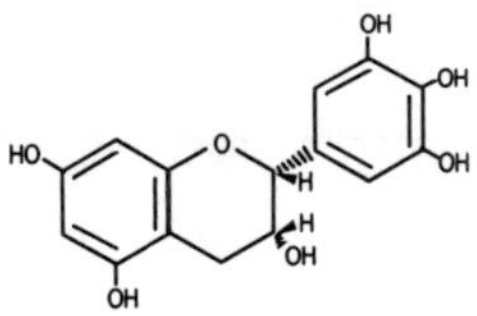

(-)-Epigallocatechin

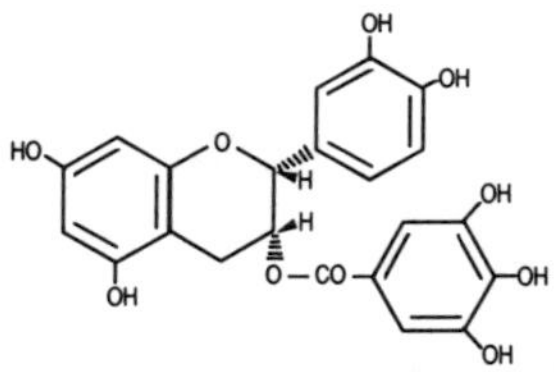

(-)-Epicatechin gallate

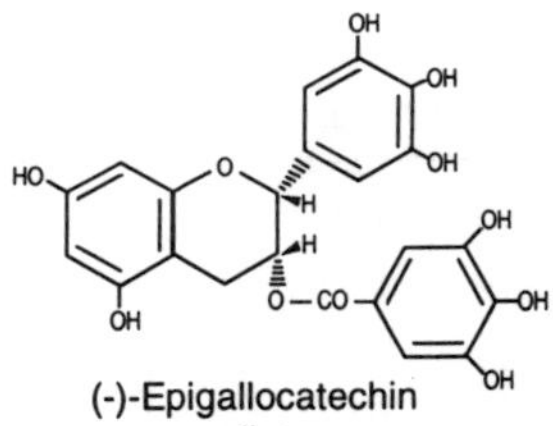

(-)-Epigallocatechin gallate

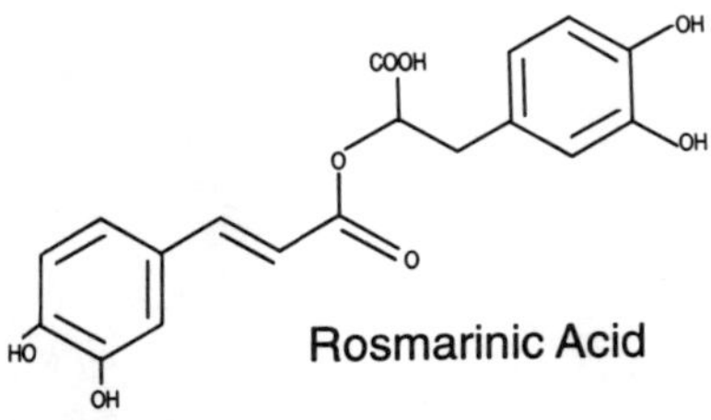

Rosmarinic Acid

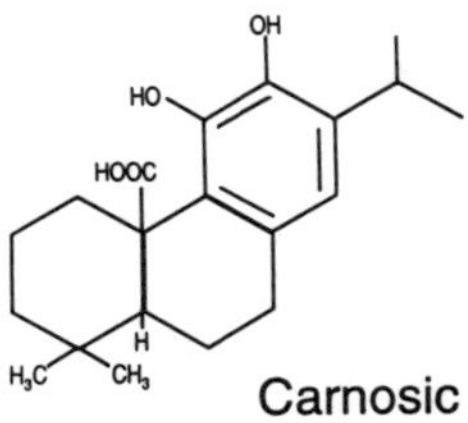

Carnosic Acid

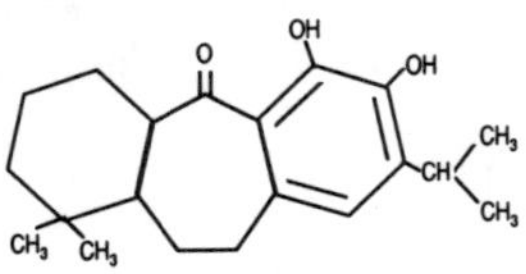

Rosmaridiphenol

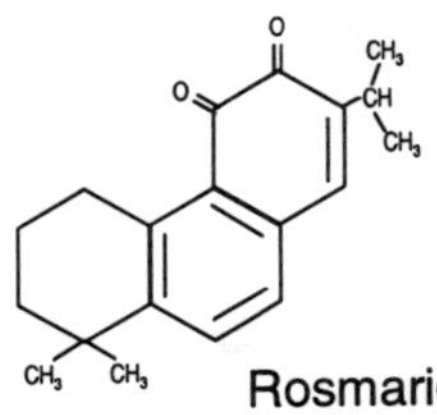

Rosmariquinone

Fig. 13.7. Some of the many identified FRIs in tea, rosemary, and soy are shown. The performance of the various natural extracts as antioxidants relates to the number of hydroxyl groups, lipid solubility, and steric and other factors.

this broad-spectrum approach. Another factor may be a difference in the visual appearance of the oil. More important is the tendency of high concentrations of some spent inhibitor radicals to polymerize and become prooxidant. Figure 13.8 illustrates the differences in the relative performance of an FRI in various oils. While the tea extract provides a positive response in all oils tested, the relative response varies. Partial hydrogenation generally improves oxidative stability of an oil. It can also change the optimum FRI formulation for stabilizing those unsaturates that survive hydrogenation. Data in Fig. 13.9 suggest that the appropriate natural FRI blend can improve stability of an oil beyond that provided by the combined effects of partial hydrogenation and the legal limit of TBHQ. Trial and error appear to be a better approach than theorizing. The commercial availability of natural FRI blends, formulated in ratios appropriate for a specific fat or oil, is the result of years of trial and error.

Ascorbic Acid. Ascorbic acid must be mentioned because it is multifunctional. Its use in lipids has been restricted by its insolubility. Ascorbyl palmitate was introduced as a synthetic approach to improving solubility. This ester has limited solubility. New technology (18) provides another approach to improving the effectiveness of ascorbic acid in lipids. This form of ascorbic acid reacts as though it were

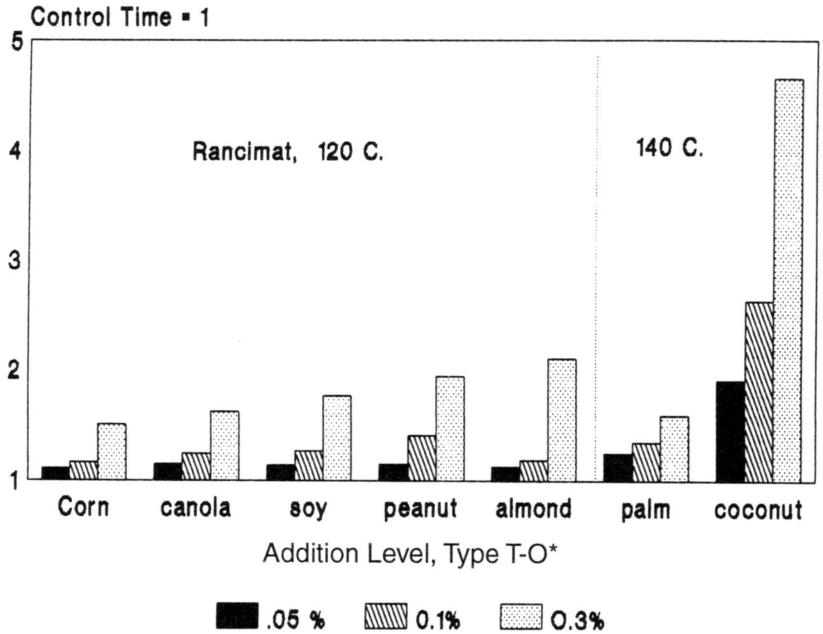

Fig. 13.8. Three levels of tea extract added to various oils show improved stability, reported as the ratio of the induction time of the fortified oil compared with the corresponding control. Note that two of the more inherently stable oils were tested at higher temperature.

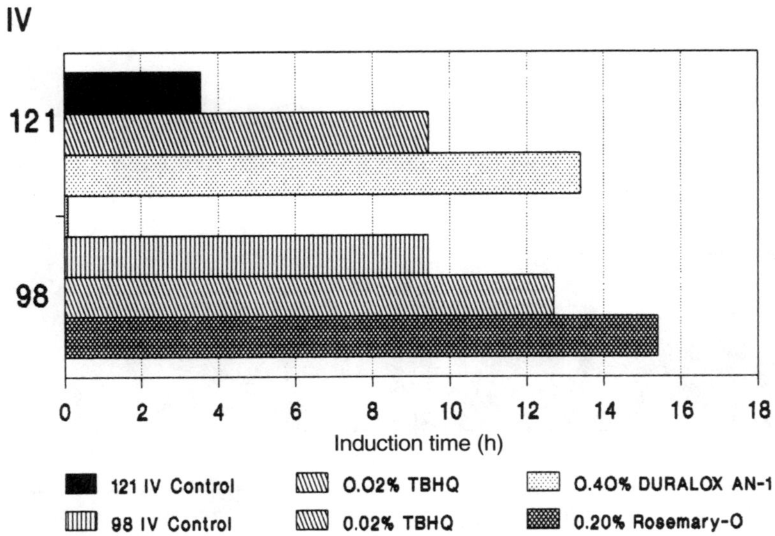

Fig. 13.9. An (RBD) canola oil with a 121 IV was treated with *tert*-butylhydroquinone (TBHQ) and with a proprietary mixture of natural inhibitors, AN-1. The control oil was also hydrogenated to 98 IV and stabilized with TBHQ or an alternate optimal free radical interceptor (FRI), oleoresin rosemary. Note that the proprietary blend in the 121 IV oil provided stability superior to that provided by hydrogenation to the lower IV and use of TBHQ (Rancimat, 120°C).

fat soluble. The benefits of combining ascorbic with phenolics in improving lipid stability are shown in Fig. 13.10. Ascorbic acid can function as a hydrogen donor, or as an oxygen absorber and as a singlet oxygen quencher. Ascorbic acid is not suggested for prolonged exposure to high temperatures such as deep fat frying. It is effective in combination with phenolics when sprayed onto the surface of oil-roasted nuts, fried and baked foods after cooking. Light exposure should be minimized.

Quenching. A theoretical oil, freshly refined and essentially devoid of free radicals, should be quite stable. Normal atmospheric oxygen, is in the triplet state, $^3O_2$, and does not normally attack fats in the absence of prooxidant initiators. It is the prooxidants factors listed above which initiate destabilization of a lipid. Light is a unique prooxidant. It induces a type of oxidation that requires careful management. Light energy impacts an exciter, usually metal-containing pigments such as chlorophyll or hemoglobin which absorbs then transfers the energy to oxygen molecules. FD&C Yellow #5 color, riboflavin, and other fluorescent compounds are also exciters. When the exciter transfers the energy to triplet state oxygen, $^3O_2$, it is converted to the singlet state $^1O_2$. This is highly reactive and attacks unsaturated fats directly.

Quenchers are molecules that can absorb energy from singlet oxygen, converting it back to the triplet state. Effective quenchers can repeatedly absorb the energy

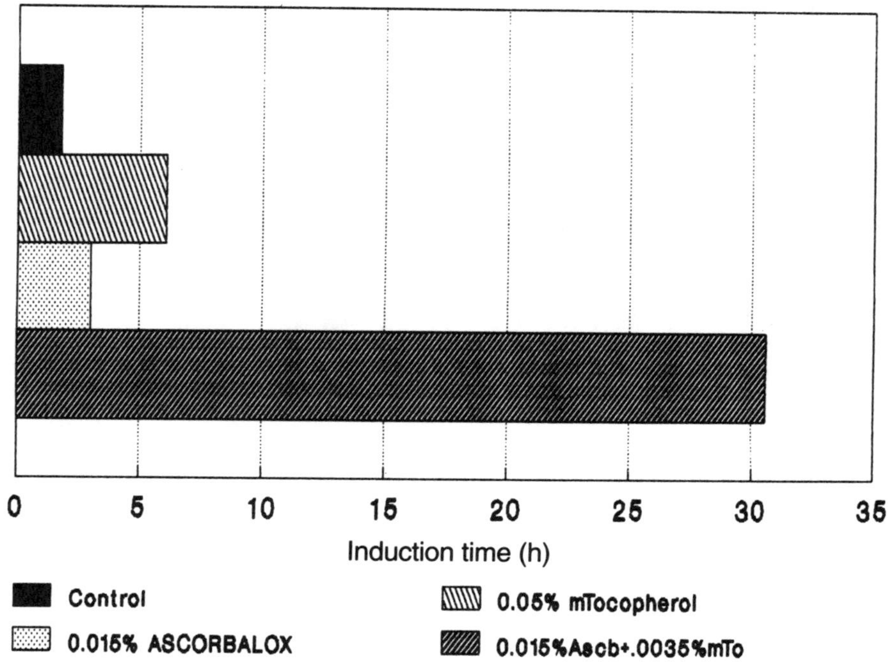

Fig. 13.10. Ratios for induction times of lard stabilized with mixed tocopherols and/or with a modified ascorbic acid, ASCORBALOX, are compared with the lard control time (Rancimat, 110°C). The free radical interceptor combination shows synergism.

(19), but eventually are altered. The relative ability of various natural carotenoid quenchers to absorb light energy is shown in Table 13.4 (19).

Ascorbic acid and tocopherol can also function as quenchers. Light levels should be restricted in processing units. Opaque packaging is a significant aid.

Chelators. Prooxidant metals can be complexed by lecithin, citric, malic and other organic acids.

TABLE 13.4
Relative Strength of Carotenoids

Carotenoid	Absorption	Color
β-Carotene	454	Orange
Zeaxanthin	454	Orange
Capsorubin	467	Red
Bixin	469	Orange-red
Capsanthin	470	Red
Lycopene	473	Red

Oxidation in Muscle Tissue

Wood smoke has long been a source of phenolics for managing lipid oxidation in cured meats and fish. A complex oxidation reaction occurs in the iron- and enzyme-catalyzed oxidation of phospholipids in muscle tissue. The term, "warmed-over flavor" (WOF), was formerly used to describe the reaction end products which can develop in meats even though reheating is not requisite. It is being replaced by "meat flavor deterioration" (MFD). Process operations, such as slicing, comminuting, or freezing, which destroy the integrity of muscle cells can initiate MFD. Oxidation progresses rapidly in further processed muscle products. Normal freezer temperatures do not effectively stop MFD development. The offensive aromas and flavors of MFD become more obvious upon cooking. The MFD mechanism is inhibited by phenolic molecules in rosemary in combination with a chelator such as phosphates (20). Data are seen in Fig. 13.11. Lipid oxidation can accelerate changes in muscle tissue color. Lipid-based free radicals may initiate protein oxidation. Oxidation of sulfhydryl linkages in muscle protein is believed to result in toughness and excessive loss of fluids.

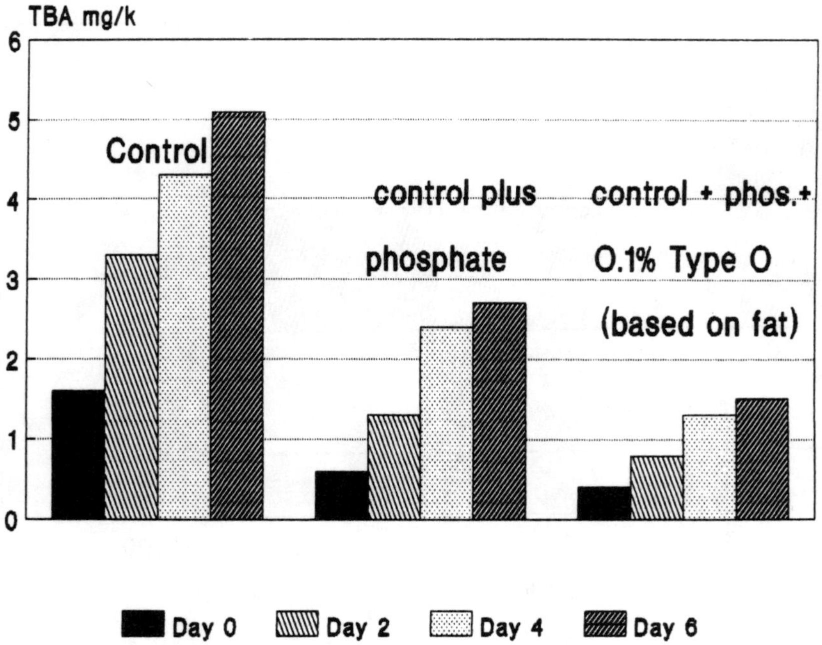

Fig. 13.11. Thiobarbituric acid reactant (TBA) levels above 2 mg/kg are indicative of off flavors in beef. The benefits of combining rosemary extract and phosphates are shown over a 6-d refrigerated storage period at 4°C. *Source:* Ref. 20.

Pigment Stabilization

Ascorbic acid, tocopherol, and spice oleoresins all contribute to the stabilization of carotenoid pigments. The ability of phenolics to retard fade is shown in Fig. 13.12. The protection probably involves intercepting intermediate free radicals, some of which are a consequence of the singlet oxygen reactions. Opaque packaging, minimal exposure to light and heat are also helpful.

Conclusions

Consumer aversion to saturated fats and trans acids formed in partial hydrogenation will lead to expanded use of phenolics generally. Complex blends of FRI will be required to manage the unusual stress of newer nutritional products based on specific polyunsaturated fatty acids. The benefits of patented (21) multicomponent systems in marine oils are shown in Fig. 13.13. Current oilseed genetic research will introduce new oils with desired changes in fatty acid ratios. New catalysts may influence the steric configuration of fatty acids in hydrogenated oils. Additional

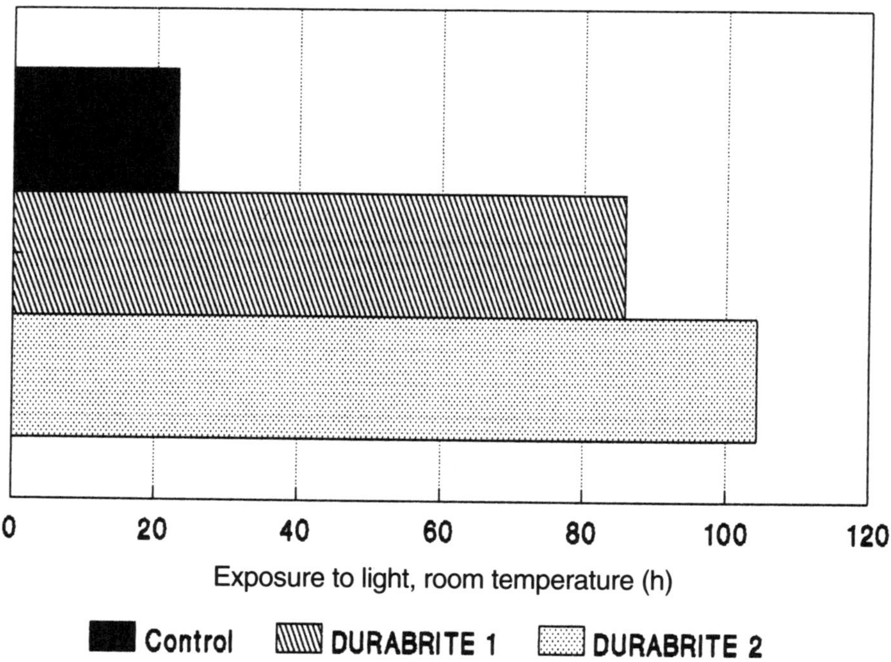

Fig. 13.12. Significant increases in stability of paprika pigment are achieved through use of either of two DURABRITE proprietary formulations. Data are reported as hours required for 33% of the perceived color to disappear.

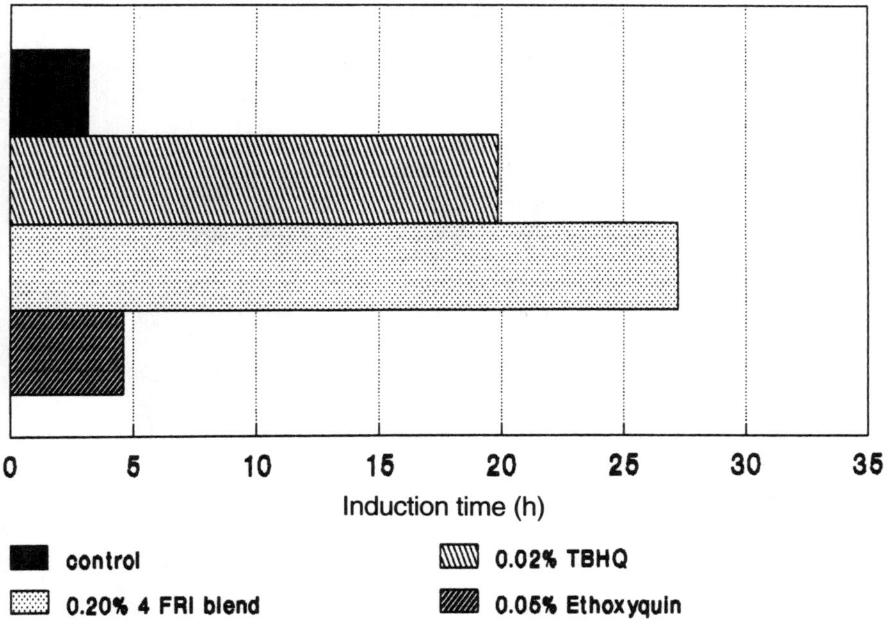

Fig. 13.13. Induction times of a menhaden oil control and of the control supplemented with *tert*-butylhydroquinone (TBHQ) or with a patented (18) 4-component DURALOX proprietary blend, or with ethoxyquin are shown (Rancimat, 80°C).

studies will be required to design optimum blends of natural inhibitors, chelators, and acidulants for these new oils. These studies should do much to further the protection of new food products against the adverse effect of oxidation.

References

1. (1985), *History of Spices, American Spice Trade Assn*, NY, p. 7.
2. Nasner, A. (1989) in *Flavor Chemistry of Lipid Foods* (Min, D.B., and Smouse, T.H., eds., American Oil Chemists' Society, Champaign, IL, p. 294.
3. Gordon, M.H. (1990) in *Food Antioxidants* (Hudson, B.J.F., ed.), Elsevier Science Publ., New York, p. 9.
4. Cort, W.M. (1974) *J. Am. Oil Chem. Soc. 51*, 322.
5. Chan, H.W.S. (1987) in *Autoxidation of Unsaturated Lipids*, Academic Press, NY, p. 9–10.
6. Gupta, M.K. (1993) *INFORM 4*, 1167–1272.
7. Grosch, W. (1987) in *Autoxidation of Unsaturated Lipids* (Chan, H.W.S., ed.), Academic Press, NY, p. 103.
8. Schuler, P. (1990) in *Food Antioxidants* (Hudson, B.J.F., ed.), Elsevier Publishing, New York, p. 139.

9. Sonntag, N.O.V. (1987) in *Bailey's Industrial Oil and Fat Products* (Swern, D., ed.), John Wiley and Sons, New York, p. 151.
10. Mukai, M., Cillard, J., and Cillard, P. (1993) *Lipids 28*, 747–752.
11. Husain, S.R., Sawada, K., Kohno, Y., and Terao, J. (1987) *J. Am. Oil Chem. Soc. 64*, 109–111.
12. Cosgrove, J.P. (1987) *Lipids 22*, 299–304.
13. Sonntag, N.V.O. (1987) in *Bailey's Industrial Oil and Fat Products* (Swern, D., ed.), John Wiley and Sons, New York, p. 72.
14. Fukuzumi, K., and Naburo, I. (1970) *J. Am. Oil Chem. Soc. 47*, 369–370.
15. Chang, S.S. (1977) *J. Food Sci. 42*, 1102–1106.
16. Xie, B. (1993) in *Proc. Natl. Sci. Council, ROC, 17*, 77–84.
17. Matsauzaki, T., and Hara, M. (1985) *Nippon Nogeikagatu Kai Shi 59*, 129.
18. Todd, P.T., U.S. Patents 4,877,635, 5,084,293.
19. Min, D.B. (1989) in *Flavor Chemistry of Lipid Foods* (Min, D.B., and Smouse, T.H., eds.), American Oil Chemists' Society, Champaign, IL, pp. 85–86.
20. Gray, J.I. (1988) in Proceedings of the 3rd International Conference on Food Additives, Food Ingr. Europe, London.
21. Chang, S., U.S. Patent, 5,077,069.
22. Todd, P.T., U.S. Patents 5,084,293,4,877,635.

Chapter 14

Vitamin Antioxidants and Disease Prevention

J.H. Weisburger

American Health Foundation, Valhalla, New York.

Introduction

Throughout the world, people are afflicted with a number of chronic diseases including coronary heart disease, hypertension and stroke, adult-onset diabetes, many types of cancer, and, of growing importance, AIDS. Extensive research on the etiology of each type of disease has indicated that most cases stem from the locally prevailing as well as the personal lifestyle (1–8). It has been shown that tobacco use, especially smoking of cigarettes or chewing of tobacco products in some parts of the world, accounts for about 35% of chronic diseases, including coronary heart disease, and cancer in the respiratory tract, pancreas, kidney, urinary bladder, and cervix. Nutritional traditions involving salted and pickled foods are associated with a high risk of hypertension and stroke, and cancer of the esophagus and stomach (9–11). Eating habits involving high-fat diets are accompanied by a risk for heart disease and cancer of the colon, pancreas, breast, prostate, ovary, and endometrium. Such diets also potentiate the effect of smoking on the lung. Importantly, it was discovered that populations who by tradition also regularly consume vegetables and fruits are at lower risk for chronic disease, everything else being equal (19–21). For example, populations of Mediterranean countries display a lower incidence of heart disease and many types of cancer; this is also true in the Southern part of the United States. In Southern areas of China and Japan, there are fewer cases of stroke and gastric cancer.

Vegetables and fruits contain a variety of micronutrients that may play a role in the protection against chronic diseases. They contain fibers, particularly soluble fibers, that together with insoluble fibers as found in bran cereals, increase intestinal health and lower the risk of heart disease and breast cancer by limiting the enterohepatic circulation of cholesterol, bile acids, and hormones (22,23). In addition, vegetables, fruits, and also tea, contain powerful antioxidants, with a polyphenol structure accounting for their beneficial effect. They also include phase I and phase II enzymes with detoxifying potential for endogenous and xenobiotic substrates (24).

In addition, vegetables and fruits contain essential micronutrients as vitamins (25–28). Vitamins are defined as complex organic substances found in many foods that are essential in small amounts for the normal function of the body. Individuals or populations who have a low intake of vitamins may suffer from deficiency dis-

Major portions of this chapter have appeared in *Hypernutritious Foods*, J.W. Finley *et al.*, eds., AGSCIENCE, Auburndale, FL, 1996. Reprinted with permission.

eases. For example, a deficiency of vitamin A affects the function of the eye, leading to blindness; a low intake of vitamin C is a cause of scurvy; vitamin B_1 in low levels is a cause of beriberi; and a low intake of niacin relates to the occurrence of pellagra. Vitamin D is an essential component in calcium availability and metabolism, and a low intake may lead to rickets. Beginning in 1940, with the development of the concept of Recommended Daily Allowances, RDA, by experts in nutrition under the auspices of the Food and Nutrition Board of the U.S. National Academy of Sciences, recommendations were made on specific amounts of each vitamin that would minimize the risk of these deficiency diseases (29). In each case, the amount selected was higher than the minimum, to provide some buffer against inadequate intake under specific conditions. These concepts were implemented by not only improving the nutritional status of individuals through personal action but also through the fortification of widely used foods with specific vitamins. For example, milk contains additional vitamins A and D, and certain breakfast cereals in the United States are fortified with varied vitamins. In the last 50 years, implementation of the RDA concept has been most successful. Deficiency diseases have disappeared, even in the lower socioeconomic groups that previously accounted for most of the cases.

Research in the last 35 years has suggested that deficiency diseases were not the only area in which vitamin supplementation might benefit the public. One pioneering study in Norway showed that smokers often had appreciably lower values of plasma vitamin A than nonsmokers (30). Part of the explanation is that individuals who smoke frequently have poor nutritional habits. In addition, however, it was found that individuals who smoke display a different biochemical pattern to metabolize chemicals. Cigarette smoke induces metabolic enzymes such as those of the cytochrome P450 system, and the phase II conjugating enzymes, such as glucuronyl transferase. Thus, vitamin A undergoes metabolism to products that no longer serve the vitamin A function. This is true for many other of the fat-soluble micronutrients, including vitamins E and D. In smokers, such metabolic reactions occur at a higher rate and hence account for higher vitamin requirements (31–35).

The Recommended Daily Allowance for vitamin E is quite low, 10 international units (IU)/d, simply because this excellent antioxidant is found in diverse foods (29). Thus, classical nutritionists comment that deficiencies of vitamin E are nonexistent. In recent years, however, research has shown that vitamin E has a number of extraordinarily beneficial effects as a specific antioxidant, acting together with vitamin C and β-carotene, in improving antioxidant defenses in the body (36–46).

A number of lifestyle-associated adverse effects stem from cell-mediated oxidative systems. For example, low density lipoprotein (LDL)-cholesterol is one of the circulating lipoproteins that act as carriers for cholesterol. It has been found that the specific mechanism underlying its adverse effect is oxidation (46–50). The oxidized LDL-cholesterol damages the vascular system. Active oxygen compounds are also generated through normal physiological reactions that can modify the genetic apparatus of the cell and lead to modified DNA, visualized as the 8-hydroxydeoxyguanylic acid (8-OHdG) component in DNA (51). It is thought that a number of carcinogenic events relate to the production of 8-OHdG in DNA. All of these reactions are lowered by antioxidants, including the antioxidant vitamins individually, or especially when acting in concert. Studies in humans and animal models have shown that supplementation with vitamin E decreases the risk of atherosclerosis and coronary heart disease (52–56). Vitamins E and C act individually or together as efficient traps for nitrite in foods, or nitrite formed by the bacterial flora in the oral cavity and in the stomach from environmental nitrate. Current concepts indicate that nitrite may be associated with risk for gastric cancer, as well as cancer of the esophagus in the Far East. Populations receiving an adequate intake, either by consuming adequate amounts of vegetables, fruits and tea, rich in nitrite-traps and antioxidants, or by taking supplements of vitamin C or E, have a lower risk of these types of cancer (57–62).

A number of vitamins are essential cofactors for specific enzyme systems (Table 14.1). Thus, it is important for optimal functioning of these varied enzymes that sufficient amounts of these vitamins be available. A number of these vitamins act not only as cofactors for enzymes but also can assist in the chemical detoxification of potentially harmful metabolites. For example, it has been shown that moderate-to-high intake of alcoholic beverages depletes a number of enzymes, particularly the water-soluble vitamins, such as vitamin B_6 and folate (63). One element in the loss of vitamin B6 could be the reaction of acetaldehyde, a key metabolite of alcohol, with pyridoxamine, forming an inactive Schiff-base (64).

The antioxidant β-carotene, a pro-vitamin A, has not been part of the recognized list of essential micronutrients. Yet, numerous studies document that carotene and vitamin A can function as effective inhibitors in neoplasia and other chronic diseases (65–83). It has been established, however, that β-carotene is converted metabolically to vitamin A. It is an excellent precursor, because β-carotene has not displayed any indication of chronic toxicity, in part because the modest intestinal absorption of carotene limits the amount circulating. On the other hand, chronic use of high levels of vitamin A has led to adverse effects, with emphasis on liver damage. For this reason, there is a recommendation to hold the intake of vitamin A to 10,000 units/d (84–86). In addition, β-carotene has antioxidant functions beyond its action as a source of vitamin A. Carotene can act as a trap for radical reactions. Such oxidative reactions lead to the introduction in carotene of an unbalanced electron structure, and for that reason, it is best to consider the use of carotene together with vitamin E and vitamin C to terminate the effect of reactive radicals through a chain reaction, resulting in the oxidation of vitamin C.

Based on these and other related considerations, it would seem important to revise the recommended daily allowances by new proposals providing amounts of essential micronutrients, with the avoidance of chronic diseases as the ultimate aim (Table 14.2). In many instances, the desirable amounts of vitamins involve higher daily intakes than the conventional RDA. If populations could be convinced to

TABLE 14.1
Functions of Vitamins

Water-soluble vitamins					
Vitamin	Active form	Functions	Enzyme cofactor	Deficiency indicator	Deficiency diseasee
Thiamine vitamin B_1	Thiamine pyrophosphate	Decarboxylation α-ketoacids, carbohydrate metabolism	Transketolase	Increased pyruvate in blood Erthrocyte transketolase	Beriberi Neuritis, cardiovascular Alcoholic polyneuropathy
Riboflavin vitamin B_2	Flavin mononucleotide Flavin adenine dinucleotide, generated with ATP	Respiratory enzymes flavoprotein catalytic systems	Xanthine oxidase dehydrogenases, oxidases, reductases	Reduced erythrocyte GSH reductase, dermatitis, anemia, neuropathy	Nonspecific syndromes (See indicators)
Pyridoxine vitamin B_6	Pyridoxal phosphate Pyridoxamine phosphate	Amino acid metabolism, decarboxylation, transamination, racemization	Transaminases, decarboxylases	Abnormal tryptophan metabolism, neuritis, seborrheitis, glossitis, stomatitis, blood homocysteine	Nonspecific syndromes (See indicators)
Cyanocobalamin Vitamin B_{12}	Methylcobalamin 5-Deoxyadenyl-cobalamin hydroxycobalamin Bound to intrinsic factor, a glycoprotein	Cell growth, duplication; methionine purine, pyrimidine RNA, DNA biosynthesis (with folate) hematological and nervous systems	Enzymes for 1-carbon and sulphydryl metabolism, in coordination with folate	Deficiency in folate metabolism, methionine biosynthesis; malabsorption syndrome; homocysteine accumulation, abnormal DNA replication	Megaloblastic erythropoiesis, or anemia, pancytopenia, neurologic syndromes, including irreversible neural damage
Folic acid pterolyglutamic acid	Tetrahydrofolates	Homocysteine to cysteine, serine to glycine, formate and histidine; organization and differentiation	Enzymes for 1-carbon and sulphydryl, purine synthesis metabolism, in concert with vitamin B12	Alcoholism lowers avail- abnormal hematopoietic system	Megaloblastic erythropoiesis, or anemia; abnormal fetal development; neural tube (*cf.* vitamin B_{12})
Pantothenic acid	Coenzyme A	2-Carbon metabolism, acetyltransfer; metabolism of carbohydrates, fatty fatty acids, biosynthesis of sterols, porphyrins	Acyltransferases	Adrenocortical deficiencies, neuromuscular degeneration (rare to find deficiencies)	Rarely observed

Nicotinic acid or amide, niacin (biosynthesis from tryptophan)	Nicotinamide adenine dinucleotide (NAD), nicotinamide adenine dinucleotide phosphate (NADP)	Coenzymes for oxidation-reduction enzymes, microsomal, mitochondrial enzymes, dehydrogenases, coordinated with flavoproteins	Oxido-reductases	Dermatitis, diarrhea, dementia (chronic alcoholism)	Pellagra
Biotin	Complex with lysine	Carboxylation of acetylcoenzyme A, carbohydrate/fat metabolism, CO_2 fixation, oxidative enzyme reactions nitrite trap	Carboxylases acetyltransfer	Exfoliative dermatitis alopecia (patients with malabsorption)	Rare
Vitamin C	Facilitates iron absorption	Several oxidation-reduction enzymes, provides terminal reductive element to other antioxidants such as β-carotene, vitamin E, sulfhydryl, and GSH transferases	Provides coordinated reductive potential to oxidation-reduction enzymes and their associated cofactors	Low plasma vitamin C; perifollicular hyper-keratosis; hemorrhages hematomas, alcohol/cigarette use, oral contraceptives, infectious diseases, surgical stress increase requirements, nitrite-related methemo-globinemia	Scurvy
			Fat-Soluble Vitamins		
β-Carotene	β-Carotene and vitamin A, carotenoids	Antioxidant, biosynthesis progesterone, traps oxi-radicals and peroxides	See Vitamin A	See Vitamin A	See Vitamin A
Vitamin A	Retinol Retinal	Antioxidant, growth and differentiation, eye, bone, reproduction, embryonic development, intercellular communication, gene expression	Rhodopsin biosynthesis, epithelial differentiation, retinol binding protein	Visual defects, night blindness, skin lesions, keratomalacia, deficient pulmonary mucus, fetal resorption, teratogenesis	Fetal or infant deaths owing to incomplete function of epithelial tissues

cont.

TABLE 14.1
Functions of Vitamins *(cont.)*

Fat-soluble Vitamins *(cont.)*					
Vitamin	Active form	Functions	Enzyme cofactor	Deficiency indicator	Deficiency disease
Vitamin D	Cholecalciferol, calciferol	Regulation of calcium and phosphate metabolism through calcifediol and calcitriol, bone synthesis, degradation; magnesium energy cycle; cell duplication; blood pressure regulation	—	Intestinal metaplasia (diarrhea), increased cancer risk, malabsorption of calcium, magnesium; demineralization	Rickets, tetany
Vitamin E	α-Tocopherol	Antioxidant; stabilizes ubiquinone; acts in concert with carotene, vitamin A, vitamin C, and selenium; prevents peroxidation, traps free radicals, nitrite; antagonizes metal-catalyzed LDL-cholesterol, fats, DNA.	—	Neurological syndromes, reproductive defects; peroxidation, myopathy, cardiac disorders, erythrocyte instability, vascular reperfusion injury	Rare, except in fetus, newborn
Vitamin K	K_1: 2-methyl-3-phytyl-1,4-naphthoquinone, phylloquinone; K_2: series of menaquinones; synthetic 2-methyl-1,4-naphthoquinone	Synthesis of blood clotting factors, prothrombins	Microsomal decarboxylase, epoxide reductase	Increased bleeding, gastrointestinal bleeding, hematuria, coagulation defects	Rare, except in newborn

TABLE 14.2
Optimal Intake of Vitamins for Chronic Disease Prevention

			Fat-Soluble Vitamins					
Category	Age(y) or condition	Protein (g)	β-Carotene mg[a]	Vitamin A (μg TE)[a]	Vitamin D (μg)[b]	Vitamin E (mg α-TE)[c]	Vitamin K (μg)
Infants	0.0–0.5	13	3	200	7.5	10–12	5
Children	4–10	24	5	400–600	8–10	30–40	20
Males	11–14	42–50	8	1500	10–12	80–120	45
	25–50	42–50	8	1500	10–12	80–120	80
	51 +	40	8	1500	10–12	80–120	65
Females	11–14	40–45	8	1500	10–12	80–120	45
	25–50	40–45	8	1500	10–12	80–120	80
	51+	40	8	1500	10–12	80–120	65
Pregnant		55–65	10	1200	10–12	100–150	65
Lactating	1st 6 mon	60–65	10	1500	15	100–150	65
	2nd 6 mon	60–70	10	2000	15	100–150	65

	Water-Soluble Vitamins								
Category	Vitamin min C (mg)	Thiamin min (mg)	Ribo-flavin (mg)	Niacin (mg NE)[d]	D-Panto-thenate (mg)	Vitamin B_6 (mg)	Folate (mg)	Biotin (mg)	Vitamin min B_{12} (μg)
Infants	30	0.3	0.4	5	5	0.3	0.25	0.1	0.3
Children	60–100	0.9	1.1	12	10	1.5	0.25	0.2	2.0–3.0
Males	300–400	2.0–3.0	2.0–3.0	40	20	4.0	0.4–0.5	0.5	10
	400	2.0–3.0	2.0–3.0	40	20	4.0	0.4–0.5	0.5	10
	400	2.0–3.0	2.0–3.0	40	20	4.0	0.4–0.5	0.5	10
Females	300–400	2.0–3.0	2.0–3.0	40	20	4.0	0.4–0.5	0.5	10
	400	2.0–3.0	2.0–3.0	40	20	4.0	0.4–0.5	0.5	10
	400	2.0–3.0	2.0–3.0	40	20	4.0	0.4–0.5	0.5	10
Pregnant	500	3.0	3.0	50	30	4.0	0.4–0.5	0.7	12
Lactating	500	3.0	3.0	50	30	4.0	0.5	0.7	12
	500	3.0	3.0	50	30	4.0	0.5	0.7	12

Source: This table is modified from Ref. (29).
[a] Retinol equivalents. 1 retinol equivalent = 1 μg retinol or 6 μg β-carotene, or 3.3 IU vitamin A activity.
[b] As cholecalciferol. 10 μg cholecalciferol = 400 IU of vitamin D.
[c] α-Tocopherol equivalents. 1 mg δ-α tocopherol = 1 α-TE.
[d] 1 NE (niacin equivalent) is equal to 1 mg of niacin or 60 mg of dietary tryptophan.

alter their lifestyle and consume on a daily regular basis the desirable 5–9 fruits and vegetables per day with emphasis on the higher amount, the preventive needs could be met through fruits and vegetables. In fact, in the history of mankind, anthropology shows that humans were gatherers of fruits and vegetables for their daily nutritional needs. This tradition has changed with the development of the agricultural industries and especially the relocation of people from rural areas to cities where the gathering of fruits and vegetables was not possible. Also, in the last century, industrialization led to increasing intakes of fatty foods, meats, and refined foods in which essential micronutrients were present in reduced amounts.

In addition, segments of populations acquired singular nutritional habits, such as a diet almost exclusively derived from corn and associated products. Such manner of imbalanced eating was a cause of deficiency diseases. In addition, consumption of even nine fruits and vegetables per day fails to meet the recommended, optimal intake of vitamin E by adults of 80–120 units/d. Thus, supplementation of vitamin E, an inexpensive product, is indicated.

Is general supplementation with vitamins necessary? Probably not, if individuals have a lifestyle providing for an adequate consumption of fruits and vegetables (see note on supplementary vitamin E, above). In most instances, however, this goal is not achieved for a number of reasons, including time for preparing meals, as well as the cost of these desirable foods. Thus, moderate supplementation, as suggested in Table 14.1, may be in order. It is important to realize that the fat- soluble vitamins require a certain amount of food, particularly some fatty foods, to ensure their complete absorption. Thus, people that use vitamin supplements should take them after their main meal, essentially fortifying the foods eaten present in the stomach, and increasing their availability to tissues and cells.

In the United States, about one third of men and women are regular users of vitamin supplements. There is less information about other countries, but it seems that Americans stand out in this regard. Within this country, there may be a socioeconomic gradient, and the groups at the lower end seem to be less likely users of vitamin supplements. Actually, that fairly sizeable part of the population might be better off with supplement use, because their nutritional habits often are poor in vegetable and fruit intake. In fact, there might be merit in public policies providing appropriate multivitamins, including adequate amounts of vitamin E, to these groups of people, perhaps as part of the supply of food stamps. This situation also applies to institutional food supplies, such as in hospitals, schools, armed services, and in general, in broad public nutrition programs. Legislation passed by the 103rd Congress in 1994, the Dietary Supplement Act, recognizes these micronutrients as part of the dietary supply, and provides for their continuing availability on the open market.

In the sale of drugs and pharmaceuticals, the areas of primary concern are safety and effectiveness. Vitamin supplements are not drugs, but are part of an informed nutritional intake. Except for infrequent reports on toxicity with excessive use of vitamins A, D and B_6, there have been few safety problems reported in vitamin use. The late Professor Pauling is said to have consumed 10 g of vitamin C per day without any obvious adverse effects; he succumbed recently to prostate cancer at the age of 93. The question of effectiveness is important. A number of field studies have shown that short-term vitamin supplementation does not seem to lower the development of cancer of the lung or cancer of the esophagus. These trials were designed more to develop information on the possible therapeutic effect of vitamins. It would seem that vitamin use should be part of a healthy lifestyle with life-long proper dietary habits, exercise and vitamin use, and emphasis on prevention. There are relatively few studies in which such use of vitamin supplementation has been explored. As noted, populations who as a rule have nutritional traditions involving regular intake of fruits, vegetables and tea display fewer of the main chronic diseases, including heart disease and cancer. Vitamins C and E act as inhibitors of nitrosation and through this mechanism should decrease the risk of gastric cancer. Yet, it is known that the intake of salted pickled foods or inhabiting an area with high geochemical nitrate for the first 20 years of life determines the eventual occurrence of gastric cancer. Hence, it seems likely that any relatively short trial with these two vitamins would fail to display evidence of lower risk. On the other hand, carotene and vitamin A, which may operate through enhancing differentiation and decreasing cell duplication, could eventually yield evidence that regular adequate intake would lower the development of clinical cancer (87–90). Experiments in animal models have also indicated that vitamin A may decrease the development of breast cancer (90). Vitamin D plays an essential role in the proper metabolism of calcium and thus, maintaining bone structure (91–95). Vitamin D analogs that show effectiveness in certain types of cancer have begun to be introduced. Vitamin B_6 has been found useful in cases of poisoning with certain hydrazines, including the drug isoniazid. Research in this laboratory deals with exploration of the relevant mechanisms.

Conclusions

Vitamins are essential micronutrients that were discovered in the first half of this century, because their low intake led to specific deficiency diseases. Introduction of the concept of the Recommended Daily Allowances and ensuring adequate intake of such micronutrients through foods or supplements has been effective in its designed goal to eliminate deficiency diseases.

The current problem is to assess the role of specific vitamins and of mixtures of the essential micronutrients in multivitamin pills to lower the risk of the current burden of chronic diseases which carries such a high cost to individuals and to society. It is clear that vitamins, as used, are safe. About one third of the American people regularly take vitamin supplements, and cases of adverse effects are extremely rare. People consuming the recommended 5–9 servings of vegetables and fruits per day are likely to have an adequate, indeed optimal, intake of vitamins and minerals and other desirable micronutrients, to prevent the major chronic diseases due to lifestyle or environmental factors. The exception would be vitamin E for which some moderate supplementation on the order of 80–120 IU/d may be desirable. Much has been learned about the role of each vitamin or sets of vitamins in terms of mechanisms of beneficial effects. Thus, there is an underlying body of evidence that adequate intake of vitamins and minerals is part of a healthy lifestyle, designed to lower the risk of major diseases.

Acknowledgments

Research in this laboratory is supported by a grant from the Tea Trade Health Research Association, contract NO1-CN35569 from the National Cancer Institute, and a gift from Texaco Foundation, Inc. Ms. Beth-Alayne McKinney assisted effectively in the development of this article.

References

1. McGinnis, J.M., and Foege, W.H. (1993) *J. Am. Med. Assoc. 270*, 2207.
2. WHO Study Group (1990) *Technical Report Series 797, Diet, Nutrition, and the Prevention of Chronic Diseases*; World Health Organization, Geneva, pp. 1–203.
3. Surgeon General's Report (1988) *Nutrition and Health, Public Health Service DHHS* (PHS) Publication No. 88-50210, Washington, D.C.
4. Levi, F., Lucchini, F., and La Vecchia, C. (1994) *Europ. J Cancer Prev.*, 109.
5. Hill, M.J., Giacosa, A., and Caygill, C.P.J., eds., *Epidemiology of Diet and Cancer*, Ellis Horwood, Chichester, Sussex, UK, pp. 1–411.
6. Hoffmann, D., Rivenson, A., Chung, F.-L., and Wynder, E.L. (1993) *Ann. N.Y. Acad. Sci. 686*, 140.
7. Weisburger, J.H., Horn, C.L., and Wynder, E.L. (1991) in *Recent Advances in Clinical Nutrition: 3. Proceedings of the Fourth International Symposium on Clinical Nutrition* (Schlierf, G., ed.), Smith-Gordon, London, pp. 83–96.
8. Williams, C.L., Bollella, M., and Wynder, E. (1994) *Atherosclerosis 108*, S117.
9. Temple, N.J., and Burkitt, D.P., eds. (1994) *Western Diseases: Their Dietary Prevention and Reversibility*, Humana Press, Inc., Totowa, NJ, pp. 1–453.
10. Wattenberg, L.W. (1992) *Cancer Res. 52*, 2085.
11. Dwyer, J.T. (1988) *Am. J. Clin. Nutr.*, 712.
12. Shibata, A., Paganini-Hill, A., Ross, R.K., and Henderson, B.E. (1992) *Br. J. Cancer 66*, 673.
13. Gao, C.-M., Tajima, K., Kuroishi, T., Hirose, K., and Inoue, M. (1993) *Jpn. J. Cancer Res. 84*, 594.
14. Steinmetz, K.A., Potter, J.D., and Folsom, A.R. (1993) *Cancer Res. 53*, 536.
15. Steinmetz, K.A., Kushi, L.H., Bostick, R.M., Folsom, A.R., and Potter, J.D. (1994) *Am. J. Epidemiol. 139*, 1.
16. Block, G., Patterson, B., and Subar, A. (1992) *Nutr. Cancer 18*, 1.
17. Trock, B., Lanza, E., and Greenwald, P. (1990) *J. Natl. Cancer Inst. 82*, 650.
18. Wynder, E.L. (1992) *J. Natl. Cancer Inst. 12*, 87.
19. Bal, D.G., and Forester, S.B. (1993) *Cancer 72*, 1005.
20. Gillman, M.W., Cupples, L.A., Gagnon, D., Posner, B.M., Ellison, R.C., Castelli, W.P., and Wolf, P.A. (1995) *J. Am. Med. Assoc. 273*, 1113.
21. Verlangieri, A.J., Kapeghian, J.C., el-Dean, S., and Bush, M. (1985) *Med. Hypotheses 16*, 7.
22. Micozzi, M.S., and Moon, T.E., eds. (1992) *Macronutrients: Investigating Their Role in Cancer*, Marcel Dekker, New York, p. 477.
23. Parke, D.V., Ioannides, C., and Walker, R., eds. (1993) *Food, Nutrition and Chemical Toxicity*, Smith-Gordon, Nishimura, pp. 1–451.
24. Sohn, O.S., Surace, A., Fiala, E.S., Richie, J., Colosimo, S., Zang, E., and Weisburger, J.H. (1994) *Xenobiotica 24*, 119.
25. Moon, T.E., and Micozzi, M.S., eds. (1989) *Nutrition and Cancer Prevention*, Marcel Dekker, New York, p. 588.
26. Sauberlich, H.E., and Machlin, L.J., eds. (1992) *Ann. N.Y. Acad. Sci. 669*, 1.
27. Gaby, S.K., Bendich, A., Singh, V.N., and Machlin L.J., eds. (1991) *Vitamin Intake and Health*, Marcel Dekker, New York, pp. 1–217.
28. Block, G. (1993) *J. Natl. Cancer Inst. 85*, 846.

29. National Research Council (1989) *Recommended Dietary Allowances*, 10th edn., National Academy Press, Washington, D.C.
30. Bjelke, E. (1975) *Int. J. Cancer 15*, 561.
31. Edes, T.E., Kwan, S.M., Buckley, C.S., and Thornton, W.H. (1992) *Int. J. Cancer 50*, 99.
32. Pamuk, E.R., Byers, T., Coates, R.J., Vann, J.W., Sowell, A.L., Gunter, E.W., and Glass, D. (1994) *Am. J. Clin. Nutr. 59*, 891.
33. Schectman, G. (1993) *Ann. N.Y. Acad. Sci. 686*, 335.
34. Tribble, D.L., Giuliano, L.J., and Fortmann, S.P. (1993) *Am. J. Clin. Nutr. 58*, 886.
35. van Poppel, G., Verhagen, H., van't Veer, P., and van Bladeren, P.J. (1993) *Cancer Epimediol. Biomark. Prev. 2*, 441.
36. Lubin, B., and Machlin L.J., eds. (1982) *Ann. N.Y. Acad. Sci. 393*, 1.
37. Knekt, P. (1993) *Ann. N.Y. Acad. Sci. 686*, 280.
38. Comporti, M., Maellaro, E., DelBello, B., and Casini, A.F. (1991) *Xenobiotica 21*, 1067.
39. Paolisso, G., Di Maro, G., Galzerano, D., Cacciapuoti, F., Varricchio, G., Varricchio, M., and D'Onofrio, F. (1994) *Am. J. Clin. Nutr. 59*, 1291.
40. Yano, T., Obata, Y., Yano, Y., Otani, S., and Ichikawa, T. (1994) *Cancer Lett. 87*, 205.
41. Longnecker, M.P., Martin-Moreno, J-M., Knekt, P., Nomura, A.M.Y., Schober, S.E., Stähelin, H.B., Wald, N.J., Gey, K.F., and Willett, W.C. (1992) *J. Natl. Cancer Inst. 84*, 430.
42. Garewal, H. (1994) *Europ. J. Cancer Prev. 3*, 101.
43. Sinha, R., Patterson, B.H., Mangels, A.R., Levander, O.A., Gibson, T., Taylor, P.R., and Block G. (1993) *Cancer Epimediol. Biomark. Prev. 2*, 473.
44. Verlangieri, A.J., and Bush, M.J. (1992) *J. Am. College Nutr. 2*, 131.
45. Bostick, R.M., Potter, J.D., McKenzie, D.R., Sellers, T.A., Kushi, L.H., Steinmetz, K.A., and Folsom, A.R. (1993) *Cancer Res. 53*, 4230.
46. Witztum, J.L., and Steinberg, D. (1991) *J. Clin. Invest. 88*, 1785.
47. Esterbauer, H., Dieber-Rotheneder, M., Striegl, G., and Waeg, G. (1991) *Am. J. Clin. Nutr. 53*, 314.
48. Jialal, I., and Gundy, S.M. (1991) *Circulation 88*, 2780.
49. Packer, L., ed. (1994) *Methods in Enzymology: Oxygen Radicals in Biological Systems, Part C & D, Vol. 233 & 234*, Academic Press, San Diego, CA, pp. 704,711.
50. Eichholzer, M., Stähelin, H.B., and Gey, K.F. (1992) *EXS 62*, 398.
51. Kensler, T.W., Simic, M.G., and Trush, M.A., eds. (1994) *Cancer Res. 54*, 1872.
52. Jacques, P.F., Sulsky, S.I., Perrone, G.A., and Schaefer, E.J. (1994) *Epidemiology 5*, 19.
53. Herbert, J.R., Hurley, T.G., Hsieh, J., Rogers, E., Stoddard, A.M., Sorensen, G., and Nicolosi, R.J. (1994) *Am. J. Epidemiol. 140*, 132.
54. DeMaio, S.J., King, S.B., Lembo, N.J., Roubin, G.S., Hearn, J.A., Bhagavan, H.N., and Sgoutas, D.S. (1992) *J. Am. Coll. Nutr. 11*, 68.
55. Ferrari, R., Ceconi, C., Curello, S., Cargnoni, A., Alfieri, O., Pardini, A., Marzollo, P., and Visioli, O. (1991) *Am. J. Med. 91*, 95.
56. Stalenhoef, A.F.H. (1994) *Nutrition 10*, 564.
57. Slater, T.F., and Block, G., eds. (1991) *Am. J. Clin. Nutr. 53*, 189.
58. Barone, J., Taioli, E., Herbert, J.R., and Wynder, E.L. (1992) *Nutr. Cancer 18*, 31.
59. La Vecchia, C., Ferraroni, M., D'Avanzo, B., Decarli, A., and Franceschi, S. (1994) *Cancer Epidemiol. Biomark. Prev. 3*, 393.

60. Xu, G.P., Song, P.J., and Reed, P.I. (1993) *Eur. J. Cancer Prev. 2*, 327.
61. Dyke, G.W., Craven, J.L., Hall, R., and Garner, R.C. (1994) *Carcinogenesis 15*, 291.
62. Wang, G-Q., Dawsey, S.M., Li, J-Y., Taylor, P.R., Li, B., Blot, W.J., Weinstein, W.M., Liu, F.-S., Lewin, K.J., Wang, H., Wiggett, S., Gail, M.H., and Yang, C.S. (1994) *Cancer Epidemiol. Biomark. Prev. 3*, 161.
63. Lieber, C.S. (1993) *Seminars Liver Diseases 13*, 136.
64. Dakshinaumurti, K., ed. (1990) *Ann. N.Y. Acad. Sci. 585*, 1.
65. Byers, T., and Perry, G. (1992) *Annu. Rev. Nutr. 12*, 139.
66. Machlin, L.J. (1994) *Nutrition 10*, 507.
67. Ziegler, R.G., Subar, A.F., Craft, N.E., Ursin, G., Patterson, B.H., and Graubard, B.I. (1992) *Cancer Res. 52*, 2060.
68. Le Marchand, L., Hankin, J.H., Kolonel, L.N., Beecher, G.R., Wilkens, L.R., and Zhao, L.P. (1993) *Cancer Epidemiol. Biomark. Prev. 2*, 183.
69. Canfield, L.M., Krinsky, N.I., and Olson, J.A., eds. (1993) *Ann. N.Y. Acad. Sci. 691*, 1.
70. Garewal, H., Meyskens, F., Friedman, S., Alberts, D., and Ramsey, L. (1993) *Prev. Med. 22*, 701.
71. Tominaga, K., Saito, Y., Mori, K., Miyazawa, N., Yokoi, K., Koyama, Y., Shimamura, K., Imura, J., and Nagai, M. (1992) *Jpn. J. Clin. Oncol., 22*, 96.
72. Shekelle, R.B., Tangney, C.C., Rossof, A.H., and Stamler, J. (1992) *Epidemiology 3*, 282.
73. Bos, R.P., van Poppel, G., Theuws, J.L., and Kok, F.J. (1992) *Int. Arch. Occupat. Environ. Health. 64*, 189.
74. Edes, T.E., and Gysbers, D.S. (1993) *Ann. N.Y. Acad. Sci. 686*, 203.
75. Hoffmann, D., Rivenson, A., Chung, F.L., and Wynder, E.L. (1993) *Ann. N.Y. Acad. Sci. 686*, 140.
76. Goodman, G.E., Omenn, G.S., Thornquist, M.D., Lund, B., Metch, B., and Gylys-Colwell, I. (1993) *Cancer Epidemiol. Biomark. Prev. 2*, 389.
77. Cardinal, A.F., van't Veer, P., Koki, F.J., Kohlmeier, L., Martin-Moreno, J.M., Huttunen, J.K., Hallen, M., Aro, A., Delgado-Rodriguez, M., and Gomez-Aracena, J. (1993) *Eur. J. Clin. Nutr. 2*, 64.
78. Greenberg, E.R. (1993) *Prev. Med. 22*, 723.
79. Harris, R.W., Key, T.J., Silcocks, P.B., Bull, D., and Wald, N.J. (1991) *Nutr. Cancer 15*, 63.
80. Stähelin, H.B., Gey, K.F., and Eichholzer, M. (1991) *Am J. Clin. Nutr. 53*, 265.
81. Mayne, S.T., Janerich, D.T., Greenwald, P., Chorost, S., Tucci, C., Zaman, M.B., Melamed, M.R., Kiely, M., and McKneally, M.F. (1994) *J. Natl. Cancer Inst. 86*, 33.
82. Mogren, H. (1994) *Nutr. Rev. 52*, 1.
83. Shibata, A., Paganini-Hill, A., Ross, R.K., Yu, M.C., and Henderson, B.E. (1992) *Cancer Causes Control 3*, 207.
84. Hathcock, J.N., Hattan, D.G., Jenkins, M.Y., McDonald, J.T., Sundaresan, P.R., and Wilkening, V.L. (1990) *Am. J. Clin. Nutr. 52*, 183.
85. Fallon, M.B., and Boyer, J.L. (1990) *J. Gastroenterol. Hepatol. 5*, 334.
86. van Dam, M.A. (1989) *Nurse Practitioner 28*, 30.
87. Zhang, L.-X., Acevedo, P., Guo, H., and Bertram, J.S. (1995) *Mol. Carcinog. 12*, 50.
88. Scita, G., and Wolf. G. (1994) *Carcinogenesis, 15*, 1043.
89. Mercier, T., Honikman-Leban, E., Chaumontet, C., Martel, P., and Shahin, M.M. (1993) *Fundament. Appl. Toxicol. 21*, 270.

90. Fraser, D.R. (1995) *Lancet 345*, 104.
91. Machlin, L.J., and Sauberlich, H.E. (1994) *Nutrition Today, 29*(1), 25.
92. Kelloff, G.J., Boone, C.W., Crowell, J.A., Steele, V.E., Lubet, R., and Sigman, C.C. (1994) *Cancer Epidemiol. Biomark. Prev. 3*, 85.
93. Bendich, A., and Butterworth, C.E., eds. (1991) *Micronutrients in Health and in Disease Prevention*, Marcel Dekker, New York, pp. 1–504.
94. Dickinson, V.A., Block, G., and Russek-Cohen, E. (1994) *J. Am. Coll. Nutr. 13*, 22.
95. Helzlsouer, K.J., Block, G., Blumberg, J., Diplock, A.T., Levine, M., Marnett, L.J., Schueplein, R.J., Spence, J.T., and Simic, M.G. (1994) *Cancer Res., 54*, 2044.
96. Public Health Service (1991) *Healthy People 2000: National Health Promotion and Disease Prevention Objectives*, U.S. Dept. Health and Human Services, Washington, D.C.

Chapter 15

Endogenous Antioxidants: Role of Antioxidant Enzymes in Biological Systems

Y.V. Yuan and D.D. Kitts

Department of Food Science, University of British Columbia, Vancouver, British Columbia, Canada.

Introduction

Enzymes involved in the detoxification of reactive oxygen species (ROS) and lipid hydroperoxides include Cu/Zn superoxide dismutase (SOD; cytoplasm), Mn-SOD (mitochondria), catalase (CAT; peroxisomes), the glutathione redox cycling enzymes: selenium-dependent glutathione peroxidase (GSH-Px) and glutathione reductase (GSSG-Red; cytoplasm and mitochondria) and finally, the nonselenium-dependent glutathione-*S*-transferases (cytoplasm). Nonenzymatic cellular antioxidants active *in vivo* include α-tocopherol, β-carotene, and ascorbyl palmitate which are present in membranes, as well as the tripeptide glutathione (GSH) present in the cytoplasm (Table 15.1). Extracellular antioxidants include plasma components such as uric acid, bilirubin, and carnosine (Table 15.1). In the absence of adequate endogenous antioxidant defenses, the propagation of free radical events can lead to the co-oxidation of nucleophilic cellular constituents as well as reaction of secondary lipid autoxidation products with nucleophilic macromolecules, such as membrane constituents, enzymes, or DNA (1,2). These events can result in the disruption of cellular membranes and cell death (cytotoxicity), ultimately leading to tissue damage. The pathological significance of lipid peroxides and free radical damage in humans continues to be demonstrated and investigated. This chapter reviews the mechanisms of endogenous antioxidant enzyme activity and its role as a defense against toxic oxygen-derived free radicals and lipid oxidation end products.

Reactive Oxygen Species

Endogenous oxygen-derived free radical species occur naturally as products of aerobic metabolism produced during normal oxidative metabolism as a result of oxidase activity (e.g., both xanthine oxidase and glucose oxidase produce $O_2^{-\bullet}$), flavoprotein dehydrogenases, mitochondrial electron transport proteins, cytochrome P_{450} activity, as well as autoxidation of thiols and hydroquinones (3). The respiratory burst of phagocytes in response to microbial infection and inflammation represent an additional source of endogenous ROS. Exogenous initiators of ROS production include

TABLE 15.1
Endogenous Antioxidant Defense Systems

Antioxidant	Location	Function
Nonenzymatic		
Albumin	plasma	binds Fe, Cu ions
Ascorbic acid	plasma	electron donor; $^1O_2$ quencher; regenerates α-tocopheryl radical
Bilirubin	plasma	free radical scavenger
β-Carotene	plasma, cell membranes	electron donor; $^1O_2$ quencher;
	free radical scavenger	
Ceruloplasmin	plasma	binds Cu ions
Ferritin	plasma	binds Fe ions
Glutathione (GSH)	plasma, intracellular cytosol, mitochondria) free radical scavenger	thiol group maintains redox potential;
Haptoglobulin	plasma	binds hemoglobin
Hemopexin	plasma	binds heme
protein sulfhydryl groups	plasma	free radical scavenger
α-Tocopherol (and β, γ, δ isomers)	plasma, cell membranes	electron donor; $^1O_2$ quencher; free radical scavenger; H^+ donor
Transferrin	plasma	binds free Fe ions
Ubiquinone	plasma	free radical scavenger
Uric acid	plasma	binds free Fe ions
Enzymatic		
Catalase (CAT)	intracellular (peroxisomes)	metabolizes H_2O_2 into H_2O and O_2
Superoxide dismutase (SOD)	plasma, milk, intracellular (cytosol, mitochondria)	dismutates $O_2^{-\bullet}$ into H_2O_2
Glutathione peroxidase (GSH-Px)	plasma, intracellular	inactivates hydroperoxides using GSH reducing equivalents
Glutathione reductase (GSSG-Red)	intracellular	regenerates GSH from GSSG
Glutathione-*S*-transferase (GST)	intracellular	conjugates xenobiotics and alkylating agents with GSH for excretion.

radiation and xenobiotic agents derived from air pollution or drugs (e.g., carbon tetrachloride, paraquat, cigarette smoke). Production of ROS occurs at the intracellular (e.g., mitochondrial), cellular (e.g., muscle and neurons) and organ (e.g., heart, liver, and lung) levels. *In vivo* production of ROS can occur *via* the single addition of electrons to molecular oxygen during reduction of O_2 to H_2O (4). For example, the superoxide radical is formed through the addition of a single electron to molecular oxygen in the following Equation [1] (5):

$$O_2 + 1e^- \rightarrow O_2^{-\bullet} \qquad [1]$$

Superoxide radical formation can also occur by electron transfer to dioxygen (O_2) from a strong reducing agent, such as a transition metal (e.g., ferrous ion) or an uncoupled electron transport system (6). The superoxide radical itself has limited reactivity, abstracting hydrogen atoms only from very strong donors such as ascorbic acid (6). The toxicity of $O_2^{-\bullet}$ is based primarily on its role as a precursor in $^\bullet$OH radical formation *via* the Haber-Weiss reaction (7):

$$O_2^{-\bullet} + Fe^{3+} \longrightarrow Fe^{2+} + O_2 \qquad [2]$$

$$2O_2^{-\bullet} + 2H^+ \longrightarrow H_2O_2 + O_2 \qquad [3]$$

$$Fe^{2+} + H_2O_2 \longrightarrow {}^\bullet OH + OH^- + Fe^{3+} \qquad [4]$$

Dismutation of the superoxide radical either spontaneously or catalyzed by SOD, yields hydrogen peroxide (Equation [3]). When H_2O_2 interacts with ferrous ion in the Fenton reaction (Equation [4]), the result is the formation of the highly reactive hydroxyl radical ($^\bullet$OH). The $^\bullet$OH radical can then abstract another electron from a neighboring compound, such as an unsaturated lipid (RH; Equation [5]), to initiate a cascade of lipid autoxidation reactions (Equations [6] and [7]):

$$^\bullet OH + RH \rightarrow R^\bullet + H_2O \quad \text{Initation} \qquad [5]$$

$$R^\bullet + O_2 \rightarrow ROO^\bullet \qquad [6]$$

$$ROO^\bullet + RH \rightarrow ROOH + R^\bullet \qquad [7]$$

([6] and [7]: Propagation/Autoxidation)

Singlet oxygen ($^1O_2$), another form of excited oxygen, is produced when O_2 absorbs energy, such as in photochemical reactions involving photons of light. This species of oxygen radical is more selective in its subsequent reactions than •OH and ROO$^\bullet$, but is less selective than $O_2^{-\bullet}$.

Oxygen Derived Free Radicals in vivo

Dietary deficiencies of enzymatic trace metal cofactors (Cu, Mn, Se, Zn) or vitamins (A, C, E) may lead to the accumulation of $O_2^{-\bullet}$ and H_2O_2, thus favoring the generation of the highly reactive hydroxyl radical $^\bullet$OH (1,8,9). Normally, the compartmentalization of cellular oxidative and antioxidant components within organelles *in vivo* facilitates the control of a balance between these two events. However, the formation of reactive lipid free radicals and hydroperoxides may result in the disruption of cell membranes due to the increased polarity of lipid autoxidation products. Thus, membrane phospholipid components will undergo degradation due to the polar $^-$OOH group of lipid hydroperoxides moving out of the relatively nonpolar environment within the fluid membrane structure. Other detrimental effects of oxidative stress *in vivo* may involve specific biological processes. For example, malondialdehyde (OHC-CH_2-CHO), a secondary product of polyunsaturated fatty acid (PUFA) autoxidation is capable of crosslinking proteins, inactivating enzymes, and interacting with cellular DNA (10). Fraga and coworkers (1) demonstrated decreased protein synthesis in rat liver tissue exposed to oxidative stress mediated by halogenated compounds. Furthermore, aging may be the result of cumulative oxidative events throughout a lifetime (5,11). Development of lipofuscin age-pigments in older animals is due to the condensation of carbonyl lipid autoxidation products with basic protein amino acid residues, similar to Maillard reaction products (12,13). Damage to DNA by $^{\bullet}OH$ or lipid free radicals resulting in alterations to bases, single or double strand breakage, crosslinking, or chromosomal aberrations may be involved in the initiation of carcinogenesis (11,14). The involvement of lipid autoxidation products in the pathogenesis of cardiovascular disease has also been suggested in reference to the elucidation of disease mechanisms (15). The link between age and the development of chronic diseases such as cancer and atherosclerosis is reflected by the fact that the progression of these biological outcomes occurs over several years. Nutritional factors and dietary habits have a significant effect on the regulation of antioxidant enzyme activity (Table 15.2) as well as on *in vivo* concentrations of several nonenzymatic antioxidants which can be influenced by the diet (e.g., glutathione, α-tocopherol).

Endogenous Antioxidant Enzymes

Superoxide Dismutase, SOD: (EC 1.15.1.1)

The superoxide radical ($O_2^{-\bullet}$) resulting from the reaction of intracellular free radicals with dioxygen or from generation during oxidative metabolism can be deactivated by the enzyme superoxide dismutase (32,33). SOD has two principal forms located within the cytosol and mitochondria. Both forms, Cu/Zn-SOD (cytosol) and Mn-SOD (mitochondria) catalyze the dismutation of the superoxide radical in two ways, resulting in hydrogen peroxide and oxygen as products as in Equations [8] and [9] below (3).

$$2O_2^{-\bullet} + 2H^+ \rightarrow H_2O_2 + O_2 \quad [8]$$

$$HO_2^{-\bullet} + HO_2^{-\bullet} \rightarrow H_2O_2 + O_2 \quad [9]$$

A third form of SOD containing Fe as a cofactor exists in some plants (4,34). Comparative biochemistry studies have shown great variation in tissue SOD activity among different organisms such as insects, rodents, and humans (35). The structure of bovine red blood cell Cu/Zn-SOD has been characterized as consisting of two identical 151 amino acid residue subunits with two active sites on opposite sides of the enzyme (4). The copper ion is situated within a deep cleft, whereas

TABLE 15.2
Nutritional Factors Influencing Antioxidant Enzyme Activity[a]

Enzyme	Tissue	Effect on activity	Nutritional factor	Reference
Catalase	Heart, liver	↑	energy-restricted diet	16–18
	Lung	↓	iron deficiency	19
	Kidney, lung	↓	low-protein diet;	20
			hyperbaric O_2	21
GSH-Px	Heart, liver, kidney	↑	energy-restricted diet	18
		↑	low-protein diet	22
	Aorta	↑	increased plasma lipids	23
	All tissues	↓	selenium deficiency	24
	Liver	↓	obesity	25
GSSG-Red	Aorta	↑	increased plasma lipids	21,23
	All tissues	↓	riboflavin deficiency	26
	Liver	↓	obesity	25
GST	Liver	↓	saturated fatty acids	27
			and fatty acid esters	28
Cu/Zn-SOD	Brain, liver, kidney	↑	energy-restricted diet	16–18
	Aorta, erythrocytes	↓	copper deficiency	4,29
Mn-SOD	Liver	↑	low-protein diet	21
	Lung	↑	increased pO_2	30
	Heart, liver	↓	fish oil diet	31

[a]See Table 15.1 for abbreviations.

zinc is buried inside the enzyme structure. Thus, the copper ion is easily displaced. Studies have shown that zinc can be replaced by other metallic cations such as cadmium, mercury, or cobalt, with only slight decreases in enzyme activity (4). On the other hand, copper cannot be replaced with another cofactor. Thus, zinc deficiency has little effect on Cu/Zn-SOD activity, whereas copper deficiency results in reduced enzyme activity (4,36). During enzyme catalysis, the copper ion is reduced by $O_2^{-\bullet}$ to yield O_2, whereupon the copper is then reoxidized to produce H_2O_2. Cu/Zn-SOD activity is rapidly lost with copper deficiency, but can be recovered when copper is restored to the diet or administered intraperitoneally. Of particular interest is the finding that Mn-SOD activity is actually higher in tissues of copper-deficient animals (37). The SOD enzymes are also sensitive to the inhibitory effects of H_2O_2 concentrations in the reaction environment (3,38). Some interaction between these two forms of SOD exist, in that the Cu/Zn- and Mn-SOD forms can compensate for each other in deficiencies (4). During organ differentiation, Mn-SOD activity changes the most (35). McElroy and co-workers (39) reported that hepatic SOD activity increased throughout gestation, and that this increase was due primarily to Cu/Zn-SOD activity. The presence of cumene hydroperoxide and D-amino acid oxidases stimulates SOD differentiation (40), whereas GSH, butylated hydroxytoluene and dithiothreitol can inhibit its differentiation (41). Other endogenous nonenzymatic antioxidants such as β-carotene, ascorbate, and α-tocopherol have been shown to have a beneficial effect on SOD differentiation. In fetal lung, SOD activity is elevated by dexamethasone, a synthetic corticosteroid (42).

Increased oxygen consumption *in vivo* has been shown to result in elevations in SOD activity (30). This protective mechanism is vital because the generation of oxygen-derived free radicals from enzymatic reactions is elevated when oxygen concentrations are high (43). The interaction of ROS metabolism with SOD activity has been hypothesized to play a principal role in the detoxification of various classes of peroxy radicals (44). The concept of the superoxide radical acting as a biochemical "sink" for metabolism-derived free radicals is based on the production of $O_2^{-\bullet}$ by free radicals with reducing power, directly reacting with molecular oxygen as in Equation [10] below:

$$RH^{\bullet} + O_2 \rightarrow R + O_2^{-\bullet} + H^+ \quad [10]$$

In the presence of SOD activity, the reaction equilibrium is displaced to the right, allowing free radical deactivation *in vivo* to occur in large part due to metabolism of the superoxide radical.

Catalase, CAT: (EC 1.11.1.6)

Catalase (CAT) activity is located intracellularly within the mitochondria and peroxisomes. Humans, guinea-pigs, pigs, and sheep have high levels of liver catalase activity in both intracellular compartments, whereas liver peroxisomal catalase activity predominates in mice and rats (45). The activity of CAT varies among tissues, with the liver and kidney having the greatest amounts, and connective tissue the least. CAT decomposes H_2O_2 to water and oxygen (Equation [11]) and also converts hydroperoxides to the corresponding alcohols in the presence of a hydrogen donor (AH_2; Equation [12]) (46):

$$2H_2O_2 \rightarrow 2H_2O + O_2 \quad [11]$$

$$ROOH + AH_2 \rightarrow H_2O + ROH + A \quad [12]$$

In Equation [11], the second molecule of H_2O_2 acts as a hydrogen donor for the deactivation of the first H_2O_2. Each enzyme molecule contains four ferriprotoporphyrin groups in its structure (MW 240,000). It is therefore not surprising that some alterations in CAT activity can be linked to reduced availability of iron (19). CAT activity increases in most tissues during development (47). The enzyme is mainly particle-bound within organelles, but is free within red blood cells (46). Furthermore, species differences have been found to exist for red blood cell (RBC) CAT activity (48). For example, human RBCs are rich in CAT activity, whereas those of avian species (e.g., duck and quail) are almost devoid of CAT activity (46,48).

Glutathione Redox Cycling Enzymes

The enzymes of the glutathione peroxidase/reductase redox cycle consist of a selenium-dependent glutathione peroxidase (GSH-Px), as well as a glutathione reductase (GSSG-Red) enzyme required to regenerate the GSH reducing equivalents. These enzymes occur in the plasma as well as intracellularly (49,50). Glutathione plays a central role in the activity of its metabolizing enzymes in addition to its activity as an intracellular and extracellular nonenzymatic antioxidant molecule.

Glutathione. Thiol (-SH) groups of proteins contribute to antioxidant capacity not only *in vivo*, but also *in vitro*, as seen in studies with model lipid peroxidation systems incubated with casein (51). Similarly, intracellular thiols, namely, glutathione (GSH; L-γ-glutamyl-L-cysteinyl-glycine), possess strong antioxidant activity (2). The γ-glutamyl linkage renders the GSH molecule resistant to proteases. The main role of GSH *in vivo* is to be a primary agent involved in deactivating electrophilic free radicals.

$$2GSH + O_2 \rightarrow GSSG + H_2O_2 \qquad [13]$$

$$O_2^{-\bullet} + GSH + H^+ \rightarrow GS^\bullet + H_2O_2 \qquad [14]$$

The ability of thiol groups such as those of glutathione to have antioxidant activity in Equation [13] is dependent on the pO_2, pH, and the percentage of the thiol groups in the anion form (2). Oxidation of GSH as an antioxidant can occur *in vivo* with oxidized glutathione (GSSG) and hydrogen peroxide being formed as products. In Equation [14], the formation of a glutathionyl radical ($GS^\bullet$) from the reaction of GSH with a superoxide radical provides not only a defense against oxygen radical damage, but also represents a potential risk for further free radical reactions. For example, if the glutathionyl radical is not subsequently reduced by another reducing equivalent, it could go on to react with susceptible cellular constituents (e.g., membrane PUFA). Thus, GSH is an effective radical scavenger under conditions in which the glutathionyl radical ($GS^\bullet$) is efficiently removed (i.e., reduced back to GSH) or the potential PUFA reactant concentrations are very low (44).

Approximately 90% of intracellular nonprotein thiol content is GSH. In the hepatocyte, 85–90% of GSH is present in the cytoplasm with the remaining 10–15% within the mitochondria. In addition to acting as a coenzyme or substrate for antioxidant enzymes (i.e., GSH-Px and GST), cellular GSH also has a protective role to shield protein thiol groups from oxidation as an intracellular redox buffer (52). The mammalian liver normally has a high concentration of reduced GSH. Approximately 0–8% of the GSH content in rat liver tissue is in the oxidized (GSSG) form, hence 0–16% of total GSH may exist in the disulfide form (52). Glutathione has been shown to undergo interorgan circulation *via* translocation from cells into the plasma (53). Metabolism of GSH within the blood is thought to involve the reduction of disulfide bonds of plasma constituents and mobilization of compounds bound by disulfide bridges to plasma proteins. These products, in turn, are used to synthesize GSSG and low molecular weight derivatives of GSH, such as disulfides. Levels of GSH in rat plasma have been reported to range from 22–27 μM.

Approximately 85% of plasma GSH is in the reduced form (53). Cellular levels of GSH are dependent on the growth, nutritional status, and hormone balance of the subject (52). Pélissier and co-workers (54) demonstrated that with a protein deficient diet (6% casein), reduced levels of GSH were observed in the small intestine and liver of rats. As an index of *in vivo* susceptibility to lipid autoxidation, these workers reported increased levels of thiobarbituric acid reactive substances in the intestinal mucosa of experimental animals. In studies varying the protein content of diets fed to rats, Hum and co-workers (55) reported an increase in hepatic GSH concentration and total liver GSH content when dietary casein was increased from 0 to 20%. A further increase in dietary protein to 40% did not result in a further increase in liver GSH content, but did reduce the relative concentration of GSH due to increased liver tissue weight (55). These workers demonstrated a strong correlation between liver GSH concentration and total GSH content with sulfur amino acid intake. In this study, the plasma concentration of free cysteine was a better predictor of liver GSH content than was plasma GSH content (55). This observation may be due to the sigmoidal relation between plasma GSH turnover and liver GSH content (55). Moreover, the plasma GSH concentration was strongly associated with the absolute turnover rate of plasma GSH. Fasting for 24–48 h can reduce liver GSH in the rat to 50–70% of that in fed counterparts (2). Liver GSH content can be altered by variations in diurnal/circadian rhythms (2). Tissue concentrations of GSH are greater at night and early morning, compared with lower concentrations measured in the late afternoon (2).

Glutathione Peroxidase, GSH-Px: (EC 1.11.1.9). Glutathione peroxidase activities catalyze the deactivation of hydrogen peroxide (Equation [15]) or organic hydroperoxides derived from unsaturated lipids (Equation [16]) using the reducing power of glutathione (GSH) (56–58). These reactions serve to protect cellular membranes from the detrimental effects of *in vivo* oxidative stress.

$$H_2O_2 + 2GSH \rightarrow 2H_2O + GSSG \qquad [15]$$

$$ROOH + 2GSH \rightarrow ROH + H_2O + GSSG \qquad [16]$$

Traditionally, GSH-Px activity refers to selenium-dependent GSH-Px activity which is localized within the mitochondria, whereas nonselenium-dependent GSH-Px activity (also known as GSH-*S*-transferase activity) is located in the cytosol (59). The GSH-Px enzyme in the mitochondria (MW = 76,000–85,000 Da) contains four selenium atoms per subunit (MW of subunits = 17,000–22,000 Da) with very high specificity for GSH. Because the active site of the enzyme holds both selenol and thiol groups (60), restricting selenium intake through a dietary deficiency of this trace mineral results in reduced GSH-Px activity (24). The tertiary structure of GSH-Px, which is characterized by the presence of reactive selenocysteinyl residues on the surface of the protein, facilitates its reaction with a variety of hydroperoxides, resulting in varied states of redox status of the enzyme (e.g., reduced or oxidized state). At physiological levels of GSH, the enzyme is largely in the reduced form. The activity of GSH-Px is greatest when the enzyme is in its reduced form. Decreased GSH-Px activity can occur with oxidation by H_2O_2.

GSH-Px has been considered a key enzyme of the *in vivo* antioxidant system under both normal conditions as well as oxidative stress (3). Activity of this enzyme varies according to species differences, interference from competing enzymatic systems, tissue distribution, and the compartmentalization of co-substrates or inhibitors. Originally found in the bovine erythrocyte (61), GSH-Px activity has been reported in human erythrocytes (62), rodent and fish liver (63–65), but is absent from mammalian skin (66). In studies with cultured fibroblasts and human endothelial cells, lower amounts of GSH-Px were required, compared with CAT or SOD for the same level of antioxidant protection (3). Inhibition of GSH-Px by ROS such as $O_2^{-\bullet}$ and hydroperoxides is possible. Enzyme activity was reduced 50% in the presence of 50 µM tertiary butylhydroperoxide (3). Moreover, GSH-Px is directly inactivated by the superoxide radical (67). GSH-Px activity is also influenced by the presence of other enzyme systems, notably catalase and glutathione-*S*-transferase. While CAT competes with GSH-Px for H_2O_2, glutathione-*S*-transferase competes with GSH-Px for hydroperoxides only. Tissue compartmental localization is another factor that will influence the competition between GSH-Px and CAT. For example, in liver tissue, CAT activity is restricted to the peroxisomes, whereas GSH-Px activity is located in cytosolic and mitochondrial compartments. Another example of an enzyme interaction with GSH-Px is prostaglandin hydroperoxidase which shares the ability to reduce hydroperoxy intermediates in the arachidonic acid cascade (68).

Glutathione Reductase, GSSG-Red: (EC 1.6.4.2). Oxidized glutathione is reduced back to its native form *via* catalysis by GSSG-Red and nicotinamide adenine dinucleotide phosphate in Equation [18] below (NADPH; 50,52):

$$\mathrm{GSSG + NADPH \rightarrow 2GSH + NADP} \qquad [18]$$

Riboflavin is an important cofactor of GSSG-Red and thus can influence the level of intracellular reduced GSH and activity of GSH-Px. Riboflavin deficiency has been linked to the susceptibility of erythrocytes to oxidant stress and lysis common in malaria (26). GSSG-Red can also be inhibited by the phenylalanine chain of insulin (69). Thus, increased levels of GSSG-Red activity have been observed in hemolysates of diabetic patients' RBC (69).

Glutathione-S-transferase, GST: (EC 2.5.1.18). The nonselenium-dependent glutathione-*S*-transferases are involved in the biotransformation (detoxification) of xenobiotics (52). This group of enzymes detoxifies potential alkylating agents by conjugation with GSH (70). GST enzymes have a high specificity for GSH as reflected by the finding that this substrate is bound with a high affinity to the active site, thus providing an enzyme-bound glutathione thiolate anion (GS^-) which is very effective for conjugate formation (2). Cytosolic GST enzymes are composed of homo- or heterodimers and thus, are classified on the basis of subunit composition and substrate specificity. These enzymes conjugate the reactive intermediates of metabolized xenobiotics with GSH. The reaction of the GSH thiol group to neutralize the electrophilic sites of a xenobiotic to yield a more water-soluble product is catalyzed by GST activity (70). The GSH conjugate products can be metabolized further by cleavage of the glutamate and glycine residues, followed by acetylation of the resulting free amino group of the cysteinyl residue to yield a mercapturic acid for excretion (52). Further, the glutathione-*S*-transferases also have GSH-Px activity (52), as evidenced by the metabolism of *t*-butyl hydroperoxide in GSH-Px-deficient animals (71). In cases of selenium deficiency, GST activity in guinea pigs is induced, thereby indicating a compensatory mechanism of this enzyme towards lipid peroxidation in the absence of GSH-Px activity. GST competes with GSH-Px for organic hydroperoxides, but not for H_2O_2 (71). Inhibition of GST activity occurs from a wide assortment of endogenous and exogenous compounds, including bilirubin (72), saturated fatty acids (e.g., stearic and palmitic acids), and fatty acid esters (27,28).

Endogenous Enzymatic Antioxidants and Disease

There is considerable controversy concerning the role of antioxidants in the prevention of chronic diseases such as cancer and atherosclerosis. Nonenzymatic antioxidants such as α-tocopherol, ascorbic acid, and probucol have been shown to reduce some of the risk factors associated with atherosclerosis (e.g., plasma lipids, oxidation of low density lipoproteins (LDL) (73,74), but do not always effectively prevent the development of the disease (75). Altered antioxidant enzyme activities are sometimes associated with certain disease states or conditions (Table 15.3). For example, increases in GSH-Px activity can provide a significant defense against the presence of lipid peroxides in aortic tissue (21), a common constituent of arterial tissue from patients suffering from atherosclerosis (83). Interpretation of the tissue-specific and antioxidant enzyme-specific changes associated with different disease states is difficult, however, and often complicated by the intricate nature in which specific antioxidant enzyme activities are regulated by adaptive or compensatory metabolic factors within the organism. Moreover, the tissue-specific nature in which significant decreases or increases in antioxidant enzyme activity occur in a disease state adds to the challenge in ascertaining whether the differences are the causative factor of injury or in response to tissue damage. Certainly, underlying metabolic factors that regulate antioxidant enzyme activity and are sensitive to the nutritional status and health of the individual play a primary role in the response of organ systems to oxidative or lipid peroxidative stress.

TABLE 15.3
Examples of Diseases or Conditions Associated with Altered Antioxidant Enzyme Activity[a]

Enzyme	Location	Effect on activity	Condition	Reference
Catalase	Heart	↑	diabetes	76
	Erythrocyte	↑	multiple sclerosis	77
	Erythrocyte	↓	increased metabolic rate	48
	Heart, kidney	↓	aging	18
Cu/Zn-SOD	Brain, heart, liver, kidney	↓	aging	18
	Heart	↓	weight loss	78
	Kidney, pancreas	↑	weight loss	78
	Colon	↓	decreased xenobiotic detoxification	79
	Erythrocyte	↑	multiple sclerosis	77
	Erythrocyte	↓	malignant lymphoma	80
	Erythrocyte	↑	types I and II diabetes	81
GSSG-Red	Heart	↑	diabetes	76
	Liver	↓	obesity	25
	Erythrocyte	↓	malaria	26
GSH-Px	Heart, liver, kidney	↓	aging	18
	Liver	↓	obesity	25
	Heart	↓	cardiomyopathy	82
	Erythrocyte	↓	skeletal muscle weakness	82
	Colon	↓	decreased xenobiotic detoxification	79

[a]See Table 15.1 for abbreviations.

References

1. Fraga, C.G., Zamora, R., and Tappel, A.L. (1989) *Arch. Biochem. Biophys. 270*, 84.
2. Reed, D.J. (1989) in *Food Toxicology: A Perspective on the Relative Risks* (Taylor, S.L., and Scanlan, R.A., eds.), Marcel Dekker, Inc., New York, pp. 169–203.
3. Remacle, J., Lambert, D., Raes, M., Pigeolet, E., Michiels, C., and Toussaint, O. (1992) *Biochem. J. 286*, 41.
4. Harris, E.D. (1992) *J. Nutr. 122*, 636.
5. Diplock, A.T. (1986) in *Proceedings of the XIII International Congress of Nutrition* (Taylor, T.G., and Jenkins, N.K., eds.), John Libbey and Co. Ltd., London, pp. 585–589.
6. Foote, C.S. (1985) in *Chemical Changes in Food During Processing* (Richardson, T., and Finley, J.W., eds.), AVI Pub. Co., Westport, CT, pp. 17–32.
7. Graf, E., Mahoney, J.R., Bryant, R.G., and Eaton, J.W. (1984) *J. Biol. Chem. 259*, 3620.
8. Zamora, R., Hidalgo, F.J., and Tappel, A.L. (1991) *J. Nutr. 121*, 50.
9. Leibovitz, B., Hu, M.-L., and Tappel, A.L. (1990) *J. Nutr. 120*, 97.
10. Addis, P.B. (1986) *Food Chem. Toxicol. 24*, 1021.

11. Simic, M.G. (1991) *Environ. Carcinogen. & Ecotoxicol. Rev. C9*, 113.
12. Pryor, W.A. (1986) in *Proceedings of the XIII International Congress of Nutrition* (Taylor, T.G., and Jenkins, N.K., eds.), John Libbey and Co. Ltd., London, pp. 589–593.
13. Reddy, K., Fletcher, B., and Tappel, A. (1973) *J. Nutr. 103*, 908.
14. Thompson, L.U. (1994) *Crit. Rev. Food Sci. Nutr. 34*, 473.
15. Steinberg, D., Parthasarathy, S., Carew, T.E., Khoo, J.C., and Witztum, J.L. (1989) *N. Engl. J. Med. 320*, 915.
16. Rao, G., Xia, E,. and Richardson, A. (1990) *Mech. Aging Dev. 53*, 49.
17. Semsei, I., Rao, G., and Richardson, A. (1989) *Biochem. Biophys. Res. Commun. 164*, 620.
18. Xia, E., Rao, G., Van Remmen, H., Heydari, A.R., and Richardson, A. (1995) *J. Nutr. 125*, 195.
19. Transwell, A.K., and Freeman, B.A. (1984) *Pediatr. Res. 18*, 871.
20. Deneke, S.M., Lynch, B.A., and Fanburg, B.C. (1985) *J. Nutr. 115*, 726.
21. Mezzetti, A., Lapenna, D., Calafiore, A.M., Proietti-Franceschilli, G., Porreca, E., De Cesare, D., Neri, M., Di Ilio, C., and Cuccurullo, F. (1992) *Arterioscler. Thromb. 12*, 92.
22. Sambuichi, E.J., Shizuka, F., and Kishi, K. (1991) *Nutr. Res. 11*, 1415.
23. Ledwozyw, A., Michalak, J., Stepien, A., and Kadziolka, A. (1986) *Clin. Chem. Acta 155*, 275.
24. Pence, B.C. (1981) *J. Nutr. 121*, 138.
25. Capel, I.D., and Dorrell, H.M. (1984) *Biochem. J. 219*, 41.
26. Das, B.S., Das, D.B., Satpathy, R.N., Patnaik, J.K., and Bose, T.K. (1988) *Eur. J. Clin. Nutr. 42*, 277.
27. Mitra, A., Govindwar, S., and Kulkarni, A.P. (1991) *Toxicol. Lett. 58*, 135.
28. Mitra, A., Govindwar, S., Joseph, P., and Kulkarni, A. (1992) *Toxicol. Lett. 60*, 281.
29. DiSilvestro, R.A. (1989) *Arch. Biochem. Biophys. 274*, 298.
30. Stevens, J.B., and Autor, A.P. (1977) *J. Biol Chem. 252*, 3509.
31. L'Abbé, M.R., Trick, K.D., and Beare-Rogers, J.L. (1991) *J. Nutr. 121*, 1331.
32. Fridovich, I. (1975) *Annu. Rev. Biochem. 44*, 147.
33. McCord, J.M., and Fridovich, I. (1969) *J. Biol. Chem. 244*, 6049.
34. Leshem, Y.Y. (1988) *Free Radical Biol. Med. 5*, 39.
35. Allen, R.G. (1991) *Proc. Soc. Exp. Biol. Med. 196*, 117.
36. L'Abbé, M.R., and Fischer, P.W.F. (1984) *J. Nutr. 114*, 813.
37. Dubick, M.A., Zidenberg-Cherr, S., Rucker, R.B., and Keen, C.L. (1988) *Toxicol. Lett. 42*, 149.
38. Pigeolet, E., Corbisier, P., Houbion, A., Lambert, D., Michiels, C., Raes, M., and Remacle, J. (1990) *Mech. Aging Dev. 51*, 283.
39. McElroy, M.C., Postle, A.D., and Kelly, F.J. (1992) *Biochim. Biophys. Acta 1117*, 153.
40. Beckman, B.S., Balin, A.K., and Allen, R.G. (1989) *J. Cell Physiol. 139*, 370.
41. Allen, R.G., Balin, A.K., Reimer, R.J., Sohal, R.S., and Nations, C. (1988) Arch. *Biochem. Biophys. 261*, 205.
42. Randhawa, P., Hass, M., Frank, L., and Massaro, D. (1986) *Pediatr. Res. 20*, 895.
43. Misra, H.P., and Fridovich, I. (1971) *J. Biol. Chem. 246*, 6886.
44. Winterbourn, C.C. (1993) *Free Radical Biol. Med. 14*, 85.
45. Holmes. R.S., and Masters, C.J. (1972) *Arch. Biochem. Biophys. 148*, 217.
46. Aebi, H. (1974) in *Methods of Enzymatic Analysis* (Bergmeyer, H.U., ed.), Vol. 2, 2nd edn., Verlag Chemie GmbH, Weinheim, pp. 673–684.

47. Allen, R.G., and Balin, A.K. (1989) *Free Radical Biol. Med. 6*, 631.
48. Godin, D.V., and Garnett, M.E. (1992) *Comp. Biochem. Physiol. 103B*, 737.
49. Harris, E.D. (1992) *J. Nutr. 122*, 625.
50. Paglia, D.E., and Valentine, W.N. (1967) *J. Lab. Clin. Med. 70*, 158.
51. McGookin, B.J., and Augustin, M. (1991) *J. Dairy Res. 58*, 313.
52. Moron, M.S., Depierre, J.W., and Mannervik, B. (1979) *Biochim. Biophys. Acta 582*, 67.
53. Anderson, M.E., and Meister, A. (1980) *J. Biol. Chem. 255*, 9530.
54. Pélissier, M.-A., Darmon, N., Desjeux, J.-F., and Albrecht, R. (1993) *Food Chem. Toxicol. 31*, 59.
55. Hum, S., Koski, K.G., and Hoffer, L.J. (1992) *J. Nutr. 122*, 2010.
56. Christopherson, B.O. (1969) *Biochim. Biophys. Acta 176*, 463.
57. Little, C., and O'Brien, P.J. (1968) *Biochem. Biophys. Res. Commun. 31*, 145.
58. Cohen, G., and Hochstein, P. (1963) *Biochemistry 2*, 1420.
59. Lawrence, R.A., and Burk, R.F. (1978) *J. Nutr. 108*, 211.
60. Blum, J., and Fridovich, I. (1978) *Arch. Biochem. Biophys. 240*, 500.
61. Mills, G.C. (1957) *J. Biol. Chem. 229*, 189.
62. Awasthi, Y.C., Beutler, E., and Srivastava, S.K. (1975) *J. Biol. Chem. 250*, 5144.
63. Braddon, S.A., Meilvaine, C.M., and Balthrop, J.E. (1985) *Comp. Biochem. Physiol. 80B*, 213.
64. Tappel, M.E., Chaudiere, J., and Tappel, A.L. (1982) *Comp. Biochem. Physiol. 73B*, 945.
65. Nakamura, W., Hosoda, S., and Hayashi, K. (1974) *Biochim. Biophys. Acta 358*, 251.
66. Kawai, S., Komura, J., Asada, Y., and Niwa, Y. (1988) *Arch. Dermatol. Res. 280*, 171.
67. Turrens, J.F. (1991) *Xenobiotica 21*, 1033.
68. Ohki, S., Ogino, N., Yamamoto, S., and Hayashi, O.J. (1979) *J. Biol. Chem. 254*, 829.
69. Long, W.K., and Carson, P.E. (1961) *Biochem. Biophys. Res. Commun. 5*, 394.
70. Habig, W.H., Pabst, M.J., and Jakoby, W.B. (1974) *J. Biol. Chem. 249*, 7130.
71. Prohaska, J.R. (1980) *Biochim. Biophys. Acta 611*, 87.
72. Ketterer, B., Meyer, D.J., and Clark, A.G. (1988) in *Glutathione Conjugation: Mechanisms and Biological Significance* (Seis, H., and Ketterer, B., eds.), Academic Press, New York, p. 96.
73. Stein, Y., Stein, O., Delplanque, B., Fesmire, J.D., and Lee, D.M. (1989) *Atherosclerosis 75*, 145.
74. Westrope, K.L., Miller, R.A., and Wilson, R.B. (1982) *Nutr. Rep. Int. 25*, 83.
75. Morel, D.W., De La Llera-Moya, M., and Friday, K.E. (1994) *J. Nutr. 124*, 2123.
76. Wohaieb, S.A., and Godin, D.V. (1987) *Diabetes 36*, 1014–1018.
77. Jensen, G.E., and Clansen, J. (1984) *J. Neurol. Sci. 63*, 45.
78. Wohaieb, S.A., and Godin, D.V. (1987) *Diabetes 36*, 169.
79. Pence, B.C. (1991) *J. Nutr. 121,* 138.
80. Bewich, M., Coutie, W., and Tudhope, G.R. (1987) *Br. J. Haematol. 65*, 347.
81. Prasartkaew, S., Bunyaratvej, A., Fucharoen, S., and Wasi, P. (1986) *J. Clin. Pathol. 39*, 1299.
82. Cohen, H.J., Brown, M.R., Hamilton, D., Lyons-Patterson, J., Avissar, N., and Leigey, P. (1989) *Am. J. Clin. Nutr. 49*, 132.
83. Piotrowski, J.J., Hunter, G.C., Eskelson, C.D., Dubick, M.A., and Bernhard, V.M. (1990) *Life Sci. 46*, 715.

Chapter 16

Antioxidant Activity of Carnosine, a Skeletal Muscle Dipeptide

E.A. Decker, W.K.M. Chan, L. Mei, G.L. McNeill-Tompkins, and S.A. Livisay

Department of Food Science, University of Massachusetts, Amherst, Massachusetts.

Introduction

Oxidative reactions are a major cause of the chemical deterioration of muscle foods. Oxidation of muscle lipids and proteins affects flavor, aroma, texture, color, and nutritional composition. Off-flavors and aromas are created due to the formation of volatile lipid decomposition products such as aldehydes, hydrocarbons, alcohols, and ketones (1). Texture can be altered in muscle foods by polymerization of proteins and lipids induced by oxidative reactions (2,3). Both pigments (e.g., myoglobin) and nutrients (e.g., α-tocopherol) are also susceptible to oxidative deterioration (4). The safety and wholesomeness of muscle foods can also be compromised by lipid oxidation reactions which produce aldehydes, epoxides and oxidized sterols because these compounds have been implicated in the development of atherosclerosis and cancer (5).

The oxidative deterioration of muscle foods is catalyzed by transition metals, heme-containing proteins, enzymes, and active oxygen species (6–10). These catalysts accelerate the oxidation of membrane lipids (11) resulting in the formation of rancidity in both low and high fat muscle food products. Because the lipid oxidation catalysts in muscle foods are water soluble, they also can accelerate myoglobin oxidation resulting in decreased shelf-life due to loss of typical red color. Oxidative reactions in muscle foods are accelerated by heat processing which releases protein-bound iron, activates heme-containing proteins, disrupts cellular membrane systems, and inactivates antioxidant enzymes (6,12) and by addition of sodium chloride which increases the prooxidant activity of iron (13,14).

Carnosine and anserine are *N*-β-alanyl-L-histidine and *N*-β-alanyl-3-methyl-L-histidine dipeptides, respectively, endogenous to skeletal muscle (Fig. 16.1). Carnosine and anserine concentrations in beef, pork, chicken, and fish range from 10 to 70 mM (Table 16.1) (15,16). White muscle fibers generally have higher anserine and carnosine concentrations than red muscle, with chicken breast and leg muscle containing 71.0 and 12.2 mM anserine and carnosine, respectively (15).

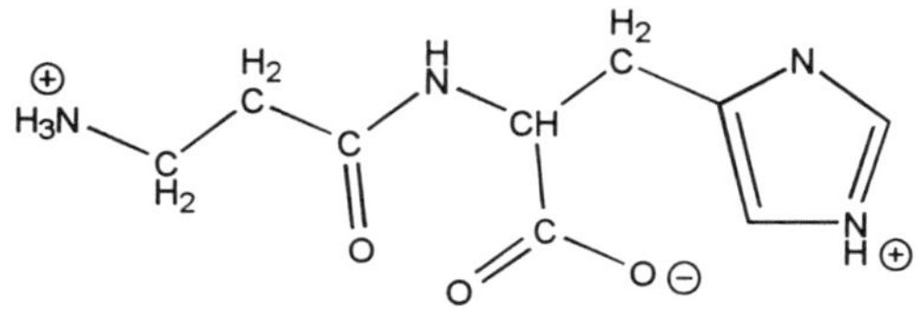

CARNOSINE

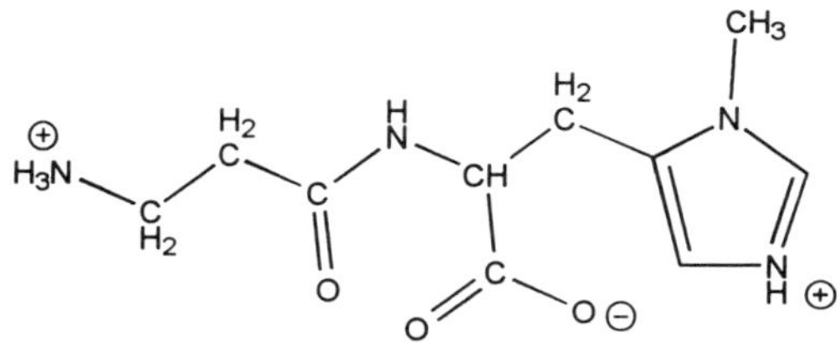

ANSERINE

Fig. 16.1. The structure of anserine and carnosine at the pH (5.0–6.5) of muscle foods.

The Biological Role of Carnosine and Anserine in Skeletal Muscle

The exact biological role of carnosine and anserine is not completely understood; however, similarities in dipeptide structures suggest similar physiological functions. Because the pK_a values for the imidazole ring of carnosine and anserine are 6.83 and 7.04, respectively, these histidine-containing dipeptides exhibit excellent buffering capacity at physiological pH values. Concentrations of anserine and carnosine are such that they can provide up to 40% of pH-buffering capacity of skeletal muscle (17). The buffering capacity of muscle has been correlated with

TABLE 16.1
The Concentration (mM) of Anserine and Carnosine in Different Skeletal Muscles

	Muscle source	Carnosine	Anserine
Chicken	Leg	2.9	9.3
	Breast	16.4	54.6
Rabbit	Leg	4.1	22.2
Atlantic salmon		0	22.2
Beef	Leg	8.8	2.8
Swine	Shoulder	9.2	1.1
Human	Quadriceps	21.3	0

Source: Refs. (15,16).

carnosine concentrations in horses, dogs, and humans (18). The role of carnosine and anserine as buffers could explain why higher concentrations are found in white muscle fibers in which high levels of anaerobic metabolism are common.

Boldyrev and co-workers (19,20) were the first to report that carnosine has membrane-protecting properties. In a system containing sarcoplasmic reticulum membranes, they demonstrated that carnosine and anserine could decrease lipid oxidation rates as determined by thiobarbituric acid reactive substance (TBARS) (20). The antioxidant activity of carnosine and anserine has also been demonstrated in systems containing phosphatidylcholine liposomes (21), linoleic acid emulsions (22), and skeletal muscle microsomes (23). Researchers found that carnosine was capable of inhibiting lipid oxidation catalyzed by iron (20,21), copper (22,23), hydrogen peroxide-activated hemoglobin (21), singlet oxygen (24), lipoxygenase (21), peroxyl radicals (22), and hydroxyl radicals (25). Antioxidant activity has been monitored by measuring a variety of lipid oxidation products including TBARS, lipid peroxides, and conjugated dienes (19,21,23). The antioxidant properties of anserine are similar to carnosine (20,22) with significant antioxidant activity occurring at concentrations comparable to those in skeletal muscle tissues (1–50 mM). Unlike many other antioxidants (e.g., ascorbic acid and α-tocopherol), carnosine has not been reported to exhibit prooxidant activity.

The antioxidant mechanism of carnosine and anserine involves both metal chelation and free radical scavenging. Carnosine is capable of chelating metals, yet its chelating activity is dependent on metal ion type (26,27). Kohen and co-workers (22) reported that oxidative damage of deoxyguanosine induced by copper and ascorbate could be inhibited by carnosine (1 mM). Decker and co-workers (23) observed that carnosine (1.0–10 mM) was capable of decreasing ascorbate oxidation catalyzed by copper. The ability of carnosine to inhibit these copper-catalyzed oxidation reactions suggests that carnosine forms a complex with copper in a manner which decreases copper's reactivity. Nuclear magnetic resonance (NMR) studies found that copper (10 μM) is chelated by carnosine (10 mM) as indicated by the loss of the C-2 and C-4 peaks of the imidazole ring (23). Carnosine is ineffective at inhibiting iron-catalyzed oxidation of ascorbate, and NMR spectroscopy studies show that carnosine (10 mM) does not complex with iron (10 μM) even though carnosine inhibits Fe-catalyzed lipid oxidation (23). Inhibition of iron-catalyzed lipid oxidation without chelation suggested that carnosine was capable of scavenging free radicals.

Electron paramagnetic resonance (EPR) studies have shown that carnosine can inactivate hydroxyl radicals generated by iron and H_2O_2 or H_2O_2 and ultraviolet (UV)-irradiation (25,28). Radicals originating from carnosine (α^N = 15.6 G (Gauss) and $\alpha^N{}_\beta$ = 18.8 G), glycine (Gly)-histidine (His) (α^N = 15.6 G and $\alpha^N{}_\beta$ = 18.6 G) and homocarnosine [γ-amino butyric acid (GABA)-His; α^N = 15.7 G and $\alpha^N{}_\beta$ = 18.9 G] were detected in the presence of hydroxyl radicals, indicating that these histidine-containing dipeptides are capable of scavenging hydroxyl radicals (28). Carnosine and anserine also actively scavenge singlet oxygen at rates ranging from 2 to 4 × 10^7 $M^{-1}\bullet s^{-1}$ (29). The quenching of singlet oxygen was suggested to be due mainly to the imidazole group of carnosine and anserine (29). Carnosine and anserine are not capable of scavenging superoxide anions as determined by the reduction of cytochrome (30) and the EPR signal intensity of a DMPO-superoxide spin adduct (31). These data indicate that carnosine is an effective scavenger of high energy free radicals such as singlet oxygen and hydroxyl radicals.

β-Alanine (β-Ala) and histidine, alone and in combination, exhibit significantly lower hydroxyl radical scavenging and antioxidant activity than equal molar concentrations of carnosine (Table 16.2). In addition, both acetyl and methyl ester derivatives of histidine exhibit reduced singlet oxygen scavenging activity compared with carnosine (32). These data suggest that the peptide bond is necessary to maximize the activity of β-Ala and His. Both the β-alanine and histidine moieties play an important role in antioxidant and free radical scavenging activity of carno-

TABLE 16.2

Ability of Carnosine and Related Peptides (25 mM) to Scavenge Hydroxyl Radicals (•OH; as Determined by Electron Paramagnetic Resonance Spectroscopy) and to Inhibit Iron-Catalyzed Oxidation of Phosphatidylcholine Liposomes (as Determined by Thiobarbituric Acid Reactive Substances; TBARS)

Amino acid or peptide	•OH scavenging activity (%)	TBARS inhibition (%)
Control	100	100
β-Ala-His (carnosine)	25.2	34.7
β-Ala-1-methyl-His (anserine)	16.8	30.2
γ-Amino butyric acid-His (homocarnosine)	31.6	73.1
Gly-His	5.1	80.9
L-Ala-His	45.2	106.9
Val-His	45.0	ND
β-Ala-Gly	157.3	ND
β-Ala-L-Ala	108.4	ND
β-Ala-Glu	187.5	ND
β-Ala-Lys	21.6	ND
β-Ala-Phe	11.6	ND
His	50.9	78.1
1-methyl-His	10.0	ND
β-Ala	244.7	98.4
γ-Amino butyric acid	169.1	96.7
Gly	157.3	96.8
L-Ala	116.9	ND
Val	171.9	ND
Phe	97.9	ND
Lys	95.2	ND
β-Ala, His	54.4	77.5
γ-Amino butyric acid, His	48.4	76.9
Gly, His	52.5	76.5

ND = not determined. *Source:* Adapted from Ref. (37).

sine. The β-alanine moiety provides unique characteristics to peptides which contain amino acids known to exhibit antioxidant activity. β-Ala-His (carnosine), β-Ala-1-methyl-His (anserine), β-Ala-Lys (lysine), and β-Ala-Phe (phenylalanine) all exhibit increased hydroxyl radical scavenging activity compared with their individual amino acids (Table 16.2). However, β-Ala linked to amino acids which do not possess antioxidant activity [e.g., β-Ala-Gly, β-Ala-L-Ala, β-Ala-Glu (glutamic acid)] and do not exhibit hydroxyl radical scavenging activity (Table 16.2), suggesting that β-Ala is not directly involved in inactivation of free radicals. β-Ala is not absolutely necessary for free radical scavenging activity because His, Gly-His, L-Ala-His, and GABA-His (homocarnosine) also possess hydroxyl radical scavenging activity (Table 16.2). However, β-Ala does impart unique antioxidant characteristics because carnosine (β-Ala-His) exhibits superior antioxidant activity in a phosphatidylcholine liposomes model system compared with histidine, Gly-His, L-Ala-His, and homocarnosine. These data indicate that both β-alanine and histidine impart unique antioxidant characteristics to carnosine. However, these data also make it obvious that the entire mechanism by which β-Ala and His contribute to the antioxidant activity of carnosine is not completely understood. Differences between the antioxidant activity of carnosine, amino acids, and related peptides could involve differences in their ability to interact with free radicals, lipid oxidation products, prooxidants, and lipid membranes. Additional research is required to elucidate how structural differences in dipeptides influence antioxidant activity.

Antioxidant Activity of Carnosine in Foods

The role of anserine and carnosine as skeletal muscle antioxidants is supported by the fact that the dipeptides inhibit lipid oxidation catalyzed by the major skeletal muscle prooxidants (iron, copper, ferryl radicals, and lipoxygenase) at the pH and temperatures expected in muscle food (20,21). Research also indicates that carnosine could be used as a food additive to increase the oxidative stability of foods. Carnosine (0.5%) more effectively inhibits oxidative rancidity in frozen (–15°C), raw, salted (33) and unsalted (Fig. 16.2) ground pork than butylated hydroxytoluene (BHT), α-tocopherol (Toc), and sodium tripolyphosphate (STP) as determined by TBARS. However, in cooked ground pork, increased concentrations of carnosine (1.5%) are required to effectively inhibit lipid oxidation (34). The reason for this is unclear; the decreased activity could be due to increased free radical or prooxidant concentrations in the cooked meats, inactivation of carnosine by Maillard reactions, or heat-induced disruption of the cellular membrane which decreases carnosine-membrane interactions.

When carnosine (0.5%) was added to frozen (–15°C), salted (2% NaCl), ground pork containing either 10 or 30% fat, antioxidant activity was found to be similar (Table 16.3). Use of carnosine in combination with rosemary extracts or mixed tocopherol isomers resulted in increased inhibition of oxidation (Table 16.3). Antioxidant combinations inhibited lipid oxidation in an additive manner

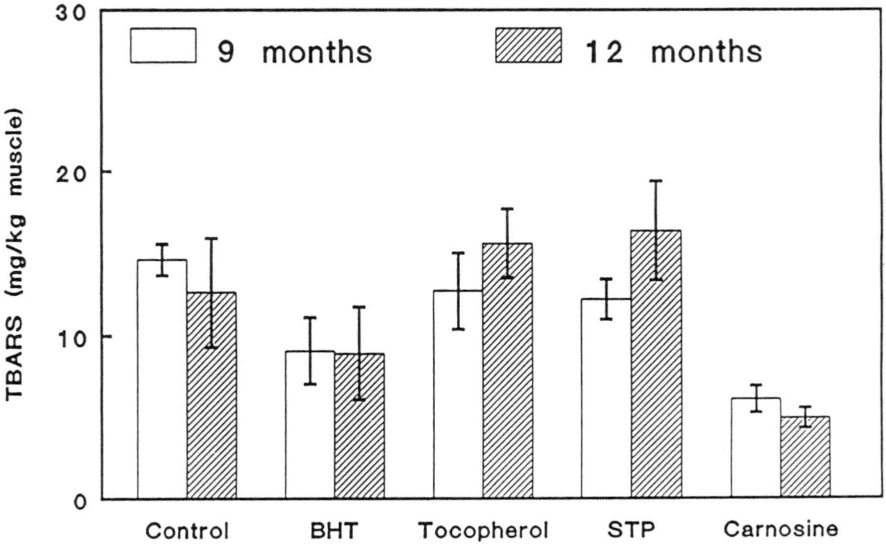

Fig. 16.2. Formation of thiobarbituric acid reactive substances (TBARS) in ground pork (20% fat) stored at –15°C. Antioxidant treatments included butylated hydroxytoluene (BHT; 0.02% of fat content), α-tocopherol (0.02% of fat content), sodium tripolyphosphate (STP; 0.5%), and carnosine (0.5%). Error bars represent standard deviations.

suggesting that the antioxidants where acting independently instead of synergistically. In ground turkey, the antioxidant activity of carnosine has also been found to be improved by mixed tocopherol isomers and ascorbyl palmitate in an additive manner but was not improved by sodium tripolyphosphate or citrate (35).

TABLE 16.3
Inhibition of TBARS (mg/kg muscle) Formation and Color Deterioration in Salted (2%) Uncooked Pork Containing Various Antioxidants After 4 wk of Frozen Storage at –15°C*

	TBARS		Color (cm)	
Treatment	10% Fat	30% Fat	10% Fat	30% Fat
Control	15.5 ± 1.0	22.0 ± 6.2	9.2 ± 0.3	10.2 ± 0.2
Carnosine (0.5%)	7.1 ± 1.5	8.5 ± 3.2	2.6 ± 0.2	2.6 ± 0.2
Rosemary (0.1% of fat)	7.3 ± 2.7	7.8 ± 2.5	6.3 ± 0.2	6.3 ± 0.3
Tocopherol (0.1% of fat)	16.5 ± 7.6	14.0 ± 4.4	7.6 ± 0.3	9.4 ± 0.2
Carnosine + rosemary	5.6 ± 2.4	6.6 ± 1.1	2.8 ± 0.2	1.2 ± 0.9
Carnosine + tocopherol	4.5 ± 0.5	8.7 ± 1.9	3.4 ± 0.2	1.5 ± 0.1

*Color deterioration was determined by sensory analysis using a 13.0 cm scale anchored by the terms red (0 cm) and brown (13.0 cm).

Carnosine also maintains the red color (as determined by sensory analysis) of stored (–15°C), salted, ground pork more effectively than BHT, Toc, and STP (33). Rosemary extract and mixed tocopherol isomers slightly improved the color-retaining properties of carnosine in 30% fat salted ground pork but not in 10% fat pork (Table 16.3). The mechanism by which carnosine prevents myoglobin oxidation is not completely understood. Carnosine is not a strong reducing agent in a model system in which reducing potential is measured by the reduction of cytochrome c (Fig. 16.3). At pH 7.0, 25 mM carnosine reduces cytochrome c at a rate of 0.6 mM/min compared with 60 mM/min for an ascorbate concentration (50 μM) which was 500 times lower. Carnosine (50 mM) can weakly (0.6 μM/min) reduce metmyoglobin at pH 7.5; however, at pH 5.0, the reduction of metmyoglobin by carnosine was not observed (Fig. 16.4). The limited ability of carnosine to catalyze the reduction of myoglobin suggests that the color-stabilizing property of carnosine is due to its ability to inhibit oxidative reactions instead of through direct interactions with myoglobin.

Carnosine also inhibits lipid oxidation in butter. Carnosine (1.5%) inhibited the photooxidation of butter as measured by the formation of lipid peroxides (Fig. 16.5A) and loss of color (Fig. 16.5B) at a level similar to BHT (0.02% of fat content). In butter stored in the dark, carnosine inhibited peroxide formation, although not as effectively as BHT (Fig. 16.6). Riboflavin-generated active oxygen species

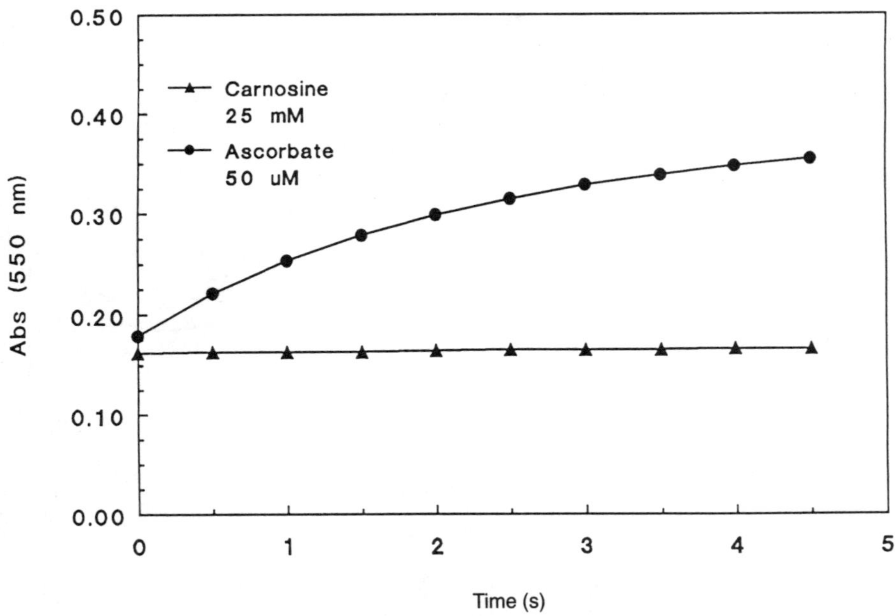

Fig. 16.3. The reduction of cytochrome c (150 mM in 0.12 M KCl, 5 mM phosphate buffer, pH 7.0) by carnosine and ascorbate.

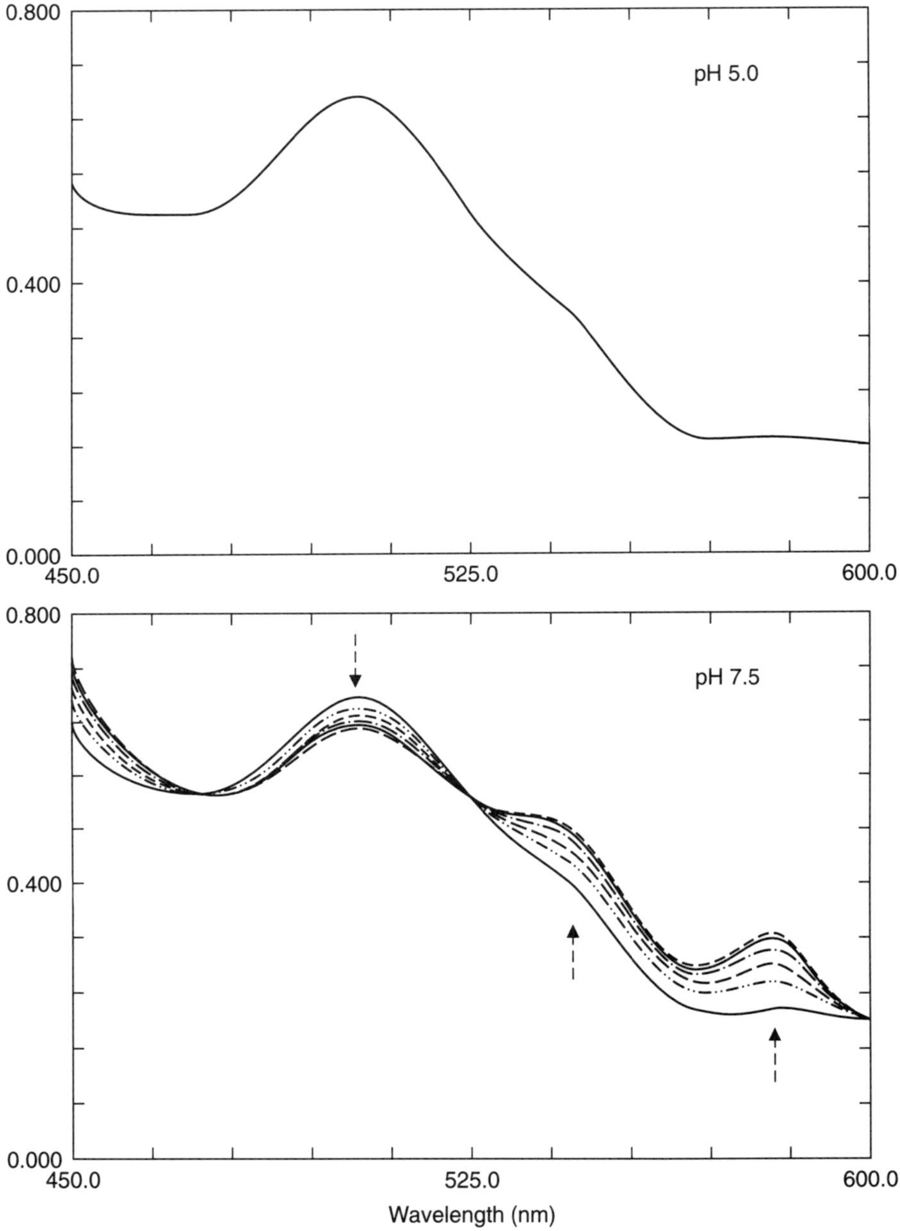

Fig. 16.4. The conversion of metmyoglobin (70 μM in 0.12 M KCl, 5 mM phosphate buffer) to oxymyoglobin by 50 mM carnosine at pH 5.0 and 7.5. Absorbance scans were taken every 4 min with arrows indicating the direction of spectral shifts with time. No detectable spectral shift was observed at pH 5.0.

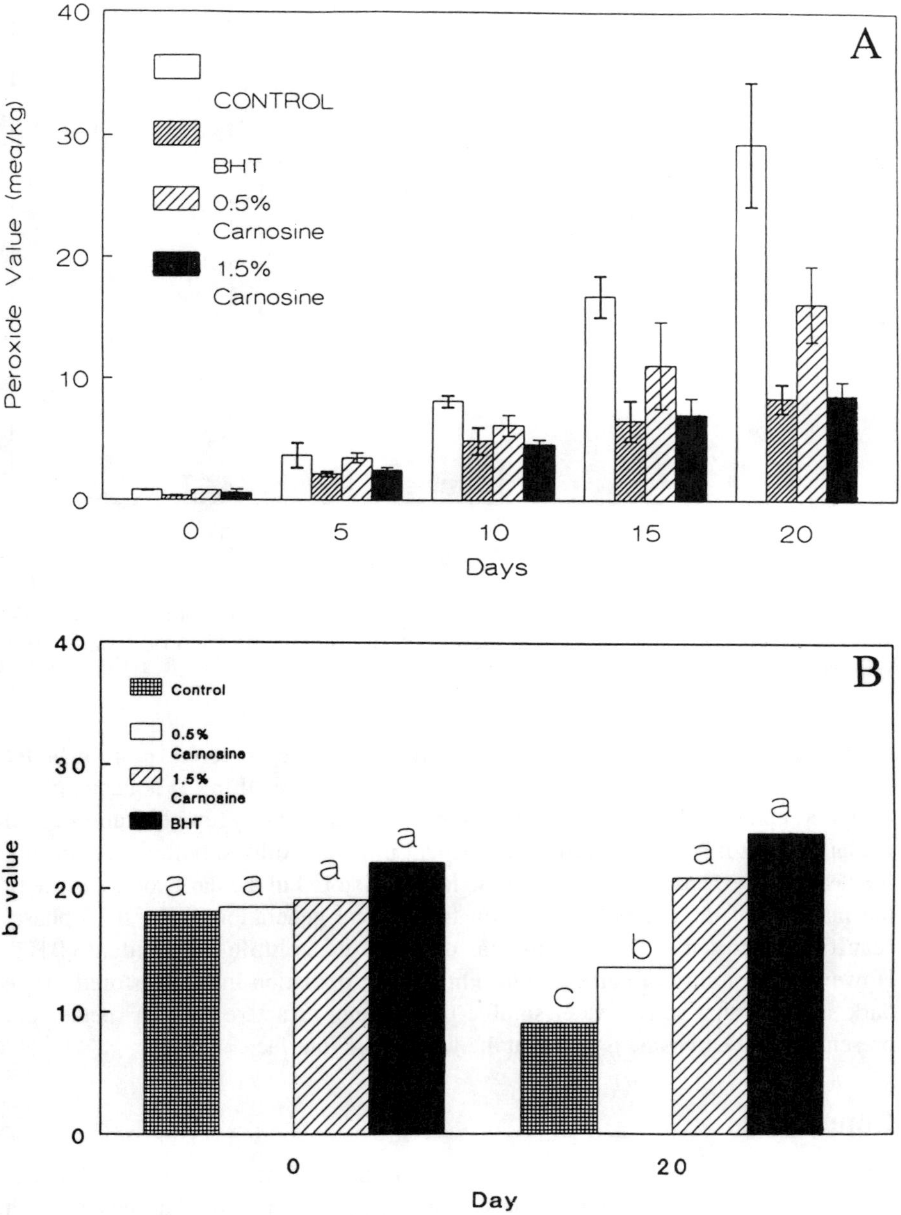

Fig. 16.5. Formation of (A) lipid peroxides and (B) loss of yellow color (Hunter colorimeter b-values) in butter containing carnosine and butylated hydroxytoluene (BHT) (0.02% of fat content) during storage (4°C) under fluorescent light (20 W/m2) at 4°C. Error bars represent standard deviations.

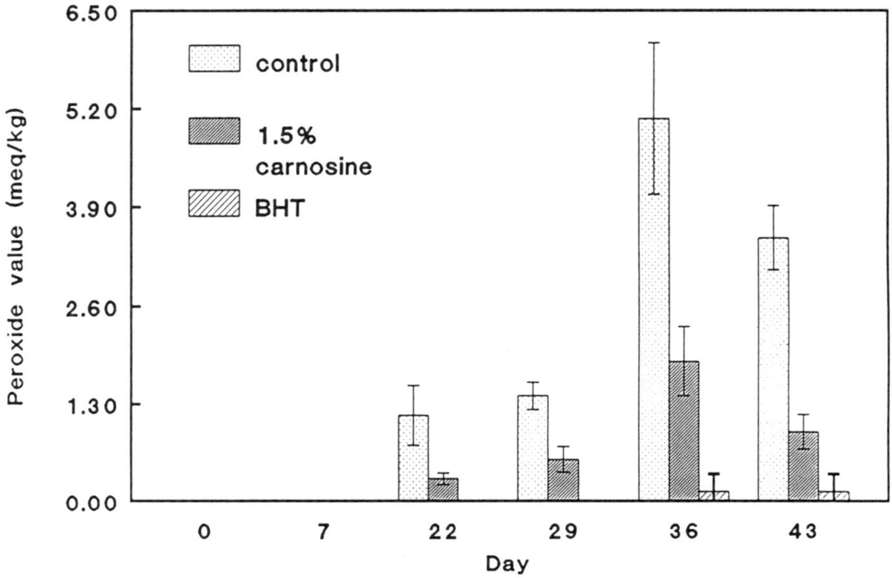

Fig. 16.6. Formation of lipid peroxides in butter containing carnosine and butylated hydroxytoluene (BHT) (0.02% of fat content) during storage at 4°C in the dark. Error bars represent standard deviations.

such as singlet oxygen are thought to be involved in the photooxidation of butter (36). Because carnosine and riboflavin would both be found in the aqueous phase of butter, carnosine's close proximity to the site of active oxygen generation could explain why it is a more effective antioxidant in photooxidized butter. Conversely, the decreased effectiveness of carnosine in butter stored in the dark could be due to the inability of the dipeptide to inhibit free radical generation in the lipid phase, resulting in lower activity than that of the lipid soluble antioxidant, BHT. However, the ability of carnosine to inhibit lipid oxidation in butter stored in the dark suggests that active water-soluble prooxidants or active oxygen species are present, or that carnosine is active at the water-lipid interface.

Conclusions

Because skeletal muscle contains high concentrations of water-soluble lipid oxidation catalysts and cellular membrane systems, it is not surprising that muscle has a biphasic antioxidant system consisting of water-soluble (e.g., anserine, carnosine, and antioxidant enzymes) and lipid-soluble (e.g., α-tocopherol, carotenoids, and ubiquinone) antioxidants. The fact that anserine and carnosine are found at higher concentrations in fast twitch (white) muscle fibers, in which anaerobic metabolism and oxidative burst are common, suggests that the dipeptides could provide a crucial line of defense against reperfusion-induced oxidation reactions which can occur *in vivo* or during food processing operations such as grinding. The higher concentration of anserine and carnosine in muscle high in white fibers could help explain why these muscles exhibit greater stability to both lipid and color oxidation.

Experimental evidence also indicates that carnosine has potential for utilization as a "natural" food antioxidant. Increasing the antioxidant defense system of the aqueous phase of skeletal muscle by increasing carnosine concentrations is effective in inhibiting both lipid and myoglobin oxidation. Carnosine also inhibits lipid oxidation in water-in-oil emulsions such as butter. The ability of carnosine to inhibit oxidative reactions in butter and muscle foods suggests that carnosine could be an effective antioxidant especially in foods susceptible to degradation by water-soluble prooxidants and active oxygen species. Currently, the high price of histidine makes the synthetic production of carnosine too impractical for utilization as a food additive. Therefore, research is required to find alternative sources of carnosine and anserine (e.g., underutilized meat by-products) if these dipeptides are to be utilized as food ingredients.

References

1. Vercellotti, J.R., Mills, O.E., Bett, K.L., and Sullen, D.L. (1992) in *Lipid Oxidation in Foods* (St. Angelo, A.J., ed.), American Chemical Society Symposium Series, Vol. 500, American Chemical Society Books, Washington, D.C.
2. Kanner, J., German, J.B., and Kinsella, J.E. (1987) *Crit. Rev. of Food Sci. Nutr. 25*, 317.
3. Decker, E.A., Xiong, Y.X., Calvert, J.T., Crum, A.D., and Blanchard (1993) *J. Agric. Food Chem. 41*, 186.
4. Faustman, C. (1993) in *Technology for Reduced Additive Food* (Smith, J., ed.), Blackie Academic and Professional, New York.
5. Addis, P.B., and Park, S.W. (1989) in *Food Toxicology: A Perspective on the Relative Risks* (Taylor, S.L., and Scanlon, R.A., eds.), Marcel Dekker, Inc., New York, p. 297.
6. Mielche, M.M., and Bertelsen, G. (1994) *Trends in Food Sci. & Technol. 5*, 322.
7. Decker, E.A., and Hultin, H.O. (1992) in *Lipid Oxidation in Foods* (St. Angelo, A.J., ed.), American Chemical Society Symposium Series, Vol. 500, American Chemical Society Books, Washington, D.C.
8. Kanner, J., Shegalovich, I., Harel, S., and Hazan, B. (1988) *J. Agric. Food Chem. 36*, 409.
9. Asghar, A., Gray, J.I., Buckley, A.M., Pearson, A.M., and Booren, A.M. (1988) *Food Technol. 42*, 102.
10. Harel, S., and Kanner, J. (1985) *J. Agric. Food Chem. 33*, 1188.
11. Wilson, B.R., Pearson, A.M., and Shorland, F.B. (1976) *J. Agric. Food Chem. 24,* 7.
12. Mei, L.Y., Crum, A.D., and Decker, E.A. (1994) *J. Food Lipids 1*, 273.
13. Osinchak, J.E., Hultin, H.O., Zajicek, O.T., Kelleher, S.D., and Huang, C.-H. (1992) *Free Radical Biol. & Med. 12*, 35.
14. Kanner, J., Harel, S., and Jaffe, R. (1991) *J. Agric. Food Chem. 39*, 1017.
15. Crush, K.G. (1970) *Comp. Biochem. Physiol. 34,* 3.
16. Plowman, J.E., and Close, E.A. (1988) *J. Sci. Food Agric. 45*, 69.

17. Davey, C.L. (1960) *Arch. Biochem. Biophys. 89*, 303.
18. Harris, R.C., Marlin, D.J., Dunnett, M., Snow, D.H., and Hultman, E. (1990) *Comp. Biochem. Physiol. 2*, 249.
19. Boldyrev, A.A., Dupin, A.M., Bunin, A. Ya., Babizhaev, M.A., and Severin, S.E. (1987) *Biochem. Int. 15*, 1105.
20. Boldyrev, A.A., Dupin, A.M., Pindel, E.V., and Severin, S.E. (1988) *Comp. Biochem. Physiol.,* 245.
21. Decker, E.A., and Faraji, H. (1990) *J. Am. Oil Chem. Soc. 67*, 650.
22. Kohen, R., Yamamoto, Y., Cundy, K.C., and Ames, B. (1988) *Proc. Natl. Acad. Sci. USA 85*, 3175.
23. Decker, E.A., Crum, A.D., and Calvert, J.T. (1992) *J. Agric. Food Chem. 40*, 756.
24. Dahl, T.A., Midden, W.R., and Hartman, P.E. (1988) *Photochem. Photobiol. 47*, 357.
25. Rubtsov, A.M., Schara, M., Sentiurc, M., and Boldyrev, A.A. (1991) *Acta Pharm. Jugoslav. 41*, 401.
26. Brown, C.E., and Antholine, W.E. (1979) *Biochem. Biophys. Res. Commun. 88*, 529.
27. Brown, C.E. (1988) *J. Theor. Biol. 88*, 245.
28. Chan, K.M., Decker, E.A., Lee, J.B., and Butterfield, D.A. (1994) *J. Agric. Food Chem. 42,* 461.
29. Egorov, S.Y., Kurella, E.G., Boldyrev, A.A., and Krasnovski, A.A., Jr. (1992) *Bioorgan. Khim. 19*, 142.
30. Aruoma, O.I., Laughton, M.J., and Halliwell, Barry (1989) *Biochem. J. 264,* 3.
31. Yoshikawa, T., Naito, Y., Tanigawa, T., Yoneta, T., and Kondo, M. (1991) *Biochim. Biophys. Acta 1115*, 15.
32. Hartman, P.E., Hartman, Z., and Ault, K.T. (1990) *Photochem. Photobiol. 51*, 59.
33. Decker, E.A., and Crum, A.D. (1991) *J. Food Sci. 56*, 1179.
34. Decker, E.A., and Crum, A.D. (1992) *Meat Sci. 34*, 245.
35. Calvert, J.T., and Decker, E.A. (1992) *J. Food Qual. 15*, 423.
36. Satter, A., and deMan, J.M. (1975) *Crit. Rev. Food Sci. Nutr. 7*, 13.
37. Chan, K.M. (1993) *Role of Carnosine in Protection Against Oxidative Processes*. Ph.D. Thesis, University of Kentucky, Lexington, KY.

Chapter 17

Isolation of a Natural Antioxidant from Shrimp Waste

S.J. Li, T.A. Seymour, and M.T. Morrissey

Oregon State University Seafood Laboratory, Astoria, Oregon.

Introduction

The West Coast shrimp fishery has maintained an annual harvest of more than 50 million pounds of shrimp since 1987 (1). More than 50% of the harvest has been landed in Oregon during this time period, although the states of Washington and California also contribute significantly to the capture. In most cases, shrimp lands at processing plants where it is cooked, peeled, packaged, and frozen for market. Cooked, peeled shrimp have an average recovery of 28–30%. The shrimp discard represents more than 30 million pounds of waste material per year on the Pacific Coast. A number of attempts have been made to utilize shrimp waste (2). These have included: extraction of pigments and flavorants (3), utilization of shell material (4), and production of shrimp meal (5). Some of these tests have led to utilization of shrimp waste materials, especially in the area of aquaculture diets. Another area of shrimp shell utilization is the production of chitosan, which has numerous applications including food processing, agriculture, biomedical use, biotechnology, water treatment, and cosmetics (6). The bulk of waste materials, however, is still underutilized and represents a valuable resource in terms of potential isolated compounds. With increasingly restrictive environmental legislation and solid-waste management regulations, it is critical that avenues be found for various aspects of waste utilization.

Antioxidants can effectively prevent lipid oxidation, which is a major cause of chemical spoilage in foods. Much attention has recently been focused on natural antioxidants because of their positive health effects against cancer and heart disease (7–9).

Although various natural antioxidants have been extracted from plant sources (10–18), little is known about antioxidants of crustacean origin. Previous studies have indicated that shelf-life of minced fish incorporated with shrimp meat was improved due to antioxidant activity from shrimp (*Pandalus jordani*) (19). Furthermore, Rosenzweig-Pasquel and Babbitt (20) reported that an ethanol extract from shrimp meat had considerable antioxidant activity.

This chapter reports isolation and purification of a natural antioxidant from shrimp waste and its stability under various test conditions.

Experimental Procedures

Shrimp Waste Samples

Shrimp waste, from the species *Pandalus jordani*, was obtained from an Oregon seafood processor during the shrimp fishing season (May through October). Samples were kept on ice and transported to the Oregon State University Seafood Laboratory in Astoria. Two hundred-gram (200-g) samples were vacuum packed, blast frozen, and stored at –20°C. Frozen samples, to be analyzed, were thawed at refrigerated temperatures.

Solvent Extraction

Extract from shrimp waste was prepared in the following manner. Fifty-gram (50-g) samples were extracted with 100 mL of organic solvents which included ethyl ether, chloroform, acetone, isopropanol, and ethanol. Mixtures were blended for 2 min using a Waring blender, and each slurry was filtered through a Buchner funnel using Whatman No. 1 filter paper. Each fraction was evaporated to dryness and redissolved in the same volume of 95% ethanol and measured for antioxidant activity. Negative controls consisted of a 95% ethanol solution. Because ethanol extracts showed the highest antioxidant activity, these fractions were further purified.

A sample of 100 g of shrimp waste was also extracted with chloroform, methanol, and water mixtures according to the method of Bligh and Dyer (21). The ability to partition in the chloroform or aqueous layer would serve to characterize the antioxidant as polar or nonpolar.

Antioxidant Activity Testing

The antioxidant activity was evaluated in a β-carotene-linoleic acid emulsion as described by Marco (22). The ability of antioxidant to prevent the oxidative destruction of β-carotene and linoleic acid emulsion was expressed as the decrease in absorbance at 470 nm. A 2-mg sample of crystalline β-carotene was dissolved in 10 mL of chloroform. One milliliter of this solution was then pipetted into a round-bottomed flask which contained 20 mg of purified linoleic acid and 200 mg of Tween 40 emulsifier. After removal of chloroform on a rotary evaporator, 50 mL of deionized water was added to the flask with vigorous stirring. A 5-mL aliquot of the aqueous emulsion which formed was then pipetted into each of a series of spectrophotometer tubes which contained 0.2-mL portions of extract solution. A zero reading was taken at 470 nm on the reaction mixture in each tube immediately after addition of the emulsion to the extract solution. The tubes were then stoppered and placed in a water bath at 50°C. Subsequent readings were taken at regular intervals.

Thin-Layer Chromatography (TLC)

Crude ethanol extract was applied to analytical silica gel thin-layer plates (Kiesel $60F_{254}$, 20 × 20 cm, 0.25-mm thickness, EM Science, Gibbstown, NJ) in a straight line 2.0 cm above the lower edge. Each plate was developed with benzene/methanol/ acetic acid (45:8:4 by vol).

Phenolic compounds were visualized by spraying plates with one of the following reagents:

1. Folin-Ciocalteu's phenol reagent, followed by an overspray of 14% sodium carbonate.
2. Ferric chloride-potassium ferricyanide reagent (1:1, vol/vol).

Plates were also sprayed with a β-carotene-linoleic acid solution. After spraying, the plates were exposed to normal room light for about 4 h. The yellow-colored band indicated the presence of antioxidant activity.

Plates were sprayed with ferric chloride solution to detect whether the active antioxidant compound had dihydroxy or trihydroxy phenolic groups.

Crude ethanol extract was purified by preparative TLC (1.0-mm thickness) using benzene/methanol/acetic acid (45:8:4). Each fraction was scraped off the TLC plates with a razor blade and measured for antioxidant activity. To check the purity of the isolated compound, analytical TLC plates were run with a more polar phase, butanol/water/acetic acid (12:5:3).

Samples prepared by the Bligh and Dyer method consisting of the methanol/ water layer were also applied to analytical TLC plates developed by benzene/ methanol/acetic acid (45:8:4, by vol). Plates were then rotated 90° and run with solvents butanol/water/acetic acid (12:5:3 by vol). Plates were sprayed with one of the following reagents to detect the presence of the phenolic and amine group, respectively:

1. Folin-Ciocalteu's phenol reagent, followed by an overspray of 14% sodium carbonate.
2. 0.1% ninhydrin in isopropanol.

High-Performance Liquid Chromatography (HPLC)

HPLC was performed on a Bio-Rad 2700 gradient pump system equipped with a Bio-Rad model 1706 ultraviolet (UV) detector (Bio-Rad, Hercules, CA). A preparative column packed with R Sil C18 HL (250 × 10 mm i.d., 5-μm particle size) was used. Five hundred milliliters of sample with TLC fraction R_f 0.05 was injected onto HPLC. The eluents used were water and acetonitrile with a gradient of 0–20% acetonitrile in 15 min and a flow rate of 2.50 mL/min. Absorbance at 280 nm was monitored. Peak fractions were collected and measured for antioxidative activity. Active fractions (retention time 8.4 min) were concentrated by a rotary evaporator and rechromatographed onto an analytical HPLC equipped with a 250 mm × 4.6 mm i.d. R Sil C18 HL column to evaluate purity. Two different conditions were used. The first analytical condition was carried out with the mobile phase of 2.5% acetic acid in water (pump A) and 2.5% acetic acid in methanol (pump B) with a gradient of 0–50% (pump B) for 30 min. A flow rate of 1.0 mL/min was used. The second condition was carried out with the mobile phase of 5.0% acetic acid in water (pump A) and acetonitrile (pump B) with a gradient of 0–20% for 15 min and a flow rate of 1.0 mL/min.

UV Spectrum

An active fraction (pH at 7.0), collected from preparative HPLC at retention time 8.45 min, was run within UV range (200–380 nm) using a Beckman Spectrophotometer DU 640 (Beckman Instruments, Fullerton, CA). The scan speed was 1200 nm/min.

Heat Treatment

Samples of ethanol extract and purified solutions from HPLC were placed in 10-mL test tubes and heated at 100°C for 0, 15, 30, 60, 120, and 240 min. Heated crude extracts were centrifuged at 10,000 × *g* for 15 min to remove precipitated substances. The tubes were then cooled to room temperature, and antioxidant activity of each sample was measured with methods previously described.

Storage Experiment

Samples of ethanol extract and purified solutions were also stored at refrigerated temperature (4°C) for 0, 5, 15, 20, and 30 d. Samples were then assayed for antioxidant activity.

Results and Discussion

Extracts of all solvents except diethyl ether improved the β-carotene-linoleic acid emulsion stability over the negative control containing only 95% ethanol solution (Fig. 17.1). Crude ethanol extract resulted in the highest antioxidant activity compared with other crude extracts. Therefore, crude ethanol extract was further analyzed by TLC and HPLC. Ethanol extracts, when analyzed by TLC in benzene/methanol/acetic acid solvents, exhibited four spots with R_f values of 0.05, 0.40, 0.48, and 0.64. Faint blue spots were visualized by spraying with Folin-Ciocalteu's phenolic reagent, and blue spots were immediately observed after spraying with ferric chloride-potassium ferricyanide reagent. Positive reactions with both indicators showed the presence of phenolic compounds. When antioxidant activity of each band was determined by measuring the decrease of the absorbance at 470 nm of β-carotene-linoleic acid emulsion, the R_f 0.05 band showed the strongest activity, whereas R_f values of 0.40, 0.48, and 0.64 gave almost no antioxidant activity (Fig. 17.2).

The separated compounds in TLC developed by benzene/methanol/acetic acid solvents were also sprayed with a solution of β-carotene-linoleic acid. It was found that only the band (R_f 0.05) maintained the yellow color on TLC plates after exposure to daylight for about 4 h, which indicated that only this band possessed antioxidant activity. The results from TLC suggest that a polar phenolic compound

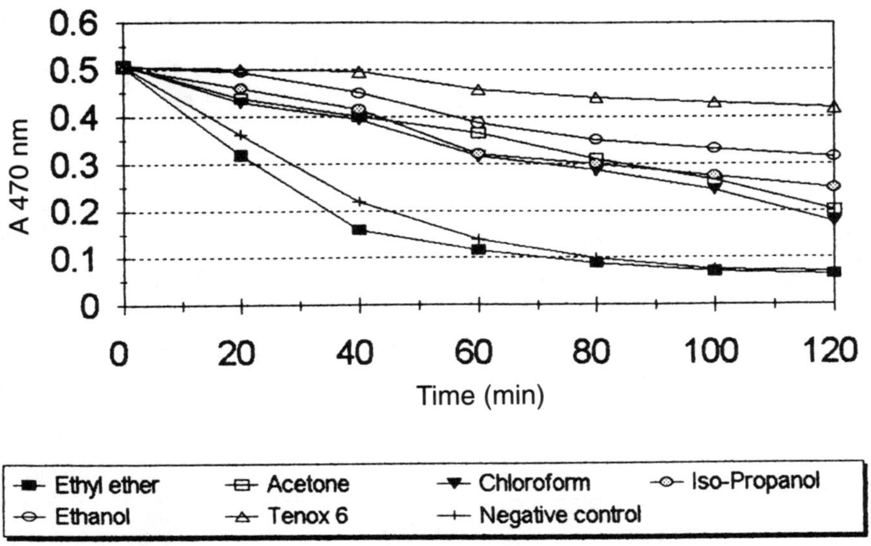

Fig. 17.1. Antioxidant activity of shrimp waste extracted with different kinds of solvents. Decrease in absorbance at 470 nm of β-carotene and linoleic acid emulsion was monitored for 120 min.

from shrimp waste was responsible for antioxidant activity. It was also observed that the methanol/water layer prepared by the Bligh and Dyer method gave one spot with R_f 0.05 using benzene/methanol/water (45:8:4, by vol) in the first dimension of two-dimensional TLC after spraying either Folin-Ciocalteu's phenol reagent or ninhydrin. When this spot was developed by the second dimension using butanol/water/acetic acid (12:5:3) solvents, two spots with R_f 0.20 and 0.32 were separated. The results indicated that an antioxidant compound was present in the polar fraction. Increased solvent strength in the second dimension separated the R_f 0.05 band into two spots. Therefore, the R_f 0.05 band was subjected to further purification by HPLC.

There were two major peaks from preparative HPLC at retention times of 8.45 and 12.53 min (Fig. 17.3), when water and acetonitrile with a gradient of 0–20% acetonitrile in 15 min were used. The fraction collected from HPLC at 8.45 min showed strong antioxidant activity (Fig. 17.4). A combination of water, and acetonitrile was used as a polar mobile phase to elute the polar fraction. Fractions were concentrated by rotary evaporator and rechromatographed on R-Sil C_{18} HPLC under two different conditions. The combination of acetic acid, water, and methanol was used as the first elution condition while the solvents of acetic acid, water, and acetonitrile were used as the second elution condition. Both conditions resulted in a single peak (Fig. 17.5). Moreover, when the active fraction was separately applied to analytical TLC plates developed with either the mobile phase of

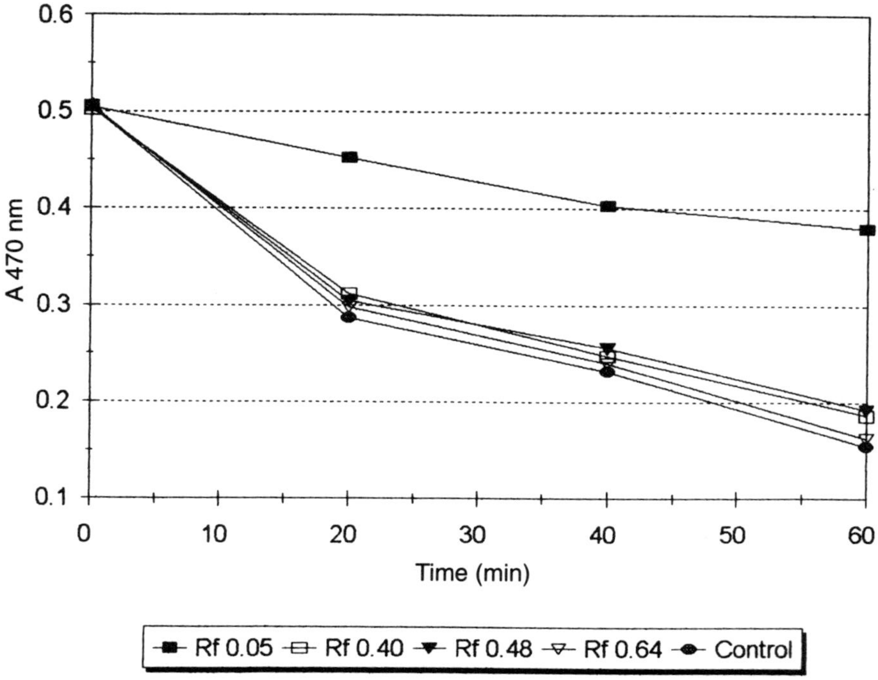

Fig. 17.2. Antioxidant activity of different R_f values of phenolic compounds separated by thin-layer chromatography (TLC) from shrimp waste. TLC plate developed with benzene/methanol/acetic acid (45:8:4, by vol). Antioxidant activity was represented by change in A 470 nm for 60 min.

butanol/water/acetic acid (12:5:3, by vol) or benzene/methanol/acetic acid (45:8:4), single spots appeared at either R_f 0.21 or 0.05, respectively. These observations confirm the purity of the active fraction collected from HPLC.

Purification of natural antioxidants by HPLC was shown by several authors (18,23,24). Reverse-phase HPLC was successfully used to purify very polar antioxidants from green barley leaves and rice hull (18,24). The combination of preparative TLC and normal-phase HPLC was adopted to purify a novel antioxidant from eucalyptus leaf waxes (23). Several natural antioxidants extracted from different sources such as rosemary, rice hull, young barley leaves, *Polygonum hydropiper* leaves, and tea have demonstrated polar properties (10,24–26).

Ferric chloride spray was used to determine whether this phenolic compound contained a dihydroxy and/or trihydroxy group. The negative reaction excluded the possibility of the existence of such a group. The UV spectrum indicated a major absorption at 268 nm and a minor peak at 323 nm (Fig. 17.6), further confirming the presence of aromatic moiety. Based on the absorbance and concentration of the purified sample, the extinction coefficient ($\varepsilon^{1cm}{}_{1\%}$) at 268 and 323 nm was calculated to be 64,000 and 7,600, respectively.

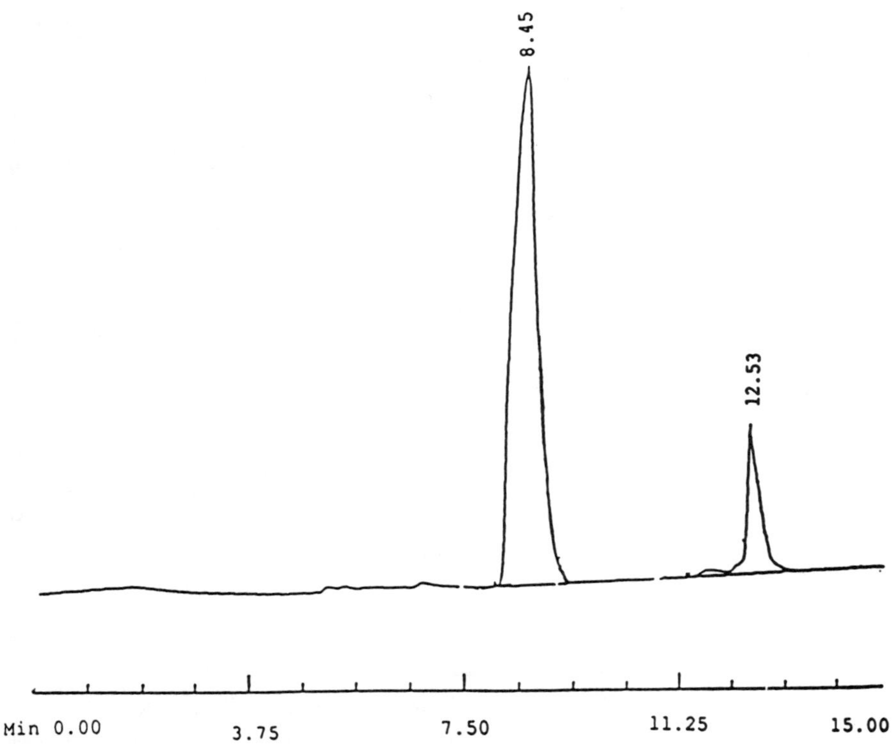

Fig. 17.3. High-performance liquid chromatography (HPLC) chromatogram of the thin-layer chromatography (TLC) fraction of R_f 0.05. The mobile solvents used were water (pump A) and acetonitrile (pump B) with a gradient of 0–20% acetonitrile in 15 min.

Babbitt *et al.* (19) reported that ethanol extracts from shrimp meat exhibited antioxidant properties. Furthermore, various solvents were used to extract antioxidant from shrimp meat. Ethanol extract was the most effective solvent (20). It was also reported that extracts of sage and rosemary made with nonpolar solvents are less effective as antioxidants (10). Our results showed that crude ethanol extract had strong antioxidant activity. However, all of those extracts showed lower antioxidant activity compared with Tenox 6, which consists of a mixture of butylated hydroxyanisole (BHA), butylated hydroxytoluene (BHT), propyl gallate, and citric acid (Fig. 17.1).

A polar phenolic compound isolated from shrimp meat with the same TLC solvent system also showed antioxidant activity, and had a strong absorption at 204 nm (20), which differed from the result presented here. Lack of major absorption at 205 or 210 nm rules out the antioxidant as a peptide. Positive reaction with ninhydrin indicated that the compound contained an amine group.

Polar phenolic compounds acting as natural antioxidants have been suggested by several authors (13,15,24–26). Hydroxytyrosol and caffeic acid from olive oil

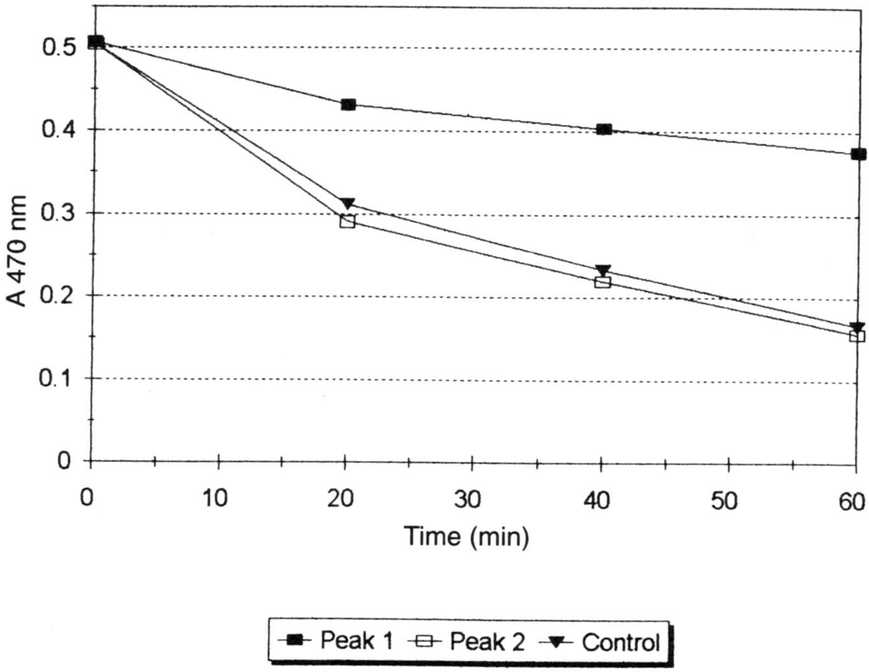

Fig. 17.4. Antioxidant activity of the collected fraction of peaks from R-Sil C_{18} high-performance liquid chromatography (HPLC). Peak 1 refers to the peak at retention time 8.45 min and peak 2 refers to the peak at retention time 12.53 min.

showed greater antioxidant activity than synthetic antioxidant BHT, whereas protocatechuic acid and syringic acid, also from olive oil, were found to have lesser antioxidant activity (15). Antioxidant activities varied with different polyphenolic compositions of different tea processing methods (26). It was well documented that water-soluble compounds, flavonoids, and flavonid glucoside possessed strong antioxidative activity (11,13,18,25). Flavonoids possess a phenolic structure, which is shared by α-tocopherol, BHA, and BHT. Recently, it was reported that the presence of phenolic compounds in grapes resulted in antioxidative effects (27). Lipid-soluble natural phenolic antioxidants, tocopherols, are the most widely distributed antioxidants in nature (28). Another phenolic antioxidant from a tropical tree, gum quaiac, showed an ability to inhibit lipid oxidation in cooked pork during refrigerated storage (29).

Although most antioxidants are phenolic compounds, another water-soluble natural antioxidant, carnosine, is a β-alanine, histidine dipeptide found in the skeletal muscle and nervous tissue (30). The antioxidant mechanism of carnosine was proposed as a combination of its ability to act as a chelator, free radical scavenger, and hydrogen donor (31). In addition, a natural antioxidant, rosmariquinone, isolated from rosemary (*Rosmarinus officinalis* L.) was superior to BHT in heated lard (32).

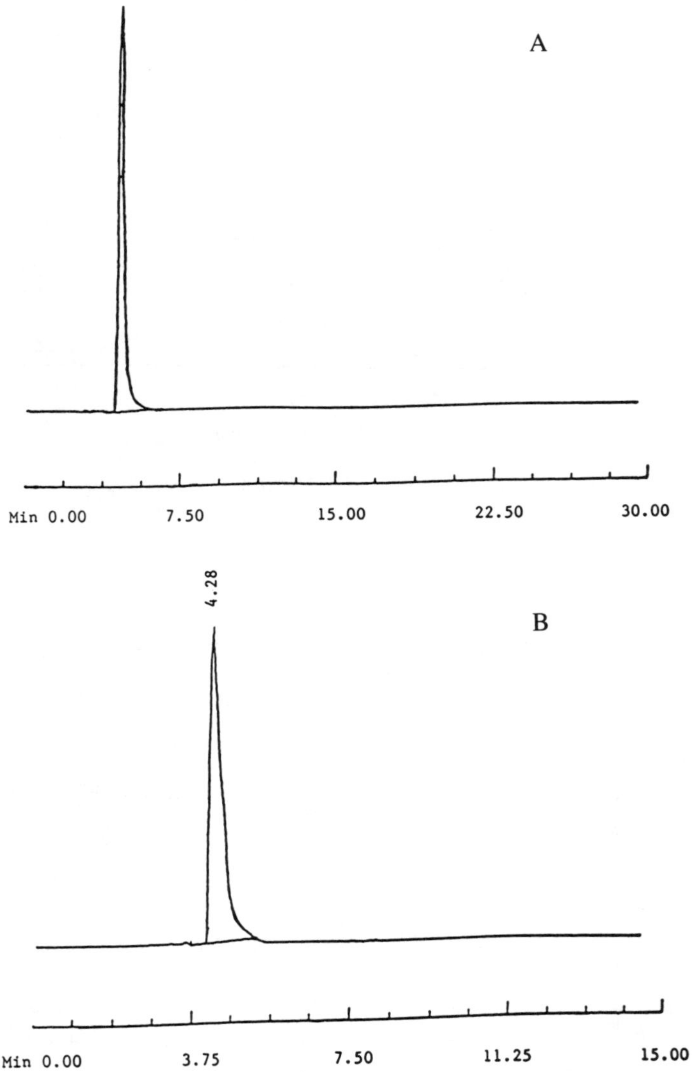

Fig. 17.5. (A) Rechromatogram of a fraction collected from preparative R-Sil high-performance liquid chromatography (HPLC) with retention time at 8.45 min. The mobile solvents used were 2.5% acetic acid in water (pump A) and 2.5% acetic acid in methanol (pump B) with a gradient of 0–50% in 30 min. (B) Rechromatogram of a fraction collected from preparative HPLC with retention time at 8.45 min. The mobile solvents used were 5.0% acetic acid in water (pump A) and acetonitrile (pump B) with a gradient of 0–20% in 15 min.

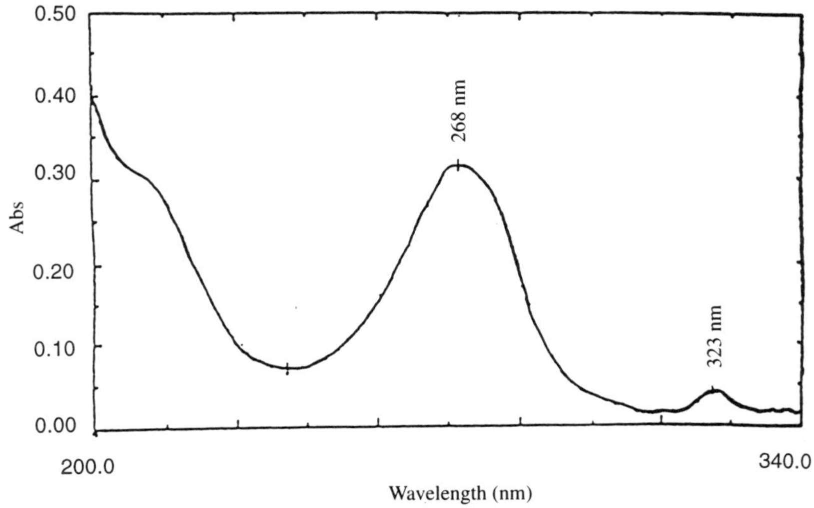

Fig. 17.6. Ultraviolet (UV) spectrum of a fraction collected from preparative high-performance liquid chromatography (HPLC) with retention time at 8.45 min.

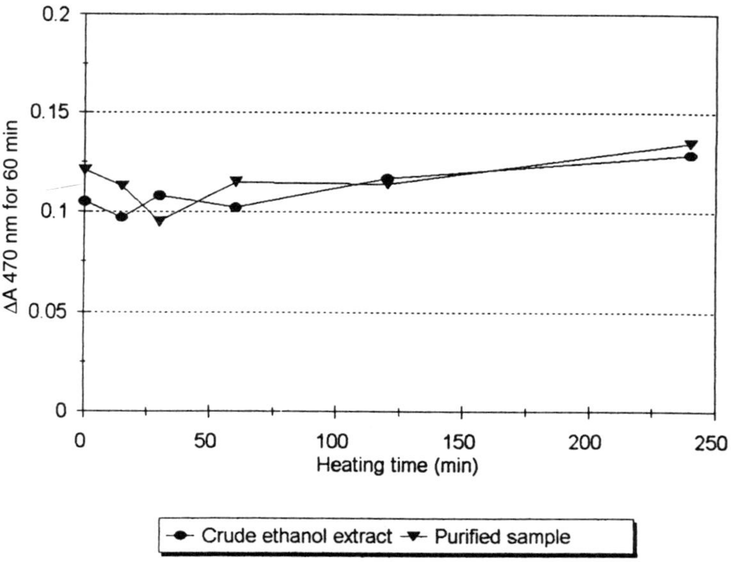

Fig. 17.7. Effects of different heating times on antioxidant activity of both crude ethanol extract and purified samples. Antioxidant activity was represented by the decrease in A 470 nm over 60 min. Samples collected from high-performance liquid chromatography (HPLC) are referred to as purified samples.

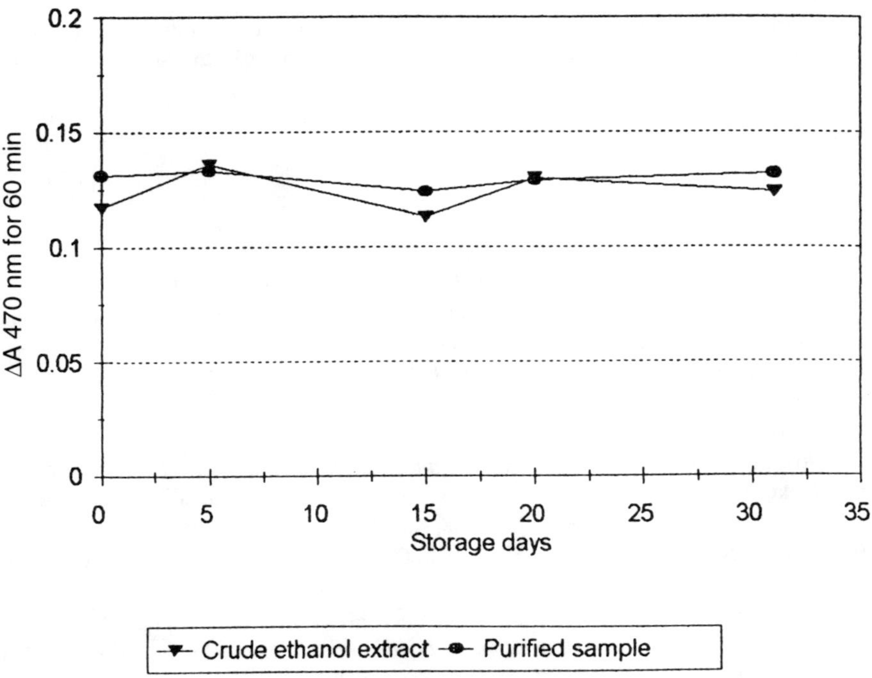

Fig. 17.8. Effect of different number of storage days at 4°C on antioxidant activity of both crude ethanol extract and purified sample. Antioxidant activity was represented by ΔA 470 nm in 60 min.

Antioxidant activity of both crude and purified samples was unchanged after heating for up to 4 h (Fig. 17.7). It was reported that antioxidant activity of extract from beef muscle heated at 60°C was not significantly different from untreated extract. However, antioxidant activity was increased 8.6-fold at 100°C due to removal of prooxidants such as iron- and heme-containing compounds by heat treatment (33). In addition, antioxidant(s) from acid whey proteins was found to be stable when heated at 90°C for 30 min (34). On the other hand, phenolic antioxidants such as BHA and BHT lose effectiveness after deep-fat frying, due to decomposition and evaporation (35,36).

When crude ethanol extract and purified samples were stored at 4°C for 1 mon, antioxidant activity changed very little (Fig. 17.8). The naturally-occurring α-tocopherol content in seaweed meal decreased with increased storage temperature (37). Furthermore, stability of α-tocopherol in a dehydrated model food system containing methyl linoleate with varying storage temperature (20, 30, and 37°C) was also studied (38), and the degradation rate of α-tocopherol increased as a function of storage temperature.

Acknowledgments

This work was supported by Grant NA26FDO139-01 from the National Oceanic and Atmospheric Administration/National Marine Fisheries Service/Saltonstall Kennedy Grant Program.

References

1. Talley, K. (1993) *Pacific Fish. 11*, 124.
2. Meyer, S.P. (1988) *Infofish Mark. Dig. 4*, 18.
3. Saito, A., and Regier, L.W. (1971) *J. Fish. Res. Board Can. 28*, 509.
4. Muzarelli, R.A., and Parisher, E.R. (1978) *Proceedings from the First International Conference on Chitin/Chitosan*, MIT Sea Grant Program, Cambridge, MA.
5. Simpson, B.D., and Haard, N.F. (1985) *J. Appl. Biochem. 7*, 212.
6. Ornum, J.V. (1992) *Infofish Int. 6*, 48.
7. Bjelke, E. (1975) *Int. J. Cancer 15*, 561.
8. Floyd, R.A. (1982) *Free Radicals and Cancer,* Marcel Dekker, Inc., New York, p. 201.
9. Knekt, P., Aromaa, A., Maatela, J., Aaran, R., Nikkari, T., Hakama, M., Hakulinen, T., Peto, R., Saxen, E., and Teppo, L. (1988) *Am. J. Epidemiol. 127*, 28.
10. Chang, S.S., Ostric-Matijasevic, B., Hsieh, O.L., and Huang, C. (1977) *J. Food Sci. 42*, 1102.
11. Pratt, D.E., and Birac, P.M. (1979) *J. Food Sci. 44*, 1720.
12. Dugan, L.R. (1980) in *Autoxidation in Foods and Biological Systems* (Simic, M.G., and Karel, M., eds.), Plenum Press, New York, p. 261.
13. Pratt, D.E., and Miller, E.E. (1984) *J. Am. Oil Chem. Soc. 61*, 1064.
14. Gopalakrishna, A.G., and Prabhakar, J.V. (1985) *J. Am. Oil Chem. Soc. 62*, 1581.
15. Papadopoulos, G., and Boskou, D. (1991) *J. Am. Oil Chem. Soc. 68*, 669.
16. Chevolleau, S., Mallet, J.F., Ucciani, E., Gamisans, J., and Gruber, M. (1992) *J. Am. Oil Chem. Soc. 69*, 1269.
17. Onyeneho, S.N., and Hettiarachchy, N.S. (1992) *J. Agric. Food Chem. 40*, 1496.
18. Osawa, T., Katsuzaki, H., Hagiwara, Y., Hagiwara, H., and Shibamoto, T. (1992) *J. Agric. Food Chem. 40*, 1135.
19. Babbitt, J.K., Law, D.K., and Crawford, D.L. (1976) *J. Food Sci. 41*, 35.
20. Rosenzweig-Pasquel, L.J.D., and Babbitt, J.K. (1991) *J. Food Sci. 56*, 143.
21. Bligh, E.G., and Dyer, W.J. (1959) *Can. J. Biochem. Physiol. 37*, 911.
22. Marco, G.J. (1968) *J. Am. Oil Chem. Soc. 45*, 594.
23. Osawa, F., and Namiki, M. (1985) *J. Agric. Food Chem. 33,* 777.
24. Ramarathnam, N., Osawa, T., Namiki, M., and Kawakishi, S. (1988) *J. Agric. Food Chem. 36*, 732.
25. Haraguchi, H., Hashimoto, K., and Yagi, A. (1992) *J. Agric. Food Chem. 40*, 1349.
26. Ho, C.T., Chen, Q., Shi, H., Zhang, K.Q., and Rosen, R.T. (1992) *Prev. Med. 21*, 520.
27. Kanner, J., Frankel, E., Granit, R., German, B., and Kinsella, J.E. (1994) *J. Agric. Food Chem. 42*, 64.
28. Nawar, W.W. (1985) in *Food Chemistry* (Fennema, O.R.P., ed.), Marcel Dekker, Inc., New York, p. 203.

29. Shahidi, F., Rubin, L.J., and Wood, D.F. (1987) *J. Food Sci. 52*, 564.
30. Crush, K.G. (1970) *Comp. Biochem. Physiol. 34*, 3.
31. Decker, E.A., and Crum, A.D. (1993) *Meat Sci. 34*, 245.
32. Houlihan, C.M., Ho, C.T., and Chang, S.S. (1984) *J. Am. Oil Chem. Soc. 62*, 96.
33. Chan, K.M., Decker, E.A., and Means, W.J. (1993) *J. Food Sci. 58,* 1.
34. Colbert, L.B., and Decker, E.A. (1991) *J. Food Sci. 56,* 1248.
35. Lin, F.S., Warner, C.R., and Fazio, T. (1981) *J. Am. Oil Chem. Soc. 58*, 789.
36. Hamama, A.A., and Nawar, W.W. (1991) *J. Agric. Food Chem. 39*, 1063.
37. Jensen, A. (1969) *J. Sci. Food Agric. 20*, 622.
38. Widicus, W.A., and Kirk, J.R. (1981) *J. Food Sci. 46*, 813.

Chapter 18

Antioxidant Properties of Maillard Reaction Products as Meat Flavor Compounds

M.E. Bailey, A.D. Clarke, Y.S. Kim, and L. Fernando

Department of Food Science and Human Nutrition, University of Missouri-Columbia, Missouri.

Introduction

An important aspect of food preservation, particularly lipid-containing foods such as meat, is oxidation which results in characteristic undesirable flavors. A specific flavor developed in cooked fresh meat during refrigerated or frozen storage is warmed-over flavor (WOF) (1) which is undesirable to most consumers. This flavor quality reduces the sale of cooked fresh meat as an easily prepared dish that would be in high demand; consequently, most precooked meat is processed by curing (using nitrite). Over 70% of pork and 30% of beef is processed by curing because of the rapid deterioration of the cooked meat flavor following cookery. Most fresh pork is cooked as small cuts such as chops from loin, steaks from shoulder or small loin or shoulder roasts. This meat is usually consumed immediately following cookery thus avoiding WOF which rapidly develops following roasting. Large roasts from the leg (ham) of pork or large loin roasts are usually avoided in the absence of large numbers of consumers served in restaurants where consumption is immediate following cookery. Even fried foods such as pork chops or pork steak and beef steak are not prepared for storage and later consumption.

Major failures have resulted from attempts to precook ground beef steak followed by refrigerated or frozen storage and reheating prior to consumption. Few precooked fresh meat products which require storage prior to heating and serving are available to the retail consumer because of the undesirability of WOF and the coincident loss of desirable meaty flavor.

Preliminary Considerations

WOF in cooked fresh meat products can be inhibited to some degree by the use of additives such as phosphates, synthesized phenolic compounds and other artificial antioxidants (2,3). With the increased need for effective antioxidants for food additives, there has been greater awareness and concern by consumers for the use of artificial additives and a greater demand for natural ingredients. The most desirable natural antioxidants for inhibiting WOF and preserving meaty flavor are formulated as Maillard reaction products (MRP). Some of these products not only prevent oxidation but also contribute desirable meat-like flavors when added to meat. The reactants for the Maillard reaction include naturally occurring ones such as sugars, amino acids, thiamine, taurine, nucleotides, and nucleosides present in proteinaceous foods such as meat.

Maillard Reaction

As explained previously (4), one series of the Maillard reaction (discovered by Louis Camille Maillard, University of Nance, France, who published results of his work between 1912 and 1916) involves the condensation of carbonyl compounds through the C-1 of aldoses and the C-2 of ketoses which rearrange to form stable intermediates (Amadori or Heynes intermediates); these in turn degrade with subsequent heating by dehydration and fission through at least three major pathways to form 1- and 3-deoxyosozones and 1-deoxyreductone (5–10). Another major leg of the Maillard reaction involving carbonyl and amine compounds is the Strecker degradation (5).

Amadori compounds degrade by heating by several different pathways to form intermediates which act as antioxidants or flavorants. Intermediates formed from 1-deoxyosone dehydration include maltol isomaltol and 5-hydroxy-3(2H)-furanone. An enol form of 1-deoxyosone (1-deoxyreductone) is degraded by fission to pyruvaldehyde, diacetyl, acetaldehyde acetoin, and other reductones which are reducing agents. These compounds form flavor molecules and antioxidants when heated with amines, although the major antioxidant pathway of the Maillard reaction involves the formation of cyclic amino reductones and polymers with antioxidant activity. Reductone is a trivial name for 3-hydroxy-2-ketopropane (similar to pyruvaldehyde).

Reductones consist of dicarbonyls formed by enolization and loss of hydrogen. They are resonance-stabilized enediols which are strong reducing agents. Hodge and Rist (11) summarized the effectiveness of amino reductones, and Evans *et al.* (12) demonstrated the excellent antioxidant activity of amino reductones because the nitrogen moiety can contribute electrophilic groups which can chelate metal ions such as copper and iron which are known for their oxidation catalysis.

Catalytic Activities

Namike and Hayaski (13) found that free radicals formed from condensation of 2 carbon fragments from sugars and amines form dialkyl pyrazine radicals which are precursors for melanoidin formation. Yamaguchi *et al.* (14) have studied extensively the antioxidant properties of melanoidins. They prepared them by heating glycine and xylose at pH 7.0 and then separating them into three molecular weight fractions. A low molecular weight (4,500 Da) fraction had the greatest antioxidant potential and was more effective than butylated hydroxyanisole (BHA), propyl gallate and erythrobates in protecting linoleic acid from oxidation. A synergetic effect was found in the use of a combination of melanoidin with BHA, butylated hydroxytoluene (BHT), propyl gallate, or natural tocopherols.

Two possible mechanisms have been proposed for the antioxidant activities of melanoidins; one is the formation of free radical species which can react with free radicals formed by oxidation of lipids, and the other is the formation of reductone (enaminol) structures. Pyrone-like structures in the melanoidin pigments may also complex and remove copper, iron, and other oxidizing trace metals (15).

Application of MRP as Food Antioxidants

German workers (16,17) were probably the first to demonstrate that MRP formed by heating glucose and glycine reduced the oxidation of margarine. Lingnert and coworkers (18,19) described the antioxidant properties of MRP in several foods. Their most important contribution was to demonstrate that the basic amino acids lysine, histidine, and arginine were the most effective amino acids for reacting with sugars to form antioxidant melanoidin mixtures. They also improved many useful analytical methodologies for surveying the antioxidant effect of MRP in processed foods.

Stabilization of Cooked Beef Flavor Quality During Refrigeration by Synthetic MRP Reaction Mixtures

Antioxidant Properties of Beef Muscle Diffusate. The water-soluble dialyzable low molecular weight diffusate from beef muscle is an ideal mixture of precursors for forming meaty flavor and MRP antioxidants for cooked beef during refrigerated storage. The diffusate works best in this capacity when heated for 2 h at 180°C and pumped into beef roasts prior to roasting. It reduces the thiobarbituric acid (TBA) values of cooked roast beef if injected at 2% prior to cooking and storage at 4°C (20). MRP formed during these procedures are undoubtedly responsible for the antioxidant properties observed.

Synthetic Flavor Mixtures. Although effective, this method is too expensive for commercial processing and can be replaced by the use of MRP prepared from synthetic ingredients which upon heating at controlled pH form synthetic meat flavor (SMF) with antioxidant properties. Bailey *et al.* (21) improved the flavor of roast beef during storage after injection of a synthetic flavor mixture prior to roasting to 70°C in a 177°C oven. The SMF was prepared by heating 0.3 M solution of glucose and histidine with 0.2 mm cysteine at 150°C for 2 h in 40% glycerol. This was used as a solvent to disperse 0.5% cysteine, 0.5% thiamine, 1.0% glycine, 3.0% autolyzed yeast, and 2% melted beef fat which was then heated at 125°C for 1 h in an oil bath. The resulting mixture was referred to as the synthetic meat flavor (SMF) which was used to improve the flavor quality of roast beef during storage at 4°C.

Stabilization of Cooked Roast Pork Loin and Chopped Steak Flavor Quality During Refrigeration by Synthetic Pork Flavor (SPF)

Preparation of SPF-I from MRP Precursors

A solution of distilled water and glycerol (6:4) containing 3.0% ribose and 3.0% histidine was refluxed in a 250-mL round bottom flask in an oil bath at 140°C for 2 h. A synthetic pork flavor (SPF-I) was formulated by adding 2% cysteine, 1.0% thiamine, 0.4% taurine, 2.0% glutamic acid, 2.0% glycine, 8.0% autolyzed yeast extract, and 1% melted pork fat in the above mixture and refluxing further at 125°C for 90 min and the excess fat removed after chilling at 4°C. This SPF-I was stable at 4°C for 3 wk.

Processing and Cooking of Pork Loin Roasts

Fresh, boneless, low-fat pork loins (USDA Choice) approximately 2.5 kg in weight were trimmed of subcutaneous fat and connective tissue and pumped to 10% of their green weights with one of four preserving solutions: (i) 10% NaCl, (ii) 10% NaCl and 4.0% sodium tripolyphosphate (STP), (iii) 10% NaCl, 4% STP and 20% SPF-I, and (iv) 10% NaCl, 4.0% STP, and 40% SPF-I. The pork roasts were tumbled under vacuum for 1 h at 10 rpm, 4°C, and cooked to well done (internal temperature of 76.7°C) in a natural gas convection oven at 177°C. Roasts were sliced in 3-mm thick slices and vacuum packaged.

Vacuum Packaging and Storage of Roasted Pork Loin Slices

Approximately 30-g slices were vacuum packaged to –0.95 bar in heat-shrinkable high oxygen barrier bags (Cryovac Div., W.R. Grace & Co., SC) using a heat seal vacuum packaging machine (Multivac, AGW, W. Germany). After packaging, samples were stored at 4°C in a refrigerator and removed for sensory analysis after 0, 3, 7, 14, 21, and 28 d of storage.

Processing and Cooking of Chopped Pork Steak

Fresh pork loin was trimmed of subcutaneous fat and connective tissue and ground through a 1/4" plate followed by grinding through a 1/8" plate using a table-top grinder. The average fat content as determined by Babcock fat analysis (22) was 8%.

Batches of 2.5 kg each were mixed with the following ingredients prior to forming into 100-g steaks with a Hollymatic 400 patty machine (Hollymatic Corp., Countryside, IL): (i) control = 1% NaCl and 0.4% STP; (ii) SMF = 1% NaCl and 0.4% STP and 2% SPF-II; (iii) SMF-NaL = 1% NaCl and 0.4% STP and 2% SPF-II and 2% sodium lactate. SPF-II was the same as SPF-I added to pork roasts prior to cooking except that the Maillard reaction product was formulated by refluxing 3% ribose and 3% histidine at 145°C for 2 h in a solution of water/monoacylglycerol/glycerol (6:2:2).

The steaks were cooked for 12 min at 177°C in a natural gas convection oven on metal racks in metal trays. The internal temperature of each steak was 70°C. Four cooked steaks were packaged in individual heat-shrinkable high oxygen barrier bags (Cryovac Div., W.R. Grace & Co.) and sealed using a heat seal vacuum packaging machine at –0.95 bar. Packages were stored in a refrigerator for up to 28 d at 4°C.

Stabilization of Cooked Chopped Beef Steak Flavor Quality with Synthetic Beef Flavor (SBF)

Preparation of Synthetic Beef Flavor (SBF-I) from MRP Precursors

Maillard reaction product (MRP) was prepared by heating 3.0% histidine and 3.0% ribose, in water/monoglyceride/glycerol 6:2:2 at pH 6.6 at 145°C for 2 h. SBF-I was formulated by refluxing (oil bath) 2% cysteine, 0.50% thiamine, 1.0% taurine, 2.0% monosodium glutamate (MSG), 2.0% glycine, 8% autolyzed yeast extract, and 1% beef tallow at 145°C for 2 h in the MRP solution. The excess fat was removed by chilling. This preparation was stable for 1 mon at 4°C.

Processing and Cooking of Chopped Beef Steak

Fresh top beef round was trimmed of subcutaneous fat and ground through a 1/4" plate followed by grinding through a 1/8" plate with a table-top grinder. The average fat content was 3.5% as determined by the Babcock procedure (22). Each batch (1 kg raw meat) was mixed with the following ingredients in a Kitchen Aid mixer for 2 min at speed level 2: (i) 1% NaCl and 0.4% STP; (ii) 1% NaCl and 0.4% STP and 2% SBF-I; (iii) 1% NaCl and 0.4% STP and 2% SBF-I and 2% sodium lactate (SMF-NaL). Samples were formed into 100-g patties with a hand patty maker. The patties were cooked for 12 min at 177°C to an internal temperature of 70°C in a natural gas convection oven on metal racks in metal trays. They were cooled and vacuum packaged in a heat-sealing vacuum machine at –0.95 bar. Packaged samples were stored at 4°C for 0, 3, and 14 d at which times they were analyzed by sensory analysis.

Sensory Analysis

At the end of each storage period, individual packages were opened; samples were trimmed to 1″ × 1″, wrapped with Saran film and reheated to 70°C in a microwave oven. These samples were served in preheated (100°C) sand baths to eight trained judges who judged them for warmed over aroma (WOA), WOF, meaty aroma and meaty flavor. All of the usual precautions of sampling and environment for good sensory techniques were followed. The quantitative descriptive analysis method of Stone *et al.* (23) was used to measure flavor quality factors. Samples were rated for each attribute on a line scale from 0 to 10 (none to strong).

Consumer samples were tested by a paired preference method. The sliced pork and chopped beef steaks were stored in vacuum packages and served to 50 consumer panelists who were selected randomly from students, clerical and technical staff, and faculty from the University of Missouri-Columbia. Soybean protein concentrate (PP 200 G) was supplied by Ralston Purina Co., St. Louis, Missouri.

Statistical Analysis

Analysis of variance methods (24) were used to evaluate treatment effects and interactions.

Results

Data are presented for the influence of synthetic meat flavor on the WOA, WOF and meaty flavor of pork roasts, pork "chopped" steak, and beef "chopped" steak.

Sensory Analysis of Precooked Pork Roast During Storage in Vacuum Package at 4°C for 28 d

Results of sensory evaluation of WOA, WOF, meaty aroma and meaty flavor of pork roast during storage at 4°C are reported in Figs. 18.1–18.4. WOA and WOF in control samples was high initially and increased in control samples during storage. The WOA and WOF of samples treated with antioxidant SPF-I at 2 and 4% were significantly ($P < 0.05$) lower in samples treated with the antioxidants, and did not increase during storage. There were few significant differences in WOA and WOF among samples receiving the various antioxidant treatments during storage for 28 d, although samples treated with SPF-I at 4% were lower in WOF than those treated at 2% SPF-I, and samples containing only phosphate were higher in WOF than samples containing SPF-I. Results of sensory evaluation of meaty aroma and meaty flavor (Figs. 18.3 and 18.4) differed from the above. Control samples had less meaty aroma and flavor during 28 d of storage at 4°C than samples treated with the various antioxidants, and values decreased during storage. Pork roast treated with SPF I at both (2 and 4%) levels had significantly ($P < 0.05$) higher scores for meaty aroma and flavor than samples treated with phosphate alone or those without antioxidants (control). There were no significant differences in the scores for samples treated with 4% SPF-I compared with those treated with 2% SPF-I, although samples containing 4% SPF-I received the highest scores for both meaty aroma and meaty flavor. It appears that pork roast treated with 2 and 4% SPF-I prior to cooking and storage at 4°C for 28 d has superior meaty flavor during storage than samples containing only 1% NaCl or samples containing 1% NaCl and 0.4% STP. The SPF-I is a highly desirable additive for preserving the meaty aroma and flavor of cooked pork roast slices during storage at 4°C for 28 d.

Consumer Testing of Pork Roast Containing SPF-I

Pork roast slices from roasts that were cooked, sliced, and stored at 4°C for 7 d were presented to 50 randomly selected consumer panelists for preference evaluation.

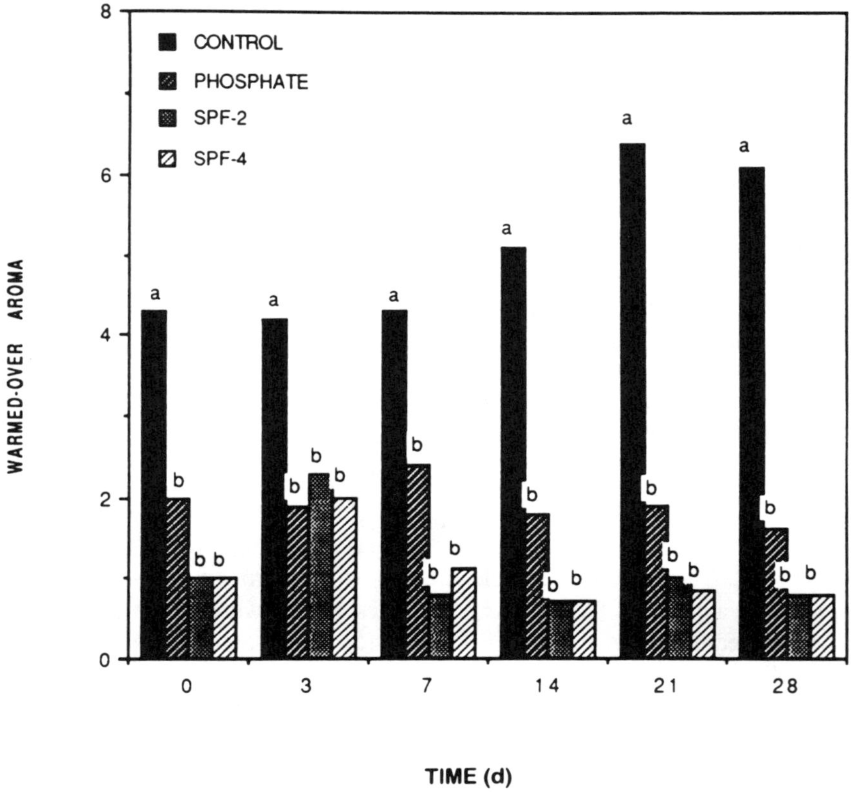

Fig. 18.1. Mean warmed-over aroma of precooked pork roast in vacuum packages during storage at 4°C. Means with different letters are significantly different ($P < 0.05$). Control = 1% NaCl; phosphate = 1% NaCl + 0.4% sodium tripolyphosphate (STP); SPI-2 = 1% NaCl + 0.4% STP + 2% synthetic pork flavor (SPF-I); SPF-4 = 1% NaCl + 0.4% STP + 4% synthetic pork flavor (SPF-I). $n = 16$.

These data are presented in Table 18.1 and indicate that the addition of SPF-I to pork roast has a significant ($P < 0.05$) effect on consumer preference, although the type of packaging was insignificant. SPF-I-treated samples were preferred 3 to 1 compared with control (untreated) samples.

Sensory Analysis of Precooked Chopped Pork Steak During Storage in Vacuum Packages at 4°C for 28 d

Results of WOF and meaty flavor of chopped pork steak during storage for 28 d are reported in Figs. 18.5 and 18.6. The WOF of control samples (Fig. 18.5) increased during storage for 28 d, and samples containing SPF-II (SMF) or SMF

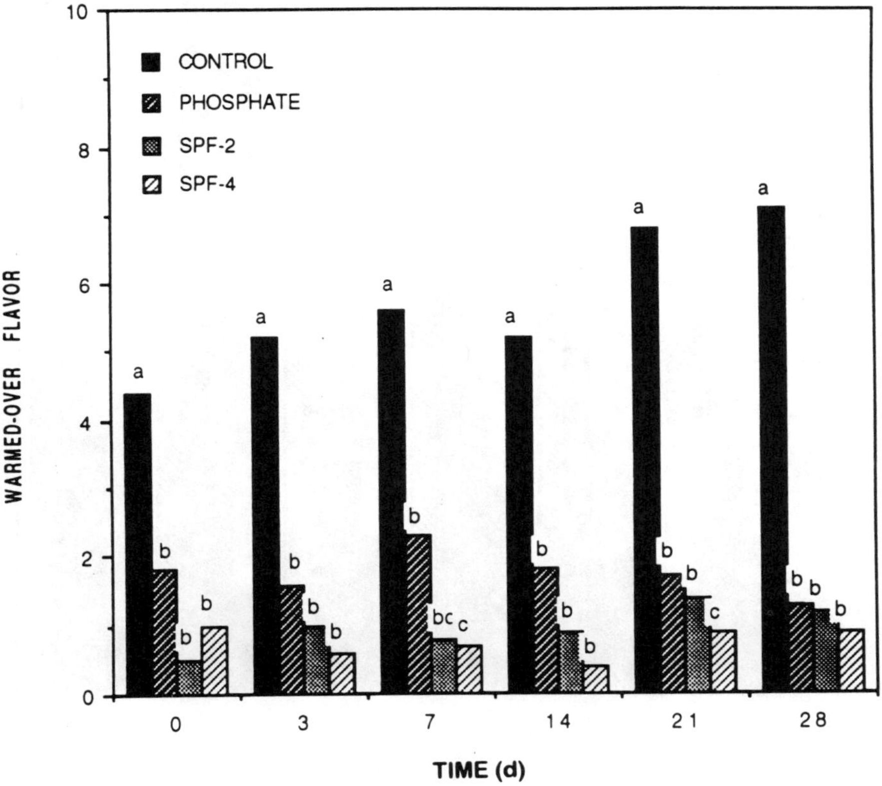

Fig. 18.2. Mean warmed-over flavor of precooked pork roast in vacuum packages during storage at 4°C. Means with different letters are significantly different ($P < 0.05$). Control = 1% NaCl; phosphate = 1% NaCl + 0.4% sodium tripolyphosphate (STP); SPF-2 = 1% NaCl + 0.4% STP + 2% synthetic pork flavor (SPF-I); SPF-4 = 1% NaCl + 0.4% STP + 4% synthetic pork flavor (SPF-I). $n = 16$.

TABLE 18.1
Percentage Preference by Consumer Panel (n = 50) for Precooked Pork Roast Treated with Synthetic Pork Flavor (SPF-I) Stored for 7 d at 4°C in Nonevacuated and Vacuum Packages

Package	Percentage preference	
	Control[a]	SPF-I[b]
Nonevacuated	24[c]	76[d]
Vacuum	26[c]	74[d]

[a]Control = 1% NaCl.
[b]SPF-I = 1% NaCl + 0.4% sodium tripolyphosphate (STP) + 2.0% SPF-I (synthetic pork flavor).
[c,d]Means in the same row bearing unlike superscripts are significantly different ($P < 0.05$).

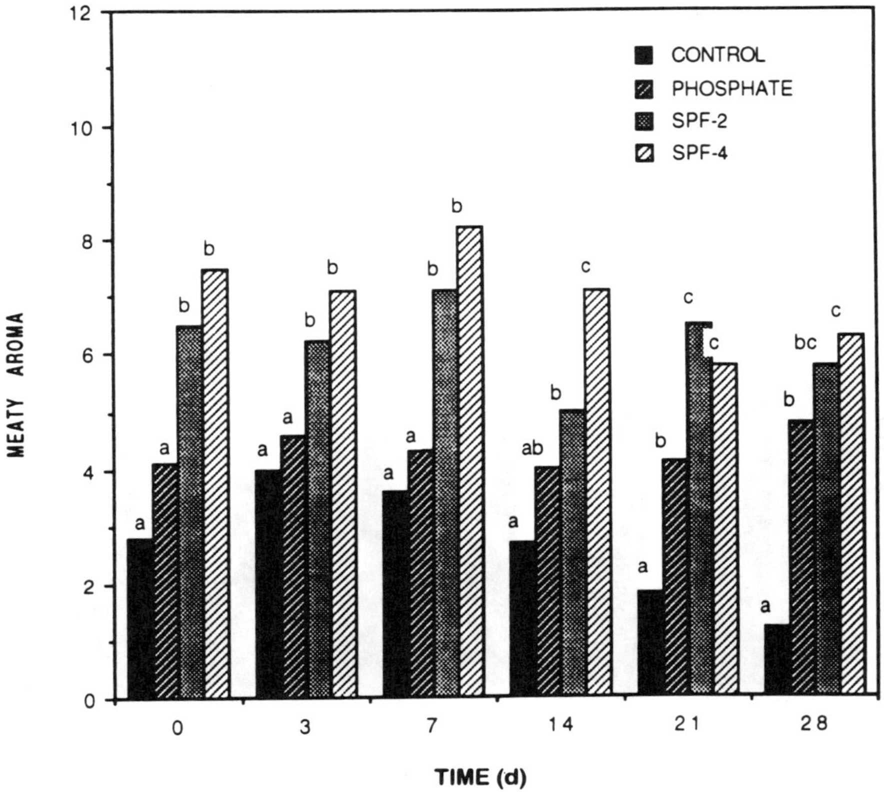

Fig. 18.3. Mean meaty aroma of precooked pork roast in vacuum packages during storage at 4°C. Means with different letters are significantly different ($P < 0.05$). Control = 1% NaCl; phosphate = 1% NaCl + 0.4% STP; SPF-2 = 1% NaCl + 0.4% STP + 2% synthetic pork flavor (SPF-I); SPF-4 = 1% NaCl + 0.4% STP + 4% synthetic pork flavor (SPF-I). $n = 16$.

with sodium lactate were significantly lower in WOF than the control samples during storage for 28 d. Samples containing both SPF-II and sodium lactate were lower in WOF than those without sodium lactate, but these values were not significantly different from those of samples containing only NaCl, STP, and SPF-II. There may be an overall microbiological advantage for adding sodium lactate. The cooked pork steaks also were evaluated for WOA and meaty aroma during storage at 4°C for 28 d, but these data are not reported because they generally confirm the flavor results reported for flavor of these samples.

Results of meaty flavor of samples treated with SPF-II and SPF-II plus NaL given in Fig. 18.6 were significantly ($P < 0.05$) higher during storage than those of the untreated controls. The NaL did not improve meaty flavor although other workers found it to be a flavor preservative. This difference may be because sodi-

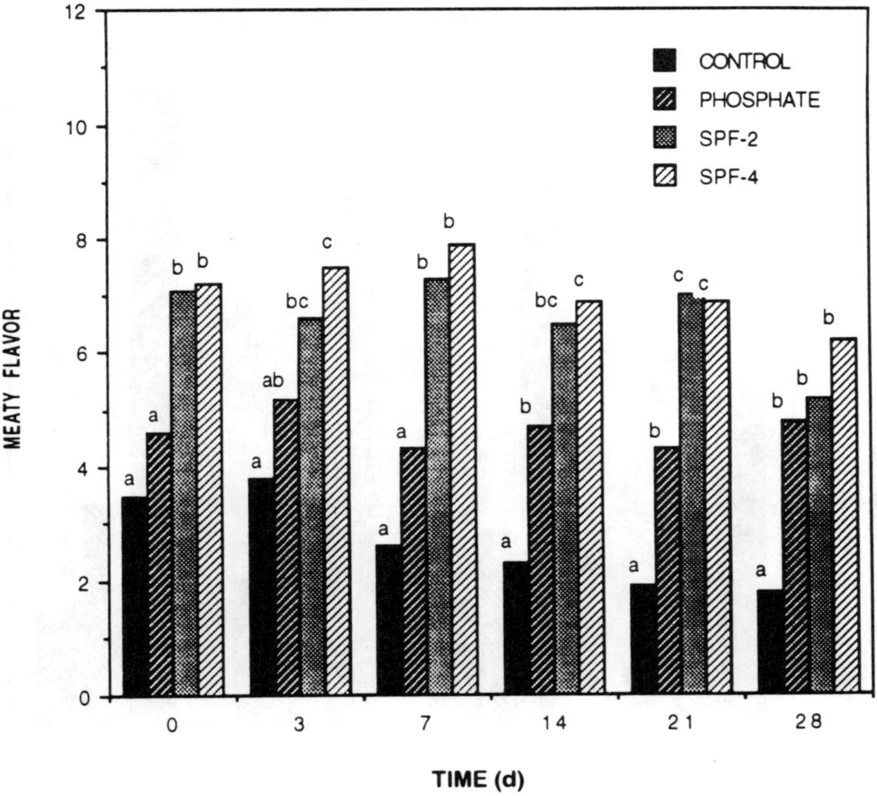

Fig. 18.4. Mean meaty flavor of precooked pork roast in vacuum packages during storage at 4°C. Means with different letters are significantly different ($P < 0.05$). Control = 1% NaCl; phosphate = 1% NaCl + 0.4% sodium tripolyphosphate (STP); SPF-2 = 1% NaCl + 0.4% STP + 2% synthetic pork flavor (SPF-I); SPF-4 = 1% NaCl + 0.4% STP + 4% synthetic pork flavor (SPF-I). $n = 16$.

um lactate adds a noticeable sour flavor to meat. Results for meaty aroma (not shown) essentially paralleled those for meaty flavor.

Sensory Analysis of Precooked Chopped Beef Steak During Storage in Vacuum Packages at 4°C for 14 d

Results of WOF and meaty flavor of chopped beef steak during storage for 14 d are reported in Figs. 18.7 and 18.8. Treatments for chopped beef steaks differed from that of chopped pork steak in that the beef samples were treated with synthetic meat flavor (SBF-I). Data in Fig. 18.7 reveal that the WOF of salt and STP-treated samples (control) increased during storage at 4°C, whereas the meaty flavor of beef samples (Fig. 18.8) receiving this treatment decreased slightly. The addition

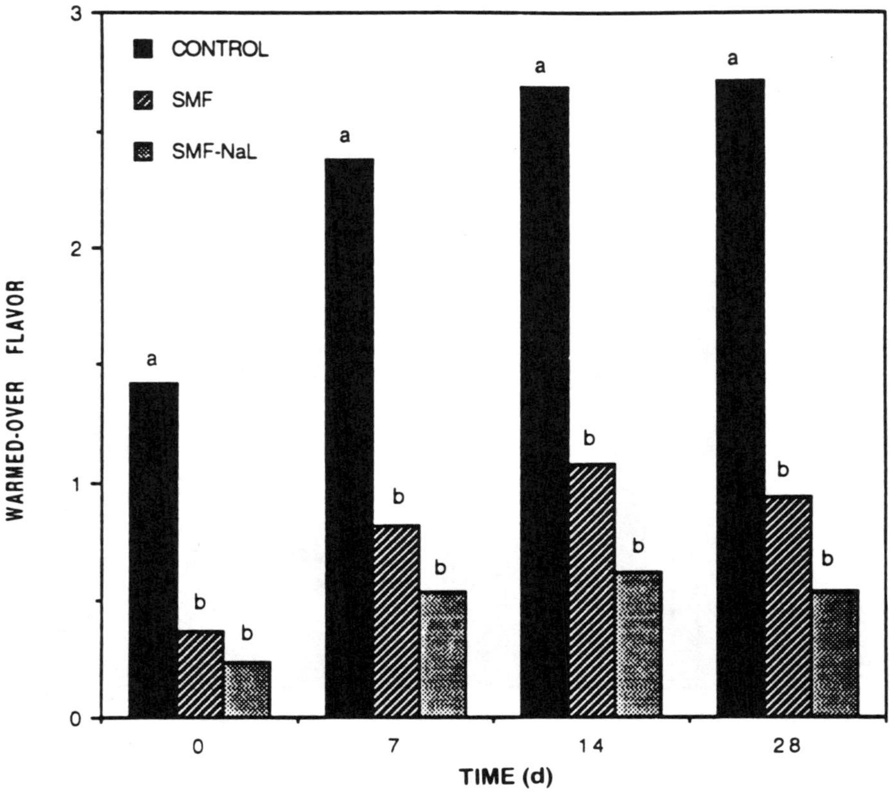

Fig. 18.5. Mean warmed-over flavor of precooked pork steak in vacuum packages during storage at 4°C. Means with different letters are significantly different ($P < 0.05$). Control = 1% NaCl + 0.4% sodium tripolyphosphate (STP); synthetic meat flavor (SMF) = 1% NaCl + 0.4% STP + 2% SPF-II (synthetic pork flavor); SMF-NaL = 1% NaCl + 0.4% STP + 2% SPF-II (synthetic pork flavor) + 2% sodium lactate. $n = 12$.

of 2% SBF-I (SMF) and SMF + NaL significantly ($P < 0.05$) inhibited WOF flavor (Fig. 18.7) during storage and significantly ($P < 0.05$) enhanced meaty flavor (Fig. 18.8) during storage. These data concerning the influence of synthetic beef flavor on WOF and meaty flavor of chopped beef steak were confirmed with results from subsequent studies of steaks containing 8% soy protein concentrate to improve texture, but not reported here because of lack of space.

Consumer Testing of Chopped Beef Steak Containing SBF-I

Table 18.2 contains data resulting from two consumer tests (50 consumers each) of cooked chopped beef steak following 3 d storage at 4°C. These results are from the analysis of samples treated with salt, SBF-I, STP, and soy protein, or without the

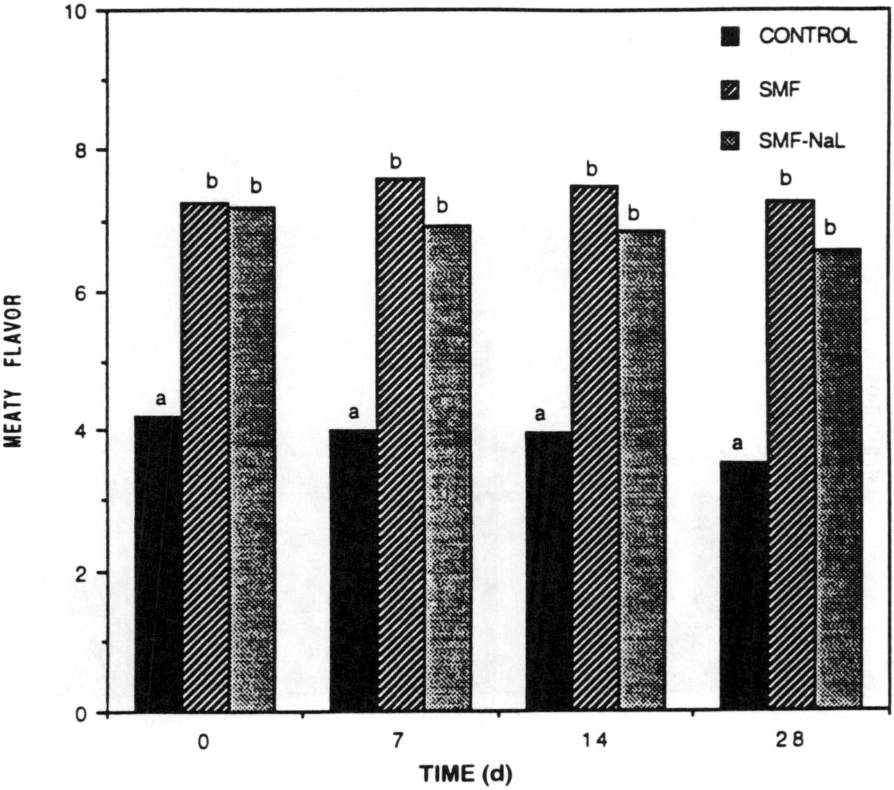

Fig. 18.6. Mean meaty flavor of precooked chopped pork steak in vacuum packages during storage at 4°C. Means with different letters are significantly different ($P < 0.05$). Control = 1% NaCl + 0.4% sodium tripolyphosphate (STP); synthetic meat lavor (SMF) = 1% NaCl + 0.4% STP + 2% SPF-II (synthetic pork flavor); SMF-NaL = 1% NaCl + 0.4% STP + 2% SPF-II (synthetic pork flavor) + 2% sodium lactate. n = 12. See Fig. 18.5 for abbreviations.

TABLE 18.2
Percentage Preference by Consumer Panel (n = 50) for Cooked Beef Steak Treated with Synthetic Beef Flavor (SPF-I) Stored for 3 d at 4°C in Vacuum Packaging

Consumer test	Percentage preference	
	Control[a]	SPF-I[b]
First	40[c]	60[c]
Second	18[d]	82[d]

[a]Control: First test; 0.5% NaCl + 0.4% sodium triphosphate (STP) + 8% soybean protein concentrate (PP 200G). Second test; 0.5% NaCl + 8% PP 200G.
[b]SBF-I: 0.5% NaCl + 0.4% STP + 8% PP 200G + 3% SBF-I.
[c,d]Percentages in the same row bearing unlike superscripts are significantly different ($P < 0.05$).

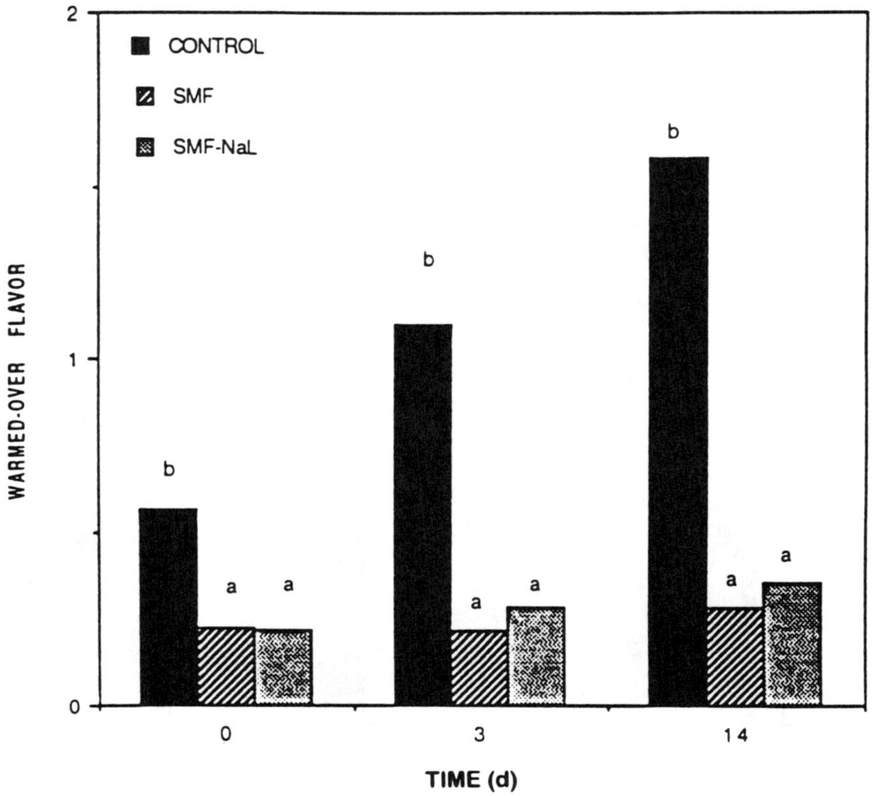

Fig. 18.7. Mean warmed-over flavor of precooked chopped beef steak in vacuum packages during storage at 4°C. Means with different letters are significantly different ($P < 0.05$). Control = 1% NaCl + 0.4% STP; SMF = 1% NaCl + 0.4% STP + 2% SBF-I (synthetic beef flavor); SMF-NaL = 1% NaCl + 0.4% STP + 2% SBF-I (synthetic beef flavor) + 1% sodium lactate. $n = 12$. See Fig. 18.5 for abbreviations.

SBF-I. In both experiments, samples treated with 3% SBF-I were more highly acceptable than samples treated with only salt, soy protein, and STP, or with salt or soy protein. There was a 4 to 1 preference for the samples containing synthetic meat flavor in the second study. From the first consumer test, it was noted that 0.4% STP had a preservative effect as judged by the acceptance scores of the consumers, but not as much as samples containing both STP and SBF-I.

Conclusions

Results of these studies lead to the conclusion that synthetic meat flavor formulated with Maillard reaction mixtures containing amino acids, sugars, taurine, thiamine, and yeast extract heated at intermediate temperatures are good antioxidants

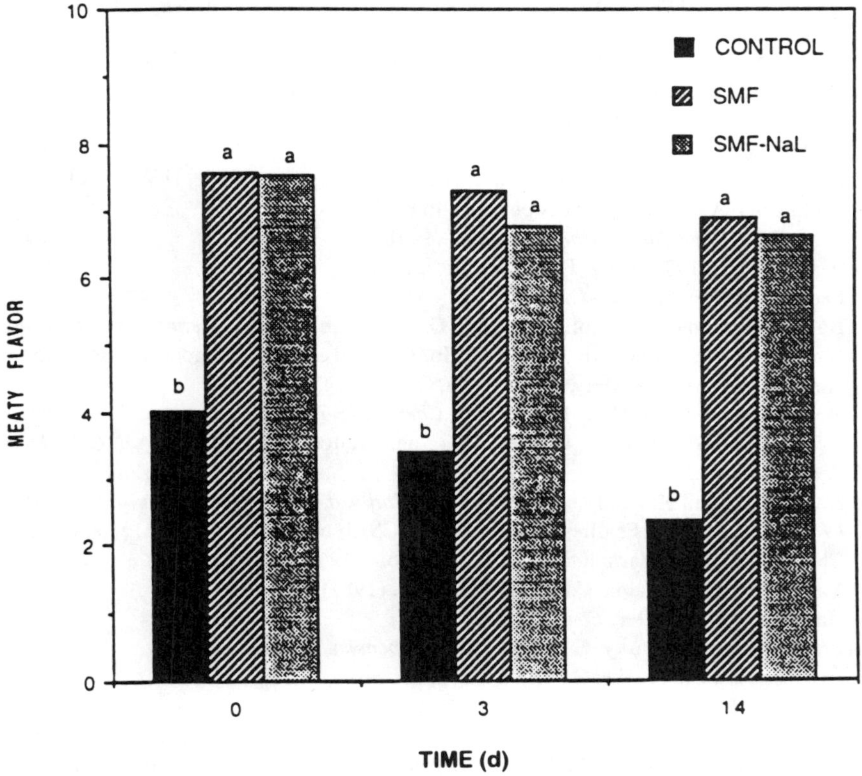

Fig. 18.8. Mean meaty flavor of precooked chopped beef steak in vacuum packages during storage at 4°C. Means with different letters are significantly different ($P < 0.05$). Control = 1% NaCl + 0.4% STP; SMF = 1% NaCl + 0.4% STP + 2% SBF-I (synthetic beef flavor); SMF-NaL = 1% NaCl + 0.4% STP + 2% SBF-I (synthetic beef flavor) + 1% sodium lactate. $n = 12$. See Fig. 18.5 for abbreviations.

for preventing WOF and preserving meatiness in precooked pork and beef during storage at 4°C for up to 28 d. These additives should have tremendous potential as flavor preservatives of pork and beef that will be consumed following cooking and storage at 4°C for short periods of time.

Acknowledgment

The editorial efforts of Elizabeth J. Bailey are gratefully acknowledged.

References

1. Tims, M., and Watts, B.M. (1958) *Food Technol. 12*, 240.
2. Bailey, M.E. (1988) *Food Technol. 426*, 123.

3. Smith. L.A., Simmons, S.L., McKeith, F.A., Bechter, P.J., and Brady, P.L. (1984) *J. Food Sci. 49*, 1636.
4. Bailey, M.E. (1983) in *The Maillard Reaction in Food Nutrition* (Waller, G.R., and Feather, M.S., eds.), *ACS Symposium Series 215*, American Chemical Society, Washington, D.C., pp. 169–184.
5. Hodge, J.E. (1953) *J. Agr. Food Chem. 1*, 928.
6. Hodge, J.E. (1967) in *Chemistry and Physiology of Flavor* (Schulz, H.W., and Libbey, L.M., eds.), AVI Pub. Co., Westport, pp. 465–491.
7. Anet, B.F. (1964) *Adv. Carbohyd. Chem. 19*, 181.
8. Feather, M.S. (1981) *Prog. Food Nutr. Sci. 5*, 37.
9. Ledel, F. (1986) *Dev. Food Sci. 13*, 569.
10. Baltes, W., Kunert-Kirchoff, J., Reise, G. (1989) in *Thermal Generation of Aroma* (Parliment, T.H., McGarrin, R.J., and Ho, C.T., eds.), ACS Symposium Series 543, American Chemical Society, Washington, D.C. pp. 143–155.
11. Hodge, J.E., and Rist, C.E. (1953) *J. Am. Chem. Soc. 75*, 316.
12. Evans, C.D., Moser, H.A., Cooney, P.M., and Hodge, J.E. (1958) *J. Am. Oil Chem. Soc. 35*, 84.
13. Namiki, M., and Hayashi, T. (1983) in *The Maillard Reaction in Foods and Nutrition* (Waller, G.R., and Feather, M.S., eds.), ACS Symposium Series 215, American Chemical Society, Washington, D.C. pp. 21–46.
14. Yamaguchi, N., Koyama, Y., and Fujimaki, M. (1981) *Prog. Food Sci. 5*, 429.
15. Hashiba, H. (1986) *Dev. Food Sci. 13*, 155.
16. Franke, C., and Iwainsky, H. (1954) *Dtsch. Lebenson. Rundsch. 50*, 251.
17. Iwainsky, H., and Franke, C. (1956) *Dtsch. Lebenson. Rundsch. 52*, 129.
18. Lingnert, H. (1980) *Food Proc. Preserv. 4*, 219.
19. Lingnert, H., Eriksson, C.E., and Waller, G.R. (1983) in *The Maillard Reaction in Foods and Nutrition* (Waller, G.R., and Feather, M.S., eds.), ACS Symposium Series 215, American Chemical Society, Washington, D.C. pp. 335–345.
20. Shin-Lee, S.Y. (1988) *Warmed-Over Flavor and Its Prevention by Maillard Reaction Products*, Ph.D. Thesis, University of Missouri, Columbia, Missouri.
21. Bailey, M.E., Clarke, A.D., Hedrick, H.B., Shin-Lee, S.Y., and Choate, G.K. (1991) *Proceedings of the 37th International Congress of Meat Science and Technology*, Kulmbach, Germany, II, pp. 684–688.
22. Official Method of Analysis of the Association of Official Analytical Chemists (1984) Method 18.045, Association of Official Analytical Chemists, Inc., Arlington, VA. p. 336.
23. Stone, H., Sidel, J.L., and Bloomquist, J. (1980) *Cereal Foods Worlds 25*, 642.
24. SAS (1988) *SAS User's Guide: Statistics, Version 6.0*, Statistical Analysis Systems Institute, Inc., Cary, NC.

Chapter 19

Controlling Oxidation and Warmed-Over Flavor in Precooked Pork Chops with Rosemary Oleoresin and Edible Film

D. Handley[a], M. Ma-Edmonds[b], F. Hamouz[b], S. Cuppett[c], R. Mandigo[d], and M. Schnepf[b]

[a]Human Ecology Department, State University of New York—Oneonta, Oneonta, NY; [b]Department of Nutritional Science and Dietetics; [c]Department of Food Science and Technology; and [d]Department of Animal Science, University of Nebraska-Lincoln, Lincoln, Nebraska.

Introduction

Warmed-over flavor (WOF) is a term first used by Tims and Watts (1) to describe the development of off flavors in cooked meat during short-term refrigerated storage. Off flavors are described as "warmed-over," "rancid," or "stale" and are detectable in cooked meats within hours of refrigerated storage. In raw meats, rancidity may become evident only after prolonged, frozen storage (2). Polyunsaturated fatty acids from polar lipids, especially phospholipids, appear to be the primary substrate for the formation of lipid oxidation reaction products that contribute to WOF (3–6). For years, nitrite, phosphate, and synthetic antioxidants have been widely used to retard lipid autoxidation and control WOF in meats (7–9). A segment of the consumer market is increasingly expressing an interest in food products that contain natural ingredients (10). This movement has led to renewed interest in the antioxidant properties of natural ingredients, especially the oleoresin extract of spices. Rosemary oleoresin (RO) contains a number of compounds which impart antioxidant activity, including rosmanol, carnosol, rosmaridiphenol, and rosemariquinone (11). A number of researchers have shown the effectiveness of RO in suppressing lipid oxidation in meat products (12–14). Since the 1960s, much research has been completed on the formation and characteristics of edible films (15,16). Renewed interest in edible films exists today because of the environmental movement, the need to find novel uses for underutilized ingredients, and the attractiveness of natural ingredients. Edible films have been shown to reduce moisture loss, microbial proliferation and deteriorative chemical and enzymatic reactions (17). Starch is one of the many ingredients used to form edible films. Hydroxypropylated amylose starch films have been found to be relatively impermeable to gas transport (16,18,19). Sodium alginate, which can complex with divalent and multivalent ions to form a coating, has been used to reduce dehydration in raw poultry patties (20), significantly reduce shrinkage of lamb carcasses (21), and reduce shrinkage and drip loss of uncooked beef steaks (22). Most research has focused on improving the quality of restructured meat products because disruption of the membrane enhances lipid oxidation. However, with the increased use of precooked meat products in convenience foods, it is important to look for ways to improve the quality of whole intact precooked meats. Therefore, this chapter illustrates the effectiveness of rosemary oleoresin and a starch/alginate film in inhibiting WOF.

Materials and Methods

Film Formulation

The edible film consisted of 2.5% Spersa-Tex CX modified starch (American Maize-Products Co., Hammond, IN) and 1.0% sodium alginate (Kelco Division of Merck and Co., Rahway, NJ). After sodium alginate was dispersed in distilled water, modified starch was slowly added and the solution was heated to boiling. An 8% calcium chloride (Fisher Scientific, St. Louis, MO) solution was used to set the film. The film and calcium chloride solutions were refrigerated at 4°C and used within 24 h.

Sample Preparation

Twenty boneless pork loins, cut into 2.54-cm chops, were purchased from a local retail grocery store. Twelve center-cut chops were chosen from each loin. Three groups of 64 chops, one group for each of the three replications, were randomly chosen from the 240 chops and stored at –20°C for a period of no more than 4 wk. The mean weight of the chops was 106.3 ± 15.7 g. Chops were removed from frozen storage 72 h prior to preparation and refrigerated at 3°C to thaw.

The following four treatments were applied to the chops: control (no RO or film); film (coated with film); RO (tumbled with a 5% RO solution); and RO/film (tumbled with a 5% RO solution and filmed). Sixteen chops were randomly assigned to each of the four treatment groups. Each group of 16 chops was tumbled separately in a Vortron tumbler (Model 40 115/1/60 3A, Beloit, WI) for 20 min. Control and film groups were each tumbled in 160 mL distilled water. The chops containing RO were each tumbled in a 160-mL 5% RO solution (Herbalox Seasoning Type P, Kalsec, Inc., Kalamazoo, MI). Immediately after tumbling, each group of chops was weighed and placed on a flat Hobart griddle (Model HG-4, Troy, OH). Chops were grilled at 163°C to an internal temperature of 71°C, grilling on each side for approximately 8 min. After grilling, chops were placed on paper towels to drain excess fat and moisture. Two groups were filmed. The chops to be filmed were immersed in the cold starch/alginate solution, drained for 10 s, and then completely immersed into the calcium chloride solution for 10 s. All chops were overwrapped with all-purpose plastic food wrap and stored at 3°C. Three replications of the experiment were completed.

Chemical Analyses

One chop per treatment per day was used for chemical analysis. Each chop was cubed and immediately submerged into liquid nitrogen. When completely frozen, the sample was ground with liquid nitrogen in a Waring blender (Model 31BL92, New Hartford, CT).

The 2-thiobarbituric acid test was performed on d 0, 3, 6, and 9 of refrigerated storage according to the method of Tarladgis *et al.* (23) as modified by Pikul *et al.* (24). Duplicate samples from each chop were analyzed.

Gas chromatographic (GC) static headspace analysis of volatiles was conducted in duplicate on d 0, 3, 6, and 9. Samples were stored at –20°C and analyzed within 2 wk. Volatile analysis was performed with a Tekmar 7000 Headspace Autosampler (Cincinnati, OH) attached to a Hewlett-Packard gas chromatograph (Model 5890, Avondale, PA) equipped with a fused silica capillary column (30 m × 0.320 mm i.d., 1.00 μm film, DB-5; J & W Co., Folsom, CA). A 5-g sample was sealed in a 20-mL glass headspace vial and equilibrated at a platen temperature of 120°C for 10 min in the headspace autosampler. After heating, samples were mixed for 2 min, stabilized for 1 min, pressurized for 0.5 min and equilibrated for 1 min. After the loop was filled and equilibrated for 1 min, the carrier gas (helium) backflushed the loop and carried the volatiles through the heated transfer line (125°C) into the GC. The released volatiles were automatically injected (injector temperature 250°C) and trapped on the GC column. The initial and final column temperatures were set at 120°C. The carrier gas was helium with a flow rate of 35 mL/min, an inlet pressure of 10 psi, and a split injection ratio of 1:50. Blanks were run between each sample to clean the column and prevent carry-over between samples. The degree of lipid oxidation was measured as the area counts for pentane, hexanal and total volatiles by a Hewlett-Packard integrator (Model 3396A). Pentane and hexanal were identified by comparing retention times with pure standards: pentane (Aldrich Chemical Co., Milwaukee, WI) and hexanal (Sigma Chemical Co., St. Louis, MO).

Sensory Analysis

Sensory evaluation was used to follow juiciness of the chops, intensity of seasoning, and intensity of WOF. A seven-member panel evaluated samples on d 0, 3, and 6 of refrigerator storage. Panelists had previous training in warmed-over flavor detection. Samples were cut from the middle of each of three chops, placed in 2-oz portion cups and coded with random three-digit numbers. Samples were heated in a microwave oven immediately before serving. Samples were presented simultaneously, and panelists were asked to evaluate samples in the randomized order indicated on the score sheets. Panelists rated three attributes of each sample: juiciness, intensity of WOF, and intensity of seasoning. An unstructured 15-cm line, anchored with descriptors 1 cm from each end, was used for evaluation. Descriptors of juiciness were dry and juicy; for WOF and seasoning intensities, the descriptors were absent and strong. All sensory panels were held in the sensory analysis room in the Department of Nutritional Science and Dietetics.

Statistical Analysis

Chemical data were analyzed as a split-plot with a 2 (film, no film) × 2 (RO, no RO) × 4 (refrigerated storage time of 0, 3, 6, and 9 d) factorial treatment design. The whole plot was randomized as a complete block design with the four treatment combinations. The blocking variable was the 9-d testing period. Analysis of variance and Fisher's Protected Least Significance Difference (LSD) were performed using statistical analysis software (SAS). Correlation coefficients were calculated between each of the variables. Statistical difference was set at $P < 0.05$.

Results and Discussion

Tumbling was chosen as the method to incorporate RO into chops because it has been shown to improve solution penetration, to have uniformity of solution dispersion, and to improve consumer characteristics (25). The overall mean weight gain of pork chops from tumbling was 4.7 ± 0.5%. The chops tumbled with the 5% RO solution absorbed 0.034% RO, based on a 7% fat content of the pork chops. This is at the lower end of the 0.04–0.2% RO recommended by Kalsec, Inc. (26) and lower than the 0.05% OR used by Lai *et al.* (27) to retard lipid oxidation in chicken nuggets.

Values of Thiobarbituric Acid Reactive Substances (TBARS)

TBARS were affected by both number of days of storage and treatment. TBARS were similar and low on d 0, had significantly increased after 3 d of storage, but did not significantly change after 6 d (except for the control). By d 9, TBARS values were the highest for all of the chops except for the RO chops which did not change significantly from d 3. A more pertinent way to look at data is to compare the treatment effect within each day. The statistically significant differences are found in Table 19.1. No differences were found on the first day but by d 3 and 6, all of the treated chops had lower values than the controls. On d 9, the lowest TBARS values were found in the chops treated with RO and RO/film, and the chops with the film alone were not different from the control chops. Other researchers have reported that RO was an effective inhibitor of lipid oxidation in ground and restructured meat products (12,14,27,28). Results from this study showed that RO was an effective inhibitor of lipid oxidation in a whole muscle product and at very low levels. The film also inhibited lipid oxidation through d 6 but not to same extent as RO. The film integrity may not have been able to prevent oxygen penetration for the total duration of the study.

Volatiles

Hexanal is one of the most potent flavor volatiles found in oxidized linoleic acid (29) and has been related to WOF (30). During the storage period of this study, hexanal values rose for the control chops but did not increase significantly over the 9-d period for the treated chops. However, the amount of hexanal detected in the treated chops was consistently lower than that of the control chops. The chops treated with both RO and film had the lowest hexanal values of all of the treatments.

Pentane is an inert short-chain hydrocarbon formed from the oxidation of linoleic acid. Pentane is not directly responsible for off-flavors, but pentane has been used as an indicator of lipid oxidation (31). Loliger (32) postulated that pentane may be a more reliable measure of oxidation than the aldehydes due to its stability because it does not undergo any further reactions. Pentane was the major volatile identified in each of the samples in this study. Over the course of the study, the only increase in pentane levels was found in the control chops with a significant increase on d 3 and 6, compared with d 6–9. However, looking at the treatment effect, differences are apparent (Table 19.1). Significantly less pentane was detected in the chops with the film than in either the control or the OR-treated chops. These results were unexpected because both hexanal and pentane are produced when linoleic acid oxidizes. The high levels of pentane found in the chops which were treated only with RO were not consistent with results found by the thiobarbituric acid (TBA) test and headspace analysis of hexanal.

Except for d 3 with the control, total volatiles did not significantly increase over time. The values for total volatile area generally follow the same pattern as for pentane (Table 19.1).

Sensory Scores

Sensory results are given in Table 19.2. For juiciness, the panelists generally rated the chops with the film higher than the chops without the film, but the difference was not significant. Little difference was seen over time. For WOF, the only significant differences were seen on d 3 when the treated chops were rated as having less WOF than the control chops. The panelists were easily able to detect a seasoning flavor in the chops that contained RO. The seasoning scores of RO- and RO/film-treated chops were significantly ($P < 0.05$) higher than the control and film-treated chops. On average, they rated the chops halfway between absent and strong. The detection of the flavor of RO may have limited the ability of the panelists to detect WOF clearly.

Correlation Coefficients

Similar results were obtained from chemical and sensory analyses. Because consistent and reliable results from a sensory panel are sometimes difficult to obtain, cor-

TABLE 19.1
Mean Chemical Test Results of Refrigerated Precooked Pork Chops Comparing Treatments Within Day[a]

Treatment	Day	Control	Film	RO	RO/Film
TBARS	0	0.54[a]	0.56[a]	0.34[a]	0.30[a]
	3	2.02[a]	1.39[b]	0.87[c]	0.90[c]
	6	2.97[a]	1.71[b]	1.20[c]	1.25[b,c]
	9	3.34[a]	3.14[a]	1.27[b]	2.02[c]
Hexanal	0	5.7[a]	5.4[a,b]	2.0[b,c]	0.4[c]
	3	16.7[a]	8.1[b]	2.4[c]	1.3[c]
	6	14.6[a]	3.6[b]	3.4[b]	1.4[b]
	9	13.3[a]	6.7[b]	3.8[b,c]	2.3[c]
Pentane	0	25.8[a]	11.3[b]	28.0[a]	6.7[b]
	3	40.0[a]	13.8[b]	30.9[c]	6.2[b]
	6	37.1[a]	10.7[b]	28.1[a]	6.7[b]
	9	29.0[a]	7.0[b]	38.2[c]	7.3[b]
Total	0	82.0[a]	44.2[b]	77.7[a]	45.9[b]
	3	117.6[a]	51.0[b,c]	59.3[b]	28.6[c]
	6	89.6[a]	39.3[b]	61.3[b]	37.3[b]
	9	79.2[a]	31.5[b]	87.6[a]	39.9[b]

[a]Means of three replications; TBARS values expressed as mg malondialdehyde/kg meat; within each row, values with different superscripts are significantly different ($P < 0.05$). *Abbreviations:* RO, rosemary oleoresin; TBARS, thiobarbituric reactive substances.

relation with chemical tests is necessary. Significant correlation coefficients were found between TBARS and hexanal ($r = 0.57$, $P < 0.01$); between WOF as determined by sensory analysis and TBARS ($r = 0.32$, $P < 0.01$); hexanal ($r = 0.39$, $P < 0.01$); and total volatiles ($r = 0.26$, $P < 0.02$).

TABLE 19.2
Mean Sensory Scores of Refrigerated Precooked Pork Chops Comparing Treatments Within Day[a]

Treatment	Day	Control	Film	RO	RO/Film
Juiciness[b]	0	5.5[a]	5.6[a]	5.3[a]	8.4[a]
	3	4.5[a]	8.8[b]	6.3[a]	7.0[a]
	6	6.3[a,b]	7.2[a]	4.9[b]	7.8[a]
WOF[c]	0	5.4[a]	5.1[a]	5.2[a]	6.3[a]
	3	7.4[a]	5.4[b]	4.9[b]	5.0[b]
	6	7.0[a]	5.3[b]	5.2[a]	6.0[a]
Seasoning[d]	0	1.0[a]	1.5[a]	7.9[b]	6.6[b]
	3	2.6[a]	1.9[a]	7.0[b]	5.1[c]
	6	1.5[a]	1.9[a]	6.8[b]	6.1[b]

[a]Within each row, values with different superscripts are significantly different ($P < 0.05$).
[b]Juiciness, 0 = very dry, 13 = very juicy.
[c]WOF, 0 = absent, 13 = intense.
[d]Seasoning, 0 = absent, 13 = intense. *Abbreviations:* RO, rosemary oleoresin; WOF, warmed-over flavor.

Conclusions

Tumbling was an effective means of incorporating RO into whole muscle meats. Even at low levels, RO was effective in controlling WOF. Sensory panelists were able to detect the RO in the pork chops but did not rate the RO as strong. The edible film reduced WOF as measured by TBARS, hexanal, and pentane. Adding RO further reduced TBARS and hexanal. TBARS and hexanal analyses were shown to be reliable indicators of WOF.

References

1. Tims, M.J., and Watts, B.M. (1958) *Food Technol. 12*, 240.
2. Pearson, A.M., and Gray, J.I. (1983) in *The Maillard Reaction in Foods and Nutrition* (Waller, G.R., and Feather, M.S., eds.), Symposium Series 215, American Chemical Society, Washington, D.C., pp. 287–302.
3. Igene, J.O., and Pearson, A.M. (1979) *J. Food Sci. 44*, 1285.
4. Wilson, B.R., Pearson A.M., and Sharland, F.B. (1976) *J. Agric. Food Chem. 24*, 7.
5. Pikul, J., Leszczynski, D.E., Bechtel, P.J., and Kummerow, F.A. (1984) *J. Food Sci. 39*, 838.
6. Allen, C.E., and Foegeding, E.A. (1981) *Food Technol. 35*, 253.
7. Sato, K., and Hegarty, G.R. (1971) *J. Food Sci. 36*, 1098.
8. Chastain, M.F., Huffman, D.L., Hsieh, W.H., and Cordray, J.C. (1982) *J. Food Sci. 47*, 1779.
9. Crackel, R.L., Gray, J.I., Booren, A.M., Pearson, A.M., and Buckley, D.J. (1988) *J. Food Sci. 53*, 656.
10. Younathan, M.T., Oon, J.K., and Yusof, B.M. (1983) *J. Food Sci. 48*, 176.
11. Houlihan, C.M., Ho, C.T., and Chang, S.S. (1985) *J. Am. Oil Chem. Soc. 62*, 96.
12. Stoick, S.M., Gray, J.I., Booren, A.M., and Buckley, D.J. (1991) *J. Food Sci. 56*, 597.
13. Barbut, S., Josephson, D., and Maurer, A. (1985) *J. Food Sci. 50*, 1356.
14. Resurreccion, A.V.A., and Reynolds, A.E., Jr. (1990) *J. Food Sci. 43*, 1776.
15. Major, C.J., and Kammermeyer, K.M. (1962) *Modern Plastics 39*, 135.
16. Roth, W.B., and Mehltretter, C.L. (1967) *Food Technol. 21*, 72.
17. Kester, J.J., and Fennema, O.R. (1986) *Food Technol. 40*, 47.
18. Jokay, L., Nelson, G.E., and Powel, E.L. (1967) *Food Technol. 21*, 1046.
19. Guilbert, S. (1986) in *Food Packaging and Preservation Theory and Practice* (Mathlouti, M., ed.), Elsevier Applied Science Publishers, London, p. 371.
20. Mountney, G.J., and Winter, A.R. (1960) *Poultry Sci. 40*, 28.
21. Lazarus, C.R., West, R.L., and Palmer, A.Z. (1976) *J. Food Sci. 41*, 639.
22. Williams, S.K., Oblinger, J.L., and West, R.L. (1978) *J. Food Sci. 43*, 292.
23. Tarladgis, B.G., Watts, B.M., and Younathan, M.T. (1960) *J. Am. Oil. Chem. Soc. 37*, 44.
24. Pikul, J., Leszczynski, D.E., and Kummerow, F.A. (1983) *J. Agric. Food Chem. 31*, 1338.
25. Addis, P.B., and Schanus, E.S. (1979) *Food Technol. 33*, 36.
26. Anonymous (1988) Technical Bulletin, Spice Oleoresin, Kalsec, Inc., Kalamazoo, MI.
27. Lai, S.M., Gray, J.I., Smith, D.M., Booren, A.M. Crackel, R.L., and Buckley, D.J. (1991) *J. Food Sci. 56*, 616.

28. Barbut, S., Draper, H.H., and Hadly, M. (1988) *J. Food Protection. 51*, 878.
29. Frankel, E.N. (1991) *J. Sci. Food Agric. 54*, 495.
30. St. Angelo, A.J., Vercelotti, J.R., Legendre, M.G., Vinnet, C.H., Kuan, J.W., James C. Jr., and Dupuy, H.P. (1987) *J. Food Sci. 52,* 1163.
31. Seo, C.W., and Joel, D.L. (1980) *J. Food Sci. 45*, 26.
32. Loliger, J. (1990) *J. Sci. Food. Agric. 52*, 119.

Chapter 20

Model Systems for Studying Pigment and Lipid Oxidation Relevant to Muscle-Based Foods

W.K.M. Chan[a], C. Faustman[a], and M. Renerre[b]

[a]Department of Animal Science, University of Connecticut, Storrs, Connecticut; and [b]Institut National de la Recherche Agronomique, Station de Recherches sur la Viande, Theix, 63122 Ceyrat, France.

Introduction

Fresh meat quality depends on color and lipid stability. Meat color changes from an acceptable cherry-red to undesirable brown when oxymyoglobin is oxidized to metmyoglobin in beef (1,2). Lipid oxidation causes rancidity which contributes to undesirable flavors in meat (3). Thus, both lipid oxidation and oxymyoglobin oxidation contribute to consumer rejection of meat and meat products. Because lipid and oxymyoglobin oxidation in meat are often concurrent, a close relationship between these processes is indicated. Meat is a complex food, and model systems have been developed to gain a fundamental understanding of oxidation processes and their interactions. *In vitro* approaches have utilized emulsion, liposome, and microsome systems. A substantial body of literature reports the use of similar approaches for studying heme protein and lipid oxidation with an emphasis on human health (4–7).

Lipid Oxidation

Lipid oxidation is characterized by initiation and propagation steps (8). Free radical species are generated from these steps and may include alkoxy, hydroxy, and peroxy radicals. In model systems, transition metals such as Fe^{2+} (9), Fe^{2+}/ascorbic acid (10), Fe^{2+}/H_2O_2 (11) and Fe^{2+}/EDTA complexes (12) have been used to initiate lipid oxidation *via* generation of hydroxyl radicals by the Fenton reaction. Enzymic systems such as cytochrome P450/P450 reductase/Fe^{3+}/NADPH (13) and xanthine oxidase/xanthine/Fe^{3+} (14) have also been used. 2,2′-Azobis(2-amidinopropane) dihydrochloride (AAPH; water soluble) and 2,2′-azobis(2,4-dimethylvaleronitrile) (AMVN; lipid soluble) (15–17) have been used to generate peroxyl radicals at a constant rate in aqueous and lipid phases, respectively. Ferryl myoglobin, which may be formed from the reaction of metmyoglobin and hydrogen peroxide, has also proved effective in initiating lipid oxidation in model systems (18–21).

A variety of procedures for measuring the extent of lipid oxidation have been published. One common method involves measurement of thiobarbituric acid reactive substances (TBARS). This assay detects the formation of malondialdehyde (MDA) and other aldehyde breakdown products of lipid oxidation (22–26). However, the TBARS assay may be useful only when lipid oxidation has progressed sufficiently to generate MDA and other aldehydes. Measurement of lipid hydroperoxide accumulation by HPLC analysis (7) and oxygen uptake (7,27) allows early detection of the lipid oxidation process. The rapid rise in luminescence formed by excited carbonyl species from lipid oxidation and rose bengal dye was also used to detect lipid oxidation (28). In addition, lipid oxidation may be measured by following formation of conjugated dienes (29), oxidized heme protein (6), and direct detection of free radicals by electron spin resonance (7,20,21). Gutteridge and Halliwell (30) published an excellent review of techniques used to measure lipid oxidation.

Heme Pigment Oxidation

The oxidation of ferrous oxymyoglobin to ferric metmyoglobin may occur spontaneously with the formation of superoxide anion and hydrogen peroxide (31). Ferrous heme protein oxidation is generally followed by spectrophotometric means. In general, a decrease in A_{580}, an absorption maxima for oxymyoglobin, and an increase in A_{630}, an absorption maxima for metmyoglobin, are consistent with oxidation. An isobestic point for both deoxymyoglobin and oxymyoglobin exists at 572 nm; the isobestic point for deoxymyoglobin, oxymyoglobin, and metmyoglobin is at 525 nm. A ratio of absorbance at 572/525 nm is related to metmyoglobin percentage (32). Investigators have proposed a variety of schemes for quantitating formation of metmyoglobin, or oxidation of oxymyoglobin, as a percentage of total myoglobin (24,25,33,34).

Oxymyoglobin used in model systems may be prepared by direct extraction from muscle tissues (35) or chemical reduction and oxygenation of commercial metmyoglobin (36). Direct extraction from muscle tissue generally involves homogenization in buffer and centrifugation to remove particulate materials. The supernatant is subjected to ammonium sulfate fractionation; myoglobin is selectively precipitated by 70–100% ammonium sulfate. The crude oxymyoglobin fraction is then further purified by ion-exchange chromatography (35). Chemical reduction of commercial metmyoglobin involves treatment with sodium hydrosulfite (dithionite) and bubbling of air to allow oxygenation. The resulting oxymyoglobin is then passed over a mixed-bed ion-exchange column to remove residual hydrosulfite (36).

Model Systems

Emulsions

An emulsion is a system containing two immiscible phases, such as fatty acids (lipid) and aqueous solution. This is a relatively simple model system for studying lipid and pigment oxidation. Within muscle foods, fatty acids are generally bound to glycerol in membrane phospholipids; free fatty acids appear more susceptible to lipid oxidation than their lipid-bound counterparts (37). Moreover, free fatty acids are present at relatively low concentrations in muscle tissues (37) compared with emulsion systems. Fatty acid emulsions are quick and easy to prepare.

The most common emulsion systems cited in the literature are linoleic acid micelles, and methyl linoleate micelles. During emulsion preparation, a mixture of fatty acids, surfactant, and aqueous solution (buffer, or myoglobin/hemoglobin in buffer solution) is vigorously mixed. Sonication is not usually required; however, it may help generate a more homogenous micelle solution. To produce a stable emulsion, surfactants must be used. These adsorb at the lipid/aqueous boundary and serve to lower interfacial tension; they are usually added during emulsion preparation to provide a physical resistance to coalescence (37). Sodium dodecyl sulfate (SDS), Triton X-100, or Tween 20 are commonly used surfactants. The net charge of the micelle may influence lipid oxidation rate depending on the types of free radical initiators used. Fukuzawa and Fujii (11) found that $Fe^{2+}SO_4$ catalyzed lipid oxidation in negatively charged SDS linoleic acid (LA) micelles, but not in positively charged tetradecyltrimethylammonium bromide (TTAB) LA micelles. They speculated that positively charged Fe^{2+} interacted with the sulfate group of SDS and facilitated the initial breakdown of lipid peroxide. The authors hypothesized that Fe^{2+} could not interact with the positively charged surface of TTAB micelles and therefore was not effective in initiating peroxidation of LA.

Nakhost and Karel (38) used an emulsion model system consisting of metmyoglobin and methyl linoleate (2:1) to evaluate the potential use of myoglobin insolubilization as an indicator of oxidative deterioration during freeze-drying. Lipid oxidation increased, whereas soluble myoglobin percentage decreased in the freeze-dried emulsion system during storage (Fig. 20.1). Myoglobin insolubilization was due to formation of myoglobin polymers. Nakhost and Karel (39) then applied findings from the emulsion model system to freeze-dried beef; they found that the extent of myoglobin insolubility and the ratio of myoglobin dimer/monomer could be used as indicators of oxidation-related changes in freeze-dried meat.

Stewart (40) used an emulsion system with oxymyoglobin and sodium oleate to study the effect of fatty acids on oxymyoglobin oxidation. The presence of oleic acid enhanced the initial rate of oxidation compared with that in the absence of oleic acid. The authors maintained that oleic acid inhibited metmyoglobin's ability to quench hydrogen peroxide by binding to hydrophobic cavities of metmyoglobin. This permitted a greater concentration of hydrogen peroxide to persist and oxidize oxymyoglobin.

The role of heme-proteins in lipid oxidation has also been studied in emulsion systems. Hirano and Olcott (41) used emulsions containing different concentrations of methemoglobin and linoleate. They found that low concentrations of heme-proteins catalyzed linoleate oxidation and hypothesized that this was due to the ability of heme-proteins to decompose peroxide with subsequent formation of chain-initiating free radicals.

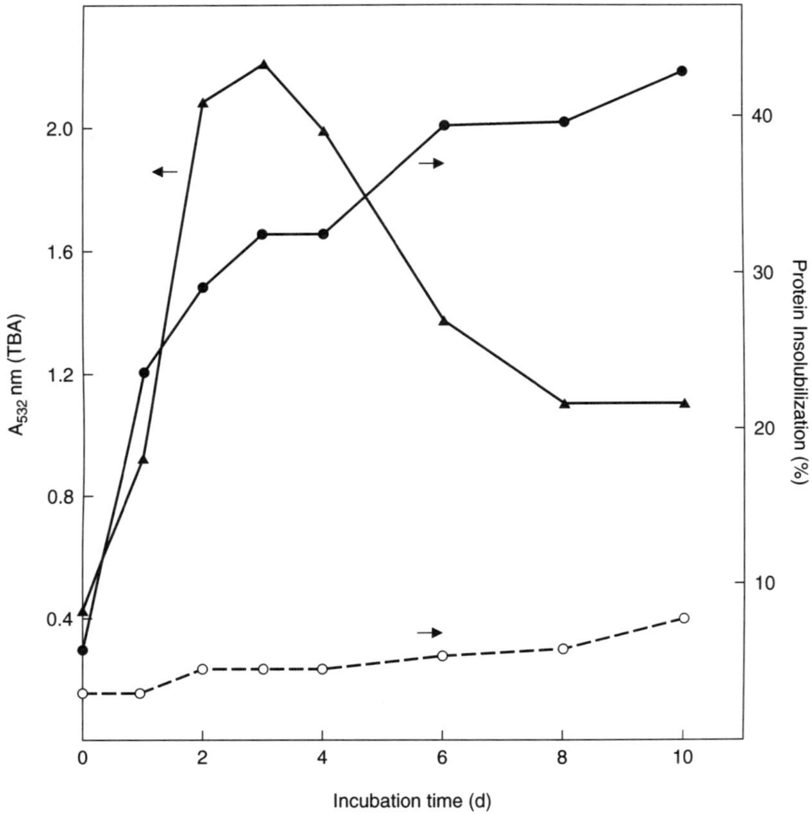

Fig. 20.1. Lipid oxidation (TBA) and protein insolubilization in freeze-dried model system of metmyoglobin (metmb) and methyl linoleate (ML) stored at 37°C. ▲, TBA; ●—●, protein insolubilization (metmb + ML); o---o, protein insolubilization (metmb without ML). Figure taken with permission (38).

Liposomes

Liposomes are phospholipid bilayer structures that serve as models of biomembranes (42). Free fatty acids are seldom found in liposomes; the phospholipids used to construct liposomes are considered the predominant lipid of biomembranes where lipid oxidation occurs. This should provide an improved *in vitro* approach over that of emulsions for modeling muscle foods. In addition, the phospholipid composition of liposomes is readily manipulated and this permits study of a variety of factors including fatty acid chain length and unsaturation, and type of polar head group. However, the liposome system may not truly represent membrane-related activity *in vivo* because the relative concentration of fatty acids and antioxidants are not necessarily those present *in vivo*. In addition, membrane-bound proteins are absent in the liposome system.

Liposomes may be classified as multilamellar large vesicles (0.1–1 μm), small unilamellar vesicles (0.015–0.025 μm) and large unilamellar vesicles (1–2.5 μm) (43). To prepare liposomes, a chloroform/methanol solution containing phospholipids is placed in a flask and the solvent removed under vacuum or a stream of nitrogen. Lipid-soluble free radical initiators (e.g., AMVN), and/or lipid soluble antioxidants (e.g., α-tocopherol), are dissolved in solvent and delivered with the phospholipid to the flasks before drying. A rotary evaporator is used to form a thin dry film. Multilamellar liposomes are formed by mixing the suspension with a vortex mixer (15), or on a table-top shaker with glass beads (44). The aqueous phase is usually a buffer containing myoglobin or hemoglobin and, when appropriate, water-soluble antioxidants (e.g., ascorbic acid). Large unilamellar liposomes may be obtained by extrusion (29,45). Small unilamellar vesicles are prepared by passing a multilamellar phospholipid dispersion through a French pressure cell (46), or by sonicating multilamellar vesicles under nitrogen (29).

Phosphatidylcholine used in liposome model systems is generally from soybean or egg yolk. Genot *et al.* (34) used *in vitro* systems with muscle phospholipid extracted from beef longissimus dorsi, psoas major and diaphragm to relate lipid oxidation with meat color stability of different muscles. Multilamellar vesicles from phospholipids extracted from turkey pectoralis muscle have also been utilized (27). The pH of liposome model systems may be manipulated to represent normal post-mortem meat (5.6), DFD (dark, firm, and dry) meat (6.4) or physiological pH (7.2) (44).

When studying lipid and heme pigment oxidation, LaBrake and Fung (29) found that the liposome vesicle size affected hemoglobin oxidation. Hemoglobin oxidation was enhanced in small unilamellar vesicles (SUV) compared with large unilamellar vesicles (LUV). The authors suggested that this was due to differences in curvature, energy, and hydrophobicity between SUVs and LUVs surfaces. Moreover, because SUVs are smaller, their surface-to-volume ratio is greater. This would permit more extensive contact with hemoglobin than in LUVs. LaBrake and Fung (29) maintained that vesicle fusion and lipid oxidation were not critical factors contributing to the differences in hemoglobin oxidation rate between SUV and LUV.

LaBrake and Fung (29) showed that no head group specificity existed for liposome-enhanced hemoglobin oxidation during incubation of phosphatidylserine and phosphatidylcholine liposomes at 37°C for 30 min (pH 7.4). Yin and Faustman (44) reported that the phospholipid head group could influence both lipid oxidation and oxymyoglobin oxidation in myoglobin-liposomes incubated at 10°C (pH 5.6). The authors showed that both lipid and oxymyoglobin oxidation increased in a manner dependent on liposome phospholipid composition, following the order phosphatidylserine (PS) > phosphatidylethanolamine (PE) > phosphatidylcholine (PC). The authors suggested that negatively charged PS liposomes may destabilize myoglobin and contribute to faster oxidation than do PE or PC liposomes which had no net charge at pH 5.6. When the fatty acid composition of PC and PE was held constant, PE-based oxymyoglobin-liposomes demonstrated greater susceptibility to oxidation than PC-based oxymyoglobin-liposomes. In addition, increasing the chain length of fatty acids within phosphatidylcholine resulted in increased oxidation of both myoglobin and lipid.

Though phospholipid and myoglobin are present in two different phases, a physical interaction between these two molecules may occur. Edward and Criddle (47) reported that myoglobin could interact with mitochondrial structural proteins *in vitro*, while Szebeni *et al.* (4) maintained that hemoglobin could interact with phospholipids through electrostatic and hydrophobic interactions. Myoglobin in muscle cells was demonstrated to localize near the I-band where mitochondria and sarcoplasmic reticulum are abundant (48). A physical interaction between myoglobin and phospholipid might cause conformational changes in both molecules which in turn could affect oxidation behavior. However, data to support such an oxidative interaction are lacking.

A relationship between oxymyoglobin/oxyhemoglobin and phospholipid oxidation was supported by results that oxymyoglobin/oxyhemoglobin oxidation was paralleled by lipid oxidation (5,44). Genot *et al.* (34) found that the phospholipid/myoglobin ratio was an important factor in determining rate of oxymyoglobin oxidation. In addition, both oxidation processes were affected by the degree of fatty acid unsaturation in phospholipids. Both lipid oxidation and myoglobin oxidation (44) or hemoglobin oxidation (5) in liposomes prepared from saturated phospholipids were much slower than in liposomes prepared from unsaturated phospholipids. These results showed that the extent of lipid oxidation in liposomes played an important role in the observed rate of heme protein oxidation.

Free radicals may be involved in lipid and heme protein oxidation (18,20). Peroxyl radicals generated in the lipid phase by AMVN, and in the aqueous phase by AAPH caused increased lipid oxidation and oxymyoglobin oxidation in oxymyoglobin/liposome systems compared with controls (without radical generators) during incubation at 37°C (Fig. 20.2). The incorporation of lipid soluble α-tocopherol, a known free radical scavenger (49), into liposome membranes inhibited both lipid oxidation and pigment oxidation (5,44). The combination of α-tocopherol and ascorbate showed a strong additive effect in delaying lipid and oxymyoglobin oxidation. However, ascorbate alone showed a prooxidant effect toward lipid and oxymyoglobin oxidation when present at high concentration (44).

Microsomes

Microsomes are small heterogenous membranous vesicles of endoplasmic reticulum and cytoplasmic membrane which contain high concentrations of polyunsaturated fatty acids and proteins (50). Microsomal membranes represent authentic biological membranes capable of biochemical function. Microsomes can be derived

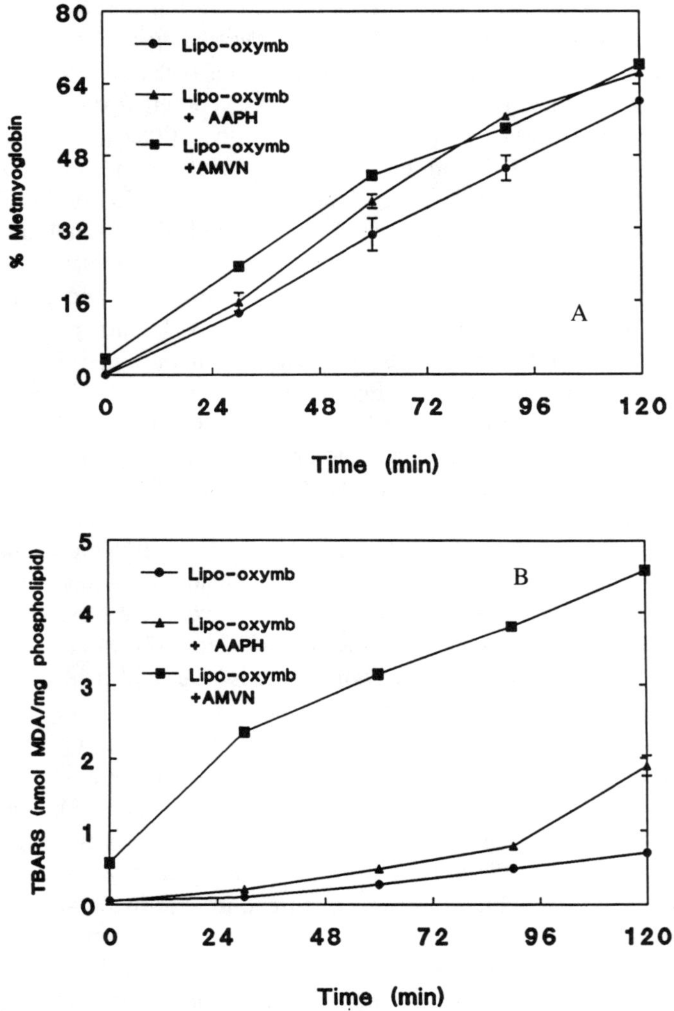

Fig. 20.2. (A) Metmyoglobin formation and (B) lipid oxidation (thiobarbituric acid reactive substances; TBARS) in phosphatidylcholine oxymyoglobin-liposomes (lipo-oxymb) incubated at 37°C (pH 5.6). Reaction was initiated by 2.2′-azobis(2-amidino-propane)dihydrochloride (AAPH; 5 mM) or 2,2′-azobis(2,4-dimethylvaleronitrile) (AMVN; 1.5 mM). Standard deviation bars are indicated (n = 3).

from muscle and thus provide a phospholipid fatty acid profile representative of that in muscle foods.

Microsome preparation can be tedious and time-consuming (19,51,52). In general, a muscle sample is first homogenized with 4 vol buffer (KCl, 0.12 M-Histidine, 5 mM buffer) at high speed in a Waring blender. The homogenate is centrifuged at

21,499 × *g* for 30 min, and the supernatant further centrifuged at 100,000 × *g* for 60 min. The sediment is treated with 0.6 M KCl-5 mM Histidine to solubilize contaminating actomyosin. The final microsome preparation is obtained by centrifugation at 100,000 × *g* for 60 min. The supernatant is discarded and the pellet resuspended in 0.12 M KCl-5 mM Histidine with a Potter-Elvehjem-type tissue homogenizer.

Antioxidants such as β-carotene or α-tocopherol may be incorporated into microsomes by either of two methods, dietary supplementation or direct addition. Dietary supplementation of experimental animals with lipid-soluble antioxidants generally results in increased tissue concentrations of the antioxidants. Endogenous α-tocopherol concentrations of muscle microsomes from pork and beef have been increased by dietary vitamin E supplementation (9,53). To incorporate lipid-soluble antioxidants directly into microsomes, antioxidants are dissolved in organic solution and homogenized with the microsomal pellet (54–56). The antioxidant-enriched microsomes are resuspended in buffer and centrifuged. Unincorporated antioxidants remain in the supernatant and are discarded. The physical orientation of antioxidants in the membrane when added by direct addition relative to incorporation *via* dietary means is not clear.

Microsomal lipid oxidation can be catalyzed by either enzymic or nonenzymic processes. Enzymic-catalyzed microsomal lipid oxidation requires cofactors such as NADPH/NADH, ADP and ferric iron, while nonenzymic-catalyzed lipid oxidation is mediated by heme proteins or transition metals (57). Microsomes may be combined with oxymyoglobin, and enzymic microsomal lipid oxidation has led to increased oxymyoglobin oxidation (22–25). Anton *et al.* (23) showed that the percentage of metmyoglobin after 40 min at 37°C was oxymyoglobin alone < oxymyoglobin + bovine muscle microsomes < oxymyoglobin + bovine muscle microsomes + cofactors (NADPH, ADP and $FeCl_3$) (Fig. 20.3). Similarly, microsomal lipid oxidation in these systems followed the same trend, suggesting an interrelationship between lipid oxidation and oxymyoglobin oxidation. Moreover, Anton *et al.* (24) observed the same reaction trend in lipid oxidation and oxymyoglobin oxidation when using mitochondrial fractions from the same muscles.

Muscle microsomes may be obtained from different species and/or muscles. The source of microsomes will affect lipid oxidation rates which in turn may affect oxymyoglobin oxidation. Yin and Faustman (44) showed that both oxymyoglobin and lipid oxidation in microsome/myoglobin systems followed the order tuna > pork > beef. This appeared strongly related to polyunsaturated fatty acid (PUFA) content (PUFA of tuna > pork > beef) and α-tocopherol concentrations (tuna < pork < beef). The lower PUFA and higher α-tocopherol contents provided beef muscle microsomes with an environment which favored a greater stability of oxymyoglobin and microsomal lipid compared with pork and tuna microsome/myoglobin systems.

Color stability of fresh beef is muscle dependent. In terms of muscles with high economic values, color stability follows the order longissimus lumborum (LL) > gluteus medius (GM) > psoas major (PM) during storage at 4°C (58,59).

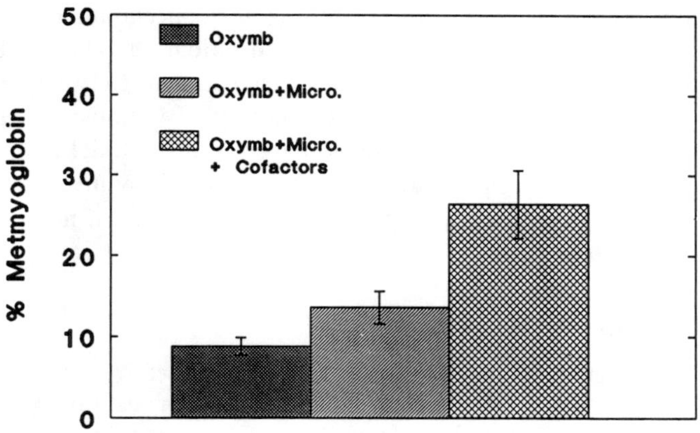

Fig. 20.3. Percentage of metmyoglobin after addition to oxymyoglobin of microsomes ± cofactors (NADPH, ADP, $FeCl_3$) with an incubation at 37°C for 40 min. Adapted with permission (23).

Studies using microsome/oxymyoglobin systems have been used to test the hypothesis that differences in lipid oxidation between these muscles contributed to color instability of different beef cuts. Anton *et al.* (23,25) isolated microsomes from fresh beef LL and PM muscles and found no difference in oxymyoglobin and lipid oxidation between the LL and PM microsome/oxymyoglobin systems. However, when microsomes were isolated from beef LL and PM muscles stored at 4°C for 8 d (25), oxymyoglobin oxidation and lipid oxidation were more pronounced in PM than LL muscle microsomes. Gatellier *et al.* (21) found differences in the phospholipid and fatty acid composition of microsomal fractions of PM and LL muscles. This could partially explain the higher oxidation rate of oxymyoglobin in PM than in LL microsome/oxymyoglobin systems. Though lipid oxidation appears to affect oxymyoglobin oxidation, whole muscle discoloration is influenced by many factors, including oxygen consumption rate, metmyoglobin reducing capacity, and microbial growth (2,58); these were not addressed in the microsome assays.

Summary—Oxidative Interactions

Oxidation of oxymyoglobin and phospholipid occur in a concomitant manner and appear interrelated. Products of oxymyoglobin oxidation include superoxide anion and hydrogen peroxide, each of which may accelerate lipid oxidation (23,24). In addition, the reaction of hydrogen peroxide with metmyoglobin appears to generate ferryl (+4) myoglobin which is a potent initiator of lipid oxidation (19). Anton *et al.* (20) reported that lipid oxidation initiated by metmyoglobin/hydrogen peroxide was more pronounced in microsomes obtained from PM than LL muscle.

The process of lipid oxidation also appears to enhance oxymyoglobin oxidation. In general, inclusion of lipid-soluble α-tocopherol within membrane fractions of muscle foods (60), or *in vitro* (44,61), results in a concentration-dependent and decreased rate of both oxymyoglobin and lipid oxidation. The mechanism by which this occurs has yet to be elucidated. Schaefer *et al.* (62) have proposed a schematic model which illustrates the complexity of various antioxidant and prooxidant reactions occurring in muscle-based foods. Model approaches for studying lipid and heme pigment oxidative interactions allow investigators to isolate specific aspects of the oxidation process which is difficult if not impossible in a complex food such as meat.

Acknowledgments

Support for this research was provided by the Cattlemen's Beef Promotion and Research Board in cooperation with the Beef Industry Council of the National Live Stock and Meat Board; Hoffmann-LaRoche, Inc.; U.S. Army RD&E Center; and the Storrs Agricultural Experiment Station, College of Agriculture and Natural Resources, University of Connecticut. We thank Dr. E. Decker for critical analysis of the manuscript. Scientific contribution no. 16250, Storrs Agricultural Experiment Station.

References

1. Faustman, C., and Cassens, R.G. (1990) *J. Muscle Foods, 1*, 217.
2. Renerre, M. (1990) *Int. J. Food Sci. Technol. 25*, 613.
3. Igene, J.O., Jennifer, A.K., Pearson, A.M., and Gray, J.I. (1979) *J. Agric. Food Chem. 27*, 838.
4. Szebeni, J., Hauser, H., Eskelson, C.D., Watson, R.R., and Winterhalter, K.H. (1988) *Biochemistry 27*, 6425.
5. Winterbourn, C.C. (1985) *Cellular and Molecular Aspects of Aging*, Alan R. Liss. Inc., New York, pp. 173–182.
6. Chen, H., Tappel, A.L., and Boyle, R.C. (1993) *Free Radical Biol. Med. 14*, 509.
7. Yoshida, Y., Kashiba, K., and Niki, E. (1994) *Biochim. Biophys. Acta 1201*, 165.
8. Kanner, J., German, J.B., and Kinsella, J.E. (1987) *CRC Critical Rev. Food Sci. Nutr. 25*, 317.
9. Monahan, F.J., Gray, J.I., Asghar, A., Haug, A., Shi, B., and Buckley, D.J. (1993) *Food Chem. 46*, 1.
10. Kagan, V.E., Serbinova, E.A., and Packer, L. (1990) *Arch. Biochem. Biophys. 282*, 221.
11. Fukuzawa, K., and Fujii, T. (1992) *Lipids 27*, 227.
12. Amici, A., Levine, R.L., Tsai, L., and Stadtman, E.R. (1989) *J. Biol. Chem. 264*, 3341.
13. Fucci, L., Oliver, C.N., Coon, M.J., and Stadtman, E.R. (1983) *Proc. Natl. Acad. Sci. USA 80*, 1521.
14. Stadtman, E.R., and Wittenberger, M.E. (1985) *Arch. Biochem. Biophys. 239*, 379.
15. Lim, B.P., Nagao, A., Terao, J., Tanaka, K., Suzuki, T., and Takama, K. (1992) *Biochim. Biophy. Acta 1126*, 178.
16. Kennedy, T., and Liebler, D.C. (1992) *J. Biol. Chem. 267*, 4658.
17. Tesoriere, L., Ciaccio, M., Bongiorno, A., Riccio, A., Pintaudi, A.M., and Livrea, M.A. (1993) *Arch. Biochem. Biophys. 307*, 217.
18. Harel, S, and Kanner, J. (1985) *J. Agric. Food Chem. 33,* 1188.
19. Kanner, J., and Harel, S. (1985) *Arch. Biochem. Biophys. 237*, 314.

20. Anton, M., Gatellier, P., and Renerre, M. (1992) *Proceedings of the 38th ICoMST*, Clermont-Ferrand, France, pp. 459–462.
21. Gatellier, P., Anton, M., and Renerre, M. (1995) *J. Agric. Food Chem. 43*, 651.
22. Lin, T.S., and Hultin, H.O. (1977) *J. Food Sci. 42*, 136.
23. Anton, M., Gatellier, and Renerre, M. (1991) *Proceedings of the 37th ICoMST*, Kulmbach, Germany, pp. 320–323.
24. Anton, M., Salgues, C., Gatellier, P., and Renerre, M. (1993) *Sci. Alim. 13*, 261.
25. Anton, M., Gatellier, P., and Renerre, M. (1993) *Proceedings of the 39th ICoMST*, Calgary, Canada, S8, P01.
26. Yin, M.C., Faustman, C., Riesen, J.W., and Williams, S.N. (1993) *J. Food Sci. 58*, 1273.
27. Genot, C., Kansci, G., and Laroche, M. (1994) *Sci. Alim. 14*, 673.
28. Nakono, M., Ito, T., Arimoto, T., Ushijima, Y., and Kamiya, K. (1994) *Biochem. Biophys. Res. Commun. 202*, 940.
29. LaBrake, C.C., and Fung, L.W. (1992) *J. Biol. Chem. 267*, 16703.
30. Gutteridge, J.M.C., and Halliwell, B. (1990) *Trends Biochem. Sci. 15*, 29.
31. Galaris, D., Buffinton, G., Hochstein, P., and Cadeaes, E. (1990) in *Membrane Lipid Oxidation* (Vigo-Pelfrey, C., ed.), CRC Press Inc., Boca Raton, pp. 269–283.
32. Hunt, M.C. (1980) 33rd Ann. Reciprocal Meat Conf., pp. 41–46.
33. Krzywicki, K. (1982) *Meat Sci. 7*, 29.
34. Genot, C., Borrel, M.N., Metro, B., Gandemer, G., and Renerre, M. (1991) *Proceedings of the 37th ICoMST*, Kulmbach, Germany, pp. 356–359.
35. Gatellier, P., Anton, M., and Renerre, M. (1993) *Meat Sci. 33*, 401.
36. Brown, W.D., and Mebine, L.B. (1969) *J. Biol. Chem. 244*, 6696.
37. Nawar, W.W. (1985) in Food Chemistry (Fennema, O.R., ed.), Marcel Dekker, Inc., New York, pp. 175–201.
38. Nakhost, Z., and Karel, M. (1983) *J. Food Sci. 48*, 1335.
39. Nakhost, Z., and Karel, M. (1984) *J. Food Sci. 49*, 1171.
40. Stewart, J.M. (1990) *Biochem. Cell Biol. 68*, 1096.
41. Hirano, Y., and Olcott, H.S. (1971) *J. Am. Oil Chem. Soc. 48,* 523.
42. Yamamoto, Y., and Niki, E. (1990) in *Membrane Lipid Oxidation* (Vigo-Pelfrey, C., ed.), CRC Press, Inc., Boca Raton, pp. 285–301.
43. New, R.R.C. (1990) in *Liposome, a Practical Approach* (New, R.R.C., ed.), IRL press, New York, pp. 1–2.
44. Yin, M.C., and Faustman, C. (1993) *J. Agric. Food Chem. 41*, 853.
45. Oshima, S., Ojima, F., Sakamoto, H., Ishiguro, Y., and Terao, J. (1993) *J. Nutr. Sci. Vitaminol. 39*, 607.
46. Barclay, L.R., Bailey, A.M.H., and Kong, D. (1985) *J. Biol. Chem. 260*, 15809.
47. Edward, D.L., and Criddle, R.S. (1966) *Biochemistry 5*, 588.
48. Kawai, H., Nishino, H., Nishida, Y., Masuda, K., and Saito, S. (1987) *Muscle & Nerve 10*, 144.
49. Burton, G.W., and Traber, M.G. (1990) *Annu. Rev. Nutr. 10*, 357.
50. Hunt, S.M., and Groff, J.L. (1990) in *Advanced Nutrition and Human Metabolism* (Gomez, J. ed.), West Publishing Company, St. Paul, p. 11.
51. Apgar, M., and Hultin, H.O. (1982) *Cryobiology 19*, 154.
52. McDonald, R., and Hultin, H.O. (1987) *J. Food Sci. 52*, 15.
53. Faustman, C. (1993) in *Technology of Reduced-Additive Foods* (Smit, J., ed.), Blackie Publ., London, pp. 160–194.

54. Vile, G.F., and Winterbourn, C.C. (1988) *FEBS Lett. 238*, 353.
55. Duthie, G.G., Gonzalez, B.M., Morrice, P.C., and Arthur, J.R. (1991) *Free Radical Res. Comms. 15*, 35.
56. Palozza, P., and Krinsky, N.I. (1992) *Arch. Biochem. Biophys. 297*, 184.
57. Kanner, J. (1992) in *Lipid Oxidation in Food* (St. Angelo, J., ed.), ACS Symposium Series, Washington, D.C.
58. O'Keefe, M., and Hood, D.E. (1982) *Meat Sci. 7*, 209.
59. Renerre, M. (1984) *Sci. Alim. 4*, 567.
60. Faustman, C., Cassens, R.G., Schaefer, D.M., Buege, D.R., Williams, S.N., and Scheller, K.K. (1989) *J. Food Sci. 54*, 858.
61. Yin, M.C., and Faustman, C. (1994) *Food Chem. 51*, 159.
62. Schaefer, D.M., Liu, Q., Faustman, C., and Yin, M.C. (1995) *J. Nutr. 125*, 1792S-1798S.

Chapter 21

Prediction of Oxidative Stability of Lipids Based on the Early Stage Oxygen Consumption Rate

A.R. Wewala

New Zealand Dairy Research Institute, Palmerston North, New Zealand.

Introduction

Flavor is widely recognized as the most important characteristic of food products and food ingredients. Control of the development of undesirable flavors is a key to the success of any food-related industry. According to Hamilton (1), lipids act as reservoirs for off-flavors. By-products of lipid deterioration impart rancidity to foods. Rancidity is considered to be based on the subjective organoleptic appraisal of the flavor quality of food and is associated with a characteristic unpalatable odor and flavor (1).

Rancidity may develop via two different lipid deterioration pathways. The rancidity caused by the chemical changes occurring from the reaction between lipids and atmospheric oxygen (i.e., lipid oxidation) is classified as oxidative rancidity or oxidized flavor (1). Lipids are not the only products in which the flavor is adversely affected by lipid oxidation. Lipid-containing food products such as potato chips (2) and dried whole milk (DWM) (3) are good examples of foods in which flavor is adversely affected by lipid oxidation during storage. Off-flavor derived from lipid *via* enzyme (lipase/esterase)-catalyzed hydrolytic reactions (i.e., lipolysis) is known as hydrolytic rancidity or lipolytic flavor.

Hydrolytic rancidity can be eliminated through good harvesting practices (*viz.*, as practiced with milk and oilseeds) and more importantly, by adopting "good manufacturing practices" during food/ingredient processing. Lipid oxidation is affected by many parameters, including the conditions of storage and handling of the lipid source (i.e., raw materials such as milk and oil seeds) and the lipid itself or the lipid-containing end-product, the initial quality of the lipid, the degree of unsaturation of the lipid, and the interactions of the lipid with other components within the lipid fraction (such as antioxidants and prooxidants because lipid is a composite product) as well as outside the lipid fraction (e.g., transition metal ions associated with the non-lipid components of complex foods). Therefore, food processors have relatively less control over oxidative rancidity.

Off-flavor resulting from the oxidation of lipids is the most common factor limiting the shelf-life of anhydrous lipid products [such as anhydrous milkfat (AMF) and vegetable oil] and/or lipid-containing dehydrated food products (such as DWM and potato chips). Lipid oxidation can cause destruction of some essential fatty acids, vitamins, and pigments. A reduction in the solubility and nutritional quality of proteins by reaction with free radicals from oxidizing lipids can also be a problem for complex foods.

Lipid Oxidation

A simplified version of the mechanism of lipid oxidation is given in Fig. 21.1.

Oxygen Consumption Studies

Lipid oxidation is the dominant mode of flavor and quality deterioration that limits the shelf-life of lipids and/or lipid-containing dehydrated foods. The reaction

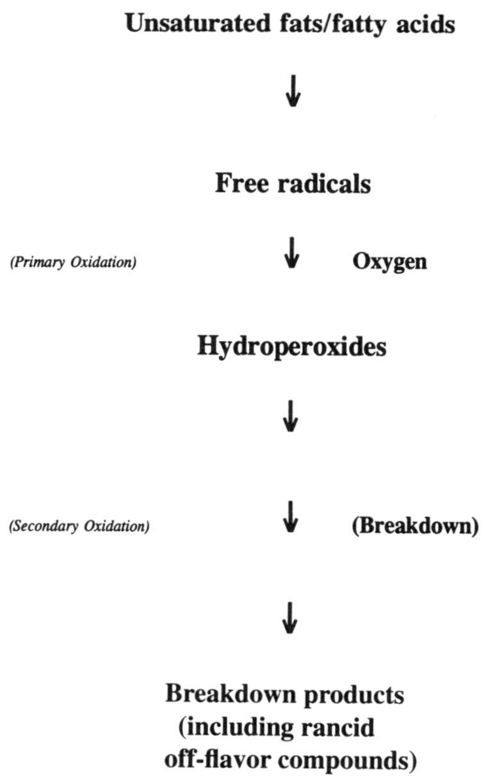

Fig. 21.1. Mechanism of lipid oxidation.

between unsaturated fats/fatty acids and oxygen is a preliminary and critical step in the lipid oxidation reaction pathway. Therefore, oxygen consumption must be an ideal parameter on which to base the oxidative stability assessment. This forms the basis for a new hypothesis and the development of a novel method for monitoring/predicting the shelf-life of lipid or lipid-containing dehydrated foods. This hypothesis is as follows:

> *The rate of oxygen consumption at an early stage of the storage life of lipids (anhydrous) and/or lipid-containing dehydrated foods is an ideal parameter for shelf-life prediction/assessment.*

The following factors from the scientific literature were used to strengthen the new hypothesis:

1. The reaction between unsaturated fats/fatty acids and oxygen is a preliminary step in the lipid oxidation reaction pathway.
2. Lipid oxidation occurs at a uniform rate during the induction period (1).
3. The induction period can be extended by incorporating antioxidants (4).

Preliminary Testing of the Hypothesis Using DWM

A preliminary investigation to test the acceptance or rejection of this hypothesis was carried out using 17 agglomerated DWM samples with different oxidative stabilities. The same quantity (350 ± 10 g) of each DWM sample was packed under atmospheric air in cans (mean volume and standard deviation of 812.7 and 4.1 mL, respectively, as measured from 24 randomly selected cans) in duplicate and stored at 30°C. The decline in the headspace oxygen content (%) was monitored by gas chromatography, several times over a period of 65 d. Headspace gas samples (350 ± 50 μL) for gas chromatography were drawn by pushing the needle of a gas-tight syringe through silicone septa glued onto the metal foil underneath the lid of the can (see Fig. 21.2).

Kinetics. The rate of decline in headspace oxygen content (%) was derived using the zero-order kinetic equation (5).

Assumptions. It was assumed that (i) the volume of the cans was constant, and (ii) the pressure decline inside the cans due to oxygen consumption and headspace gas sampling was negligible. Figure 21.3 shows the decline in headspace oxygen content with time. Very good linear relationships ($R^2 > 0.98$) between the oxygen content and time were obtained.

The oxygen consumption rates of the DWM samples were then compared with the oxidized flavor scores obtained for the 6-mon sensory evaluation; descriptive sensory analyses of the reconstituted milks (50 g DWM in 350 g water) were undertaken using a trained panel. The trend toward an increase in the oxidized flavor intensity with increasing rate of oxygen consumption can be seen clearly in Fig. 21.4.

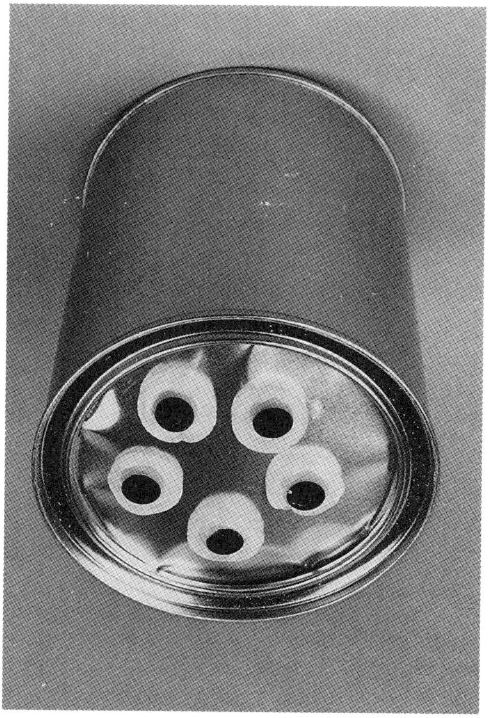

Fig. 21.2. Can of milk powder showing the septa glued onto its metal foil to facilitate headspace gas sampling.

When the oxidized flavor data were plotted against the oxygen consumption rates, an acceptable linear relationship with an R^2 value of 0.743 was obtained. The R^2 value was further improved to approximately 0.8 when the data were fitted into a quadratic model. The results of this trial using DWM are summarized in Table 21.1.

Encouraged by the success of the milk powder trial, the following aspects relevant to the other methods of predicting shelf-life were reviewed before using the oxygen consumption methodology to evaluate the oxidative stability of lipids.

TABLE 21.1
Summarized Data from the Initial Testing of the Hypothesis Using DWM[a]

Number of DWM samples	Oxygen consumption rate [μL/(d • 350 g DWM)]	Oxidized flavor score[b] (after 6 mon at 30°C)
2	≤60	<4
11	66–84	4.2–5.1
4	≥85	>6

[a]DWM = Dried whole milk. [b]Mean flavor scores on 0–10 scale (where 0 = absent, 2 = threshold, 4 = weak, 6 = moderate, 8 = strong, 10 = intense) of eight or more panelists trained for descriptive sensory evaluation.

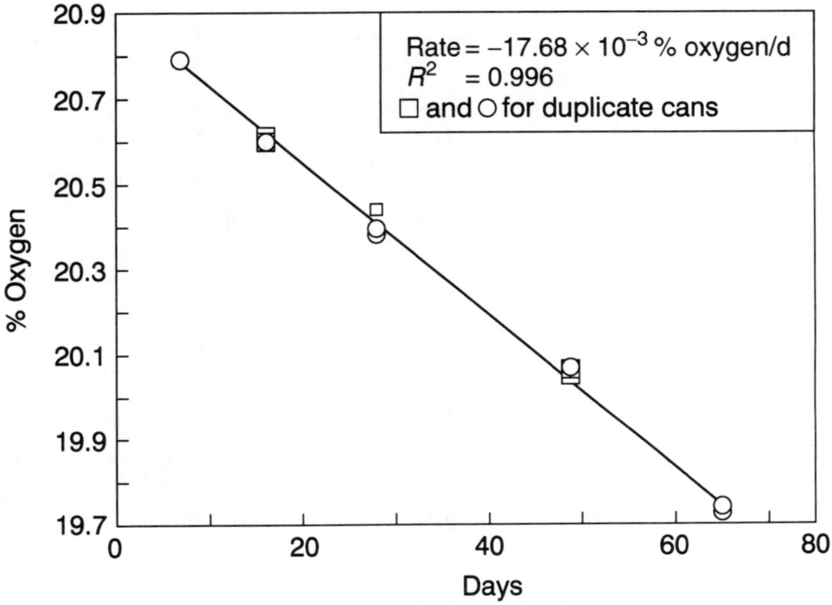

Fig. 21.3. Rate of change of the headspace oxygen content for one of the dried whole milk samples.

Accelerated Shelf-Life Testing (ASLT) Methods

The ASLT methods currently available for predicting/monitoring the oxidative stability of lipids are inadequate. They are based on temperature acceleration and primarily on induction period (IPd) measurement (see Table 21.2).

Each method is described in detail below:

- **Schaal Oven Test:** Lipid is held at 63 or 70°C in an open dish and examined at regular intervals to make a judgement on the keeping quality based on smell, taste, or peroxide value (PV).
- **Active Oxygen Method:** Oxygen is bubbled through lipid held at 98°C and the PV is monitored regularly to determine the IPd.

TABLE 21.2
Accelerated Shelf-Life Testing Methods

Older methods	Modern methods
Schaal Oven Test	Rancimat
Active Oxygen Method (Swift Test)	Oxidative Stability Instrument (OSI)
Sylvester Test	Oxidograph
FIRA-Astell Apparatus	

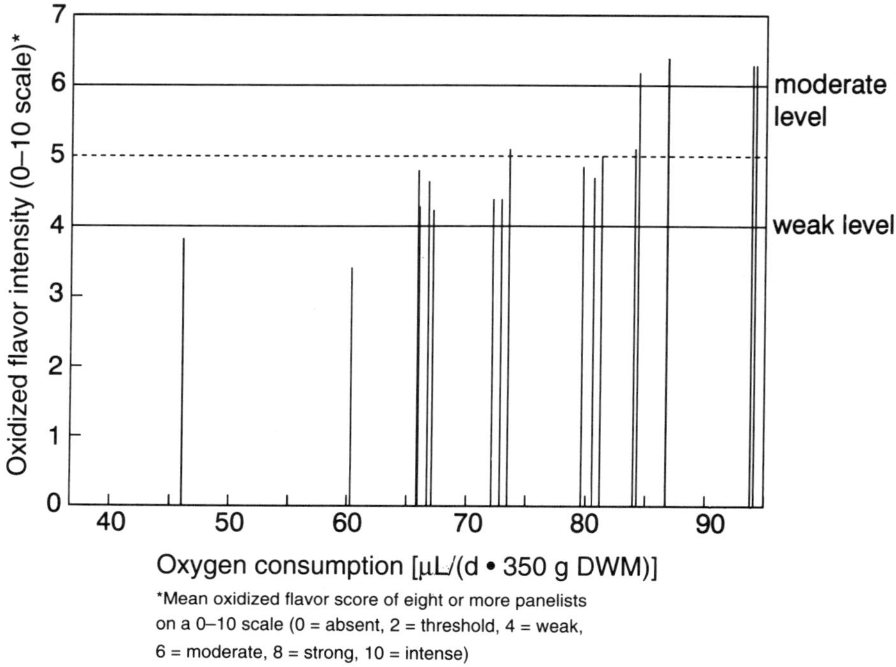

Fig. 21.4. Rate of oxygen consumption and the oxidized flavor intensity at the 6-mon evaluation (DWM = dried whole milk).

- **Sylvester Test:** Lipid is held at 100°C in a closed vessel and the pressure depression, which is a result of the decline in oxygen concentration due to the reaction between oxygen and fat, is monitored to determine the IPd.
- **FIRA-Astell Apparatus:** This apparatus, developed by the Leatherhead Food Research Association and commercially manufactured and marketed by Astell Company, is an improved and automated version of the Sylvester test. However, this equipment is no longer commercially available.
- **Rancimat:** Oxidation is carried out in the Rancimat (Metrohm, Herisau, Switzerland) at very high temperatures (>100°C) by bubbling air through the liquid (molten) lipid. The effluent gas containing secondary oxidation products is fed into a tube containing distilled water, and the conductivity of the resulting solution is measured between two platinum electrodes. The electrical signal from the electrode is amplified and fed to a strip-chart recorder. The IPd determination is based on a sudden, large change in conductivity.
- **Oxidative Stability Instrument:** The OSI (Omnion, Inc., Rockland, MA) is basically a Rancimat from a different manufacturer.
- **Oxidograph:** The Oxidograph (Mikrolab Aarhus A/S, Hojbjerg, Denmark) is a new apparatus for measuring the IPd of fats. It works on a principle similar to that of the FIRA-Astell apparatus. A sample of lipid under 100% oxygen in

a reaction vessel is heated to a high temperature (>100°C) in an aluminum block. A transducer measures the pressure change inside the reaction vessel resulting from oxygen uptake by the lipid and sends signals to a chart recorder. The IPd determination is based on a sudden, comparatively large depression in pressure.

Drawbacks of ASLT Methods. In all ASLT methods measuring the IPd, oxidation is practically carried out at temperatures >100°C. Timms and Roupas (6) have studied the oxidation of milkfat, with and without adding butylated hydroxyanisole (BHA), at different temperatures ranging from 20 to 80°C, and have shown a distinct discontinuity in the Arrhenius plots at approximately 60°C. The activation energies above and below 60°C are different, regardless of the presence or absence of BHA, which indicates a change in the milkfat oxidation reaction pathway at approximately 60°C. A change in the lipid oxidation reaction order is also possible at temperatures >60°C.

In a series of chemical reactions leading to a final product, the rate of formation of the final product or the overall reaction rate can be determined by one or two reactions in the reaction pathway. There are several reaction steps with different rate constants and activation energies in the lipid oxidation pathway (7). In a review of the influence of temperature on the ASLT of lipids, Kochhar (8) has suggested that, at ambient and subambient temperatures, the rate-limiting reaction is the propagation reaction:

$$ROO^{\bullet} + RH \rightarrow ROOH + R^{\bullet}$$

and that, at high temperatures, a different reaction:

$$ROO^{\bullet} + C{=}C \rightarrow ROO\text{-}C\text{-}C^{\bullet}$$

dominates the rate of chain propagation.

When all of the above factors are considered, the IPd measurements made at temperatures >60°C may not be relevant to the shelf-life of lipid under ambient storage temperatures. This led to the investigation of the oxygen consumption methodology as an alternative method for the shelf-life prediction of lipids.

Application of the Oxygen Consumption Methodology to Lipids

AMF was selected as the lipid substrate for evaluating the oxygen consumption methodology. The objectives of this preliminary investigation were (i) feasibility assessment, and (ii) correlation of the oxygen consumption rate with the other generated data.

Five good and poor (i.e., oxidized) quality AMF or decolorized AMF samples were subjected to the initial investigation of the oxygen consumption rate of lipids.

Each lipid sample was packed under atmospheric air in glass vials in duplicate, sealed with crimp-top septa, wrapped with aluminum foil to avoid exposure to light (see Fig. 21.5), and stored at 40°C in an incubator. The decline in the head-space oxygen content was monitored during storage.

The milkfat samples were evaluated for flavor and odor using a minimum of two expert panelists. The temperature of the milkfat at the time of flavor evaluation was approximately 40°C. The panelists were requested to comment on any objectionable flavors and odors present in the milkfat samples.

The oxygen consumption rate of the oxidized AMF sample was very high compared with those of the good quality milkfat samples (see Table 21.3). An extremely high oxygen consumption rate was shown by the poor quality decolorized AMF sample. The oxygen consumption data were consistent with the quality of the five milkfat samples.

Historically, PV has been used as a measure of the flavor quality and, in some cases, the shelf-life of lipids. The milkfat samples stored at 40°C under atmospheric oxygen were tested for PV on d 5 and several subsequent times. The decolorized AMF sample that was extremely oxidized showed a much higher initial PV than the remaining samples (see Table 21.4). Two other samples exhibited very similar PV at d 5 (i.e., 0.62 and 0.67 mEq oxygen/kg lipid) regardless of the presence or absence of oxidized flavor. Therefore, the extent of peroxidation cannot be regarded as an acceptable method for discriminating between good and oxidized lipid samples. On some rare previous occasions, oxidized flavors have been detected in milkfat samples having PV of approximately 0.3 mEq oxygen/kg lipid (A.R. Keen, 1993, personal communication). Coppen (4) has also commented that the PV can

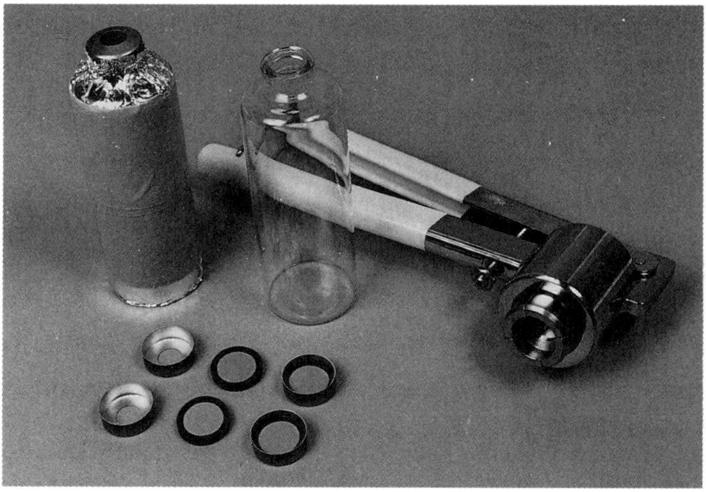

Fig. 21.5. A photograph showing an empty glass vial, crimp-top septa, crimper and a vial wrapped first with aluminum foil and then with masking tape.

TABLE 21.3
Oxygen Consumption Rates of Anhydrous Milkfat (AMF) Stored under Atmospheric Air at 40°C

Sample	Oxygen consumption rate [µL/(d • 35 g lipid)]		
	Replicate 1	Replicate 2	Mean
AMF			
Good quality	4	7	6
Poor quality	36	46	41
Decolorized AMF			
Good quality 1	4	7	5
Good quality 2	5	14	9
Poor quality	74	90	82

be misleading and it is possible for a rancid sample to have a low PV. However, very similar trends between the rates of oxidized flavor development and peroxidation have been documented for DWM (3). Although the flavor data and oxygen consumption rates given in Table 21.4 show very similar trends, the peroxidation rates are not consistent with them. This is due solely to the poor quality or extremely oxidized sample of decolorized AMF. A good linear relationship (R^2 = 0.974) between the rates of oxygen consumption and peroxidation was observed when the data, excluding the anomalous case, were subjected to a regression analysis.

Hamilton (1) has stated that oxidized flavors are noticeable in lipids that have passed the induction point (IPt). It was not implied from this statement that oxidized flavors should be absent in fat that is yet to reach the IPt. However, the use of the IPt as a reference point by Hamilton leads to the presumption that the oxidized flavor development occurs in the vicinity of the IPt. Data from the literature

TABLE 21.4
Summary of Oxygen Consumption and Peroxidation Rates and Other Relevant Data for Milkfat Stored at 40°C under Atmospheric Air

Sample	PV units[a] at d 5	Peroxidation rate (PV units/d)	Off-flavor at d 0	Oxygen consumption rate [µL/(d • 35 g lipid)]
AMF[b]				
Good quality	0.31	41×10^{-3}	None	6
Poor quality	0.67	85×10^{-3}	Oxidized	41
Decolorized AMF				
Good quality 1	0.25	47×10^{-3}	None	5
Good quality 2	0.62	55×10^{-3}	None	9
Poor quality	1.65	39×10^{-3}	Extremely oxidized	82

[a]Peroxide value (PV) units = mEq oxygen/kg lipid.
[b]AMF = Anhydrous milkfat.

(4) suggest that the PV at the IPt is much higher (approximately 20 mEq oxygen/kg lipid) than the PV encountered in this study (see Table 21.4). Presumably none of the samples had reached the IPt even on d 65, when the final PV analyses were undertaken.

With the exception of the Schaal Oven test, all other ASLT methods, including the modern methods using automated apparatus such as the Rancimat or Oxidograph, base shelf-life prediction on IPd measurement. The data generated in this study indicate that the end of the shelf-life of milkfat with reference to oxidized flavor development is prior to the IPt. Therefore, the validity of shelf-life prediction methods that are based on the IPd is suspect.

The novel method for monitoring/predicting the shelf-life, which is based on the early stage oxygen consumption rate, does not require taking the substrate as far as the IPt. Theoretically, it should be feasible to predict the IPd by measuring the rate of oxygen consumption. Shelf-life in relation to oxidized flavor development in milkfat probably has no real link with the IPd.

Evaluation of the Performance of the Rancimat. The two AMF samples (i.e., good and poor quality) used in this study were also included in a simple exercise of evaluating the performance of the Rancimat. The timing of this evaluation coincided with the oxygen consumption study, and the Rancimat results along with other relevant data are given in Table 21.5.

There were obvious flavor differences between the two AMF samples. The poor quality sample had oxidized flavors at an easily recognizable intensity. The supplier of this sample also recognized the problem and identified it as "Oxidized AMF." Because oxidized lipids should not be used as ingredients in food manufacturing, with reference to consumer requirements, the poor quality sample had either reached or passed the end of its shelf-life at the time this study was initiated.

TABLE 21.5
Comparison of Rancimat Data with Rates of Oxygen Consumption and Peroxidation and Flavor Data

Sample	Rancimat IPd[a] (min)	Oxygen consumption rate at 40°C [μL/(d • 35 g lipid)]	Peroxidation rate at 40°C (PV units[b]/d)	Off-flavors on d 0
AMF[c]				
Good quality	192 (168,216)[d]	6	41×10^{-3}	None
Poor quality	208 (197,219)[d]	41	85×10^{-3}	Typical oxidized flavor

[a]IPd = Induction period.
[b]Peroxide value (PV) units = mEq oxygen/kg lipid.
[c]AMF = Anhydrous milkfat.
[d]Individual readings of duplicate measurements.

The rates of oxygen consumption and peroxidation confirmed the state of oxidation of the poor quality AMF sample.

However, the Rancimat data indicated similar oxidative stabilities for both samples, or perhaps even slightly greater oxidative stability for the oxidized AMF sample. That is, the Rancimat failed to recognize the oxidative status of the poor-quality AMF sample. Neither of the samples was expected to have reached the IPt. As previously discussed, the IPt probably has no relationship to oxidized flavor development, and the IPd measurement is not relevant to shelf-life prediction. These results confirm the unreliable nature of the Rancimat or any other ASLT method based on the principle of IPd measurement.

Improvements Made to the Oxygen Consumption Methodology

At the development stage of the oxygen consumption test, a number of difficulties were experienced with various types of septa. Poor resealability of the penetrations made by the syringe needle, oxygen consumption due to oxidation of the polymer material from which the septa were made, and lack of a tight seal around the lip of the glass vial were the major concerns. After a series of investigations, the suitability of *Gold seal septa with Pharma-Fix Liner* (Alltech Associates, Inc., Deerfield, IL) was established. These septa were:

- made of butyl rubber for good resealability of needle penetrations;
- their inside surface was lined with polytetrafluoroethylene (PTFE) for chemical inertness; and
- they had a built-in circumferential rubber ring to form a tight seal against the lip of the glass vial.

Another serious difficulty experienced was the interference due to a slower rate of decline in the oxygen content in empty glass vials used as blanks than in the glass vials containing lipids. The rate of decline in oxygen content in the blanks was substantially increased when the glass vials were acid washed with the intention of removing any traces of transition metal ions that could catalyze lipid oxidation. Brimberg (9), utilizing previously published literature, suggested that hydrogen free radicals formed by homolytic fission of water molecules adsorbed onto the active sites of the glass surface could react with oxygen to form hydrogen peroxide. The interference, caused by the activated sites of the glass wall, with the measurement of the oxygen consumption rate of lipids was practically eliminated by the use of brand new glass vials that had not been washed previously.

Effectiveness of Commercial Antioxidants

At this stage, considerable improvements to the oxygen consumption test methodology had been made. A study was undertaken using milkfat as the substrate to investigate the effectiveness of three commercial brands of antioxidants, two of them at two different concentrations. The milkfat samples incorporated with antioxidants were packed in vials under atmospheric oxygen and then stored at 40°C. The effectiveness of the antioxidants as measured from the reduction in oxygen consumption rates is shown in Table 21.6.

The antioxidant system containing ascorbyl palmitate (25%) as the active ingredient was very effective in retarding the oxidation of milkfat at both the concentrations tested. A similar effectiveness was shown by the antioxidant formulation containing a mixture of BHA (20%), propyl gallate (6%), and citric acid (4%). The antioxidant containing mixed tocopherols (70%) was not as effective, especially at the higher concentration. Although tocopherols are widely accepted as effective antioxidants, prooxidative effects of α-tocopherol in linoleic acid (10) and arachidonic acid (11) dispersed in aqueous media are well established. Hwang *et al.* (12) have shown prooxidative effects of α-tocopherol incorporated into squid visceral oil at concentrations ranging from 100 to 1000 ppm. The decline in antioxidative properties with increasing concentration of the mixed tocopherols (see Table 21.6) may be interpreted as a change of phase from antioxidative to prooxidative behavior.

The tocopherol content of the milkfat sample used in this study was not measured. The typical tocopherol content of milkfat is 33 ppm (range 25–55 ppm), nearly all of which is in the α-tocopherol form (A. MacGibbon, 1994, personal communication). In all cases except for the antioxidant containing mixed tocopherols, the endogenous α-tocopherol of the milkfat might have enhanced the activity of the added antioxidants through synergism. The protection provided by the antioxidants, except for the antioxidant containing mixed tocopherols, might have been less if the test substrate was devoid of its own antioxidants.

The two most effective antioxidants showed similar trends in a re-evaluation, based solely on the oxygen consumption rates, using a different milkfat sample as the substrate (see Table 21.7). However, a definite prooxidant behavior, with oxygen consumption rates greater than that of the control (i.e., no added antioxidant), was exhibited at both concentrations by the antioxidant containing mixed tocopherols. The prooxidant effect of the mixed tocopherols was even greater at the higher concentration.

According to Huang *et al.* (13), in most cases cited in the scientific literature in which prooxidant activity of high concentrations of α-tocopherol was established, the measurement of the extent of oxidation had been based on PV determination. When the influence of α-tocopherol on lipid oxidation was studied by incorporating different concentrations of α-tocopherol in tocopherol-stripped corn oil or corn-oil-in-water emulsion, Huang *et al.* (13) made conflicting observations depending on which oxidation product was measured to monitor oxidation. With reference to the formation of conjugated dienes, α-tocopherol exhibited prooxidant activity at concentrations of 500–1000 ppm. However, α-tocopherol at concentrations of 100–1000 ppm showed antioxidative activity when oxidation was monitored using hexanal data. The liberation of hexanal occurs at a later stage than the formation of conjugated dienes in the lipid oxidation reaction pathway; hence

TABLE 21.6
Evaluation of the Effectiveness of Commercial Brands of Antioxidants Using Milkfat as the Substrate

Antioxidant		Oxygen consumption rate at 40°C [μL/(d • 35 g lipid)]				
Active ingredient	Concentration of the active ingredient (ppm)	Replicate 1	Replicate 2	Mean	Reduction in oxygen uptake (%)	Oxidized flavor score[a] after 70 d at 40°C
None (control)	—	11.0	10.8	10.9	0	10
Ascorbyl palmitate	150	1.4	1.3	1.4	88	7
Ascorbyl palmitate	200	2.0	1.5	1.8	84	7
Mixed tocopherols	140	5.8	4.9	5.3	51	8
Mixed tocopherols	280	7.2	6.9	7.0	36	9
Mixture of BHA,[b] propyl gallate, and citric acid	64 19.2 12.8	1.7	1.8	1.8	84	6

[a]Flavor scores on 0–10 scale (where 0 = absent, 2 = threshold, 4 = weak, 6 = moderate, 8 = strong, 10 = intense) of two or more expert panelists.
[b]BHA = Butylated hydroxyanisole.

TABLE 21.7
Comparison of the Data Obtained for Two Experiments Evaluating Antioxidants

Antioxidant		Reduction in oxygen uptake (%)	
Active ingredient	Concentration (ppm)	Experiment 1	Experiment 2
None (control)	—	0	0
Ascorbyl palmitate	150	88	82
Ascorbyl palmitate	200	84	83
Mixed tocopherols	140	51	–4[a]
Mixed tocopherols	280	36	–13[a]
Mixture of BHA,[b] propyl gallate, and citric acid	64 19.2 12.8	84	91

[a]Negative values indicate oxygen uptake greater than that of the control.
[b]BHA = Butylated hydroxyanisole.

hexanal liberation may have a closer resemblance to the development of oxidized flavor. Based on this assumption, Huang *et al.* (13) suggested that high concentrations of tocopherol may have a desirable effect on flavor stability.

This hypothesis could have been verified if the milkfat samples that consumed more oxygen than the control (see Table 21.7) had been evaluated for flavor. However, the flavor data for Experiment 1 on antioxidants (see Table 21.6) showed an increase in the oxidized flavor intensity as the concentration of mixed tocopherols was increased. This observation was consistent with the oxygen consumption data. The observation of decreasing antioxidant activity with increasing tocopherol concentration generates some doubts about the hypothesis of Huang *et al.* (13).

Conclusions

All of the data from studies on DWM and milkfat showed that early stage oxygen consumption evaluation methodology is very effective for the prediction of the shelf-life of lipids (anhydrous) or lipid-containing dehydrated foods. Because it is based on simple but proven scientific principles, the oxygen consumption methodology should also be applicable for the oxidative stability assessment of a large variety of lipids and lipid-containing dehydrated foods in which microbial spoilage is not an issue. Examples of these foods include vegetable oils of different origin, biscuits, chocolates, potato chips, cheese-based and other snack foods, peanuts and other prepared nutty foods, spray-dried cheese powders, spray-dried soup products, and dehydrated fish and meat products. This method may also be applicable to lipid-containing medium or high moisture food products in which microbial spoilage is not the dominant mode of deterioration as a consequence of sterilization or UHT treatment to curtail microbial growth.

Acknowledgments

The technical assistance of Mr. A.H. Dodge and valuable discussions with Dr. A.R. Keen are greatly appreciated.

References

1. Hamilton, R.J. (1989) in *Rancidity in Foods* (Allen, J.C., and Hamilton, R.J., eds.), 2nd edn., Elsevier Applied Science, London, pp. 1–21.
2. Quast, D.G., and Karel, M. (1972) *J. Food Sci. 37*, 584.
3. Wewala, A.R., and Dowland, N.H. (1990) in *Brief Communications and Abstracts of Posters of the XXIII International Dairy Congress*, October 8–12, 1990, Montreal, Vol. 1, Canadian National Committee of the International Dairy Federation, Ottawa, p. 256.
4. Coppen, P.P. (1989) in *Rancidity in Foods* (Allen, J.C., and Hamilton, R.J., eds.), 2nd edn., Elsevier Applied Science, London, pp. 83–104.
5. Labuza, T.P., and Bergquist, S. (1983) *J. Food Sci. 48*, 712.
6. Timms, R.E., and Roupas, P. (1982) *Lebensmittel-Wissenschaft und Technologie 15*, 372.
7. Labuza, T.P. (1971) *CRC Crit. Rev. Food Technol. 2*, 355.
8. Kochhar, S.P. (1988) *Influence of Temperature on Accelerated Stability Testing of Oils and Fats: A Literature Survey, Scientific and Technical Surveys*, No. 161, Leatherhead Food Research Association, Leatherhead, Surrey.
9. Brimberg, U.I. (1993) *J. Am. Oil Chem. Soc. 70*, 249.
10. Cillard, J., Cillard, P., Cromier, M., and Girre, L. (1980) *J. Am. Oil Chem. Soc. 57*, 252.
11. Bazin, B.J., Cillard, J., Koskas, J.P., and Cillard, P. (1984) *J. Am. Oil Chem. Soc. 61*, 1212.
12. Hwang, L.S., Lin, C.-C., and Fujimoto, K. (1994) *INFORM 5*, 474.
13. Huang, S.-W., Frankel, E.N., and German, J.B. (1994) *INFORM 5*, 466.

Chapter 22

EPR Studies of Plant Polyphenols

W. Bors[a], C. Michel[a], K. Stettmaier[a], and W. Heller[b]

[a]Inst. Strahlenbiologie; and [b]Inst. Biochemische Pflanzenpathologie, GSF Forschungszentrum für Umwelt und Gesundheit Neuherberg, D-85764 Oberschleissheim, Germany.

Introduction

Plant polyphenols are secondary metabolites comprising such diverse structures as phenolic acids (1), hydroxycoumarins (2–4), hydroxylated anthraquinones (5–8), anthrones (9), xanthones (10,11), the large group of flavonoids (12), and the rather unusual macrocyclic bis-biphenyls (e.g., marchantins) from liverwort (13). To a large extent, substances belonging to each of these structural groups have been shown to act as antioxidants or cytotoxic agents.

The basic mechanisms for antioxidant and cytotoxic activities involve the formation of radicals derived from these polyphenols, i.e., semiquinones or, more generally, aroxyl radicals. This is a consequence of scavenging of oxygen radicals, most likely peroxyl radicals, as the predominant chain carriers during lipid peroxidation (14–16):

$$Ph(OH)O^- + ROO^\bullet + H^+ \rightarrow Ph(OH)O^\bullet + ROOH \qquad [1]$$

The cytotoxicity of such compounds, in contrast, might be explained by metal-catalyzed autoxidation of the polyphenol to form an aroxyl radical, which subsequently transfers an electron to oxygen to generate a superoxide anion and is oxidized to a quinone itself (17,18):

$$Ph(OH)O^- + Me^{n+} \rightarrow Ph(OH)O^\bullet + Me^{(n-1)+} \qquad [2]$$

$$Ph(OH)O^\bullet + O_2 \rightarrow Ph(=O)_2 + O_2^{\bullet-} + H^+ \qquad [3]$$

[where $Ph(OH)O^-$, $Ph(OH)O^\bullet$, and $Ph(=O)_2$ are phenolate, semiquinone, and quinone, respectively]. This process has been thoroughly investigated with flavonoids (19). While reaction [3] also occurs during the so-called "futile redox cycling" of quinones, e.g., anthracycline antitumor drugs (20–22), reaction [2], in effect, is the opposite because superoxide generation is initiated by an *oxidation* process.

While the kinetics of such reactions can be optimally investigated by applying the technique of pulse radiolysis with spectrophotometric observation (23,24), it is quite obvious that more detailed information on the structures of these polyphenol radicals can be obtained by the technique of electron paramagnetic (or spin) resonance (EPR/ESR) spectroscopy (25–27). Furthermore, the formation of oxygen radicals during autoxidation can be verified by EPR spectroscopy combined with the spin trapping technique (28). In this chapter we describe applications of both approaches during the study of plant polyphenols, focusing on our own work on flavonoids and marchantins.

Experimental

While most model phenolic compounds, plant phenolic acids, and quite a number of flavonoid aglycones can be purchased from commercial sources, others have been obtained as extracts from plants in a more or less purified state (as indicated below, contamination by other phenolic structures may hamper the identification of defined radical species considerably). Horseradish peroxidase, the enzyme of choice to generate aroxyl radicals *in situ*, is readily available.

EPR spectra of polyphenol radicals are generally recorded at about 9.7 GHz (X-Band). Two types of parameters are normally evaluated: (i) the coupling constants (hyperfine splitting constants), denoting the resonance interactions of the delocalized electron with neighboring atoms and (ii) the g-factor.

EPR Spectra of Polyphenol Aroxyl Radicals

Early studies generally resorted to autoxidation in alkaline solutions to form EPR-detectable radicals (29–31). In the case of simple caffeic acid (3,4-dihydroxycinnamic acid) derivatives, this yields quite distinct radical spectra which can be identified readily, enabling taxonomic screening of *Lycopodium* varieties for their content of these types of substances (30); in each case, however, only catechol structures in the form of their semiquinones can be recognized because phenoxyl radicals derived from monophenolic compounds are usually too unstable and thus are produced at steady-state concentrations which are too low for EPR spectroscopy.

Flavonoids (Scheme 22.1) have similarly been investigated by EPR after autoxidation in strongly alkaline solutions, adding up to 80% DMSO to further stabilize the radicals (31). The coupling constants measured in this investigation generally pointed to the catechol group in the B-ring as the predominant radical-generating site. In the case of (+)-catechin, further hydroxylation in the 2′ and 6′ positions occurred upon autoxidation, and these secondary radicals were also identified by EPR spectroscopy (32). The 2,3-*cis* configuration, (-)-epicatechin, forms unstable intermediates, and only the final rearrangement products, catechinic acid semiquinones, are observed (32). Two flavanones, besides 10 hydroxycoumarin derivatives, were the subject of an EPR study, in which the phenols were oxidized by Ce^{4+} in acidic solutions (2). Under these conditions, aroxyl radicals are produced which are not necessarily *o*- or *p*-semiquinones. A considerable number of synthetic flavonoids with B-ring pyrogallol structure were studied by Jensen in his thesis (33), again using alkaline autoxida-

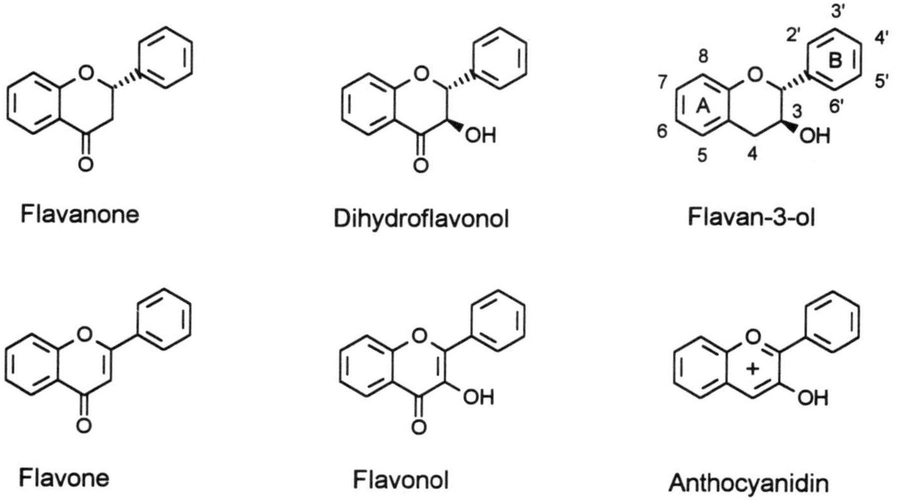

Scheme 22.1

tion. The data are listed in a very comprehensive handbook on EPR spectra of quinone- and quinol-derived radicals (34) and are therefore not presented in Table 22.1. A recent study on synthetic flavonoids with B-ring pyrogallol structure also applied autoxidation in alkaline solutions to generate the radicals (35).

To avoid unphysiological pH-conditions, we decided to perform the horseradish peroxidase/ hydrogen peroxide reaction in slightly alkaline solutions (pH 8.5, which still kept the compounds in solution) to generate the flavonoid aroxyl radicals *in situ* (36) (Fig. 22.1). We could basically confirm the coupling constants reported by Kuhnle *et al.* (31) (Table 22.1), thus verifying the B-ring catechol group as the principal radical site. Yet, the data were unequivocal only for the flavanones and dihydroflavonols investigated. Flavones and flavonols, whose 2,3-double bond enables strong electron delocalization over all three ring systems (24), exhibited unstable radical structures. During the recording period or after longer reaction times, the spectra of some of the flavonol-derived radicals changed considerably, indicating conversion of the primarily formed radicals, and thus making identification of individual radicals rather difficult (see Table 22.1). This dynamic behavior is demonstrated for quercetin in Fig. 22.2: only very rapid scanning reveals the distinct spectrum of the B-ring semiquinone, whereas normal scanning speed for higher resolution merely reflects an unidentifiable mixture of different radical species.

Applying the technique of "spin stabilization" to the EPR investigations of flavonoids, i.e., complexing the semiquinone structures with Zn^{2+} or Mg^{2+}, gave results in contrast to those for catecholamines (37–40). As shown in Scheme 22.2, formation of this complex may stabilize the semiquinone radical structure. The consequence for some flavonoids, however, is an enhanced nucleophilic attack leading to the dissociation of the C2-C1' bond (36). In contrast to our results, an earlier study

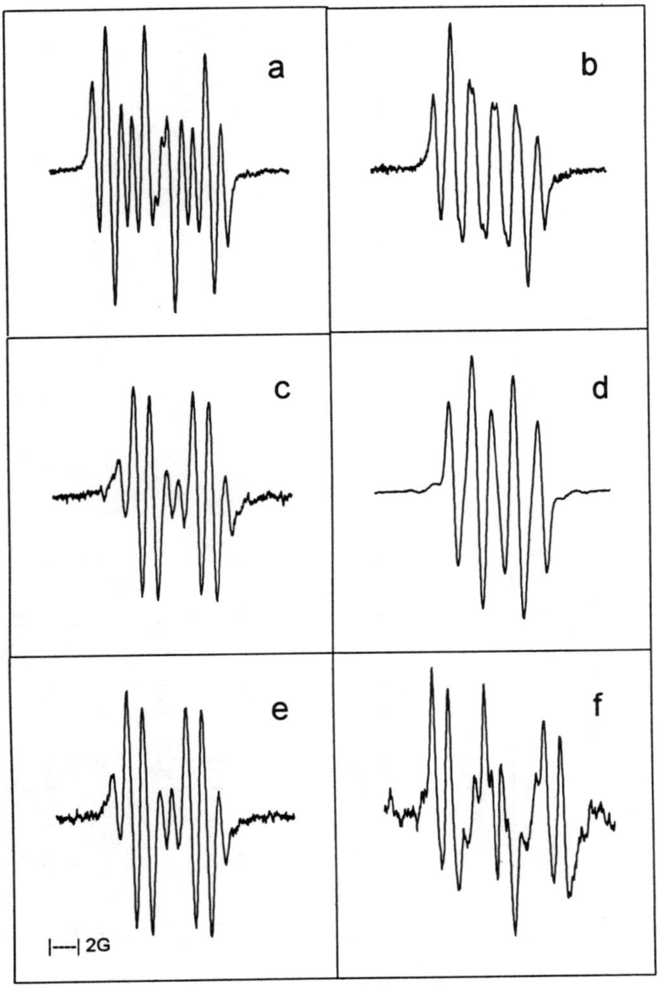

Fig. 22.1. EPR spectra of flavonoid semiquinones (radicals generated by horseradish peroxidase/hydrogen peroxide at about pH 8.5; concentration of substrates 0.1 mM, HRP 6900 units/mL, H_2O_2 1 mM; EPR settings: modulation amplitude 0.4G, scan time 84 s). (A) eriodictyol, (B) luteolin, (C) dihydrofisetin, (D) fisetin, (E) dihydroquercetin, (F) quercetin.

reported the stabilization of the semiquinone of myricetin in the presence of Mg^{2+} g (41).

Because both flavonoid and ascorbate radicals can be easily monitored by EPR spectroscopy and the interaction of these redox-active compounds is kinetically highly complex (42), we were prompted to study these reactions by both

TABLE 22.1
Coupling Constants of Flavonoid Radicals

	Substitution pattern								Coupling constant [G][a]								
Name	3	5	6	7	2′	3′	4′	5′	a_2	a_3	a_5	a_6	a_8	a_2'	a_5'	a_6'	Ref.
Flavan:																	
Catechin[b]	OH	OH	H	OH	H	OH	OH	H	1.9	—	—	—	—	1.23	1.08	3.45	31
Flavanones:																	
Chrysin[c]	H	OH	H	OH	H	H	H	H	—	0.1	—	0.82	1.13	—	—	—	2
Eriodictoyl[b]	H	OH	H	OH	H	OH	OH	H	2.25	—	—	—	—	1.2	1.08	3.4	31
Eriodictoyl[d]	H	OH	H	OH	H	OH	OH	H	2.3	—	—	—	—	0.8	0.8	3.5	34
Hesperidin[c]	H	OH	H	Orut[c]	H	H	OCH3	H	—	0.15	—	0.9	1.15	—	—	—	2
Dihydroflavonols:																	
Dihydrofisetin[b]	OH	H	H	OH	H	OH	OH	H	1.15	—	—	—	—	1.13	1.05	3.4	31
Dihydrofisetin[d]	OH	H	H	OH	H	OH	OH	H	0.9	—	—	—	—	0.9	0.9	3.4	34
Dihydroquercetin[b]	OH	OH	H	OH	H	OH	OH	H	1.2	—	—	—	—	1.15	1.08	3.4	31
Dihydroquercetin[d]	OH	OH	H	OH	H	OH	OH	H	0.9	—	—	—	—	0.9	0.9	3.4	34
Dihydrobinetin[b]	OH	H	H	OH	H	OH	OH	OH	1.55	—	—	—	—	0.825	—	0.825	31
Flavons:																	
Substance 8[f]	H	H	H	H	OH	OH	OH	H	—	0.2	—	—	—	—	0.82	4.85	33
Luteolin[b]	H	OH	H	OH	H	OH	OH	H	—	1.25	—	—	—	1.6	1.4	2.6	31
Luteolin[d]	H	OH	H	OH	H	OH	OH	H	—	1.4	—	—	—	1.0	1.0	2.8	34
Substance 7(a)[f]	H	OH	H	OH	OH	OH	OH	H	—	0.25	—	—	—	—	0.85	5.0	33

Flavonols:																	
Fisetin[b]	OH	H	H	OH	H	OH	OH	H	—	—	0.25	—	—	1.4	0.75	2.75	31
Fisetin[d]	OH	H	H	OH	H	OH	OH	H	—	—	—	—	—	1.4	1.4	2.4	34
Rutin	Orut[e]	OH	H	OH	H	OH	OH	H	—	—	—	—	—	0.95	1.05	3.0	†
3-Methylquercetin[b]	OCH_3	OH	H	OH	H	OH	OH	H	—	—	—	—	—	1.4	1.4	2.8	31
5-Methylquercetin[b]	OH	OCH_3	H	OH	H	OH	OH	H	—	—	—	—	—	1.4	0.75	2.75	31
7-Methylquercetin[b]	OH	OH	H	OCH3	H	OH	OH	H	—	—	—	—	—	1.45	0.7	2.8	31
Quercetin[b,g]	OH	OH	H	OH	H	OH	OH	H	—	—	—	—	—	1.45	0.7	2.7	31
Robinetin[b]	OH	H	H	OH	H	OH	OH	OH	—	—	0.2	1.12	1.08	0.92	—	0.92	31
Myricetin[b]	OH	OH	H	OH	H	OH	OH	OH	—	—	—	—	0.95	—	—	0.95	31
Substance 7(b)[f]	OH	OH	H	OH	OH	OH	OH	H	—	—	—	—	—	—	0.85	5.0	33

[a]Subscripts of the coupling constants denote the hydrogen atoms at the respective C-atoms—the assignments of a_2' and a_5' are interchangeable (31).
[b]Radicals produced by autoxidation in strongly alkaline solutions (62 mM NaOH) of 4:1 dimethylsulfoxide/water (31).
[c]Radicals produced by Ce^{4+} oxidation in acidic solution (2).
[d]Results from oxidation by horseradish peroxidase/hydrogen peroxide at pH 8.5–9.0 (34).
[e]Rut = rutinose (rhamnosyl-glucose).
[f]Radicals from synthetic flavonoids produced by alkaline autoxidation at pH 9 (33).
[g]Corresponding data for quercetin from our own investigations are not listed, as at least three different radical spectra have been observed [cf. Ref. (34), Fig. 22.2].
†, this work.

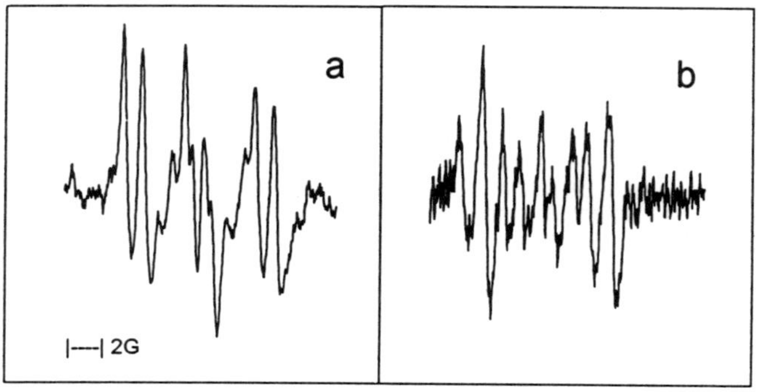

Fig. 22.2. EPR spectra of quercetin aroxyl radicals: (A) scan time 2.5 s, (B) scan time 84 s (for other conditions, see Fig. 22.1).

pulse radiolysis and EPR spectroscopy. The EPR studies allowed us to verify that even fast radical-radical recombination reactions are reversible and regenerate radicals on the EPR time-scale (43):

$$Fl(=O)_2 + AscH^- \rightarrow Fl(OH)O^\bullet + Asc^{\bullet-} \quad [4]$$

$$DHA + Fl(OH)O^- \rightarrow Fl(OH)O^\bullet + Asc^{\bullet-} \quad [5]$$

Due to the very rapid scavenging of the respective radicals by the excess of the reduced reactant, i.e.:

$$Fl(OH)O^\bullet + AscH^- \rightarrow Fl(OH)O^- + Asc^{\bullet-} + H^+ \quad [6]$$

$$Asc^{\bullet-} + Fl(OH)O^- + H^+ \rightarrow AscH^- + Fl(OH)O^\bullet \quad [7]$$

following reactions [4] and [5], respectively, either the flavonoid or the ascorbate radical should be observable exclusively; however, this was not consistently the case.

Starting from dehydroascorbate (DHA) and a flavonoid phenolate anion, reaction [5] occurred only with some flavonoids without any obvious correlation to struc-

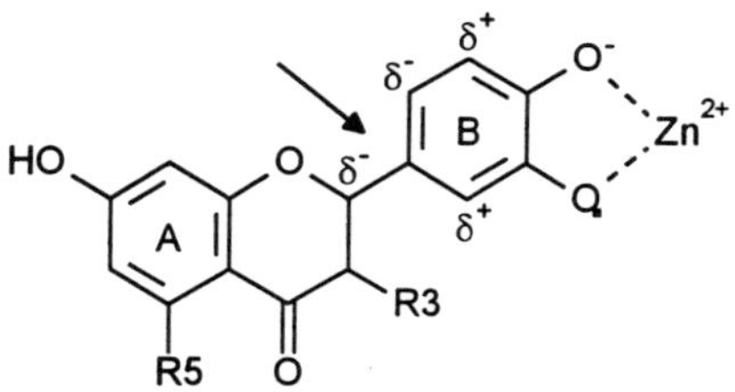

Scheme 22.2.

ture or redox potential (42). The presence of flavonoid quinones, inferred in reaction [4], is only circumstantial, and we had to resort to model naphtho- and anthraquinones to observe the ascorbate radical, in analogy to the experiments of Pethig *et al.* (44). Despite the ambiguity concerning "$Fl(=O)_2$" in reaction [4], it was interesting to note that for those flavonoids not capable of forming B-ring *o*-quinones, e.g., apigenin, kaempferol, and morin, formation of the ascorbate radical was far more pronounced and lasted over longer periods of time (43). Further complications in these investigations arose from the presence of hydrogen peroxide affecting the kinetics of the respective radicals as implicated by the effect of catalase in this system. Furthermore, the formation of ascorbate radicals may be stimulated by some flavonoids in the absence of peroxidase by an as yet unknown mechanism (43).

Recently, we investigated novel catecholic plant phenols, marchantins, and related substances isolated from liverwort (45) (see Scheme 22.3). Marchantins exist as nonplanar macrocyclic ring systems in which four aromatic rings are linked together by both ether and ethyl bridges (13,46). When the radicals were generated by horseradish peroxidase/hydrogen peroxide at pH 8.5, only the EPR spectrum of the semiquinone radical of the model lignan compound nordihydroguaiaretic acid could be

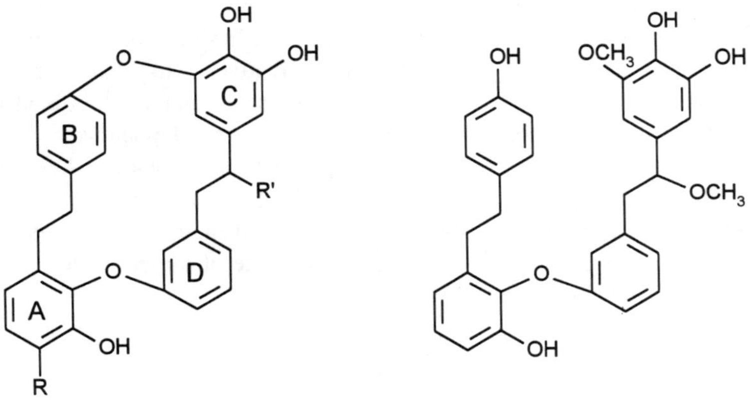

Marchantins* Paleatin B

*Substance	R	R′
Marchantin A	H	H
Marchantin B	OH	H
Marchantin D	H	OH

Scheme 22.3.

assigned unambiguously. For marchantin B, which contains two catechol moieties in the opposite rings A and C (see Scheme 22.3), evaluation of the radical structure proved considerably more difficult because several spectra seemed to be superimposed upon each other. Marchantins A, D have only one catechol group and paleatin B a methoxy group in the *o*-position to this catechol group instead of an ether bond with the neighboring dihydrostilbene moiety and represents an open-chain structure. All three compounds gave rather unspecific EPR spectra which could not be properly analyzed. Complex formation with Zn^{2+} was also attempted and found to be successful only for those compounds which had already shown a reasonable spectral resolution in the absence of the complexing ion (45).

EPR/Spin Trapping Results

As mentioned earlier, EPR spectroscopy of spin adducts obtained from unstable radical intermediates, e.g., $O_2^{\bullet-}$, allowed us to study the autoxidation mechanism as proposed in reaction [3]. This approach was attempted repeatedly with flavonoids, and the interpretations of the spin adduct spectra of the oxygen-derived radicals were generally in agreement with this mechanism (41,47). Moreover, the autoxidative and cytotoxic effectiveness correlated well with the electrochemical redox potentials (18). In a similar experiment, we found traces of the OH-adduct of DMPO after autoxidation of marchantin B (45). This compound has previously been shown to be cytotoxic (13) and to be one of the most effective antioxidative agents in an arachidonic acid autoxidation assay (48). Thus, the mechanism outlined in reactions [2] and [3] may also be valid for this class of plant polyphenols.

The technique of EPR/spin trapping was also applied to study the scavenging of reactive oxygen species by polyphenols (49–52), but due to the difficulties inherent with quantitation of EPR data, this yielded merely a phenomenological description (53,54). Nevertheless, reliable knowledge of radical yields is essential to calculate kinetic parameters.

Prospects

It is obvious that EPR spectroscopy is well suited for identification of the structures of semiquinone radicals derived from plant polyphenols, provided these radicals are the predominant species occurring and are sufficiently stable. Concerning *in vivo* studies, the technique is feasible for simple phenolic acids (30) and hydroxylated naphthoquinones (55) even in crude plant extracts. Screening of plant apoplasts or vacuoles for other polyphenol-derived radical species and possibly monitoring their appearance after stress events (56,57), however, is a difficult task, fraught with artifacts. Thus, few attempts were undertaken to demonstrate that polyphenol radical species may be detected by the EPR technique in plants themselves (58,59), and identification, structural, functional or site-specific correlations remain ambiguous. Nevertheless, taking the known limitations into consideration,

EPR spectroscopy may be developed into a useful method to study plant polyphenol reactions *in situ.*

References

1. Pratt, D.E. (1993) *Toxical. Industr. Health 9*, 63.
2. Dixon, W.T., Moghimi, M., and Murphy, D. (1975) *J. Chem. Soc., Perkin II,* 101.
3. Hoult, J.R.S., Moroney, M., and Paya, M. (1994) *Meth. Enzymol. 234*, 443.
4. Paya, M., Goodwin, P.A., Delasheras, B., and Hoult, J.R.S. (1994) *Biochem. Pharmacol. 48*, 445.
5. Ashnagar, A., Bruce, J.M., Dutton, P.L., and Prince, R.C. (1984) *Biochim. Biophys. Acta 801*, 351.
6. Dabestani, R., Hall, R.D., Sik, R.H., and Chignell, C.F. (1990) *Photochem. Photobiol. 52*, 961.
7. Mian, M., Fratta, D., Rainaldi, G., Simi, S., Mariani, T., Benetti, D., and Gervasi, P.G. (1991) *Anticancer Res. 11*, 1071.
8. Malterud, K.E., Farbrot, T.L., Huse, A.E., and Sund, R.B. (1993) *Pharmacology 47*, 77.
9. Hayden, P.J., Free, K.E., and Chignell, C.F. (1994) *Mol. Pharmacol. 46*, 186.
10. Minami, H., Kinoshita, M., Fukuyama, Y., Kodama, M., Yoshizawa, T., Sugiura, M., Nakagawa, K., and Tago, H. (1994) *Phytochemistry 36*, 501.
11. Ashida, S., Noguchi, S.F., and Suzuki, T. (1994) *J. Am. Oil Chem. Soc. 71*, 1095.
12. Bors, W., Heller, W., Michel, C., and Stettmaier, K. (1996) in *Handbook on Antioxidants* (Cadenas, E., and Packer, L., eds.), Marcel Dekker, New York, pp. 409–466.
13. Asakawa, Y. (1990) in *Bryophytes: Their Chemistry and Chemical Taxonomy* (Zinsmeister, H.D., and Mues, R., eds.), Clarendon Press, Oxford, pp. 369–410.
14. Hsieh, R.J. and Kinsella, J.E. (1989) *Adv. Food Nutr. Res. 33*, 233.
15. Bors, W., Erben-Russ, M., Michel, C., and Saran, M. (1990) in *Free Radicals, Lipoproteins & Membrane Lipids* (Crastes de Paulet, A., Dousté-Blazy, L., and Paoletti, R., eds.), Plenum Press, New York, pp. 1–16.
16. Barclay, L.R.C. (1993) *Can. J. Chem. 71*, 1.
17. Cohen, G., Heikkila, R.E., and MacNamee, D. (1974) *J. Biol. Chem. 249*, 2447.
18. Aver'yanov, A.A. (1981) *Biochemistry USSR 46*, 210.
19. Hodnick, W.F., Milosavljevic, E.B., Nelson, J.H., and Pardini, R.S. (1988) *Biochem. Pharmacol. 37*, 2607.
20. Kalyanaraman, B., Perez-Reyes, E., and Mason, R.P. (1980) *Biochim. Biophys. Acta 630,* 119.
21. Lown, J.W., and Chen, H.H. (1981) *Can. J. Chem. 59*, 390.
22. Powis, G., Hodnett, E.M., Santone, K.S., See, K.L., and Melder, D.C. (1987) *Cancer Res. 47*, 2363.
23. Patterson, L.K. (1987) in *Radiation Chemistry. Principles & Applications* (Farhataziz and Rodgers, M.A.H., eds.), V.C.H. Verlag, Weinheim, pp. 65–96.
24. Bors, W., Heller, W., Michel, C., and Saran, M. (1990) *Meth Enzymol. 186*, 343.
25. Mason, R.P., and Chignell, C.F. (1982) *Pharmacol. Rev. 33*, 189.
26. Klotz, D., Jülich, T., Wax, G., and Stegmann, H.B. (1989) in *Landolt-Börnstein Zahlenwerte und Funktionen aus Naturwissenschaften und Technik, Neue Serie* (Madelung, O., ed.), Vol. 17g, Springer, Berlin, pp. 69–394.

27. Kalyanaraman, B. (1990) *Meth Enzymol.186*, 333.
28. Schaich, K.M., and Borg, D.C. (1980) in *Autoxidation in Food and Biological Systems* (Simic, M.G., and Karel, M., eds.), Plenum Press, New York, pp. 45–70.
29. Holton, D.M., and Murphy, D. (1980) *J. Chem. Soc., Perkin II*, 1757.
30. Pedersen, J.A., and Ollgaard, B. (1982) *Biochem. System. Ecol. 10*, 3.
31. Kuhnle, J.A., Windle, J.J., and Waiss, A.C. (1969) *J. Chem. Soc. B*, 613.
32. Jensen, O.N., and Pedersen, J.A. (1983) *Tetrahedron 39*, 1609.
33. Jensen, O.N. (1982) Ph.D. Thesis, University of Aarhus, Denmark.
34. Pedersen, J.A. (1985) *Handbook of EPR Spectra from Quinones and Quinols*, CRC Press, Boca Raton.
35. Cotelle, N., Bernier, J.L., Hénichart, J.P., Catteau, J.P., Gaydou, E., and Wallet, J.C. (1992) *Free Radical Biol. Med. 13*, 211.
36. Bors, W., Heller, W., Michel, C., and Stettmaier, K. (1993) in *Free Radicals: From Basic Science to Medicine* (Poli, G., Albano, M., and Dianzani, M.U., eds.), Birkhäuser, Basel, pp. 374–387.
37. Stegmann, H.B., Bergler, H.U., and Scheffler, K. (1981) *Angew. Chem. 93*, 398.
38. Felix, C.C., and Sealy, R. (1981) *Photochem. Photobiol. 34*, 423.
39. Stegmann, H.B., Dao-Ba, H., Stolze, K., and Scheffler, K. (1985) *Z. Anal. Chem. 322*, 430.
40. Kalyanaraman, B., Premovic, P.I., and Sealy, R.C. (1987) *J. Biol. Chem. 262*, 11080.
41. Hodnick, W.F., Kalyanaraman, B., Pritsos, C.A., and Pardini, R.S. (1988) in *Oxygen Radicals in Biology and Medicine* (Simic, M.G., Taylor, K.A., Ward, J.F., and von Sonntag, C., eds.), Plenum Press, New York, pp. 149–152.
42. Bors, W., Michel, C., and Schikora, S. (1995) *Free Radical Biol. Med. 19*, 72.
43. Bors, W., Michel, C., and Stettmaier, K., in press.
44. Pethig, R., Gascoyne, P.R.C., McLaughlin, J.A., and Szent-Györgyi, A. (1983) *Proc. Natl. Acad. Sci. USA 80*, 129.
45. Schwartner, C., Michel, C., Stettmaier, K., Wagner, H., and Bors, W. (1996) *Free Radical Biol. Med. 20*, 237.
46. Taira, Z., Takei, M., Endo, K., Hashimoto, T., Sakiya, Y., and Asakawa, Y. (1994) *Chem. Pharmacol. Bull. 42*, 52.
47. Canada, A.T., Giannella, E., Nguyen, T.D., and Mason, R.P. (1990) *Free Radical Biol. Med. 9*, 441.
48. Schwartner, C., Bors, W., Michel, C., Müller-Jakic, B., Nenninger, A., Asakawa, Y., and Wagner, H. (1995) *Phytomedicine 2*, 113.
49. Zhao, B., Li, X., He, R., Cheng, S., and Wenjuan, X. (1989) *Cell Biophys. 14*, 175.
50. Sichel, G., Corsaro, C., Scalia, M., di Bilio, A.J., and Bonomo, R.P. (1991) *Free Radical Biol. Med. 11*, 1.
51. Culcasi, M., Pietri, S., Carrière, I., d'Arbigny, P., and Drieu, K. (1993) in *Ginkgo biloba Extract (EGb 761) as a Free Radical Scavenger* (Ferradini, C., Droy-Lefaix, M.T., and Christen, Y., eds.), Elsevier, Paris, pp. 153–162.
52. Okuda, T. (1993) in *Polyphenolic Phenomena* (Scalbert, A., ed.), INRA Editions, Paris, pp. 221–235.
53. Yordanov, N.D. (1994) *Appl. Magnet. Reson. 6*, 241.
54. Nagy, V. (1994) *Appl. Magnet. Reson. 6*, 259.
55. Pedersen, J.A. (1978) *Phytochemistry 17*, 775.

56. Heller, W., Rosemann, D., and Sandermann, H. Jr. (1991) in *Proc. 2. Statusseminar der PBWU zum Forschungsschwerpunkt 'Waldschäden'* (Reuther, M., Kirchner, M., and Rösel, K., eds.), GSF-Bericht 26, 173.
57. Heller, W., Ernst, D., Langebartels, C., and Sandermann, H. Jr. (1995) in *Polyphenols '94* (Brouillard, R., Jay, M., and Scalbert, A., eds.), INRA Editions, Paris, pp. 67–78.
58. Troup, G.J., Hutton, D.R., Hewitt, D.G., and Hunter, C.R. (1994) *Free Radical Res. 20*, 63.
59. Crawford, R.M.M., Lindsay, D.A., Walton, J.C., and Wollenweber-Ratzer, B. (1994) *Phytochemistry 37*, 979.

Chapter 23

Application of FTIR/ATR Differential Spectroscopy for Monitoring Oil Oxidation and Antioxidant Efficacy

J. Sedman, A.A. Ismail, A. Nicodemo, S. Kubow, and F.R. van de Voort

Department of Food Science and Agricultural Chemistry, Macdonald Campus of McGill University, Ste. Anne de Bellevue, Quebec, Canada.

Introduction

Mid-infrared (IR) spectroscopy is a simple, yet powerful, technique for the chemical characterization of fats and oils. Due to the wealth of detail in the IR spectra of fats and oils, IR spectroscopy can be used both to determine bulk properties, such as the iodine value and saponification number, and to monitor chemical changes taking place as an oil undergoes hydrogenation or oxidation. However, the only widespread application of IR spectroscopy in the analysis of fats and oils is the determination of *trans* content, which is an official method of the American Oil Chemists' Society (1). This may be largely attributed to the limited utility of IR spectroscopy as a routine analytical tool in the past due to both sample handling difficulties and the limitations of traditional dispersive IR instrumentation. During the past two decades, however, the practical capabilities of IR spectroscopy have been greatly extended as a result of the development of Fourier transform infrared (FTIR) spectroscopy together with advances in data analysis and sample handling techniques. As a result, a large number of the chemical methods routinely used in the analysis of fats and oils can potentially be replaced by FTIR methods (2). This chapter will describe the general utility of FTIR spectroscopy and the attenuated total reflectance (ATR) sampling technique in the analysis of fats and oils and will then focus on the application of FTIR/ATR differential spectroscopy in monitoring the oxidation of edible oils in the presence and absence of various antioxidants.

FTIR/ATR Spectroscopy

FTIR spectroscopy is based on interferometry and thus has a number of significant advantages over traditional dispersive infrared spectroscopy. These include: (i) a dramatic improvement in signal-to-noise ratio; (ii) a significant reduction in scan time (an FTIR spectrometer can record the entire spectrum of a sample in a 1-s scan); and (iii) higher energy throughput. FTIR spectroscopy also offers powerful data manipulation capabilities, such as spectral subtraction, co-addition of scans to improve signal-to-noise ratio, spectral smoothing and interpolation, baseline correction, resolution enhancement techniques for the separation of overlapping bands (e.g., Fourier self-deconvolution and derivative spectroscopy), and peak height/area measurements. In the past, the high cost of FTIR spectrometers impeded their use as a routine analytical tool. However, during the past five years, FTIR instrumentation has dropped into the price range of a quality ultraviolet-visible spectrophotometer with no sacrifice in performance.

Major advances in sample handling technology have taken place in conjunction with the development of FTIR spectroscopy. Among these is the development of the horizontal attenuated total reflectance (ATR) sampling accessory, which is schematically represented in Fig. 23.1. In an ATR measurement, the sample is placed in contact with a crystal of a high-refractive index material, known as an internal reflection element (IRE), and radiation from the infrared source is launched into the IRE at an angle such that it undergoes multiple internal reflection as it travels down the crystal (3). This gives rise to an evanescent wave at the surface of the IRE which decays exponentially as it propagates away from the surface of the IRE through the sample. The distance from the surface at which the intensity of the evanescent wave decays to $1/e$ (e = evenset wave) of its value at the surface is defined as the depth of penetration, d_p. The evanescent wave is attenuated by the absorption of radiation by species on or near the surface of the IRE. The measurement of this attenuation as a function of wavelength yields the infrared spectrum of these species. The effective pathlength in an ATR cell is given by the product of the number of internal reflections and the depth of penetration, d_p, given by:

$$d_p = \frac{\lambda}{2\pi n_1[\sin^2(\theta) - (n_2/n_1)]^{1/2}} \quad [1]$$

where λ is the wavelength of the radiation, n_1 is the refractive index of the IRE material, n_2 is the refractive index of the medium surrounding the IRE, and θ is the angle at which the incident light strikes the interface. The effective pathlength can thus be altered by varying the angle of incidence as well as by the choice of the IRE material; zinc selenide and germanium are the most common materials used. It should be noted that the depth of penetration, and hence the effective pathlength, increases on going from the high-frequency to the low-frequency end of the spectrum. Therefore, the relative intensities of the peaks in the ATR spectrum of a sample will not be the same as those in a spectrum recorded for the same sample in a transmission cell.

High-quality spectra can be obtained from edible oils applied directly in their neat form onto the ATR crystal, as illustrated in Fig. 23.2. Solid fats can be handled in an analogous manner if the ATR crystal is heated and thermostated to a temperature above the melting point of the fat. Thus, the ATR technique provides a simple means of obtaining FTIR spectra of fats and oils.

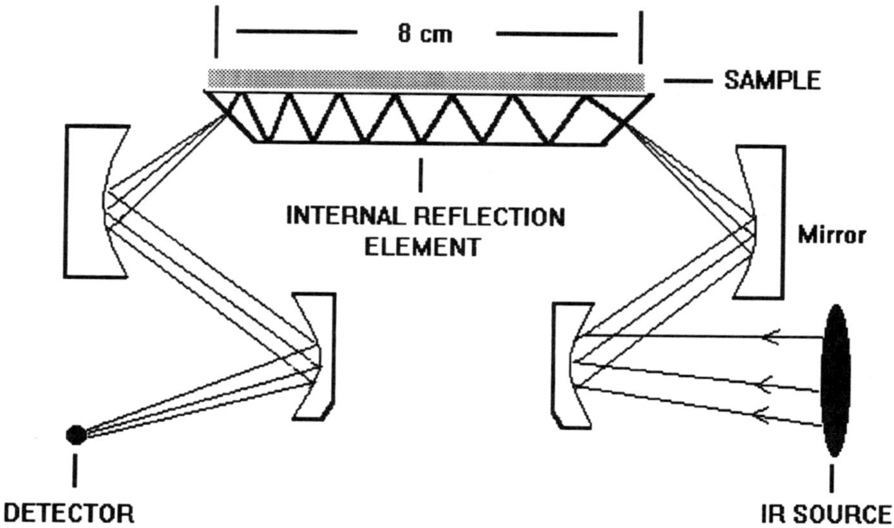

Fig. 23.1. Schematic diagram of a horizontal attenuated total reflectance (ATR) sampling accessory.

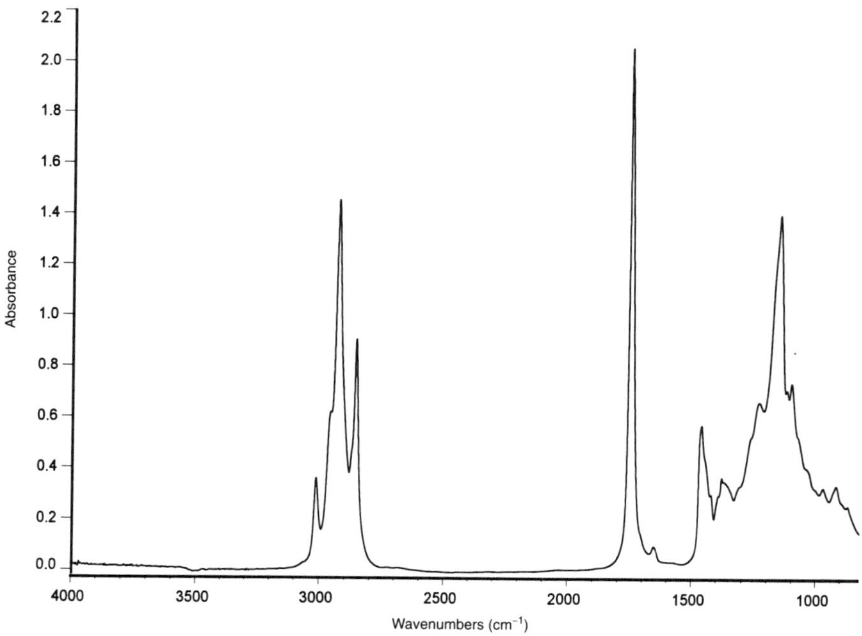

Fig. 23.2. FTIR/ATR spectrum of safflower oil recorded from the surface of a ZnSe crystal with θ = 45° and 8 internal reflections.

Applications of FTIR Spectroscopy in the Analysis of Fats and Oils

As mentioned above, the determination of *trans* content by IR spectroscopy is an AOCS official method for edible oils. The method is based on the measurement of the characteristic absorption of isolated *trans* bonds at 10.3 μ (967 cm^{-1}). While the earlier AOCS method employed a dispersive IR spectrometer, a number of researchers have described the advantages of employing FTIR spectrometers for this analysis (4–6). These include higher accuracy and a significant reduction in total analysis time (2.5 min/sample) in comparison with the traditional AOCS method, as well as amenability to automation.

Afran and Newbery (7) have demonstrated the use of FTIR/ATR spectroscopy to measure total unsaturation, and van de Voort *et al.* (8) have described an FTIR/ATR method for the simultaneous determination of both iodine value (IV) and saponification number (SN). In the latter work, calibration of the FTIR spectrometer was based on the partial-least-squares (PLS) regression technique (9) and the use of pure triglycerides as calibration standards, rather than preanalyzed oils. The calibration obtained was used to analyze commercially available fats and oils with a wide range of IV and SN values. The samples were analyzed in their neat form on a heated (65°C) ATR crystal; the time taken for analysis and prediction of both IV and SN was on the order of 2 min/sample, and the results were in good agreement with the chemically determined values for these samples. Subsequently, a similar method was developed for use with a flow-through transmission cell, and the system was recalibrated using PLS to provide results in terms of both % *cis* and % *trans* as well as IV and SN (10).

Another potential area of application of FTIR spectroscopy is in the assessment of oil quality. Lanser *et al.* (11) and Ismail *et al.* (12) have described FTIR methods for the determination of free fatty acids in crude and processed oils, respectively. Van de Voort *et al.* (13) have investigated the feasibility of employing FTIR spectroscopy to assess the oxidative status or forecast the oxidative stability of an oil. These authors constructed a spectral library by recording the FTIR spectra of oils spiked with various compounds representative of common oil oxidation products. *Tert*-butyl hydroperoxide was selected to represent hydroperoxides, the primary oxidation products of fats and oils. Alcohols, saturated aldehydes, and α,β-unsaturated aldehydes, which have all been reported as major secondary oxidation products (14), were all represented in the spectral library by C_6 homologues, with α,β,γ,δ-unsaturated aldehydes represented by *trans*, *trans*-2,4-decadienal, a major decomposition product found in oxidized polyunsaturated fats and oils. Although ketones are minor products in oxidized oils, a C_6 allylic ketone was included in the spectral library to investigate the extent of overlap between the aldehyde and ketone absorptions. Water and oleic acid were also included in view of their possible presence in oils, particularly under hydrolysis conditions. The functional group frequencies of these reference compounds are tabulated in Table 23.1, and the corresponding absorption bands are illustrated in Figs. 23.3 and 23.4. Examination of Table 23.1 shows that each of the various types of oxidation prod-

TABLE 23.1
Peak Positions of the Functional Group Absorptions of Reference Compounds Representative of Products Formed in Oxidized Oils

Compound	Vibration	Frequency (cm^{-1}) at peak maximum
Water	ν **OH**	3650 and 3550
	δ **HOH**	1625
Hexanol	ν R**OH**	3569
tert-Butyl hydroperoxide	ν RO**OH**	3447
Hexanal	ν R**HC**=O	2810 and 2712
	ν RH**C=O**	1727
2-Hexenal[a]	ν R**HC**=O	2805 and 2725
	ν RH**C=O**	1697
	ν R**C=C**H-HC=O	1640
	δ R**C=CH**-HC=O	974
2,4-Decadienal[a]	ν R**HC**=O	2805 and 2734
	ν RH**C=O**	1689
	ν R**C=C**H-HC=O	1642
	δ R**C=CH**-HC=O	987
4-Hexen-3-one[a]	ν R**C(=O)**HC=CHR	1703 and 1679
	ν RC(=O)H**C=C**HR	1635
	δ RC(=O)H**C=CH**R	972
Oleic acid	ν RCO**OH**	3310
	ν R**C(=O)**OH	1711

[a]All double bonds in the *trans* form.

ucts gives rise to discernible and characteristic absorptions in the FTIR spectrum. Similar absorption bands were detected in the spectra of oils oxidized under accelerated conditions and monitored in real time by FTIR spectroscopy (13). On the basis of the results of this study, the authors proposed a quantitative approach whereby the oxidative state of an oil could be determined through calibrations developed with oils spiked with appropriate compounds representative of the functional groups associated with typical oxidative end products. These concepts were subsequently put into practice with the development of a calibration for the determination of peroxide value (15), a chemical measure of hydroperoxides, representing the primary oxidation products which first appear when an oil undergoes oxidation. A similar approach is being taken to develop a parallel method for evaluating anisidine value, a measure of secondary oxidation products which arise subsequently as a consequence of hydroperoxide breakdown.

Monitoring of Oil Oxidation by FTIR/ATR Spectroscopy

FTIR/ATR spectroscopy has been shown (13) to provide a simple, convenient, and dynamic means for monitoring the chemical changes taking place as an oil undergoes oxidation. An FTIR/ATR oil oxidation experiment typically involves spreading the

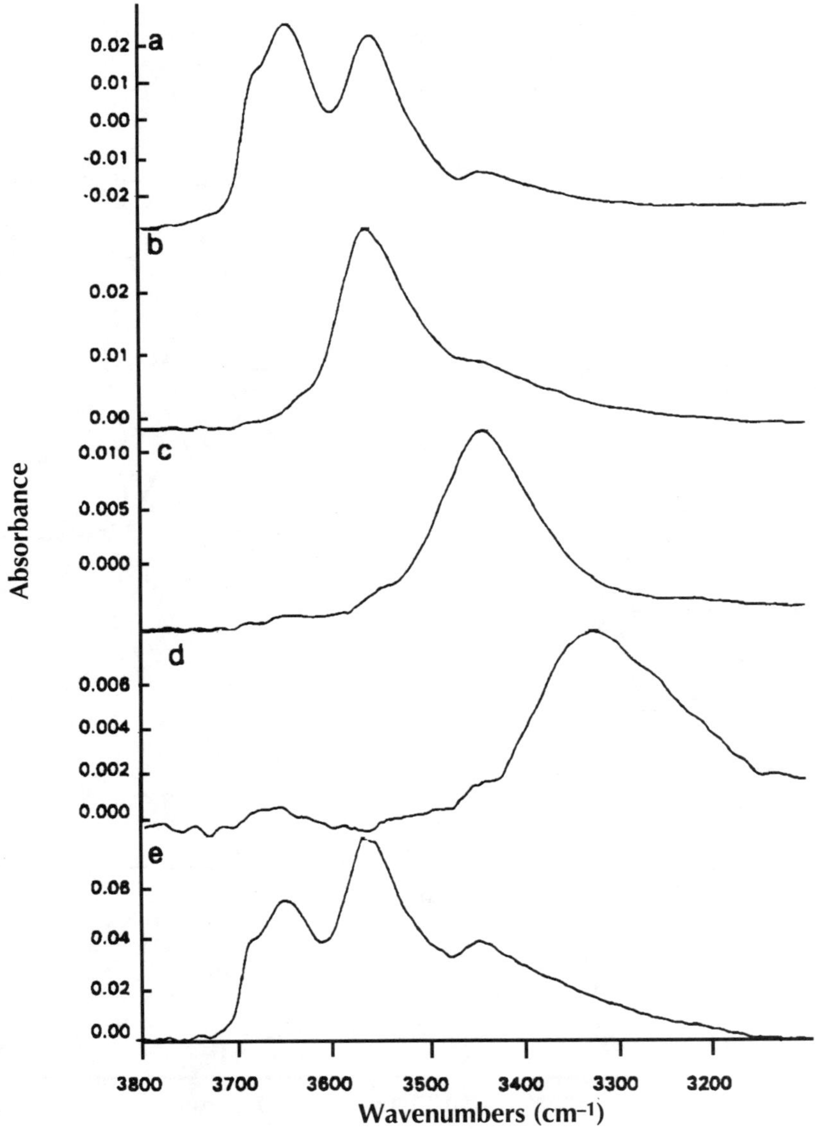

Fig. 23.3. The OH stretching region (3800–3100 cm^{-1}) in the FTIR/ATR spectra of oxidation reference compounds obtained by ratioing the single-beam spectrum of olive oil spiked with the reference compound against the single-beam spectrum of pure olive oil: (A) H_2O; (B) hexanol; (C) *tert*-butyl hydroperoxide; (D) oleic acid; (E) spectrum obtained by co-adding spectra A–D, illustrating band overlap in this region. All reference compounds were added at 2% (w/w), except for H_2O, which was added to saturation levels.

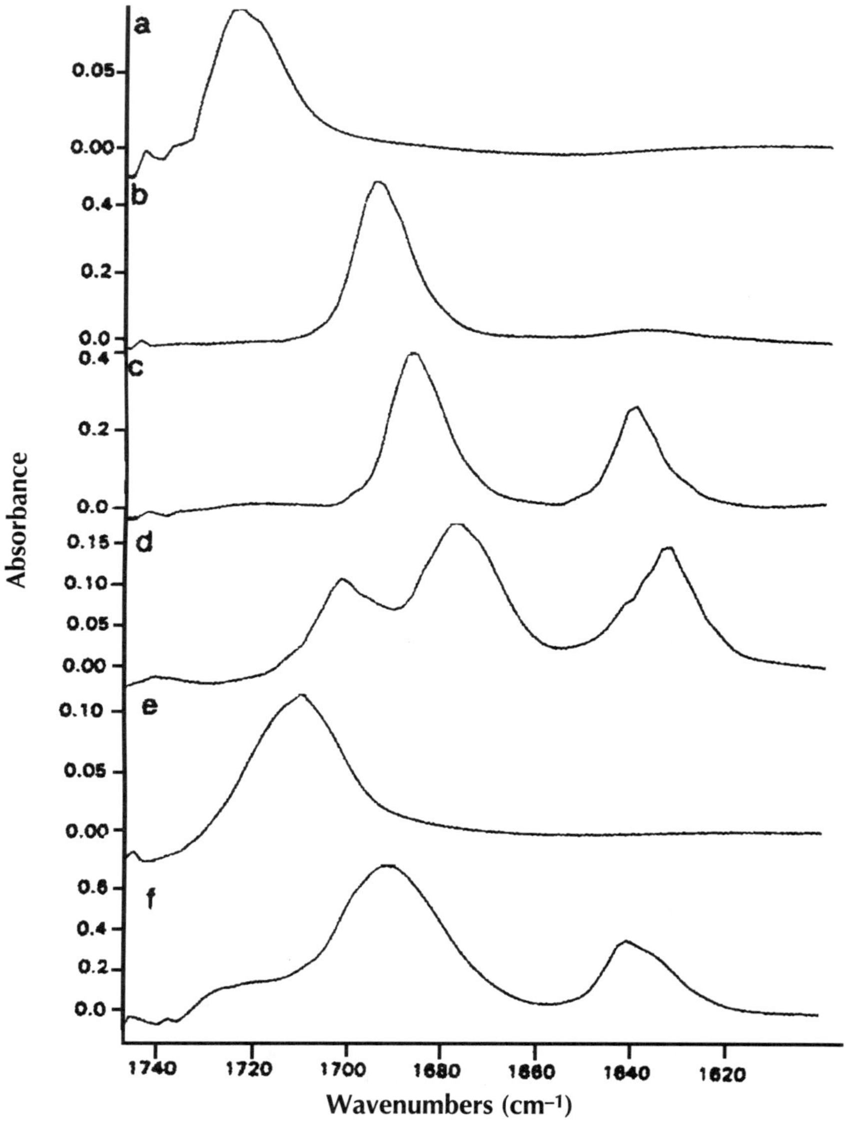

Fig. 23.4. The C=O stretching region (1750–1600 cm^{-1}) in the FTIR/ATR spectra of oxidation reference compounds obtained by ratioing the single-beam spectrum of olive oil spiked with the reference compound against the single-beam spectrum of pure olive oil: (A) hexanal; (B) *trans*-2-hexenal; (C) *trans, trans*-2,4-decadienal; (D) *trans*-4-hexen-3-one; (E) oleic acid; (F) spectrum obtained by co-adding spectra A–E, illustrating band overlap in this region. All reference compounds were added at 2% (w/w).

oil sample on the surface of a heated ATR crystal, where the oil will undergo accelerated oxidation due to the combination of higher temperature and the relatively large surface area of the sample exposed to air (see Fig. 23.1). One simply measures the changes in the FTIR spectrum of the oil as a function of time by means of spectral ratioing, which limits one's observations to the spectral changes taking place relative to the spectrum of the oil at time zero. The changes observed correspond primarily to the growth of absorption bands associated with primary and secondary oxidation products and the decrease in the characteristic absorption bands of *cis* double bonds. In the experiments described below, the spectrometer was programmed to automatically record and store spectra at 40-min intervals, measure absorbances at prespecified wavelengths, and accumulate these absorbance values, along with the time at which the spectrum was recorded, in a spreadsheet file for subsequent data analysis. A dynamic plot of absorbance values vs. time could also be displayed on screen during the course of the experiment, thus allowing real-time monitoring of oil oxidation.

For readers unfamiliar with FTIR spectroscopy, the technique of spectral ratioing, or what we term differential spectroscopy, which allows one to monitor only the *changes* in an oil as it undergoes oxidation, may require further explanation. The concept of spectral ratioing arises in FTIR spectroscopy because most FTIR spectrometers are single-beam instruments. In a single-beam instrument, the raw spectrum obtained for a sample (I_S) consists of the emittance spectrum of the infrared source on which are superimposed the absorption bands of the sample as well as those of air in the optical path. To eliminate the contributions of the source and the air background, this single-beam spectrum of the sample is digitally ratioed against a spectrum recorded with no sample in the beam (I_0), yielding the absorbance spectrum of the sample [$A_S = -\log(I_S/I_0)$]. In the case of differential spectroscopy, the single-beam spectrum of a sample is ratioed against the single-beam spectrum of a reference sample; this spectral ratioing operation then eliminates the spectral features common to the sample and the reference, yielding a difference spectrum directly. In the case of monitoring oil oxidation, the spectrum of the oil undergoing oxidation is ratioed against that of the fresh oil, resulting in only the spectral differences between the oils being recorded. The power of FTIR spectroscopy lies in its ability to carry out this operation very accurately because wavelength accuracy is maintained through the use of an internal reference laser, eliminating wavelength drift as a possible source of error when two spectra recorded at different times are ratioed. Due to this capability to accurately ratio one spectrum against another, very small differences between spectra can be detected that would not be apparent from visual inspection of the spectra.

The utility of the spectral ratioing technique can be clearly illustrated by some experimental results obtained by oxidizing safflower oil on an ATR crystal. The FTIR/ATR spectrum of safflower oil is presented in Fig. 23.2, illustrating the dominant spectral features of edible oils: the CH stretching absorptions (i.e., CH_2, CH_2/CH_3, and *cis*-C=CH stretching absorptions) observed in the region from 3100 to 2800 cm^{-1}, the carbonyl C=O absorption of the ester linkage at approximately 1745 cm^{-1}, and the bands associated with the fingerprint region (1500–1000 cm^{-1}). Figure 23.5 shows the differential spectra obtained when safflower oil was heated on an ATR crystal at 76°C for 1, 8, and 16 h; these spectra have been ratioed against the spectrum recorded at time zero to eliminate all spectral features that are unaffected by the oxidation of the oil. It is apparent from these ratioed spectra that the major changes accompanying oxidation of the oil occur in the following four regions of the spectrum.

The OH Stretching Region (3600–3200 cm^{-1}). Figure 23.6 shows a detailed view of the changes in the 3600–3200 cm^{-1} region for the same experiment as in Fig. 23.5. The broad band centered at 3444 cm^{-1} is the O-H stretching vibration of hydroperoxides, a peak assignment established by early work on the oxidation of methyl linoleate (16). In raw spectra (i.e., ratioed against an air background spectrum), this band would not be clearly discernible due to its overlap with an overtone absorption of the oil centered at 3473 cm^{-1}. However, by using differential spectroscopy, and under the experimental conditions employed here,

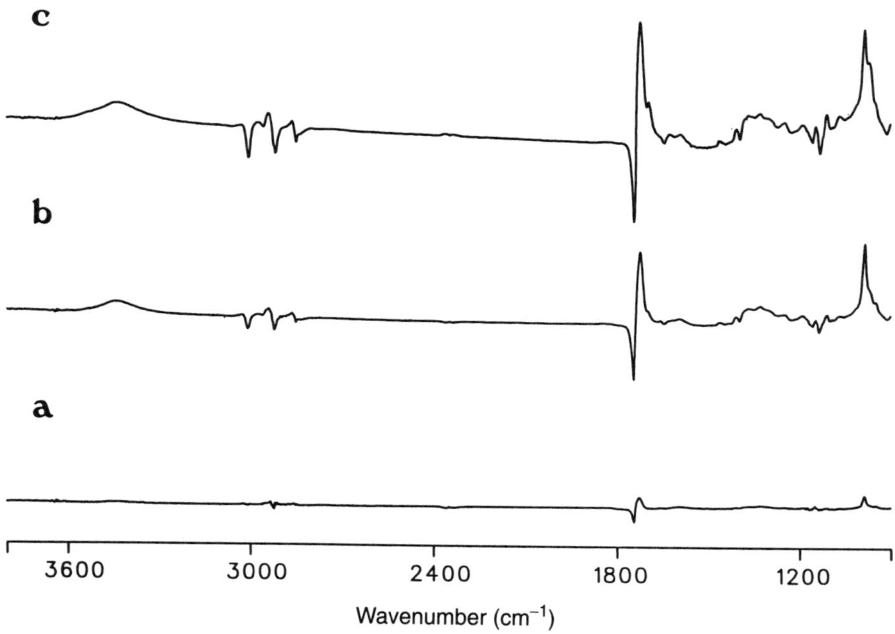

Fig. 23.5. FTIR/ATR spectra of safflower oil heated to 76°C on the surface of a 45° ZnSe ATR crystal: (A) t = 16 h; (B) t = 8 h; (C) t = 1 h. The spectra have been ratioed against the spectrum recorded at t = 0.

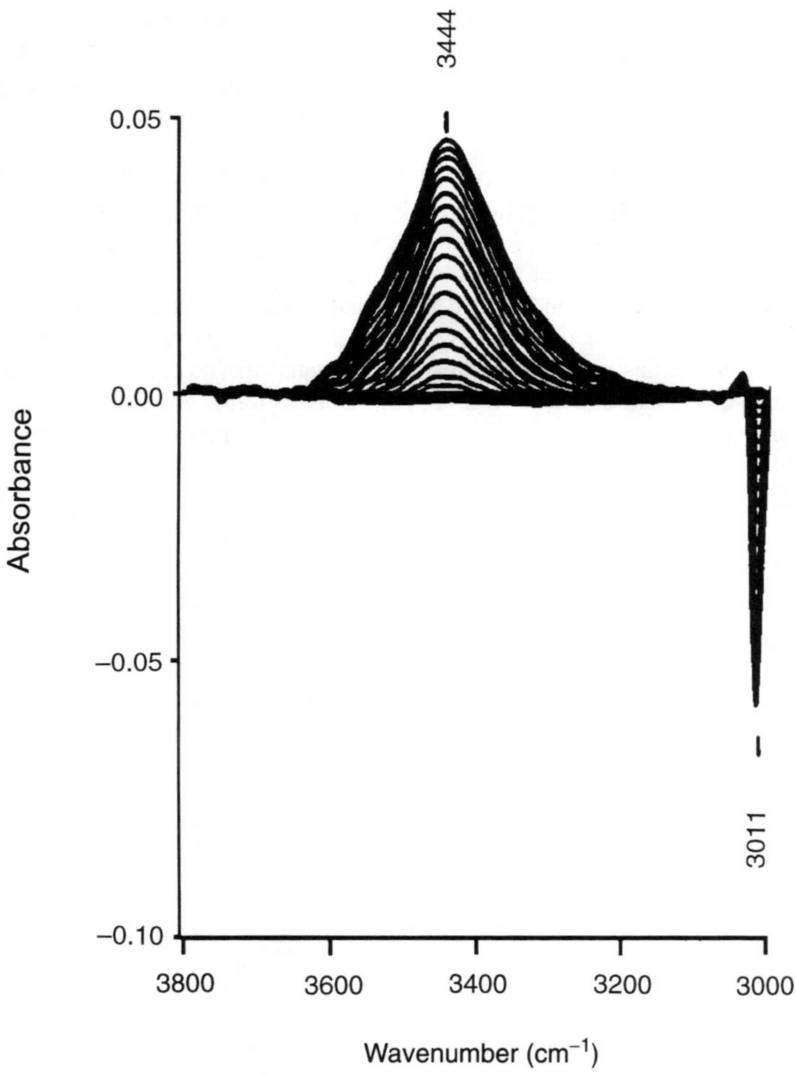

Fig. 23.6. Spectral overlay plot illustrating changes in the 3800–3000 cm^{-1} region of the FTIR/ATR spectrum of safflower oil heated to 76°C on the surface of a 45° ZnSe ATR crystal as a function of time. The overlaid spectra were recorded at 30-min intervals and have been ratioed against the spectrum recorded at $t = 0$.

the formation of hydroperoxides can be unambiguously tracked by measuring the absorbance at 3444 cm^{-1} as a function of time. This will not be the case under more severe conditions leading to the breakdown of the hydroperoxides to alcohols or the release of free fatty acids, because alcohols and free fatty acids also exhibit broad O-H stretching absorption bands that overlap with the hydroperoxide band on the high- and low-frequency side, respectively. Thus, if any asymmetry is observed in the hydroperoxide absorption band, the absorbance at 3444 cm^{-1} can no longer be considered a reliable measure of hydroperoxide formation.

The Cis C-H Stretching Region (3020–3000 cm^{-1}). The progressive increase in the intensity of the hydroperoxide band in Fig. 23.6 is accompanied by the growth of a negative band at 3008 cm^{-1}, which represents a decrease in the intensity of the C-H stretching band of *cis* C=C-H groups as a function of time. This decrease is due to the loss of *cis* double bonds that occurs upon formation of hydroperoxides and shows an excellent linear relationship with the increase in the hydroperoxide band (Fig. 23.7). Thus, this negative band in the differential spectra can be employed to monitor hydroperoxide formation and is extremely useful for tracking purposes under all experimental conditions because, unlike the hydroperoxide band itself, it is not subject to interference from overlapping absorptions.

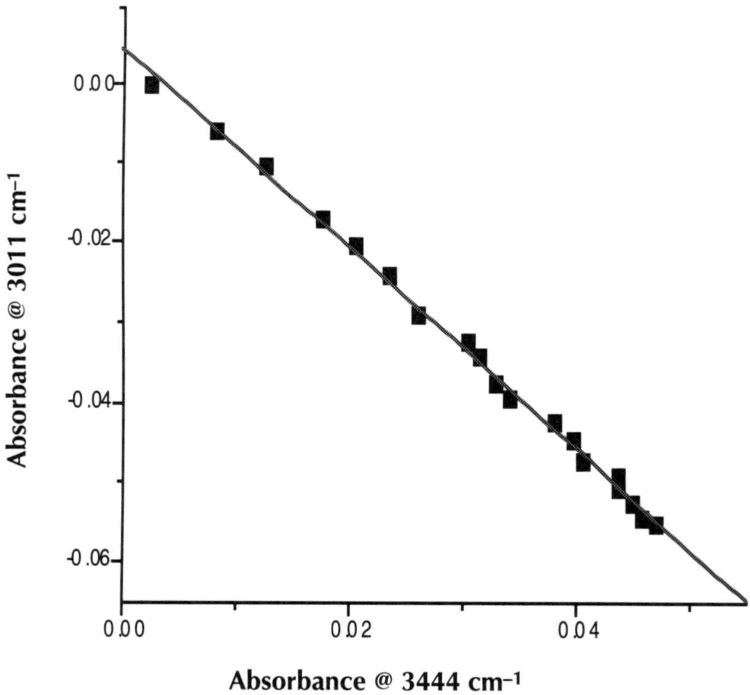

Fig. 23.7. Plot of the peak height of the hydroperoxide absorption band, measured at 3444 cm^{-1} relative to a baseline point at 3750 cm^{-1}, vs. that of the *cis* C=C-H stretching band, measured at 3008 cm^{-1} relative to a baseline point at 3100 cm^{-1}, for the spectra in Fig. 23.6 ($R = -0.998$).

The C=O Stretching Region (1730–1650 cm⁻¹). Figure 23.8 illustrates the changes taking place in the 1730–1650 cm^{-1} region of the spectrum, in which C=O stretching bands are observed, as autoxidation proceeds. The intense carbonyl absorption of the triglyceride ester linkage centered at 1744 cm^{-1} does not ratio out perfectly in the differential spectra, due to the digitization noise that results upon ratioing intense bands, and has been excluded from Fig. 23.8. New bands appearing at 1726 and 1698 cm^{-1} as oxidation proceeds have been attributed to the formation of aldehydes (13), which are major secondary oxidation products, formed as a result of the breakdown of hydroperoxides. However, it is important to note that hydrogen bonding between hydroperoxides and the ester carbonyl groups of the oil is expected to cause a shift of the carbonyl absorption to a lower frequency. In fact, the spectra of oils spiked with *tert*-butyl hydroperoxide (TBHP), a stable hydroperoxide that does not promote oil autoxidation (14), exhibit a shoulder on the 1744-cm^{-1} ester carbonyl absorption band (Fig. 23.9B). When the spectrum of the unspiked oil is subtracted from these spectra, a band at 1725 cm^{-1} is observed (Fig. 23.9C) whose intensity is proportional to the concentration of TBHP in the oil.

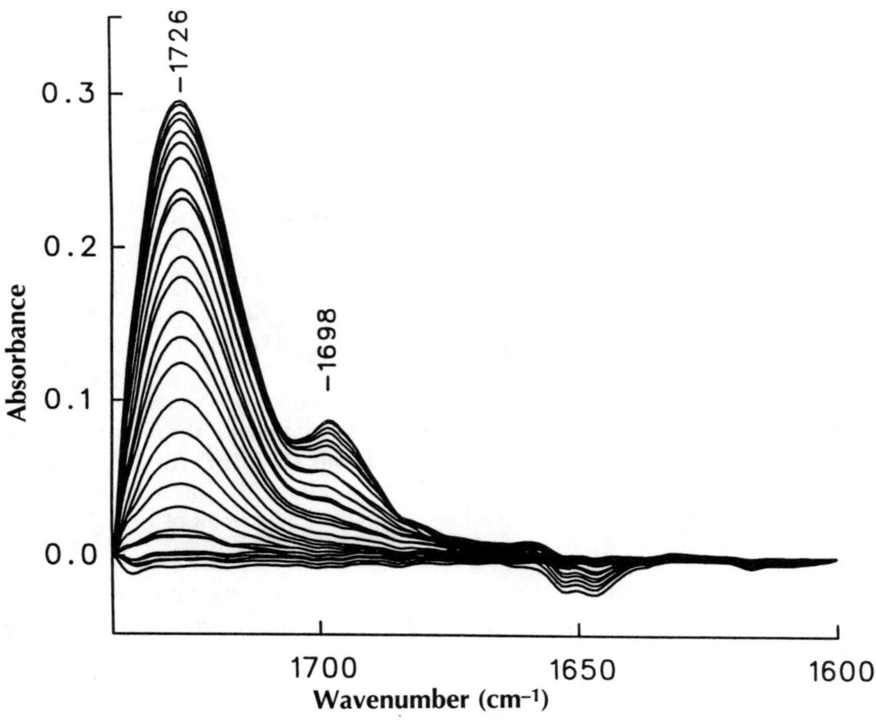

Fig. 23.8. Spectral overlay plot illustrating changes in the 1730–1600 cm^{-1} region of the FTIR/ATR spectrum of safflower oil heated to 76°C on the surface of a 45° ZnSe ATR crystal as a function of time. The overlaid spectra were recorded at 30-min intervals and have been ratioed against the spectrum recorded at $t = 0$.

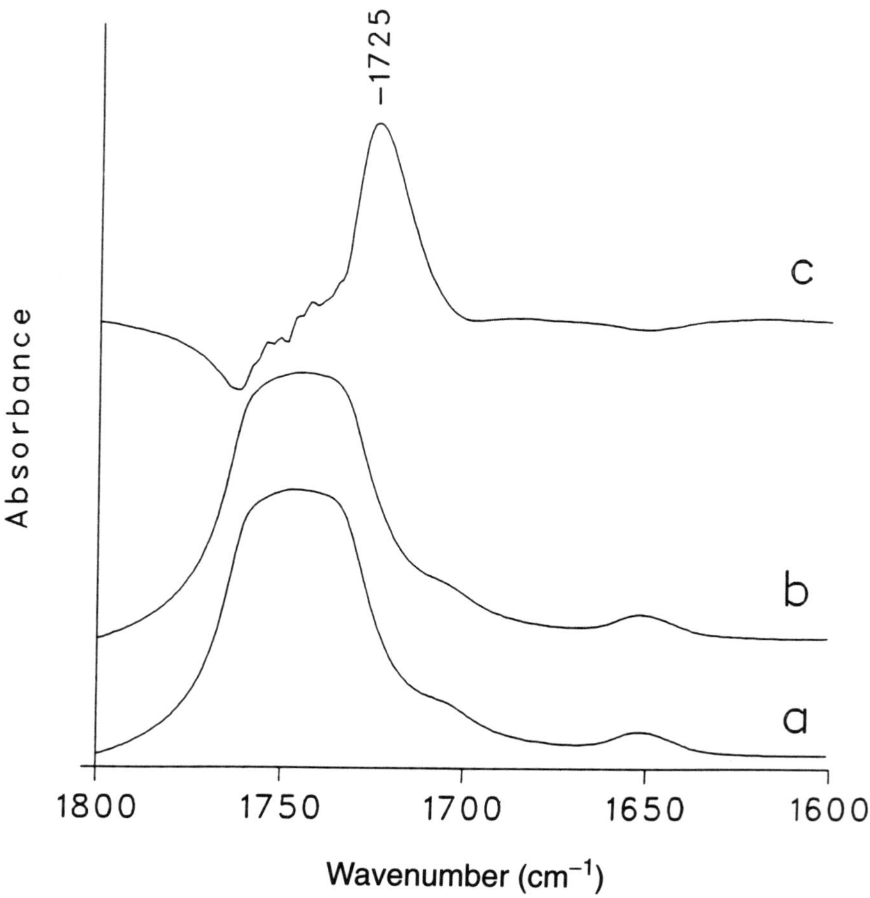

Fig. 23.9. Effect of hydrogen bonding between *tert*-butyl hydroperoxide (TBHP) and the triglyceride ester carbonyl groups on the ester carbonyl absorption band: (A) TBHP-free safflower oil; (B) the same oil spiked with 1% TBHP; (C) difference spectrum obtained by subtracting spectrum (A) from spectrum (B). The spectra have been offset for clarity, and spectrum (C) has been multiplied by a factor of 10.

This observation indicates that the effects of hydrogen bonding on the ester carbonyl absorption band are a complicating factor in the interpretation of spectral changes in this region.

The Trans C=C-H Bending Region (1000–950 cm^{-1}). Figure 23.10 shows that major changes occur in the 1000–950 cm^{-1} region of the infrared spectrum of safflower oil as the oil undergoes oxidation. Bands in this region are due to the C=C-H bending vibrations of *trans* double bonds. Hydroperoxides containing isolated *trans* bonds exhibit an absorption maximum at 969 cm^{-1}, whereas those con-

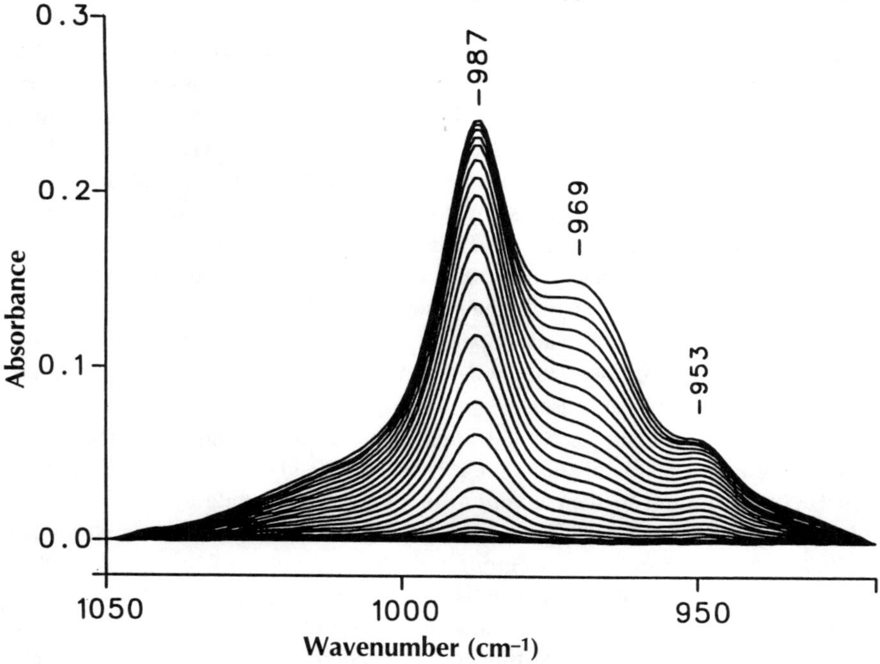

Fig. 23.10. Spectral overlay plot illustrating changes in the 1050–900 cm^{-1} region of the FTIR/ATR spectrum of safflower oil heated to 76°C on the surface of a 45° ZnSe ATR crystal as a function of time. The overlaid spectra were recorded at 30-min intervals and have been ratioed against the spectrum recorded at $t = 0$.

taining *cis*, *trans*- and *trans*, *trans*-conjugated double bonds give rise to absorption maxima at ~985 cm^{-1} (13). Thus, the overlaid differential spectra in Fig. 23.10 demonstrate the formation of *trans* hydroperoxides; the relative contributions of conjugated and isolated *trans* bonds to the absorption in this region cannot be easily estimated because of extensive band overlap.

All of the four regions mentioned above can potentially be useful in the monitoring of antioxidant performance. However, because the changes in the carbonyl region are due to both the effects on the ester linkage carbonyl band of changes in hydrogen bonding and the formation of carbonyl-containing secondary oxidation products, the interpretation of spectral features in this region is not straightforward. Accordingly, this region was not considered in the work described below on the FTIR evaluation of antioxidant efficacy.

Evaluation of Antioxidant Performance by FTIR/ATR Differential Spectroscopy

As indicated, FTIR/ATR differential spectroscopy provides a rapid and convenient means of monitoring the oxidation of an oil under controlled conditions and, as such, also provides a simple means of evaluating antioxidant performance. The oil chosen for illustration is menhaden oil, a highly unsaturated fish oil monitored at 65°C. Three synthetic primary chain-breaking antioxidants, butylated hydroxyanisole (BHA), *tert*-butylhydroquinone (TBHQ), and propyl gallate (PG), were added to the oil at various concentrations to assess their relative efficacy in retarding autoxidation. In these experiments, a 250-μL sample of antioxidant-containing oil was pipetted onto the heated ATR crystal, and its FTIR spectrum was immediately recorded (t = 0). Spectra were subsequently recorded at 40-min intervals and ratioed against the spectrum recorded at $t = 0$ to eliminate the spectral features of the starting oil, thus allowing the spectral changes accompanying oxidation to be clearly observed. Time-course oil oxidation profiles were then obtained by plotting the absorbances at selected frequencies vs. time of heating.

Figure 23.11 illustrates typical time-course oxidation plots for menhaden oil containing PG at levels of 0.01 and 1%. In Fig. 23.11A, the peak height at 3444 cm^{-1}, corresponding to the maximum of the hydroperoxide absorption band, is plotted vs. time of heating. This plot clearly demonstrates the prolongation of the induction period when the concentration of PG is increased from 0.01 to 1.0%. At the lower level, the induction period is ~5 h, whereas at the higher level, no oxidation of the oil is observed for the duration of the experiment (50 h). Similar information can be obtained by plotting the peak height of the *cis* C=C-H stretching absorption (measured at 3008 cm^{-1}) as a function of time (Fig. 23.11B); the decrease in this band is due to *cis* → *trans* isomerization as hydroperoxides are formed. The corresponding increase in the *trans* absorption band, measured from the absorbance at 971 cm^{-1}, as a function of time is shown in Fig. 23.11C, and the relationship between the *cis* and *trans* absorbance changes for spectra of the oil containing PG at the 0.01% level is shown in Fig. 23.11D. The *cis* and *trans* plots both show an induction period of ~5 h, followed by a rapid decrease and increase, respectively. However, the plot for the *cis* absorption peak reaches a plateau, whereas there is a subsequent decrease in the *trans* plot. This effect arises because both *cis, trans*- and *trans, trans*-conjugated hydroperoxides as well as isolated *trans* isomers contribute to the absorbance measured at 971 cm^{-1}, and thus the breakdown of *cis, trans*- and *trans, trans*-conjugated hydroperoxides as oxidation proceeds may give rise to a decrease in the absorbance at 971 cm^{-1}. Hence, in the initial stages of oxidation, the general *trans* measurements are quite useful; however, their interpretation becomes more complex as oxidation becomes more extensive, and thus these measurements are less suitable for monitoring antioxidant performance than measurements of either the hydroperoxide or *cis* C=C-H stretching absorption bands.

Similar experiments were subsequently performed with menhaden oil containing BHA and TBHQ at levels of 0.01, 0.1, and 1%. The plots obtained for the change in the hydroperoxide absorption band during the first 35 h of heating the BHA-containing oils are presented in Fig. 23.12, again demonstrating an increase in the induction period with increasing antioxidant concentration: the level of *cis* depletion at 80 h

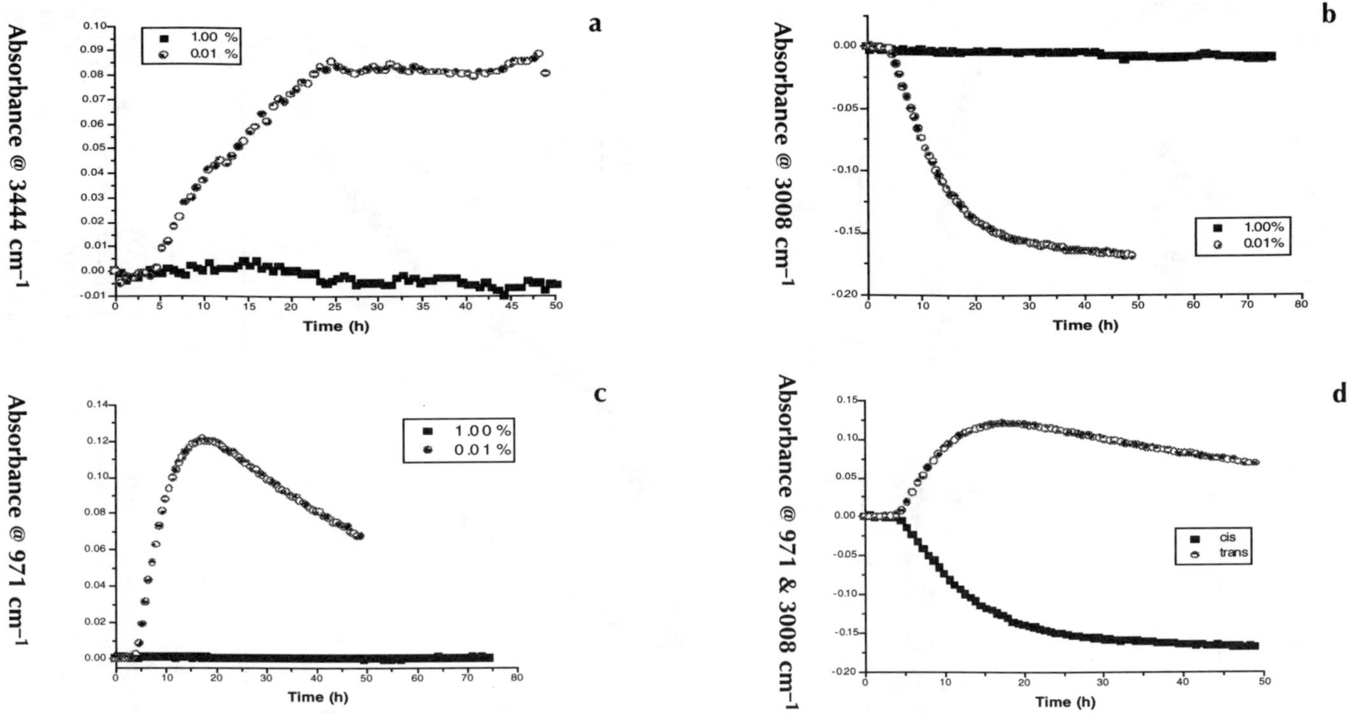

Fig. 23.11. Time-course oxidation plots obtained by FTIR/ATR monitoring of menhaden oil containing propyl gallate (PG) at levels of 0.01 (●) and 1% (■) at 65°C: (A) peak height of the hydroperoxide absorption band, measured at 3444 cm^{-1} relative to a baseline point at 3750 cm^{-1}; (B) peak height of the *cis* C=C-H stretching absorption, measured at 3008 cm^{-1} relative to a baseline point at 3100 cm^{-1}; (C) peak height of the *trans* C=C-H bending absorption, measured at 971 cm^{-1} relative to a baseline point at 920 cm^{-1}; (D) relationship between the *cis* (■) and *trans* (●) absorbance changes in spectra of the oil containing PG at the 0.01% level.

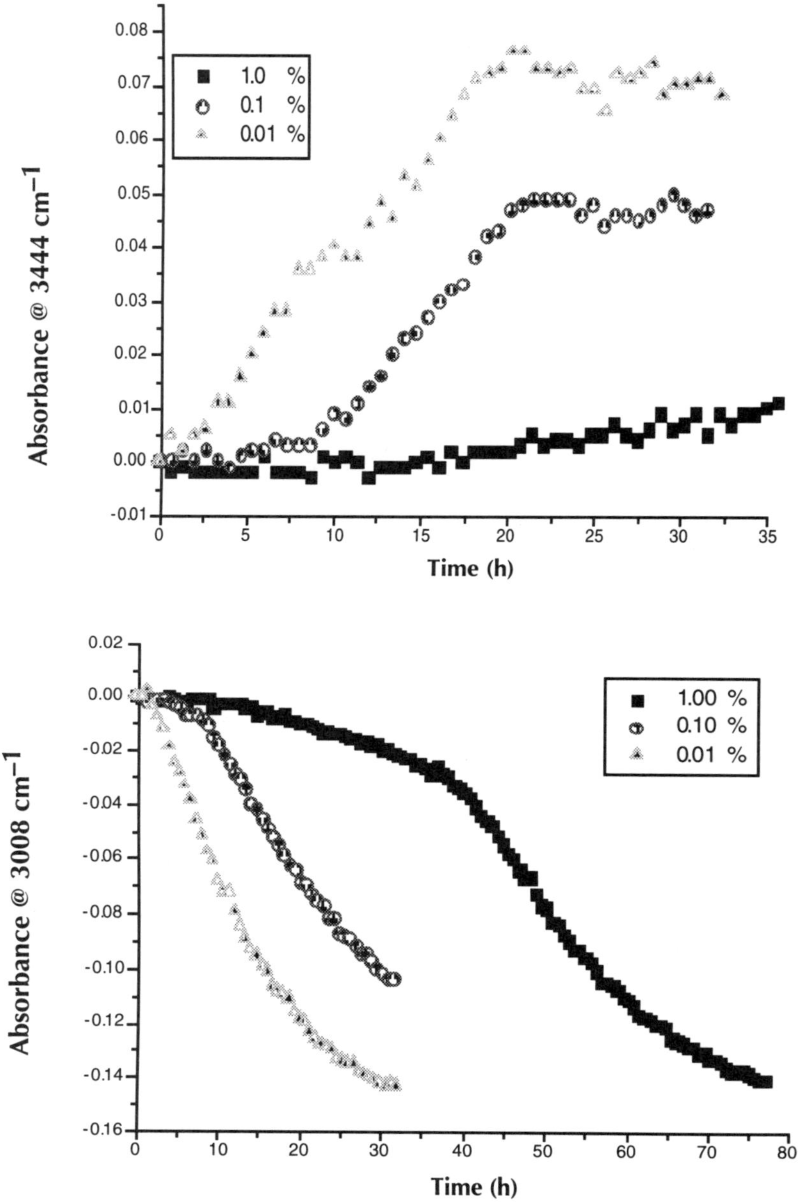

Fig. 23.12. Time-course oxidation plots obtained by FTIR/ATR monitoring of menhaden oil containing butylated hydroxyanisole (BHA) at levels of 0.01 (Δ), 0.1 (●), and 1% (■) at 65°C: (A) peak height of the hydroperoxide absorption band, measured at 3444 cm^{-1} relative to a baseline point at 3750 cm^{-1}; (B) peak height of the *cis* C=C-H stretching absorption, measured at 3008 cm^{-1} relative to a baseline point at 3100 cm^{-1}.

for the oil containing 1.0% BHA is comparable to that at 30 h for the oil containing 0.01% BHA. The superior antioxidant performance of TBHQ is apparent from the plots in Fig. 23.13. In this case, the plots for the *cis* absorption band (Fig. 23.13B) show an induction period of ~15 h for the oil containing 0.1% TBHQ, whereas no decrease in the *cis* absorption was observed throughout the 120-h heating period in the case of the oil containing 1.0% TBHQ.

By combining the time-course plots for the three antioxidants (Fig. 23.14), one potentially has a simple means by which the performance of the antioxidants can be compared. Although such comparisons are useful, they are valid only if the data are obtained under identical conditions (e.g., temperature of the ATR crystal, spectral collection/processing parameters), and care must be taken to minimize a number of sources of variability and error. Of primary concern is instrumental drift, which can be expected to occur due to the extended time course of the oil monitoring experiments. Drift will manifest itself in the recorded spectra as a progressive tilting of the spectral baseline. These effects can be minimized by measuring all absorbances relative to a local single-point baseline as close as possible to the absorption band of interest. This procedure was found to be more reliable than either baseline correction across the entire spectrum or the use of a two-point local baseline. Another consideration is oxygen tension, which is a function of the surface area/sample thickness ratio; thus, it is imperative that the amount of sample on the ATR crystal be consistent between experiments. The last major consideration is the alignment of the ATR sampling accessory, because an alignment shift can change the effective pathlength of the ATR cell. Such changes are not a source of error *per se* because they will not alter the shape of the oxidation profiles obtained, but they limit the absorbance values measured to be relative rather than absolute unless accessory alignment is scrupulously maintained.

The sample experiments and results presented demonstrate that, under carefully controlled experimental conditions, FTIR/ATR differential spectroscopy affords a simple means of monitoring antioxidant performance. Alternatively, an oil may be heated in a reservoir at a controlled rate of air input and circulated through a heated transmission flow cell. This approach is somewhat more complex experimentally but affords superior control over the experimental conditions. It also allows oil monitoring experiments to be conducted at more elevated temperatures without significant evaporative loss of antioxidant or volatile oxidation products. It must be kept in mind that the oxidative process is very complex and that the oxidative end product distribution is a function of the oil type and oxidation conditions. As such, the measurements discussed in our examples provide only a rough guide as to what one may expect to see. Thus, whenever a new set of experimental conditions or a different oil is considered, a careful examination of the spectra recorded throughout the course of the oxidation experiment is required in order to make a suitable choice of wavelengths for use in oxidation monitoring.

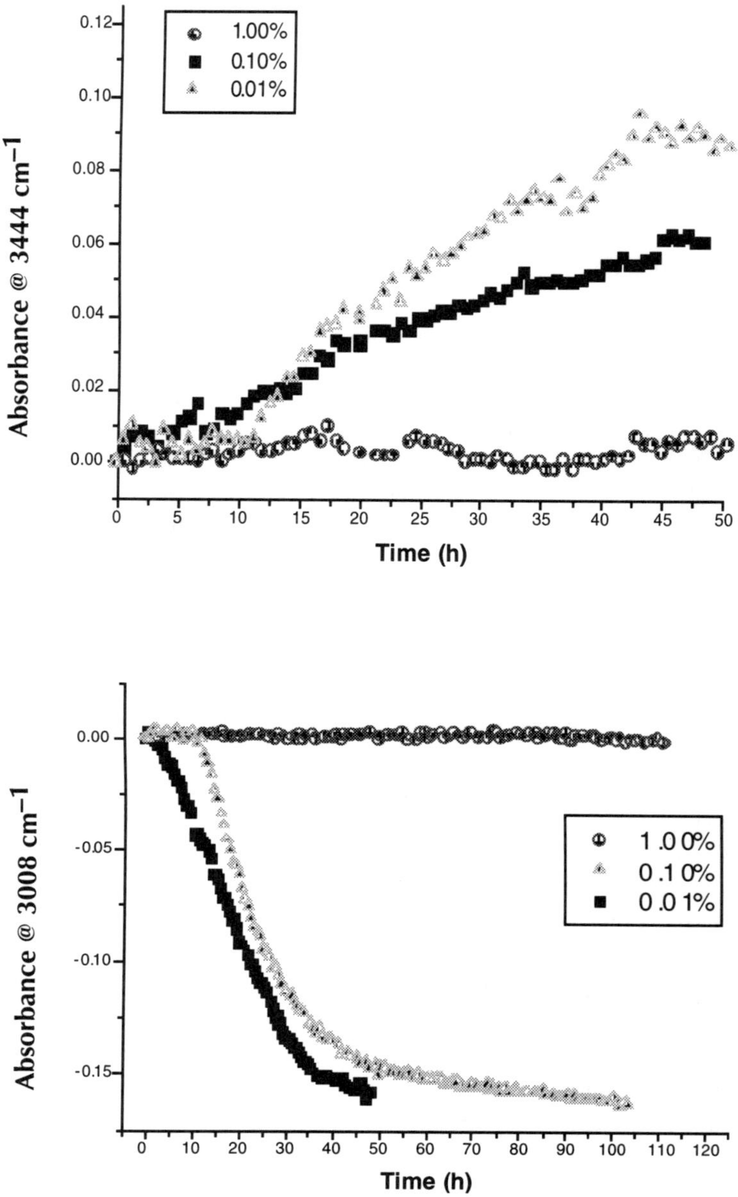

Fig. 23.13. Time-course oxidation plots obtained by FTIR/ATR monitoring of menhaden oil containing *tert*-butylhydroquinone (TBHQ) at levels of 0.01, 0.1, and 1% at 65°C: (A) peak height of the hydroperoxide absorption band, measured at 3444 cm^{-1} relative to a baseline point at 3750 cm^{-1}; (B) peak height of the *cis* C=C-H stretching absorption, measured at 3008 cm^{-1} relative to a baseline point at 3100 cm^{-1}.

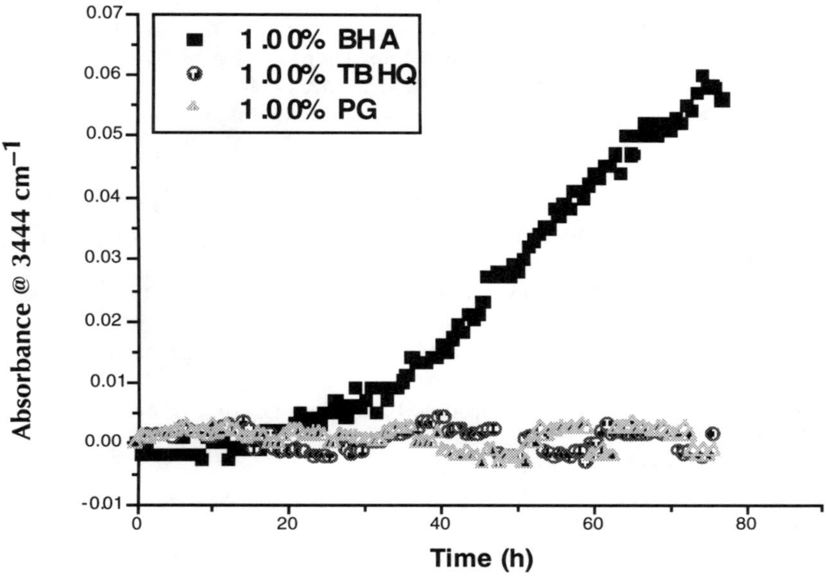

Fig. 23.14. Combined time-course oxidation plots for propyl gallate (PG) (△), *tert*-butylhydroquinone (TBHQ) (●), and butylated hydroxyanisole (BHA) (■) added to menhaden oil at the 1% level, obtained by plotting the peak height of the hydroperoxide absorption band, measured at 3444 cm^{-1} relative to a baseline point at 3750 cm^{-1}, vs. time of heating.

Conclusion

FTIR spectroscopy is a powerful tool by which one can monitor oxidative changes in edible fats and oils and a simple means by which to assess the efficacy of antioxidants. In particular, FTIR/ATR differential spectroscopy provides the researcher with access to detailed comparative and selective time-course data which provide information on both the primary and secondary oxidation products as they appear, eliminating the need for tedious chemical analyses.

Acknowledgment

The authors wish to thank the Natural Sciences and Engineering Research Council of Canada for its support of this work.

References

1. *Official Methods and Recommended Practices of the American Oil Chemists' Society* (1989) 4th edn., American Oil Chemists' Society, Champaign, IL.
2. van de Voort, F.R. (1994) *INFORM 5*, 1038–1042.

3. Harrick, N.J. (1967) *Internal Reflection Spectroscopy*, Interscience, New York.
4. Lanser, A.C., and Emken, E.A. (1988) *J. Am. Oil Chem. Soc. 65*, 1483–1487.
5. Sleeter, R.T., and Matlock, M.G. (1989) *J. Am. Oil Chem. Soc. 66*, 121–127.
6. Ulberth, F., and Haider, H.-J. (1992) *J. Food Sci. 57*, 1444–1447.
7. Afran, A., and Newbery, J.E. (1991) *Spectroscopy 6*, 31–34.
8. van de Voort, F.R., Sedman, J., Emo, G., and Ismail, A.A. (1992) *J. Am. Oil Chem. Soc. 69*, 1118–1123.
9. Fuller, M.P., Ritter, G.L., and Draper, C.S. (1988) *Appl. Spectrosc. 42*, 217–227.
10. van de Voort, F.R., Ismail, A.A., and Sedman, J. (1995) *J. Am. Oil Chem. Soc. 72*, 873–880.
11. Lanser, A.C., List, G.R., Holloway, R.K., and Mounts, T.L. (1991) *J. Am. Oil Chem. Soc. 68*, 448–449.
12. Ismail, A.A., van de Voort, F.R., Emo, G., and Sedman, J. (1993) *J. Am. Oil Chem. Soc. 70*, 335–341.
13. van de Voort, F.R., Ismail, A.A., Sedman, J., and Emo, G. (1994) *J. Am. Oil Chem. Soc. 71*, 243–253.
14. Frankel, E.N. (1982) *Prog. Lipid Res. 22*, 1–33.
15. van de Voort, F.R., Ismail, A.A., Sedman, J., Dubois, J., and Nicodemo, T. (1994) *J. Am. Oil Chem. Soc. 71*, 921–926.
16. Dugan, L.R., Beadle, B.W., and Henick, A.S. (1949) *J. Am. Oil Chem. Soc. 26*, 681–685.

Chapter 24

Measurement of Lipid Oxidation and Evaluation of Antioxidant Activity

F. Shahidi and U.N. Wanasundara

Department of Biochemistry, Memorial University of Newfoundland, St. John's, Newfoundland, Canada.

Introduction

Lipid oxidation has been recognized since antiquity as a challenging problem in the storage of fats and oils and lipid-containing foods. Characteristic changes associated with oxidative deterioration of vegetable oils and animal fats include development of unpleasant tastes and odors as well as changes in color, viscosity, specific gravity and solubility (1,2). Several authors (2–4) have reviewed the mechanisms involved in lipid oxidation and subsequent effects of lipid oxidation in foods.

Autoxidation is a natural process that takes place between molecular oxygen and unsaturated fatty acids. Autoxidation of unsaturated fatty acids occurs *via* a free radical process whose basic steps are initiation, propagation, and termination. Initiation starts with the abstraction of a hydrogen atom adjacent to a double bond in a fatty acid (RH) and this may be catalyzed by light, heat, or metal ions to form a free radical. The resultant alkyl free radical ($R^{\bullet}$) reacts with atmospheric oxygen to form an unstable peroxy free radical which may in turn abstract a hydrogen atom from another unsaturated fatty acid to form a hydroperoxide (ROOH) and a new alkyl free radical. The new alkyl free radical initiates further oxidation and contributes to the chain reaction. The chain reaction (or propagation) may be terminated by formation of non-radical products resulting from the combination of two radicals species.

The mechanism of lipid autoxidation has been postulated by Farmer *et al.* (5), Boland and Gee (6), and Bateman *et al.* (7). The propagation step in the autoxidation process includes an induction period in which hydroperoxide formation is minimal (2,8). The rate of oxidation of fatty acids increases in relation to their degree of unsaturation. The relative rate of autoxidation of oleate, linoleate, and linolenate is in the order of 1:40–50:100 on the basis of oxygen uptake and 1:12:25 on the basis of peroxide formation (9). Therefore, oils that contain relatively high amounts of polyunsaturated fatty acids (PUFA) experience stability problems. The breakdown products of hydroperoxides such as alcohols, aldehydes, ketones, and hydrocarbons generally possess offensive off-flavors. These compounds may also interact with other food components and bring about changes in their functional and nutritional properties (10). A generalized scheme for autoxidation of food lipids which also illustrates some of its possible consequences is provided in Fig. 24.1.

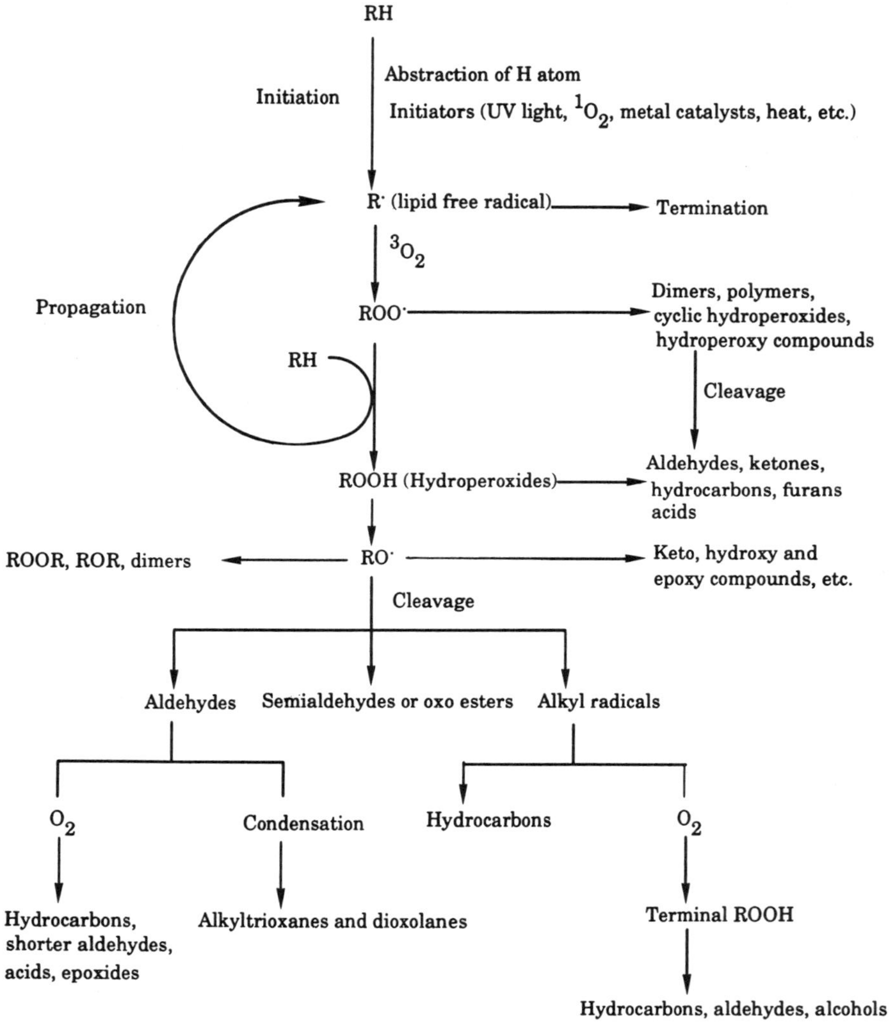

Fig. 24.1. Generalized scheme for autoxidation of unsaturated lipid fatty acids and its consequences.

Methods of Measuring Oxidative Rancidity in Fats and Oils

There are various methods available for measurement of lipid oxidation in foods. Changes in chemical, physical, or organoleptic properties of fats and oils during oxidation may be monitored to assess the extent of lipid oxidation. However, there is no uniform/standard method for detecting all oxidative changes in all food systems. The methods available to monitor lipid oxidation in foods and biological systems may be divided into two groups. The first group measures primary changes, and the second determines secondary changes that occur in each system. Primary changes are generally measured by monitoring (i) loss of unsaturated fatty acids, (ii) oxygen uptake by weight gain or other methods, (iii) hydroperoxide values, and (iv) conjugated diene value. Secondary changes are followed by quantitation of (i) carbonyl compounds (as their dinitrophenylhydrazone or by gas chromatography), (ii) malonaldehyde and other aldehydes [thiobarbituric acid (TBA) test], (iii) hydrocarbons (ethane or pentane content), and (iv) fluorescence products (1-amino-3-iminopropane derivatives). The method of choice depends on a number of factors including the nature and history of the oxidized oil, the type of information required, the time available, and the test conditions. Nonetheless, it is advisable to use a combination of methods to assess both primary and secondary oxidative changes in oils. However, the results must be in agreement with sensory perception and acceptability of foods.

Primary Changes

Changes in Reactants. Methods that measure primary changes of lipids may be classified as those that quantify loss of reactants (unsaturated fatty acids), addition of oxygen, or formation of primary lipid oxidation products (hydroperoxides). These methods are more suitable for measuring low levels of oxidation in uncooked products at low temperatures (11). The measurement of changes in fatty acid composition is not widely used in assessing lipid oxidation because it requires total lipid extraction and conversion into derivatives suitable for gas chromatographic analysis; separation of lipids into neutral, glycolipid, phospholipid, and other classes may also be necessary. However, it has been proven that this method serves as a useful technique to identify which class of lipids and fatty acids is involved in the oxidative changes (11,12) and also to assess lipid oxidation simulated by different metal complexes that give different products (13). On the other hand, changes in fatty acid composition cannot be used in more saturated oils because this indicator reflects only the changes that occur in unsaturated fatty acids during oxidation. Therefore, oxidative changes in marine oils and highly unsaturated vegetable oils may be monitored using this indicator. Similarly, changes in iodine value due to loss of unsaturation during accelerated oxidation studies may be used as an index of lipid oxidation (14).

During oxidation of lipids, the oxygen above the lipid surface slowly reacts with it; thus changes in the oxygen pressure may be measured quantitatively. This is the principle used in the Sylvester test in which the oil is subjected to high temperatures (100°C) in a closed system. The drop of pressure in the system is quantified, using Oxidograph apparatus available from a Danish supplier, as oxidation proceeds (15).

Weight Gain. It is generally accepted that the addition of oxygen to lipids and the formation of hydroperoxides are reasonably quantitative during initial stages of autoxidation. Therefore, the measurement of the induction period from weight gain data is theoretically sound. In this method, oil samples (about 2.0 g) are weighted into petri dishes; traces of water are removed by placing the samples overnight in a vacuum oven at 35°C over a desiccant. Samples are then reweighed and stored in an oven at a set temperature. The weight gain of the samples may be recorded at different time intervals.

Olcott and Einset (16) reported that marine oils exhibit a fairly sharp increase in their weight at the end of the induction period and are rancid by the time they gain 0.3–0.5% in weight (at 30–60°C). Ke and Ackman (17) reported that this method is simple, has a satisfactory reproducibility, and may be used to compare oxidation of lipids from different parts of fish. Recently, Wanasundara and Shahidi (18) used this method to compare storage stability of canola oil as affected by added natural and synthetic antioxidants and were able to compare relative activity of the antioxidants employed. However, surface exposure of the sample to air is an important variable in determining the rate of oxidation. Therefore, use of containers of equal size in which to store samples is very important in conducting such experiments.

The weight-gain method also suffers from certain disadvantages: (i) the weighing frequency hinders monitoring of fast kinetics (a higher frequency would involve nocturnal weighing), and low or moderate temperatures require long analysis times for stable samples; (ii) discontinuous heating of the sample (which must be cooled before weighing) may give rise to nonreproducible results, thus the heating and cooling intervals must be accurately controlled; (iii) the method involves intensive human participation; and (iv) the working conditions (sample size, shape of the container, and temperature) influence the results. Nevertheless, this method offers advantages such as low instrumentation cost and unlimited capacity for sample processing.

Hydroperoxides. In the oxidation of fats and oils, the initial rate of formation of hydroperoxides exceeds their rate of decomposition; however, this is reversed at later stages. Therefore, monitoring the amount of hydroperoxides as a function of time will indicate whether a lipid is in the growth or decay portion of the hydroperoxide concentration curve. This information can be used as a guide for considering the acceptability of a food product with respect to the extent of product deterioration. By monitoring the induction period before the appearance of hydroperoxides, one can assess the effectiveness of added antioxidants on the stability of a food.

Peroxide Value. The classical method for quantitation of hydroperoxides is the determination of "peroxide value" (PV). The hydroperoxide content, generally referred to as PV, is determined by an iodometric method. This is based on the titration of the iodine released from potassium iodide by the peroxides in a biphasic system with a thiosulfate solution as given below.

$$ROOH + 2H^+ + 2I^- \rightarrow I_2 + ROH + H_2O$$
$$I_2 + 2S_2O_3^{2-} \rightarrow S_4O_6^{2-} + 2I^-$$

Potential drawbacks of this method are absorption of iodine at unsaturation sites of fatty acids and liberation of iodine from potassium iodide by oxygen present in the solution to be titrated (19). Results may also be affected by the structure and reactivity of peroxides as well as reaction temperature and time. The official iodometric method Cd 8-53 (20) for determination of PV is applicable to all normal fats and oils, but it is highly empirical and any variation in procedure may affect the results. The official method also fails to adequately measure low PV because of difficulties encountered in determination of the titration end point. Therefore, the official method has been modified in an attempt to increase the sensitivity for determination of low PV. The modification involves the replacement of the titration step with an electrochemical technique in which the liberated iodine is reduced at a platinum electrode maintained at a constant potential with this method. PV ranging from 0.06 to 20 have been determined in this manner, but it is essential to deaerate all solutions to prevent further formation of peroxides.

Several other chemical methods have also been suggested for monitoring PV. Colorimetric methods based on the oxidation of Fe^{2+} to Fe^{3+} and determination of Fe^{2+} as ferric thiocyanate, and a procedure using 2,6-dichlorophenol-indophenol are reported in the literature (21). In studies on the oxidation of biological tissues and fluids, measurement of fatty acid hydroperoxides is more common than measuring their decomposition products. Fatty acid hydroperoxides can be analyzed by high-performance liquid chromatography (HPLC), or their corresponding hydroperoxy acid reduction products may be determined by gas chromatography-mass spectrometry (GC–MS) (22,23). Fluorescence methods have also been developed to determine hydroperoxides by allowing them to react with substances such as luminol and dichlorofluorescein which form fluorescent products (19). Although determination of peroxide value is common, its usefulness is generally limited to the initial stages of lipid oxidation.

Active Oxygen and Oil Stability Index/Rancimat Methods. The Active Oxygen Method (AOM), also referred to as the Swift test of the American Oil Chemists' Society, is a commonly used accelerated method for assessing oxidative stability of fats and oils. This method is based on the principle that aging and rancidification of a fat is greatly accelerated by aeration in a tube held at a constant elevated temperature. The peroxide value reached by the AOM at which a fat will be rancid by organoleptic evaluation varies with the nature of the fat (24). Even though this method has been used extensively over the years, its inherent deficiencies and difficulties have also been identified, including the following: (i) the end point is determined by the amount of peroxides in the oxidized oil; peroxides are unstable and decompose readily to more stable secondary products; (ii) during the rapid oxidation phase, the reaction is extremely susceptible to variations in the oxygen supply.

Automated versions of the AOM apparatus, known as the Oil Stability Instrument (OSI), Rancimat, and Oxidograph are now available. The Rancimat method uses a commercial apparatus marketed by Metrohm, Ltd. The OSI, a computer-assisted instrument developed by Archer Daniels Midland (ADM), is now produced commercially by Omnion Inc. (Rockland, MA). These methods may be considered as automated AOM because both employ the principle of accelerated oxidation. However, the OSI and Rancimat tests measure the changes in conductivity caused by ionic volatile organic acids, mainly formic acids, automatically and continuously, whereas in the AOM, peroxide values are determined. These organic acids are stable oxidation products which are produced when an oil is oxidized by a stream of air bubbled through it. As in the AOM, the OSI and Rancimat tests proceed slowly at first because during the induction period, little acid is released. The end point is selected as the point at which the rapid rise in conductance begins. The Rancimat became available in the early 1980s and is capable of running only six samples simultaneously; however, OSI is capable of running up to twenty-four samples at a time.

Jabe *et al.* (25) reported that the newly developed OSI method is superior to the AOM in many respects: (i) in the AOM, the end point does not determine the induction period, but is merely related to it, whereas the OSI end point determines the induction period precisely; (ii) the AOM provides a single data point, whereas OSI provides continual data points; (iii) the AOM relies on the analysis of unstable primary reaction products, whereas the OSI is based on the analysis of stable secondary products; (iv) in the AOM, the end point is determined during the rapid oxidation phase which is oxidant dependent, highly variable, and difficult to reproduce, whereas the OSI end point is determined at the end of the induction period which is relatively insensitive to oxidant flow; (v) the AOM depends on a manually obtained end point, whereas OSI has an instrumental automatic end point control; and (vi) the AOM is manual, labor-intensive and time-consuming, but OSI is automated. Despite the high cost of the apparatus, OSI and Rancimat are currently regarded as the methods of choice for examination of fat stability by the industry.

Conjugated Dienes. Oxidation of polyunsaturated fatty acids is accompanied by an increase in the ultraviolet absorption of the product. Lipids containing methylene-interrupted dienes or polyenes show a shift in their double bond position during oxidation due to isomerization and conjugate formation (26). The resulting conjugated dienes exhibit intense absorption at 234 nm; similarly conjugated trienes absorb at 268 nm. Farmer and Sutton (27) indicated that the absorption increase due to the formation of conjugated dienes and trienes is proportional to the uptake of oxygen and formation of peroxides during the early stages of oxidation. St. Angelo *et al.* (28,29) studied the autoxidation of peanut butter by measuring the PV and absorption increase at 234 nm due to the formation of conjugated dienes. Shahidi *et al.* (30) and Wanasundara *et al.* (31) found that conjugated dienes and PV of marine (seal blubber and cod liver) and vegetable (canola and soybean) oils correlated during their oxidation. These authors concluded that the conjugated diene method may be used as an index of stability of lipids in place of, or in addition to PV. However, carotenoid-containing oils may give high absorbance values at 234–236 nm, due to the presence of double bonds in the conjugated structures of carotenoids. The conjugated diene method is faster than PV determination, is much simpler, does not depend upon chemical reactions or color development, and requires a smaller sample size.

Parr and Swoboda (32) described an alternate spectroscopic method to determine lipid oxidation of stored oils. In this assay, hydroperoxides of polyenoic fatty acids as well as hydroxy and carbonyl compounds derived from them are converted to more conjugated chromophores by two chemical reaction steps, first reduction and then dehydration (Fig. 24.2). These yield "conjugable oxidation product (COP)" which are measured and expressed as COP values. The first step of the analytical procedure involves reduction by sodium borohydride, which results in the disappearance of the characteristic ultraviolet absorption of the carbonyl compounds of oxidized polyenoic fatty acids (oxodienes). The decrease in the absorption at 275 nm is known as oxodiene value.

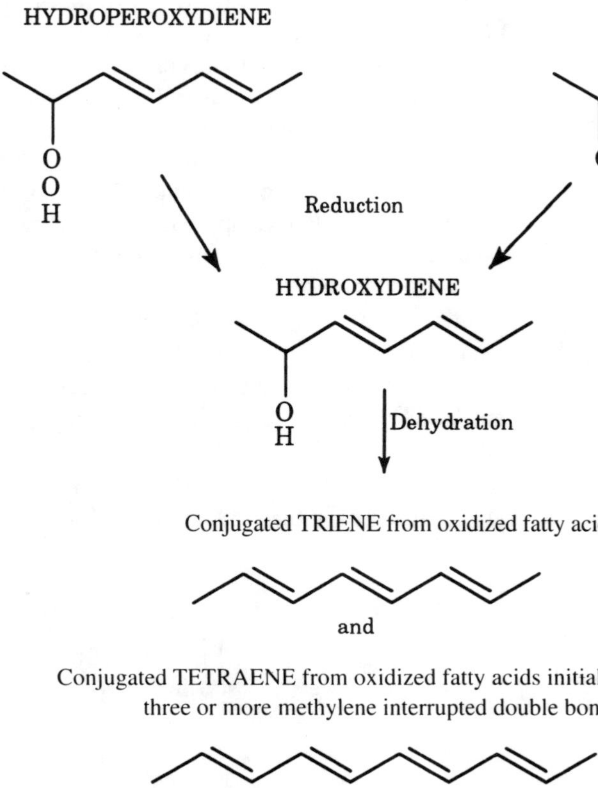

Fig. 24.2. Chemical reaction steps in the assay of conjugable oxidation products.

Secondary Changes

The primary oxidation products (peroxides) of fats and oils are transitionary intermediates that decompose into various secondary products. Measurement of secondary oxidation products as an index of lipid oxidation is more appropriate because secondary products of oxidation are generally flavor-active, whereas primary oxidation products are colorless and flavorless. Secondary oxidation products include aldehydes, ketones, hydrocarbons, and alcohols. The following sections describe common methods used for measuring secondary oxidation products of lipids.

The 2-Thiobarbituric Acid (TBA) Value. One of the oldest and the most frequently used tests for assessing lipid oxidation in foods and other biological systems is the TBA test. The extent of lipid oxidation is reported as the TBA value and is expressed as milligrams of malonaldehyde (MA) equivalents per kilogram sample or as μmol MA equivalents/g sample. Malonaldehyde is a relatively minor product of oxidation of polyunsaturated fatty acids which reacts with the TBA reagent to produce a pink-colored complex with an absorption maximum at 530–532 nm (33). The adduct is formed by condensation of two molecules of TBA with one molecule of MA (Fig. 24.3). Dahle *et al.* (34) postulated a mechanism for the formation of MA and indicated that only peroxides which possess unsaturation β or γ to the peroxide group are capable of undergoing cyclization with the ultimate formation of MA. Such peroxides may be produced from fatty acids containing three or more double bonds (34). Other products of lipid oxidation, such as aldehydes, alkenals, and 2,4-alkadienals, may also react with the TBA reagent to form a pink-colored complex with the same absorption maximum as the MA-TBA complex (35). Therefore, the term "thiobarbituric acid-reactive substances" (TBARS) is now commonly used in place of TBA value (36–38).

There are certain limitations when using the TBA test for evaluation of the oxidative state of foods and biological systems because of their chemical complexity. Dugan (24) reported that sucrose and some compounds in wood smoke react with the TBA reagent to give a red color which interferes with the TBA test. Baumgartner *et al.* (39) also found that a mixture of acetaldehyde and sucrose subjected to the TBA test produced a 532-nm absorbing pigment identical to that produced by MA and TBA. Modifications of the original TBA test have been reported by Marcuse and

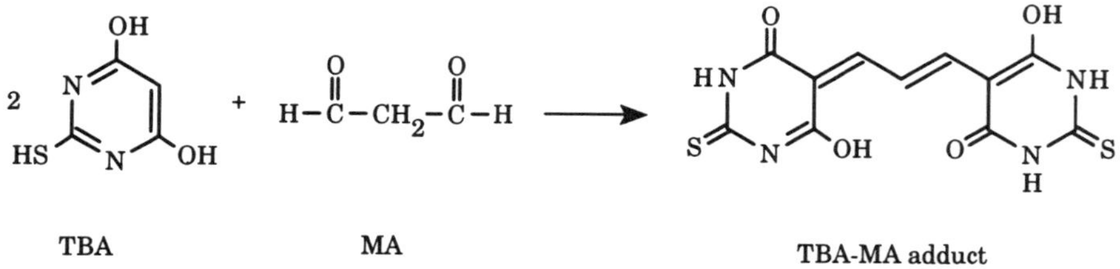

Fig. 24.3. Reaction of 2-thiobarbituric acid (TBA) and malonaldehyde (MA).

Johansson (35), Ke and Woyewoda (40), Robbles-Martinez *et al.* (41), Pokorny *et al.* (42), Shahidi *et al.* (43), Thomas and Fumes (44), and Schmedes and Holmer (45). However, it has been suggested that TBARS provide an excellent means for evaluating relative oxidative status of a system as affected by storage or processing variables (46). Nonetheless, it is preferable to quantitate the extent of lipid oxidation by a complementary analytical procedure so as to verify the results.

Several attempts have been made to establish a relationship between TBA values and the development of undesirable flavors in fats and oils. It has been shown that flavor threshold values correlate well with TBA values of vegetable oils such as those of soybean, cottonseed, corn, safflower (19), and canola (8).

Oxirane Index Value. The oxirane oxygen or epoxide groups are formed during autoxidation of fats and oils. The epoxide content is determined by titrating the oil sample with HBr in acetic acid, in the presence of crystal violet, to a bluish-green end point. This method has been standardized by the American Oil Chemists' Society in their tentative method Cd 9-57 (47). However, this test is not sensitive and lacks specificity. The HBr may also attack α,β-unsaturated carbonyls and conjugated dienols, and the reaction is not quantitative with some *trans*-epoxides. Fioriti *et al.* (48) have found that picric acid was the best of several acidic chromophores in its reaction with epoxides. Despite a nonquantitative reaction, the product concentration followed Beer's Law. This method has been found to be particularly well suited for the determination of epoxides in heated fats and oils in which the oxirane content is often less than 0.1%.

p-Anisidine Value. *p*-Anisidine value is used to measure secondary products of lipid oxidation. This method determines the amount of aldehydes (principally 2-alkenals and 2,4-alkadienals) in animal fats and vegetable oils. Aldehydes in an oil and the *p*-anisidine reagent react under acidic conditions (49; method number 2.504). The proposed reaction of *p*-anisidine with aldehydes to form a yellowish product is shown in Fig. 24.4. List *et al.* (50) have reported a highly significant correlation between *p*-anisidine values and flavor acceptability scores of salad oils processed from undamaged soybeans.

TOTOX Value. The *p*-anisidine value (*p*-AnV) is often used in the industry in conjunction with PV to calculate the so-called total oxidation or TOTOX value:

$$\text{TOTOX value} = 2\text{PV} + p\text{-AnV}$$

The TOTOX value is often considered to have the advantage of combining evidence about the past history of an oil (as reflected in the *p*-AnV) with its present state (as evidenced in the PV). Therefore, determination of TOTOX value has been conducted extensively to estimate oxidative deterioration of food lipids (51). However, despite its practical advantages, TOTOX value does not have any sound scientific basis because it combines variables with different dimensions. Recently, Wanasundara

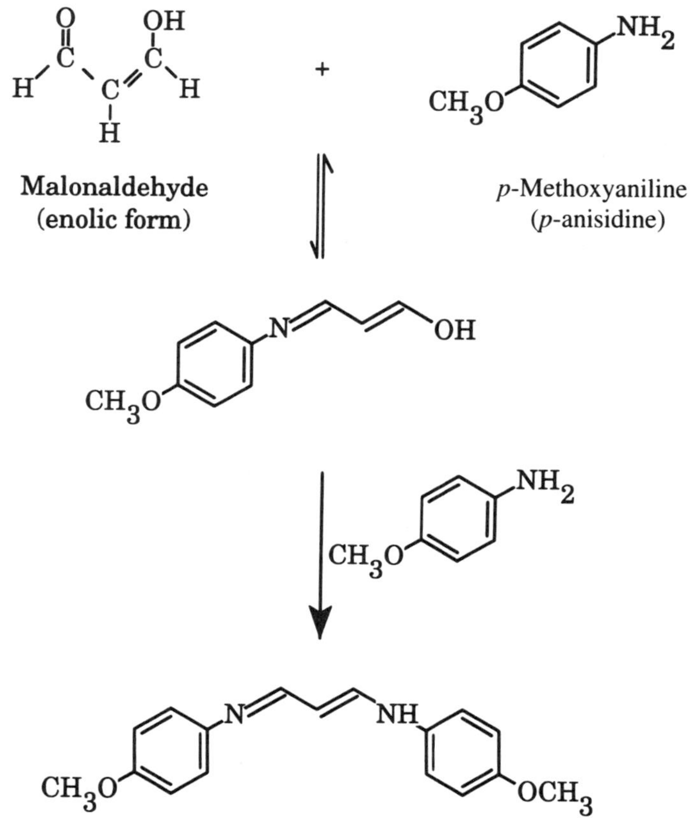

Fig. 24.4. Possible reactions between *p*-anisidine reagent and malonaldehyde.

and Shahidi (52) have defined $TOTOX_{TBA}$ as 2PV + TBARS because determination of *p*-AnV may not always be as feasible as the determination of TBARS.

Carbonyls. An alternative approach for monitoring the extent of lipid oxidation in fats and oils is to measure the total or individual volatile carbonyl compounds formed from degradation of hydroperoxides. One of the more reliable methods for total carbonyl analysis is based on the absorbance of the quinoidal ion, a derivative of aldehydes and ketones. This ion is formed from the reaction of 2,4-dinitrophenylhydrazine (2,4-DNDH) with an aldehyde or ketone, followed by the reaction of the resulting hydrozones with alkali as shown in Fig. 24.5. Many variations of this spectroscopic method have been reported (53,54). Each method offers an alternative solvent, wavelength, or work-up to analyze the quinoidal ion.

The analysis of individual carbonyl compounds is another method which has recently gained popularity. Hexanal, one of the major secondary products formed during the oxidation of linoleic acid of oils (55), as well as other aldehydes, has

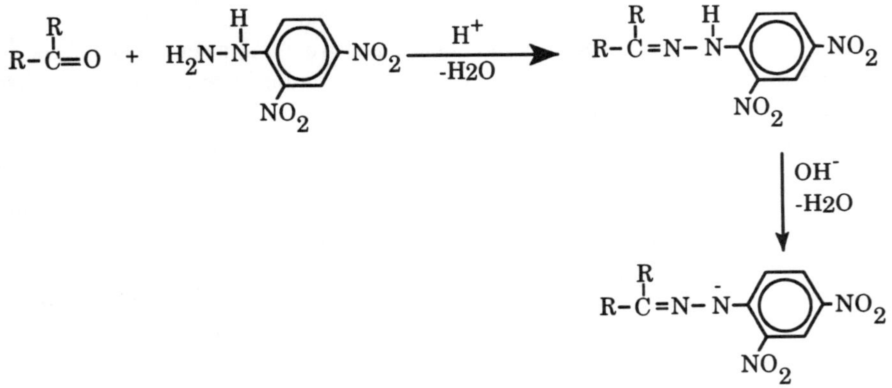

Fig. 24.5. Reaction steps in the production of hydrazones from carbonyls and 2,4-dinitrophenyl hydrazine.

been used to follow lipid oxidation in food products. Shahidi *et al.* (43) reported that a linear relationship existed between hexanal content, sensory scores, and TBA numbers of cooked ground pork, while St. Angelo *et al.* (56) established a similar correlation for cooked beef. O'Keefe *et al.* (57) used hexanal as an indicator to assess oxidative stability of meat from broiler chicken fed fish meal. Supplementation of high amounts of fish meal to the diet increased the hexanal content of the thigh meat during storage. However, recent studies in our laboratories showed that during oxidation of marine oils, rich in polyunsaturated fatty acids of the ω-3 type, large amounts of propanal are formed and that a good correlation exists between the content of propanal and TBARS values (58). Therefore, it is essential to use appropriate indicators when assessing the stability of food lipids. We recommend that hexanal be used when the oils under investigation are rich in ω-6 fatty acids whereas propanal would serve as a reliable indicator when oils high in ω-3 fatty acids are considered.

Hydrocarbons and Fluorescent Products. Studies of oxidized methyl linoleate and soybean oil (59) have revealed that saturated hydrocarbons could be detected when aldehydes are either absent or undetectable. Snyder *et al.* (60) reported that ethane, propane, and pentane are predominant short-chain hydrocarbons formed through thermal decomposition of soybean oil. Correlations of flavor acceptability scores and pentane content, as determined by gas chromatographic techniques, have been used to assess rancidity of fats and oils (61). Significant correlations existed between the amount of pentane produced and the number of rancid descriptions of aged vegetable oils (62). Correlation of headspace pentane concentrations and sensory scores of stored freeze-dried pork samples was reported by Coxon (11).

Another secondary change that occurs during autoxidation of biological systems is the formation of fluorescent products from the reaction of MA with amino compounds such as proteins and nucleotides (63). This method has been used in determining the extent of lipid oxidation in biological tissues. Dillard and Tappel (64,65) have established that fluorescent compounds with a general structure of 1-amino-3-iminopropane may develop through the reaction of an amino group with carbonyl compounds, mainly malonaldehyde (Fig. 24.6).

Buttkus and Rose (66) reported that the development of fluorescence depends not only on the formation of condensation products between malonaldehyde and free amino groups, but also on the nature of the substituents of the latter compounds. Different excitation and emission maxima were observed for different condensation products. Advantages of the fluorescence method as a means of measuring lipid oxidation were reported by Dillard and Tappel (64,65). This method can detect fluorescent compounds at part per billion levels and was found to be 10 to 100 times more sensitive than the TBA assay.

Measurement of Frying Fat Deterioration

Deep frying is a popular method for food preparation, especially in fast food restaurants. Although used primarily as a heat exchange medium to cook food, the oil used for deep frying contributes to the quality of fried products. In the process of deep fat frying, a complex series of chemical reactions takes place. These reactions are characterized by a decrease in the total unsaturation content of the fat with an increase in the content of free fatty acids, cyclic fatty acids (Fig. 24.7), foaming, color, viscosity, formation of polar materials, and polymeric compounds. As these reactions proceed, the functional, sensory, and nutritional quality of frying fats is changed and may reach a point at which high-quality foods can no longer be prepared. The question is, how does one know when the frying fat is no longer usable?

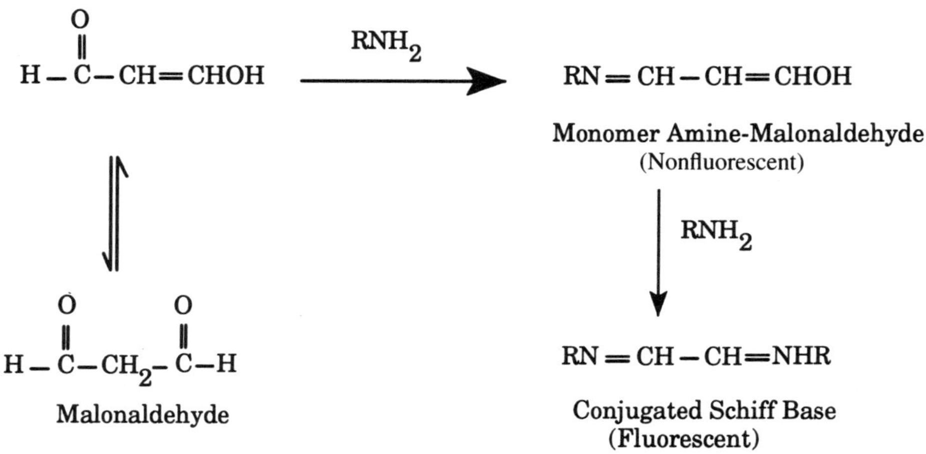

Fig. 24.6. Production of fluorescent chromophores from the reaction of lipid oxidation products and amines.

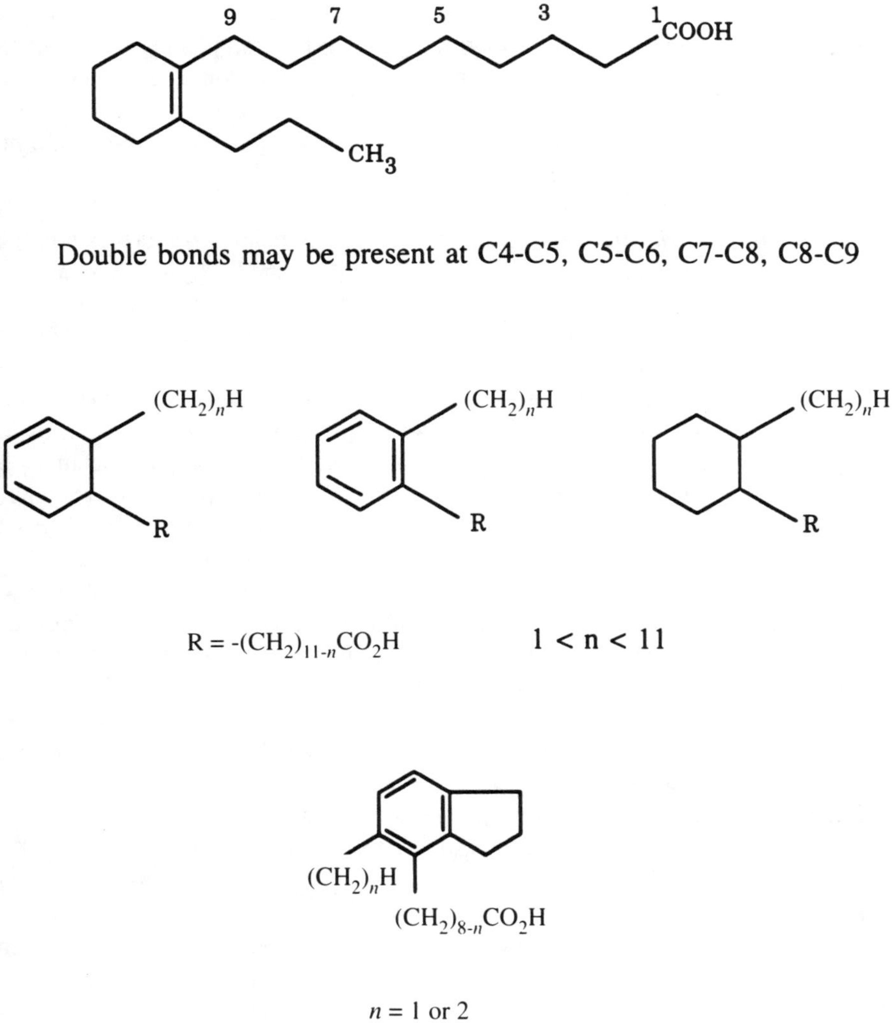

Fig. 24.7. Structures of cyclic fatty acids formed during frying.

Quality evaluation of frying fats may be carried out in many ways. The first attempt to define a deteriorated frying fat was made by the German Society for Fat Research in 1973 (67). It was recommended that "a used frying fat is deteriorated if, without doubt, its odor and taste are unacceptable; or if in case of doubtful sensory assessment, the concentration of petroleum ether-insoluble oxidized fatty acids in it is 0.7% or higher and its smoke point is lower than 170°C; or if the concentration of petroleum ether insoluble oxidized fatty acids is 1.0% or higher." Although sensory evaluation in any food operation is the most important quality assessment, taste evaluations are unreliable for routine quality control. It is always preferred to have a quantitative method for which a rejection point could be established by sensory means. Peroxide values provide an indication of frying fat quality if they are used in a very specific way. However, peroxides generally decompose at about 150°C and hence, at frying temperatures (usually 180–190°C), no accumulation of peroxides occurs. Free fatty acids from frying fats can be determined by direct titration. However, Fritsch (68) has shown that, in most deep fat frying operations, the amount of free fatty acids produced by hydrolysis is too small to affect the quality of the food. However, industrially, frying oil quality is usually checked by measurement of color and/or free fatty acid content to inform an operator when a fat is ending its useful life. The foaming characteristics of used fats would also lead one to the same conclusion.

A quick colorimetric test kit is now available for measuring oil quality (69). Robern and Gray (70) have developed a spot test to measure free fatty acids in which drops of used fat are placed on a glass covered with silica gel containing a pH indicator to give a three-color test scale of blue, green, and yellow. This may indicate the amount of free fatty acids in a sample. Northern States Instrument Corp. (Lino Lakes, MN) has developed an instrument which measures the dielectric constant of insulating liquids. The instrument is a compact unit, which is relatively inexpensive and simple to operate, requiring only a few drops of oil for each measurement. For evaluation of frying fats, the instrument must first be calibrated with a fresh oil sample that is used in the frying operations.

Determination of total polar materials in frying fats appears to be emerging as a practical method for assessing the useful life of fats and oils subjected to frying; it is an official method in Europe (67). Total polar materials are determined by dissolving the fat in a relatively non-polar solvent such as toluene or benzene and running it through a silica gel column which adsorbs the polar compounds. After evaporation of the solvent, the non-polar fat can be weighed and the total polar materials estimated by difference, or the total polar materials can be determined directly by eluting them from the column with ether or a mixture of chloroform and methanol. Sebedio *et al.* (71) showed that polar and non-polar fractions of fried oils can be quantitatively estimated by using the Iatroscan thin-layer chromatography–flame ionization detection (TLC–FID) system with Chromarod SII. This method requires only a very small amount of sample and is much faster than silicic acid column separation.

Recent Developments for Quantitation of Lipid Oxidation

Lipid oxidation in foods and biological systems has conventionally been studied by monitoring either primary or secondary oxidation products. Over the last twenty years, advances in pulse radiolysis (72) and electron spin resonance (ESR; 73) techniques have facilitated the detection and study of short-lived free radical intermediates. ESR spectroscopy selectively detects species with an unpaired electron, such as free radicals. The technique depends on the absorption of microwave energy (which arises from the promotion of an electron to a higher energy level) when a sample is placed in a variable magnetic field. A major limitation in the detection of free radicals by ESR is the requirement that radical concentrations remain higher than 10^{-8} M. Radical lifetimes in solution are very short (<1 ms), and steady-state concentrations generally remain well below 10^{-7} M. Several approaches have been developed to overcome this problem, either by enhancing the rate of radical production or diminishing the rate of its disappearance. These techniques include rapid freezing, lyophilization, or spin trapping (74). Although application of ESR as a precise method to study lipid oxidation in animal tissues and other biological systems is commonplace, its application to foods is relatively new.

Yen and Duh (75), Brand-Williams *et al.* (76), and Chen and Ho (77) have reported that determination of free radical inhibitory ability of different antioxidants can be achieved by using very stable free radicals such as 1,1-diphenyl-2-picrylhydrazyl (DPPH). The mechanism of the reaction of antioxidant with a DPPH radical is given below:

$$(\text{DPPH})^{\bullet} + \text{HO-R-OH} \rightarrow (\text{DPPH}):\text{H} + \text{HO-R-O}^{\bullet}$$

$$\text{HO-R-O}^{\bullet} + (\text{DPPH}) \rightarrow (\text{DPPH}):\text{H} + \text{O=R=O}$$

DPPH, a radical with a deep violet color, receives a proton from the antioxidant and converts to a colorless protonated DPPH molecule. Using this reagent, the free radical-scavenging ability of the antioxidant can be determined by spectrophotometric methods.

Infrared (IR) spectroscopy has also been used for measurement of rancidity; it is of particular value in recognition of unusual functional groups and in studies of fatty acids with *trans* double bonds. Production of hydroperoxides during oxidation of lipids gives rise to an absorption band at about 2.93 μm, whereas the disappearance of a band at 3.20 μm indicates the replacement of a hydrogen on a double bond, or polymerization. It is also suggested that the appearance of an additional band at 5.72 μm, due to C=O stretching, indicates the formation of aldehydes, ketones, or acids. Furthermore, changes in the absorption bands in the 10–11 μm region indicates *cis*, *trans*-isomerization and probably formation of conjugated linkages. Determination of oxidative deterioration of lipids using the IR method is simple, rapid, and requires only small amounts of sample (20 mg). Application of Fourier transform infrared (FTIR) and nuclear magnetic resonance (NMR, 78) to determine both primary and secondary oxidation products is reported elsewhere in this monograph.

Recently, Burkow *et al.* (79) reported that hypochlorite-activated chemiluminescence could provide a useful method for evaluation of antioxidants in edible oils. Due to high sensitivity and ability to detect small changes in the degree of oxidation, this method provides a useful means to evaluate effects of antioxidants on oils at low storage temperatures (about 35°C) within 24 h. Chemiluminescence generally originates from electrically excited stages such as singlet molecular oxygen in lipid peroxidation (80,81). The chemiluminescence method has now been tested for estimating the degree of deterioration of edible oils containing antioxidants (82) as well as for shelf-life dating of fish samples (83).

References

1. Enser, M. (1987) *Food Sci. Technol. Today, 1*, 151.
2. Labuza, T.P. (1971) *CRC Crit. Rev. Food Technol. 2*, 355.
3. Frankel, E.N. (1980) *Prog. Lipid Res. 19*, 1.
4. Kanner, J., German, J.B., and Kinsella, J.E. (1987) *CRC Crit. Rev. Food Sci. Nutr. 25*, 317.
5. Farmer, E.H., Bloomfield, G.F., Sundaralingam, A., and Sutton, D.A. (1942) *Trans. Faraday Soc. 38*, 348.
6. Boland, J.L., and Gee, G. (1946) *Trans. Faraday Soc. 42*, 236.
7. Bateman, L., Hughes, H., and Morris, A.L. (1953) *Discuss. Faraday Soc. 14*, 190.
8. Hawrysh, Z.J. (1990) in *Canola and Rapeseed: Production, Chemistry, Nutrition and Processing Technology* (Shahidi, F., ed.), Van Nostrand Reinhold, New York, p. 99.
9. Hsieh, R.J., and Kinsella, J.E. (1989) *Adv. Food Nutr. Res. 33*, 233.
10. Sherwin, E.R. (1978) *J. Am. Oil Chem. Soc. 55*, 809.
11. Coxon, D. (1987) *Food Sci. Technol. Today, 1*, 164.
12. Gray, J.I., and Monahan, F.J. (1992) *Trends Food Sci. Technol. 3*, 320.
13. Gultteride, J.M.C., and Halliwell, B. (1990) *Trends Biochem. Sci. 15*, 129.
14. Hudson, B.J.F. (1983) *Rancidity of Foods* (Allen, J.C., and Hamilton, J., eds.), Applied Sci. Pub., London, p. 47.
15. Sylvester, N.D., Lampitt, L.H., and Ainsworth, A.N. (1942) *J. Soc. Chem. Ind. 61*, 165.
16. Olcott, H.S., and Einest, E. (1958) *J. Am. Oil Chem. Soc. 35*, 161.
17. Ke, P.J., and Ackman, R.G. (1976) *J. Am. Oil Chem. Soc. 53*, 636.
18. Wanasundara, U.N., and Shahidi, F. (1994) *J. Am. Oil Chem. Soc. 71*, 817.
19. Gray, J.I. (1978) *J. Am. Oil Chem. Soc. 55*, 539.
20. *Official Methods and Recommended Practices of the American Oil Chemists' Society*, 1990 (Firestone, D., ed.), 4th edn., American Oil Chemists' Society, Champaign.
21. Lips, A., Chapman, R.A., and McFarlane, W.D. (1943) *Oil Soap 20*, 240.
22. Hughes, H., Smith, C.V., and Mitchell, J.R. (1983) *Anal. Biochem. 130*, 431.
23. Hughes, H., Smith, C.V., Tsoko-Kuhn, J.O., and Mitchell, J.R. (1986) *Anal. Biochem. 152*, 107.
24. Dugan, L.R. (1955) *J. Am. Oil Chem. Soc. 32*, 605.
25. Jabe, T.A., Matlock, M.G., and Sleeter, R.T. (1993) *J. Am. Oil Chem. Soc. 70*, 1055.
26. Logani, M.K., and Davies, R.E. (1980) *Lipids 15*, 485.
27. Farmer, E.H., and Sutton, D.A. (1946) *Trans. Faraday Soc. 42*, 228.
28. St. Angelo, A.J., Ory, R.L., and Brown, L.E. (1972) *Am. Peanut Res. Edu. Assoc. 4*, 186.
29. St. Angelo, A.J., Ory, R.L., and Brown, L.E. (1975) *J. Am. Oil Chem. Soc. 52*, 34.
30. Shahidi, F., Wanasundara, U.N., and Brunet, N. (1994) *Food Res. Inter. 27*, 555.
31. Wanasundara, U.N., Shahidi, F., and Jablonski, C.R. (1995) *Food Chem. 52*, 249.
32. Parr, L.J., and Swoboda, P.A.T. (1976) *J. Food Technol. 11*, 1.
33. Tarladgis, B.G., Pearson, A.M., and Dugan, L.R. (1964) *J. Sci. Food Agric. 15*, 602.

34. Dahle, L.K., Hill, E.G., and Holman, R.T. (1962) *Arch. Biochem. Biophys. 98*, 253.
35. Marcuse, R., and Johansson, L. (1973) *J. Am. Oil Chem. Soc. 50*, 387.
36. Shahidi, F., Rubin, L.J., Diosady, L.L., and Wood, D.F. (1985) *J. Food Sci. 50*, 274.
37. Ke, P.J., Cervantes, E., and Robles-Martinez, C. (1984) *J. Sci. Food Agric. 35*, 1248.
38. Wanasundara, U.N., and Shahidi, F. (1993) *J. Food Lipids 1*, 15.
39. Baumgartner, W.A., Baker, N., Hill, V.A., and Wright, E.T. (1975) *Lipids 10*, 309.
40. Ke, P.J., and Woyewoda, A.D. (1979) *Anal. Chem. Acta 106*, 279.
41. Robbles-Martinez, C., Cervantes, E., and Ke, P.J. (1982) *Can. Tech. Report Fish Aquatic Sci.*, No. 1089.
42. Pokorny, J., Valentova, H., and Davidek, J. (1985) *Die Nahrung 29*, 31.
43. Shahidi, F., Yun, J., Rubin, L.J., and Wood, D.F. (1987) *J. Food Sci. 52*, 546.
44. Thomas, M.C., and Fumes, J. (1987) *J. Food Sci. 52*, 575.
45. Schmedes, A., and Holmer, G. (1989) *J. Am. Oil Chem. Soc. 66*, 813.
46. Gray, J.I., and Pearson, A.M. (1987) *Advances in Meat Research: Restructured Meat and Poultry Products* (Pearson, A.M., and Dutson, T.R., eds.), Van Nostrand Reinhold, New York, p. 219.
47. *Official and Tentative Methods of the American Oil Chemists' Society*, (1981) 3rd edn., American Oil Chemists' Society, Champaign.
48. Fioriti, J.A., Bentz, A.P., and Sims, R.J. (1966) *J. Am. Oil Chem. Soc. 43*, 37.
49. Standard Methods for the Analysis of Oils, Fats and Derivatives (1987) (Paquot, C., and Hautfenne, A., eds.), 7th edn., Blackwell Scientific Publishers Ltd., Oxford.
50. List, G.R., Evans, C.D., Kwolek, W.K., Warner, K., and Bound, B.K. (1974) *J. Am. Oil Chem. Soc. 51*, 17.
51. Rossell, J.B. (1983) in *Rancidity in Foods* (Allen, J.C., and Hamilton, J., eds.), Applied Sci. Pub., London, p. 21.
52. Wanasundara, U.N., and Shahidi, F. (1995) *J. Food Lipids 2*, 73.
53. Pool, M.F., and Klose, A.A. (1951) *J. Am. Oil Chem. Soc. 28*, 215.
54. Yukawa, N., Takamura, H., and Matoba, T. (1993) *J. Am. Oil Chem. Soc. 70*, 881.
55. Frankel, E.N., Neff, W.E., and Selke, E. (1981) *Lipids 16*, 279.
56. St. Angelo, A.J., Vercellotti, J.R., Legengre, M.G., Vinnelt, C.H., Kuan, J.W., Janies, C., and Duppy, H.P. (1987) *J. Food Sci. 52*, 1163.
57. O'Keefe, S.F., Proudfoot, F.G., and Ackman, R.G. (1995) *Food Res. Int. 28*, 417.
58. Wanasundara, U.N., and Shahidi, F. (1995) Paper presented at the Canadian Section of American Oil Chemists' Society's Annual Meeting, Guelph, ON, November 15–16.
59. Selke, E., Moser, H.A., and Rohwedde, W.K. (1970) *J. Am. Oil Chem. Soc. 47*, 393.
60. Snyder, J.M., Frankel, E.N., and Selke, E. (1985) *J. Am. Oil Chem. Soc. 62*, 1675.
61. Jarvi, P.K., Lee, G.D., Erickson, D.K., and Butkus, E.A. (1971) *J. Am. Oil Chem. Soc. 48*, 121.
62. Warner, K., Evans, C.D., List, G.R., Boundly, B.K., and Kwolek, W.F. (1974) *J. Food Sci. 39*, 761.
63. Bidlack, W.R., and Tappel, A.L. (1973) *Lipids 8*, 203.
64. Dillard, C.J., and Tappel, A.L. (1971) *Lipids 6*, 715.
65. Dillard, C.J., and Tappel, A.L. (1973) *Lipids 8*, 183.
66. Buttkus, H., and Rose, R.J. (1972) *J. Am. Oil Chem. Soc. 50*, 387.
67. Guhr, G., and Waibel, J. (1979) *Fette Seifen Anstrichm. 75*, 449.
68. Fritsch, C.W. (1981) *J. Am. Oil Chem. Soc. 81*, 511.
69. Blumenthal, M. (1985) *J. Am. Oil Chem. Soc. 65*, 482.

70. Roben, H., and Gray, L. (1981) *Can. Inst. Food Sci. Technol. J. 14*, 159.
71. Sebedio, J.L., Astorg, P.O., Septier, A., and Grandgirard, A. (1987) *J. Chromatogr. 405*, 371.
72. Simic, M.G. (1980) in *Autoxidation in Food and Biological Systems* (Simic, M.G., and Karel, M., eds.), Plenum Press, New York, p. 17.
73. Schaich, K.M., and Borgi, D.C. (1980) in *Autoxidation in Food and Biological Systems* (Simic, M.G., and Karel, M., eds.), Plenum Press, New York, p. 45.
74. Davies, M.J. (1987) *Chem. Phys. Lipids 44*, 149.
75. Yen, G.C., and Duh, P.D. (1994) *J. Agric. Food Chem. 42*, 629.
76. Brand-Williams, W., Cuvelier, M.E., and Berset, C. (1995) *Lebensm. -Wiss. u. -Technol. 28*, 25.
77. Chen, C.W., and Ho, C.T. (1995) *J. Food Lipids 2,* 35.
78. Wanasundara, U.N. (1993) *Stabilization of Canola Oil by Naturally Occurring Antioxidants*, M.Sc. Thesis, Memorial University of Newfoundland, St. John's, Canada.
79. Burkow, I.C., Moen, P., and Overbo, K. (1992) *J. Am. Oil Chem. Soc. 69*, 1108.
80. Neeman, I., Joseph, D., Biggeley, W.H., and Seliger, H.H. (1985) *Lipids 20*, 729.
81. Cash, G.A., George, G.A., and Bartley, J.P. (1987) *Chem. Phys. Lipids 43*, 265.
82. Burkow, I.C., Vikersveen, L., and Saarem, K. (1995) *J. Am. Oil Chem. Soc. 72*, 553.
83. Miyazawa, T., Kikuch, M., Fujimoto, K., Endo, Y., Cho, S.-Y., Usuki, R., and Keneda, T. (1991) *J. Am. Oil Chem. Soc. 68*, 39.

Chapter 25

Application of Proton Nuclear Magnetic Resonance (^{1}H NMR) Spectroscopy for Assessment of Oxidative Stability of Fats and Oils

F. Shahidi and U.N. Wanasundara

Department of Biochemistry, Memorial University of Newfoundland, St. John's, Newfoundland, Canada.

Introduction

Autoxidation of unsaturated fats and oils is a major concern for processing industries and consumers alike because it is directly related to cost, nutrition, flavor, safety, and storage of products (1,2). Extensive research has been conducted to elucidate the mechanism and to devise methods to control oxidation of food lipids. Various oxidative products and their possible interaction with food components and biological compounds have been studied (3,4). The oxidation of oil occurs at sites of unsaturation and proceeds *via* a free radical chain mechanism (1) consisting of initiation, propagation, and termination steps.

Chemical, instrumental, and sensory techniques have been employed to assess the extent of autoxidation, photooxidation, and thermal degradation of edible oils (5). The content of hydroperoxides, the primary products of lipid oxidation, is often used as an indicator to monitor oxidation during the early stages of storage of oils (6). However, hydroperoxides, once formed, decompose rapidly during storage and upon heating. Thus, peroxide value may not necessarily show the actual extent of lipid oxidation (7). Measurement of conjugated dienes (at 234 nm) and trienes (at 268 nm) as rapid physical methods has been suggested for assessing oxidative stability of vegetable oils (8). However, the most widely used classical method for determination of lipid oxidation in foods is the 2-thiobarbituric acid (TBA) test (6). This test measures the concentration of secondary oxidation products such as malonaldehyde and other TBA reactive substances (TBARS). The *p*-anisidine value (*p*-AnV) also measures secondary products of lipid oxidation, namely carbonyl compounds (9). The *p*-AnV is often used together with PV to calculate the so-called total oxidation or TOTOX value, defined as 2PV + *p*-AnV. The TOTOX value is said to have the advantage of combining evidence about the history of an oil (as reflected in the *p*-AnV) with its present state (as evidenced in the PV). Therefore, determination of TOTOX value is used extensively to assess the oxidative deterioration of lipids (10). Each method of evaluation of oil stability has its own limitations as discussed elsewhere in this monograph. Although sensory methods are considered to be the most sensitive for assessing the oxidative state of food lipids, their use is not practical for routine analysis (6). Therefore, a simple, quick, nondestructive method for quality control of products leaving a processing plant and evaluation of the oxidative state of edible oils is required. A method which could simultaneously evaluate both primary and secondary changes during storage/oxidation of food lipids is desired.

NMR Methodology for Assessment of Oxidative Deterioration of Fats and Oils

High resolution nuclear magnetic resonance spectroscopy (NMR) makes it possible to determine various types of hydrogen atoms (protons, ^1H) in triacylglycerol (TAG) molecules because hydrogen atoms in a strong magnetic field absorb energy from radio frequency, depending on the environment in which they are placed in a molecule. During oxidation of food lipids, changes occur in the environment in which protons in an oxidizing TAG molecule are located. These changes may be monitored by employing ^1H NMR spectroscopy as originally described by Saito and Nakamura (11), Saito and Udagawa (12), and Wanasundara and Shahidi (13). For this purpose, the oil is dissolved in $CDCl_3$, and the NMR spectrum of the oil is recorded (see Fig. 25.1). The sharp signal at the extreme right side of the spectrum (high applied field) is due to tetramethylsilane (TMS) added to the solution to serve as an internal standard. The spectrum shows eight groups of signals labeled *a* to *h*. These signals are assigned as follows: *a*, hydrogens directly attached to double-bonded carbons (olefinic protons) and the methine proton in the glyceryl moiety (δ 5.1–5.4); *b*, hydrogens in the two methylene groups in the glyceryl moiety (δ 4.0–4.4); *c*, hydrogens in the CH_2 groups attached to two double-bonded carbon atoms (diallylmethylene protons) ($=HC\text{-}CH_2\text{-}CH=$; δ 2.6–2.9); *d*, hydrogens in the three CH_2 groups alpha to the carboxyl groups (α-CH2; δ 2.2–2.4); *e*, hydrogens in the CH_2 groups attached to saturated carbons and double-bonded carbon atoms ($\text{-}CH_2\text{-}C=$; δ 1.8–2.2); *f*, hydrogens in the CH_2 groups attached to the saturated carbon atoms ($=C\text{-}CH_2\text{-}\underline{CH_2}$; δ 1.45–1.8); *g*, hydrogens in the CH_2 groups bonded to two saturated carbon atoms ($[CH_2]_n$; δ 1.1–1.45); and *h*, hydrogens in the three terminal CH_3 groups (δ 0.7–1.0). The relative number of protons in each group is calculated based on the integration of methylene protons of the glyceryl moiety (δ 4.0–4.4) of the TAG (four protons in the two methylene groups of the TAG moiety) molecules. The area per proton is expressed as

$$\text{Area per proton} = \text{Area of } b\text{-type protons}/4$$

Because area per proton is known, one may calculate the number of protons belonging to each and every individual signal by dividing the integration number

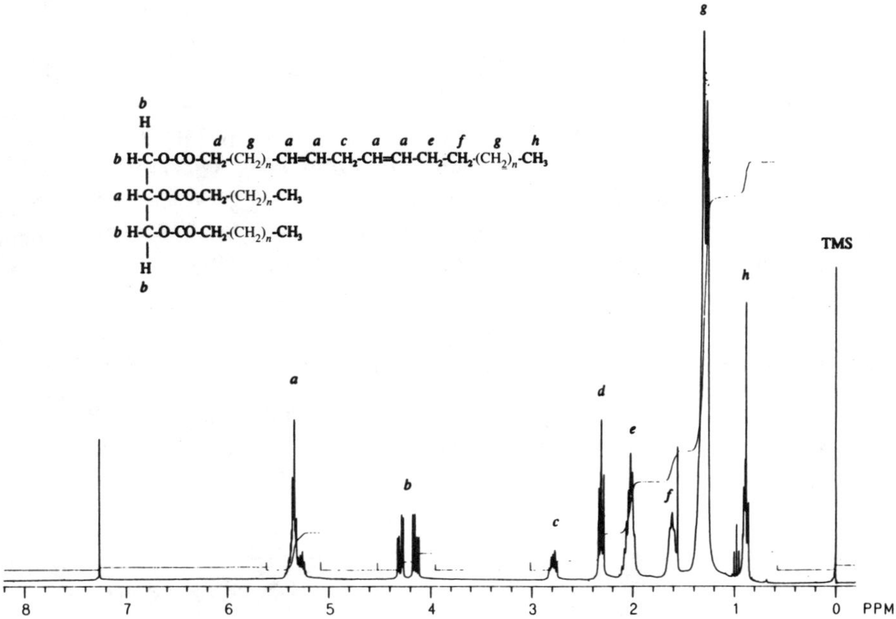

Fig. 25.1. ^{1}H Nuclear magnetic resonance spectrum of oxidized canola oil [peaks at δ 0.00 and 7.26 are for tetramethylsilane (TMS) and $CHCl_3$ protons as impurities in $CDCl_3$, respectively)].

of each signal by the area per proton. For example, the total number of diallylmethylene protons equals the Area of *c*-type protons/(the Area of *b*-type protons/4).

Table 25.1 shows the changes in relative proportion of the number of each type of proton during oxidation of canola and soybean oils stored at 65°C (oils were not stripped of their naturally occurring antioxidants). During a 30-d storage

TABLE 25.1
Relative Changes in the Total Number of Olefinic, Diallylmethylene, and Aliphatic Protons of Canola and Soybean Oils During Accelerated Storage at 65°C

Storage time	Olefinic protons		Diallylmethylene protons		Aliphatic protons	
(d)	Canola	Soybean	Canola	Soybean	Canola	Soybean
0	7.12	8.12	2.18	4.00	79.28	75.64
5	6.76	8.04	1.90	3.92	80.94	79.44
10	6.37	7.60	1.86	3.80	83.32	80.48
15	6.00	7.24	1.54	3.40	84.19	80.64
20	5.57	7.08	1.36	3.36	85.62	84.89
25	5.36	6.52	1.12	2.84	86.88	85.24
30	5.21	5.88	0.99	2.60	88.18	86.00

period, the relative number of olefinic protons (-HC=CH-; δ 5.1–5.4, changed from 7.12 to 5.21 for canola oil and from 8.12 to 5.88 for soybean oil) and diallylmethylene protons (=C-CH_2-C=; δ 2.6–2.9, changed from 2.18 to 0.99 for canola oil and from 4.00 to 2.60 for soybean oil) protons decreased and the total number of aliphatic (CH_3 + $[CH_2]_n$ + CH_2-CH_2-C= + CH_2-C= + α-CH_2; δ 0.6–2.5, changed from 79.3 to 88.2 for canola oil and from 75.6 to 86.0 for soybean oil) protons increased. During autoxidation of fats and oils, diallylmethylene protons are attacked first by free radicals followed by intramolecular rearrangement of the olefinic protons (12). Thus, the relative number of diallylmethylene and olefinic protons decreases.

Data Manipulation and Correlation with Other Indices

The ratios of aliphatic to olefinic (R_{ao}) and aliphatic to diallylmethylene (R_{ad}) protons are easily calculated. These ratios increase steadily during the storage and oxidation of oils (Fig. 25.2). Numerical values of R_{ao} and R_{ad} may be plotted against

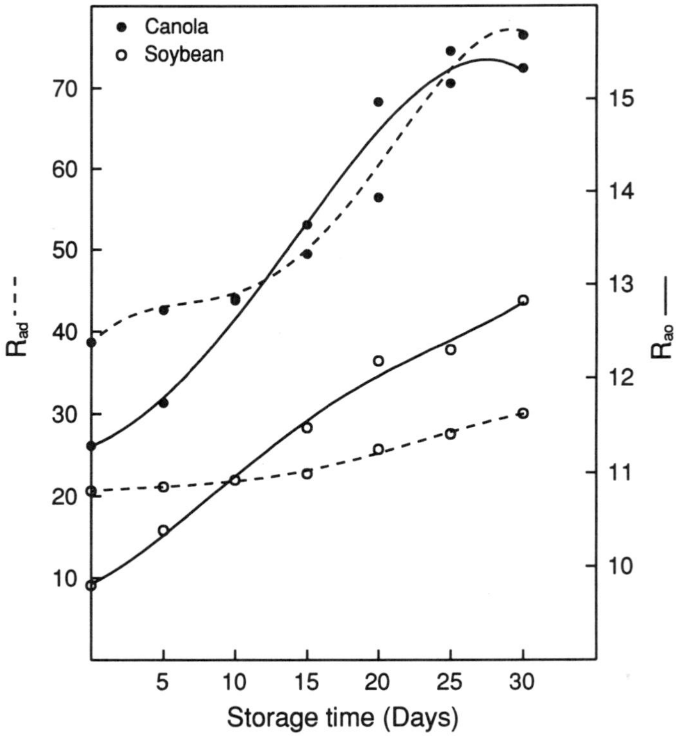

Fig. 25.2. Changes in the ratios of aliphatic to diallylmethylene protons (R_{ad}) and aliphatic to olefinic protons (R_{ao}) of canola and soybean oils.

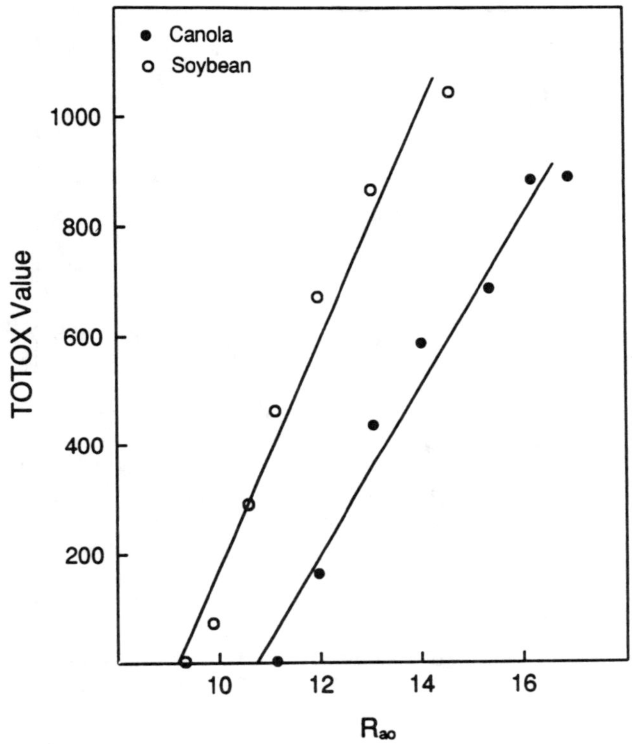

Fig. 25.3. Relationship between total oxidation (TOTOX) values and the ratio of aliphatic to olefinic (R_{ao}) protons of oxidized canola and soybean oils.

corresponding TOTOX values for both canola and soybean oils (Figs. 25.3 and 25.4, respectively). A significant ($P < 0.05$) correlation existed between R_{ao} or R_{ad} and TOTOX values. Correlation coefficients were 0.984 for R_{ao} and 0.933 for R_{ad} of canola oil, and 0.985 for R_{ao} and 0.969 for R_{ad} of soybean oil. Linear regression equations of these relationships were as follows:

$$TOTOX_{Canola} = 155R_{ao} - 1662$$

$$TOTOX_{Canola} = 16R_{ad} - 430$$

$$TOTOX_{Soybean} = 2088R_{ao} - 1920$$

$$TOTOX_{Soybean} = 73R_{ad} - 1300$$

Shahidi *et al.* (14) have further shown that significant ($P < 0.05$) linear correlations exist between R_{ao} or R_{ad} and TOTOX values for oxidized seal blubber and

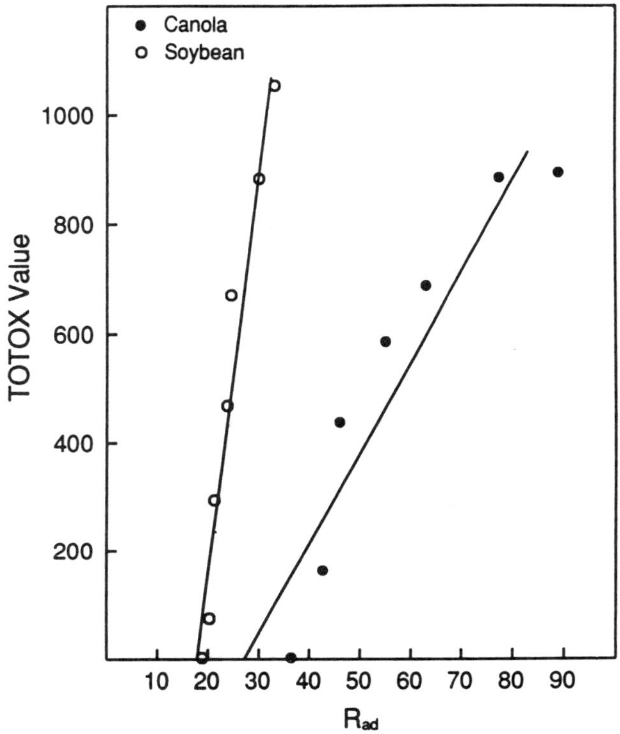

Fig. 25.4. Relationship between total oxidation (TOTOX) values and the ratio of aliphatic to diallylmethylene (R_{ad}) protons of oxidized canola and soybean oils.

cod liver oils (Figs. 25.5 and 25.6). Correlation coefficients were 0.931 and 0.945 for R_{ao} and R_{ad} for seal blubber oil, and 0.975 and 0.994 for R_{ao} and R_{ad} for cod liver oil, respectively. Therefore, NMR methodology may also be used to monitor oxidation of oils rich in polyunsaturated fatty acids. This method is particularly useful for assessing oxidation of lipids during later stages of storage when peroxide values start to decline due to decomposition of hydroperoxides.

Saito and Nakamura (11) have shown that the ratio of olefinic to aliphatic protons measured by NMR decreases continuously as long as the oxidative reaction proceeds. They suggested that the NMR technique could be useful for measuring oxidative deterioration of polyunsaturated fatty acid-containing oils, even at stages beyond the point at which peroxide value reached its maximum. Saito and Udagawa (12) have used this method to evaluate oxidative deterioration of brown fish meal and suggested that NMR methodology is suitable for comparing the storage conditions of the fish meal as well as estimating the effect of antioxidants in fish meals and oils. These authors reported good correlations between peroxide values and NMR data. However, in our studies, we found that linear relationships

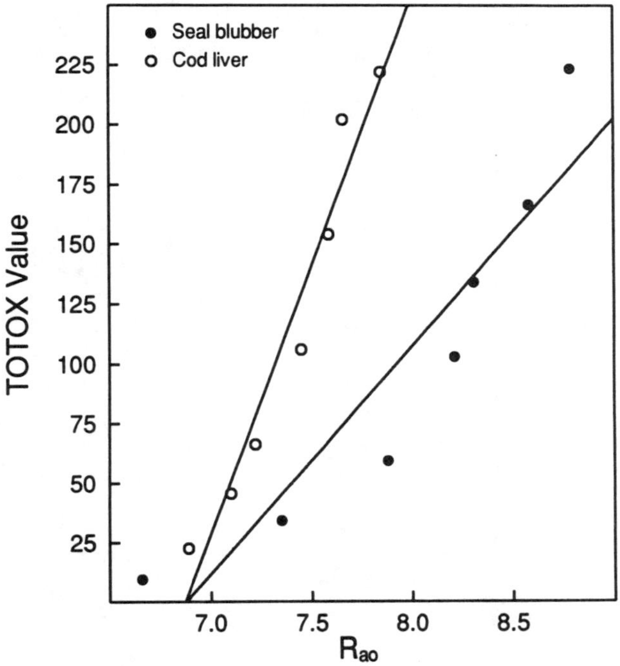

Fig. 25.5. Relationship between total oxidation (TOTOX) values and the ratio of aliphatic to olefinic (R_{ao}) protons of oxidized seal blubber and cod liver oils.

between peroxide value and NMR data were not as suitable as those of TOTOX values and NMR data. It is obvious that TOTOX values correlate better with R_{ao} and R_{ad} than do peroxide values because both TOTOX and NMR data estimate overall changes that occur in fatty acid profiles as reflected in both the primary and secondary oxidation products of lipids. Thus, NMR methodology offers a rapid, nondestructive, and reliable technique for estimating the oxidative state of edible oils during processing and storage.

References

1. Labuza, T.P. (1971) *CRC Crit. Rev. Food Sci. Technol. 2*, 355.
2. Frankel, E.N. (1980) *Prog. Lipid Res. 19*, 1.
3. Horton, A.A., and Fairhurst, S. (1987) *CRC Crit. Rev. Toxicol. 18*, 27.
4. Kanner, J., German, J.B., and Kinsella, J.L. (1987) *CRC Crit. Rev. Food Sci. Nutr. 25*, 317.
5. Hawrysh, Z.J. (1990) in *Canola and Rapeseed, Production, Chemistry, Nutrition, and Processing Technology* (Shahidi, F., ed.), Van Nostrand Reinhold, New York, p. 99.
6. Gray, J.I. (1978) *J. Am. Oil Chem. Soc. 55*, 539.
7. Sherwin, E.R. (1978) *J. Am. Oil Chem. Soc. 55*, 809.

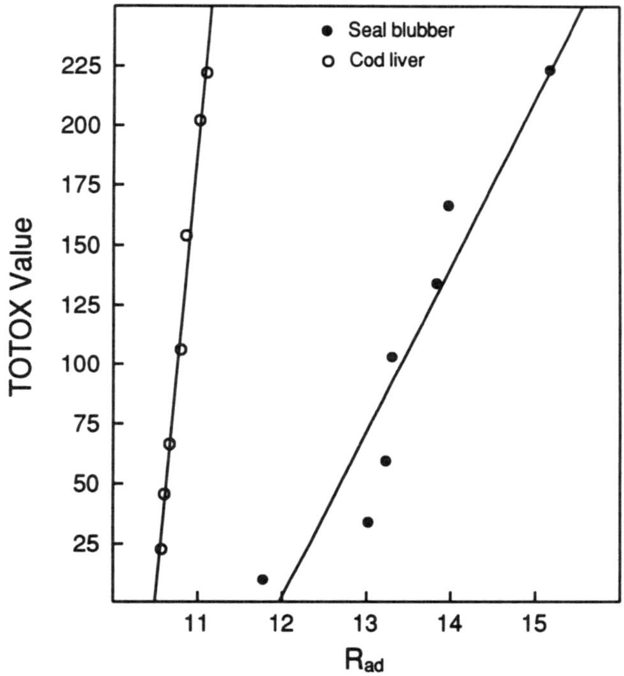

Fig. 25.6. Relationship between total oxidation (TOTOX) values and the ratio of aliphatic to diallylmethylene (R_{ad}) protons of oxidized seal blubber and cod liver oils.

8. St. Angelo, A.J., Ory, R.L., and Brown, L.E. (1975) *J. Am. Oil Chem. Soc. 52*, 34.
9. *Standard Methods for the Analysis of Oils, Fats and Derivatives* (1987) (Paquot, C., and Hautfenne, A., eds.), 7th edn., Blackwell Scientific Pub. Ltd., Oxford.
10. Rossell, B. (1991) *Lipid Technol. 3*, 122.
11. Saito, H., and Nakamura, K. (1990) *Agric. Biol. Chem. 54*, 533.
12. Saito, H., and Udagawa, M. (1992) *J. Sci. Food Agric. 58*, 135.
13. Wanasundara, U.N., and Shahidi, F. (1993) *J. Food Lipids 1*, 15.
14. Shahidi, F., Wanasundara, U.N., and Brunet, N. (1994) *Food Res. Inter. 27*, 555.

Index

A

Accelerated shelf life testing (ASLT) methods, 335–337
Active oxygen method (AOM), 112, 335
  drawbacks of, 383
  compared with OSI and Rancimat methods, 384
Active oxygen species, role in diseases, 97
Aging process
  and endogenous antioxidant defenses, 76
  free radical theory, 86
  and phytochemicals, 76–77
Alkaloids, plant antioxidants, 108
Amadori compounds, *see also* Maillard reaction products
  degradation to antioxidants and flavorants, 297
AMF, *see* Anhydrous milkfat
Amines, antioxidant activity of, 108
Amino acids
  antioxidants in cereals and legumes, 32–33
  antioxidative activity of, 6, 108
  prooxidant effect, 6, 32–33, 108
Amino reductones, antioxidants activity of, 297
Anserine, 8, 271–274
Anhydrous milkfat (AMF), application of oxygen consumption method, 337–341
p-Anisidine value, measurement of secondary products of lipid oxidation, 387
Antioxidant activity, assessment of lipid oxidation, 9
Antioxidant assays, radical scavenging methods, 205
Antioxidant defense systems
  and aging, 76
  in plants, 98
  vegetable extract studies, 77–86
Antioxidants, *see also* specific antioxidants
  definition, 1, 13
  in cereals and legumes, 25–53
  criteria for use in food systems, 13–14
  endogenous, *see* Endogenous antioxidants, Endogenous antioxidant enzymes
  effectiveness of different commercial, 341–344
  food safety and quality, 1, 3
  in grapes and wine, *see* Proanthocyanidins
  health benefits from consumption of, 1, 3
  in herbs and spices, 64–73
  mechanism, 3
  natural sources, 4–9
  in oilseeds, 98–111, 113–126
    methods of screening compounds, 111–113
  radical trapping mechanisms of,
  role in plant defense systems, 4
  in shrimp waste, 283–292
  synthetic, *see* Synthetic antioxidants
  in vegetable extracts, 77–82
Ascorbic acid, *see* Vitamin C
Ascorbyl palmitate, 238–241
Autoxidation, *see also* Lipid peroxidation
  FTIR/ATR differential spectroscopy, 358–377
  NMR methodology, 398–403
  mechanism, 1–2, 12, 379, 397
  primary changes, 381–385
  secondary changes, 386–390

B

Barley, antioxidants in, 36–38
Bean varieties, antioxidants in, 52–53
Biacalein, lipid peroxidation inhibitor, 180–181, 183
Butylated hydroxyanisole (BHA)
  comparison with FRI, 231
  comparison with condensed tannins, 208–210
  comparison with crude tea catechins, 214
  comparison with tocopherol, 232

effectiveness, 227
possible carcinogenic properties, 12
Butylated hydroxytoluene (BHT)
comparison with FRI, 231
comparison with condensed tannins, 208–210
comparison with tocopherol, 232
effectiveness, 227
possible carcinogenic properties, 12

C

Cancer
antigenotoxicity of rosemary antioxidants, 91–93
risk reduction through consumption of plant foods, 76–77
Canola/Rapeseed (*Brassica napus, B.campestris*), antioxidants in, 113–114
Capsaicin, 70
Capsaicinol, 70
Carbonyl analysis, 388–389
Carnosic acid
antigenotoxicity effect, 91–93
antimutagenic test in bacteria, 91
antioxidant properties in lipid and nonlipid systems, 90–91
antitumor promoting activity, 93–95
conversion to carnosol, 19
rosemary constituent, 19, 89
Carnosine, 8
antioxidative activity in foods, 275–281
lipid oxidation inhibition in butter, 277, 280
in photooxidized butter, 277, 280
prevention of myoglobin oxidation, 277
antioxidative membrane-protecting properties, 273
Carnosol
antigenotoxicity of, 90–93
antimutagenicity test in bacteria, 91
antioxidant activity, 90–91
antitumor promoting activity, 93–95
rosemary constituent, 89
β-Carotene
antioxidant and nutritional benefits, 109, 134–136, 247
functions, 247, 249
provitamin A role, 134, 247
Carotenes
carotenoid composition of various, 137
commercial sources and uses, 137–138
enriched red palm oil, 141–142
quenching of $^1O_2$, 16
Carotenoid pigments, stabilization of, 242
Carotenoids
antioxidant role in oilseeds, 109
antioxidants in cereals and legumes, 34–35
natural food sources of, 5
in palm oil, 133–142, 147
nutritional benefits, 134–136
processing methods, 136–142
provitamin A role, 134
quenchers, 240
Cassumunin A, B and C, anti-inflammatory activities, 73
Catalase, role in plants, 106
Catechins, *see also* Tea polyphenols
antioxidant potency, 214–215
antioxidant effect on marine oils, 218–219
chemical structure, 213–214
chemoprotective effects, 73
cytoprotective effects, 190
DPPH radical-scavenging by, 216
lipid oxidation-inhibition by, 218
lipoxygenase-inhibition by, 218
natural food sources of, 5
superoxide-scavenging ability, 216–217
Cereals, antioxidants found in legumes and, 25–55; *see also* specific cereals
Chain-breaking acceptor (CB-A) antioxidants, mechanism, 14
Chain-breaking electron donor (CB-D) antioxidants, mechanism, 14
Chalcones, antioxidant activity of, 101
Chelators, 13, 240
Chemiluminescence method, evaluation of antioxidants in edible oils, 393–394

Chia (*Salvia hispanica* L.), antioxidants in, 116
Chili pepper (*Capcicum frutescence* L.), antioxidant in, 70
Chlorophyll derivatives, antioxidant activity of, 35, 108
Chronic diseases, optimal vitamin intakes and prevention of, 245–253
Condensed tannins, antioxidant activity, 204–211
Conjugable oxidation products assay, 385
Conjugated diene method, index of lipid stability, 384–385
Corn (*Zea mays* L.), antioxidants in, 38–40, 125
Coronary artery disease, effect of flavonoids, 190–194
Cottonseed (*Gossipium hursutum* L.), antioxidants in, 116–117
Curcumin, antitumor and anti-inflammation activity, 73
(+)-Cyanidanol-3, comparison with butylated hydroxyanisole, 183

D

2′-Deoxyribose, suppression of oxidation by vegetable extracts, 77–79
Dihydrocapsaicin, 70
1,1-Diphenyl-2-picrylhydrazyl radical, *see* DPPH
Diosmetin, cytoprotective effects, 190
Diosmin, vascular protectant, 190
Diterpenes, antioxidant activity, 19–22
DPPH
  mechanism of antioxidant reaction with, 393
  radical scavenging assay, 205
Dried whole milk (DWM), oxygen consumption studies, 333–335
DWM, *see* Dried whole milk

E

Edible (starch/alginate) films
  pork chops warmed-over flavor inhibition by, 311–316
Electron paramagnetic resonance (EPR) spectroscopy
  studies of plant polyphenols, 346–354
    spectra of aroxyl derivatives, 347–354
Electron spin resonance (ESR) spectroscopy, quantitation method of lipid oxidation, 392–393
Emulsions, model systems of lipid and pigment oxidation, 320–322
Enzyme antioxidants, 9; *see also* specific enzymes
  in oilseeds, 105–107
  role in biological systems, 258–268
    catalase, 263
    glutathione, 264–265
    glutathione peroxidase, 265–266
    glutathione reductase, 266
    glutathione-S-transferase, 266–267
    riboflavin, 266
    superoxide dismutase, 261–263
  role in chronic diseases prevention, 267–268
(–)-Epigallocatechin gallate (EGCG)
  green tea polyphenol, 206, 213
  relative antioxidant potency among catechins, 214–215

F

Fats and oils, asssessment of oxidative stability by NMR spectroscopy, 397–404
Fatty acids, and lipid oxidation assessment, 381
FIRA-Astell apparatus, description, 336
Fish, shelf-life dating method, 394
Flavanones, 19, 27
Flavonoids, 18–19, 26–28, 98–102, 174–197
  antioxidant potency, 18, 98, 100–101
  antioxidant mechanisms, 19, 28, 98, 176–177
  antitoxicity, 187–190
  dietary intake, 174
  effect on lipid peroxidation and oxy-radical production, 179–187
  enzyme-modifying actions, 176
  health benefits of, 176

and coronary heart disease, 190–194 influence on ROS production by phagocytic cells, 177–179
ischemia reperfusion, 190–194
natural sources of, 5
in oilseeds, 98–102
structural features affecting antioxidant activity of, 19
structures and occurence of, 26–27, 98, 174–176
effects on vitamin C, 176, 193–194
Flavones, 19, 27
Flaxseed (*Linum usitassimum* L.), antioxidants in, 115–116
Fluorescent products, lipid oxidation method, 389–390
Food industry
criteria for "ideal antioxidant," 13–14
interest in polyphenolic antioxidants, 88
interest in natural antioxidants, 14, 89
Food lipid oxidation
autoxidation scheme, 379–380
methods of measuring, 380–394, 397–404
primary and secondary changes,
PUFA levels and oxidative stability, 379
Free radical chain, mechanism of autoxidation, 1–2
Free radical interceptors (FRI), 224–243
effectiveness factors, 227
mechanism, 228–229
substrate specificity, 230–233
synergistic combinations, 231–236
ascorbic acid and phenolics applications, 238–239
Free radicals, role in diseases and tissue injuries, 2
Free radical theory of aging, 86
French Paradox, possible role of proanthocyanidins and health, 154–155, 192
FRI, *see* Free radical interceptor
Frying fat, measurement of deterioration, 390–392
FTIR/ATR differential spectroscopy
advantages over dispersive infrared spectroscopy, 358–359
antioxidant performance evaluation by, 371–377
applications in analysis of fats and oils, 361–362
horizontal attenuated total reflectance (ATR) technique, 359
oil oxidation monitoring by, 362, 365–371

G

German Society of Fat, definition of deteriorated frying fat, 391
Ginger (*Zingiber officinale* Roscoe), antioxidants in, 66, 68
Glutathione (GSH), 107
Glutathione peroxidase, 265–266
Glutathione reductase, 266
Glutathione-S-transferase, 266–267
Grape seed extract proanthocyanidins, *see* Proanthocyanidins
Green tea polyphenols
antimutagenic and anticarcinogenic effects, 213–214
antioxidative effect, 214–215
catechins, 213 *see* Catechins
composition of, 206, 213, 215–216
scavenging activities, 214

H

Heme pigment, oxidation, 320–328
Heme-proteins, role in lipid oxidation, 321
Herbs, with antioxidant effects, 65; *see also* specific herbs
Hexanal
flavor volatile related to warmed-over flavor, 315
oxidation of linoleic acid oils, 388–389
HPLC analysis, 320
Hydrocarbons
correlations of pentane and sensory scores in oils, 389
Hydroperoxides
autoxidation process, 12–13
effect of flavanoids, 177
formation, 382

in photo-oxidation, 13
primary oxidation products, 2
quantitation, *see* Peroxide value
4-Hydroxynonenal (4-HN), secondary oxidation product, 3
Hydroxyl radical, scavenging properties of vegetable extracts, 82–83

I

Infrared (IR) spectroscopy, applications to rancidity measurement, 393
IPd measurement, *see* Accelerated shelf-life testing methods
Ischemia reperfusion, flavonoid action, 190–194
Isoflavones, 102

J

Japanese diet, vegetable consumption and health benefits, 77, 86

L

Legumes, antioxidants in cereals and, 25–55; *see also* specific legumes
Lignans, antioxidant properties, 102
Linoleic acid miscelles, emulsion model system for lipid oxidation studies, 321
Lipid oxidation
assessment, 90
effects on fat and oil characteristics, 379
health concerns, 89, 97
mechanism, 319, 332, 379
autoxidation and photo-oxidation, 12
methods for assessing, 9, 319–320, 380–394
model systems for studying in muscle-based foods, 319–328
prevention by antioxidants, 88–89
Lipid peroxidation
effect of flavonoids, 179–187
mechanism, 181–182
Lipid stability
optimizing with natural inhibitors, 224–243
prediction based on oxygen consumption rate, 331–334
Liposomes, muscle foods models of lipid and pigment oxidation, 322–324
Low density lipoproteins (LDL)
effect of flavonoids, 190–192
oxidation damage, 246–247

M

Maillard reaction, *see also* Maillard reaction product
description, 297
Maillard reaction products (MRP)
antioxidative activity of, 111–112, 297–301
synthetic beef flavor (SBF), 300–301
synthetic meat flavor (SMF) as synthetic MRP, 298
synthetic mixtures, 298
synthetic pork flavor (SPF), 298–300
Malonaldehyde (MDA), 386
reactive secondary oxidation product, 3
Marjoram (*Origanum majorana* L.), antioxidants in, 66
Meat products, *see* Muscle-based foods
Meaty flavor loss of cooked meats, *see also* Warmed-over flavor
inhibition, 296–297
Medicinal plants, effect on lipid peroxidation, 183
Melanoidins
antioxidative activity, 111, 297–298
prevention of WOF and preservation of meatiness, 301–308
Methyl linoleate miscelles, emulsion model for studying lipid and pigment oxidation, 321
Microsomes, muscle foods models of lipid and pigment oxidation, 324–327
Milkfat oxygen consumption methodology studies
evaluation of commercial antioxidants, 341–344
oxidative stability of anhydrous milkfat (AMF), 337–341

Millet, antioxidants, 40
MRP, *see* Maillard reaction products
Muscle-based foods, model systems of pigment and lipid oxidation, 319–328
Mustard (*Brassica juncea*), antioxidants in, 114–115
Myricetin, inhibition of lipid peroxidation, 184

N

Natural antioxidants, 1–9; *see also* specific antioxidants
  consumer preference in food products, 311
  isolated from shrimp waste, 283–292
Natural inhibitors, *see* Free radical interceptors (FRI)
NMR methodology, and lipid oxidation, 398–403

O

Oat, antioxidants, 40–44
Oils, PUFA content and oxidative instability, 379
Oilseeds, natural antioxidants from, 113–126; *see also* specific oilseeds
  alkaloids, 108
  amines, 108
  amino acids, 108
  chlorophyll derivatives, 108
  derived during processing, 110–111
  enzymes, 106
  glutathione, 107
  phenolic compounds, 98–105
  screening methods, 111–113
  superoxide dismutase, 107
Olive oil (*Olea europaea* L.), antioxidants in, 117
Oolong tea, antioxidants, 213, 215
Oregano, antioxidative compounds in, 66
Oxidative Stability Instrument, 336
Oxidative stress, in aging and disease processes, 76
Oxidograph, apparatus measuring IPd of fats, 336–337
Oxirane value, 387
Oxodiene value, 385
Oxygen, singlet, *see* Singlet oxygen
Oxygen bomb calorimetry, accelerated oxidation test, 112
Oxygen consumption methodology, prediction of lipid shelf-life, 337–344
Oxygen pressure, measurement of lipid oxidation, 381
Oxygen uptake/absorption, accelerated oxidation test, 112
Oxymyoglobin oxidation, lipid oxidation interactions: model systems studies, 319–328

P

Palm oil (*Elais guineensis* Jacq.)
  antioxidants in, 125
  carotenoids, 125, 133–142
  composition of crude and kernel, 133
  processing of carotene-enriched red, 141–142
  tocols, 125, 133–134, 142–147
    nutritional benefits, 135–136
Peanut (*Arachis hypogaea*), antioxidants in, 54–55, 117–118
Peas, antioxidants, 53–54
Pentane, lipid oxidation indicator, 315
Pepper (*Piper nigrum* L.), antioxidant activity of, 70–71
Peptides, 6–8
Peroxidases, function in plants, 106
Peroxide value (PV)
  frying fat quality indicator, 392
  measure of flavor quality and lipid shelf-life, 338
  methods for monitoring, 383
  quantitation method for hydroperoxide, 382–383
Peroxyl radical formation, 12–13
Phagocytosis, and reactive oxygen species generation, 177–179
Phenolic acids *see* Phenolic compounds
Phenolic compounds
  in cereals and legumes, 25–26
  flavonoids *see* Flavonoids

in grapes and wine, *see* Proanthocyanidins
health benefits of, 6
natural food sources, 5
in oilseeds, 98–105; *see also* specific oilseeds
peroxy radical trapping antioxidant activity, 17–18
role in plant defense systems, 4–5
structure and antioxidant activities, 26, 102–105
Phospholipids
antioxidants, 8–9, 31–32, 110
commercial source, 8
and oxymyoglobin oxidative interactions: model systems for studying, 319–328
Photo-oxidation in foods, mechanism, 13
Phytates *see* Phytic acid
Phytic acid, 33–34
antioxidant activity, 8, 109–110
Phytoestrogens, sources and health benefits of dietary, 168
Pigments, *see* Carotenoids
Plant polyphenols, 346
EPR spectroscopy studies of, 346–354
green tea *see* Green tea polyphenols
Polyunsaturated fatty acids (PUFA), autoxidation of, 25
Pork, warmed-over flavor in
inhibition by rosemary oleoresin and edible film, 311–317
inhibition by synthetic meat flavor compounds, 298
Proanthocyanidins, in grapes and wine, 150–170
antioxidant capacity of wine, 159–164
biological activity in cell culture, 164–165
biological implications, 157–159
chromatographic methods of analysis, 153–154
estrogenic potential, 168–170
free radical scavenging activity in cell culture, 165–168
potential health effects, 154–159
role in wine flavor and aging potential, 150
structure and occurence, 150–152
Prooxidants, 229
Propanal, oxidation of ω-3 fatty acids, 389
Proton Nuclear Magnetic Resonance (^{1}H NMR) spectroscopy, assessment of oxidative stability, 397–404
PV, see Peroxide value

Q

Quenchers, 239–240
Quenching, and lipid stabilization, 239–240
Quercetin, 28
anticancer agent, 170
cytotoxicity and lack of bioavailability, 165–166, 168, 170
extraction from grape seeds, 153
estrogenic activity, 168–170
inhibition of lipid peroxidation, 180, 182
inhibition of reactive oxygen species production, 178–179
mechanism of antiradical action of, 182–183
mechanism of antithrombotic action, 193–194

R

Rancidity, see also Warmed-over flavor
control by antioxidants, 3
and evolution of food oxidation management, 224–225
Rancidity, hydrolytic
cause and prevention, 331
Rancidity, oxidative
cause and food quality consequences, 331–332, 379
methods of measuring in foods, 380–394
Rancimat test
assessment of lipid peroxidation in foods, 90, 112
description, 336, 383–384
evaluation, 340–341
hydrolytic, 331
mechanism, 382

oxidative, 331
Reactive oxygen species (ROS)
in vivo production, 258–261
oxidative stress, aging and disease, 261
endogenous antioxidant enzymes, 261–268
phagocytic generation inhibition by flavonoids, 177–179
scavenging and inhibition by flavonoids, 177
Recommended Daily Allowance (RDA)
need to revise optimal vitamin intakes to prevent chronic diseases, 247
use in eliminating deficiency diseases, 246
Red palm oil, quality, 141–142
Red pepper (*Capcicum annuum* L.), antioxidants, 70
Reductones
antioxidative effect of, 111
in Maillard reaction, 297
Rice (*Oryzae sativa* L.), antioxidants, 44–46, 125–126
Rosemarinic acid, 89
Rosemary (*Rosmarinus officinalis* L.) *see also* Carnosic acid, Carnosol, Rosemarinic acid, Rosemary extract, Rosemary oleoresin
antioxidants, 65–66
implications for food and health, 88–95
purification and characterization, 89
Rosemary extract (RE-S)
antigenotoxicity effects, 91–93
antimutagenicity in bacteria, 91
antioxidant activity, 19–20, 89–91
anti-tumor promoting activity, 93–95
Rosemary oleoresin (RO)
antioxidant constituents of, 311
lipid oxidation suppression mechanism, 311, 314
study of warmed over flavor inhibition by, 311–316
Rutin
antioxidant activity, 186
mechanism of antiradical action, 182–183
mechanism of antithrombotic action, 193–194
Rye, antioxidants, 46

S

Sage, antioxidant activity, 19
Schaal oven test, 112
method description, 335
Screening methods, antioxidants in oilseeds, 111–113
Selenium, antioxidative activity with enzyme antioxidants, 9
Sesame (*Sesamum indicum* L.), antioxidants, 72, 118–122
Sesamol, 72, 120
Sesamolin, 72, 120–121
Semisynthetic hydroxyethyl flavonoids, antioxidant activity, 184–185
Shelf-life of foods
dating of fish samples by chemiluminescence method, 394
and oxygen consumption method, 331–344
Shrimp (*Pandalus jordani*) waste, isolation of natural antioxidant from, 283–292
Silybin
antitoxic effects, 187
comparison with butylated hydroxytoluene, 185
prevention of CCl_4-induced lipid peroxidation, 188
protection of xanthine dehydrogenase/oxidase ratio, 192–193
Silybum marianum, silynarin
antitoxicant effects, 187
inhibition of lipid peroxidation, 180
Singlet oxygen
formation in photo-oxidation process, 13
high reactivity of, 13
quenching by carotenes, 16, 34
quenching by tocopherols, 14
Sorghum, antioxidants, 47
Soybean (*Glycene max.* L.), antioxidants, 49–52, 122–125
Soybean isoflavones, antioxidant potency, 180
Spices *see also* specific spices
antioxidant activity, 21, 65–73

Sterols, 35, 110
Superoxide anion
phagocytic formation and effects, 177–178
inhibition by flavanoids, 178–179
Superoxide dismutase (SOD), antioxidant function in plants, 107
Superoxide radical scavenging, by vegetable extracts, 83–86
Sylvester Test, description of, 336
Synthetic antioxidants, *see* BHA, BHT and TBHQ
consumer concerns, 12, 25
Synthetic meat flavor (SMF)
antioxidative meat applications studies, 298–309
preparation from MRP precursors, 298
Synthetic pork flavor (SPF-1), *see* Synthetic meat flavor

T

Tannins, phenolic antioxidants in oilseeds, 105; *see also* Condensed tannins
TBARS, *see* Thiobarbituric acid reactive substances
Tea polyphenols, 213–221 *see also* Green tea polyphenols
antimutagenic and anticarcinogenic activities, 213–214
antioxidative effect, 214–215
catechins, 214–215
composition of, 215
DPPH radical-scavenging, 216
lipid oxidation-inhibition, 218–219
lipoxygenase-inhibition, 218
major types of manufactured teas, 213
superoxide-scavenging, 216–217
theaflavins, 214, 221
therubigens, 213
TBHQ (tert-Butylhydroquinone), effectiveness, 227
Theaflavins, 213–215
Thearubigens, 213
2-Thiobarbituric acid (TBA) value, 386–387
correlation of flavor threshold values of fats and oils with, 387
Thiobarbituric acid reactive substances (TBARS), method to measure lipid oxidation, 319–320
Thyme (*Thymus vulgaris* L.), antioxidants in, 66
Tocols, 105, 133–147
in cereals and legumes, 28–31
factors affecting relative antioxidant activity, 29
in palm oil, 134, 142–145
nutritional benefits, 134–136
role in biological membranes, 29
structures of, 28–29
vitamin E activity, 28–31
Tocopherols, 14–15, 28–31
antioxidant mechanisms, 14–15, 29, 105
comparison with tea catechins, 214
enhancement of antioxidative activity by synergists, 30–31
factors affecting relative antioxidative activity, 29
quencher, 240–241
structure and antioxidative activity mechanism, 105–106
Tocotrienols, 28, 31
Totox value, estimation of food lipids oxidative deterioration, 387–388, 397
Triticale, antioxidant content, 47–48
Tumor initiation and formation
beneficial effects of spices/herbs on, 73
protective effect of phenolic antioxidants, 93
rosemary components as antitumor promoting agents, 93–95
Turmeric (*Curcuma domestica* L. , C. longa L.) antioxidants, 68–70

V

Vegetable extracts
active oxygen radical scavenging ability, 79, 82–86
antioxidative activities of specific, 77–82
Vegetables
disease prevention function of phytochemicals from, 76–77

importance in Japanese diet, 76, 86
Vitamin A
antioxidant properties and health benefits, 135–136
biological role, 134
functions, 249
recommended intake, 247
Vitamin antioxidants, 9
chronic disease prevention and optimal intakes of, 245–253
Vitamin C, 108–109
antioxidant activity, 35–36
functions, 247, 249
interaction with flavonoids, 176, 193–194
pigment stabilization, 242
plant sources, 5
Vitamin E (tocopherols and tocotrienols)
antioxidative properties and health benefits, 135–136
content and isolation from palm oil, 142, 144–145
economic feasibility assessment, 145–147
functions, 250
natural food sources of, 5
recommended dietary allowance, 246
Vitamins
intake and disease prevention, 245–253; *see also* specific vitamins

W

Warmed-over aroma (WOA)
effects of synthetic meat flavor on, 300–301
Warmed-over flavor (WOF)
development in stored cooked meats, 296, 311
inhibition by additives, 296
inhibition by Maillard reaction products (MRP), 296–309 inhibition in pork chops by rosemary oleoresin, 311–317
and muscle tissue oxidation, 241
Weight-gain method, measurement of lipid oxidation, 381–382
Wheat, antioxidant content, 48–49
Wine proanthocyanidins, *see also* Proanthocyandins
chromatographic methods for analysis, 153–154
content of various wines and grape seeds, 152
potential health effects, 154–153
role in flavor and aging potential of wines, 150
Wood smoke, management of lipid oxidation in muscle foods, 241

X

Xanthine dehydrogenase/xanthine oxidase ratio
protective effect by quercetin, 192–193
protective effect by silybin, 192–193

Z

Zingiberaceae, antioxidants in, 66–70